SECOND EDITION

D0025897

Life Choices

HEALTH CONCEPTS AND STRATEGIES

SECOND EDITION

Life Choices

HEALTH CONCEPTS AND STRATEGIES

Lori Waite Turner

Frances Sienkiewicz Sizer

Eleanor Noss Whitney

Barbara Braxton Wilks

WEST PUBLISHING COMPANY

Saint Paul   New York   Los Angeles   San Francisco

Copyeditor:	Mary Berry, Naples Editing Services
Cover Image:	"Creole Dancer," Henri Matisse. © 1992 Succession H. Matisse/ARS, New York.
Cover Design:	Pollock Design Group
Interior Design:	K. M. Weber
Composition:	Carlisle Communications
Illustrations:	Cyndie Clark-Huegel, Wayne Clark, John Waller, and Judy Waller
Cartoons:	Gary Carroll, Robert Celander, and William Celander
Indexer:	JoAnne Naples, Naples Editing Services

WEST'S COMMITMENT TO THE ENVIRONMENT

In 1906, West Publishing Company began recycling materials left over from the production of books. This began a tradition of efficient and responsible use of resources. Today, up to 95 percent of our legal books and 70 percent of our college texts are printed on recycled, acid-free stock. West also recycles nearly 22 million pounds of scrap paper annually—the equivalent of 181,717 trees. Since the 1960s, West has devised ways to capture and recycle waste inks, solvents, oils, and vapors created in the printing process. We also recycle plastics of all kinds, wood, glass, corrugated cardboard, and batteries, and have eliminated the use of styrofoam book packaging. We at West are proud of the longevity and the scope of our commitment to our environment.

Production, Prepress, Printing and Binding by West Publishing Company.

Library of Congress Cataloging-in-Publication Data

Life choices : health concepts and strategies / Lori Turner . . . [et al.].—2nd ed.
    p.   cm.
   Rev. ed. of: Life choices / Frances Sienkiewicz Sizer and Eleanor Noss Whitney with Dana Knighten Cowley.   1988.
  ISBN 0-314-93384-0 (Annotated Instructor's Edition)
  ISBN 0-314-93383-2 (Student's Edition)
  1. Health behavior. 2. Health. I. Turner, Lori Waite.
II. Sizer, Frances Sienkiewicz. Life choices.
RA776.9.L54 1992
613—dc20

                91–41650
 CIP

Acknowledgments

Page 45, Copyright © by The New York Times Company. Reprinted by permission.**Page 76, Table S3-1.** Adapted from C. L. Whitfield, *Healing the Child Within* (Deerfield Beach, Fla.: Health Communications, 1987), pp. 2–3.
Pate 78, Table S3-2. Adapted from C. L. Whitfield, *Healing the Child Within* (Deerfield Beach, Fla.: Health Communications, 1987), pp. 2–3.
Page 171, Department of Exercise, University of South Carolina
Page 193, Permission of *Executive Edge Newsletter*, P.O. Box 58171, Boulder, CO 86322-8171, (800) 365-1847

(continued following index)

To Brad—so glad you are
a child of mine.

Lori

To Bill, for his good ideas. Thanks.

Fran

For my youngest friends, Bradley,
Will, and Elizabeth: May your
futures be bright in a
welcoming world.

Ellie

To my students who have enriched
my life over the years.

Barbara

Lori Waite Turner, MS, RD, attended Florida State University where, in 1980, she received her BS in Food and Nutrition with a minor in Physical Education. In 1983 she completed her MS in Dietetics and Nutrition at Florida International University.

She has worked for Capitol Foods of Atlanta, Georgia where she marketed a computerized menu system to health care institutions. She has served as a Therapeutic Dietitian at Kennestone Hospital in Marietta, Georgia; as Chief Clinical Dietitian for Doctors' Hospital in Coral Gables; Florida, and as a Nutrition Consultant for a Cardiac Rehabilitation program, also in Coral Gables. She presently teaches Concepts of Positive Living, an introductory personal health course, at Tallahassee Community College in the Department of Health Education and Nutrition.

She has authored instructor's manuals, test banks, and student study guides that accompany several nutrition, health, and fitness textbooks including *Essential Life Choices, Understanding Nutrition, 5th edition, Nutrition: Concepts and Controversies, 5th edition, Understanding Normal and Clinical Nutrition, 3rd edition,* and *The Fitness Triad.* She has authored several articles for the *Nutrition Clinics* monograph series: *Very-Low-Calorie Diets, The Calcium Controversy—Nature Vs. Nurture,* and *Weight Maintenance and Relapse Prevention.* She has also authored a user's manual to accompany a nutrition analysis computer software program. She is a member of the American School Health Association.

Frances Sienkiewicz Sizer, MS, RD, attended Florida State University where, in 1980, she received her BS, and in 1982, her MS in nutrition. She has counseled clients in the University's stress-reduction clinic and served as nutrition consultant to schools and alcoholism programs in Florida. She coauthors the textbooks *Nutrition: Concepts and Controversies,* now in its fifth edition, *Essential Life Choices: Health Concepts and Strategies,* a short version of this book, *The Fitness Triad,* and *Making Life Choices,* a high school textbook. She has published in *Shape* magazine, in the health newsletter *Healthline,* and in the *Journal of Chemical Senses.* She is vice-president and a founding member of Nutrition and Health Associates, an information resource center in Tallahassee, Florida, where she currrently devotes her time to studying and writing in the areas of nutrition and health.

Eleanor Noss Whitney, PhD, has a BA in biology and English (Harvard University, 1960), and a PhD in biology (Washington University, St. Louis, 1970). She served as a member of the faculties at Florida A and M University and Florida State University between 1970 and 1982, and has authored and coauthored many textbooks on nutrition, health, and environmental subjects since 1977. Notable among them are *Understanding Nutrition* (with S. R. Rolfes), *Nutrition: Concepts and Controversies* (with F. S. Sizer), *The Fitness Triad* (with L. K. DeBruyne and F. S. Sizer), and *Life Choices.* Dr. Whitney now devotes full time to research, writing, and consulting, primarily in environmental biology and lifestyle changes needed for a sustainable future. She is president of Nutrition and Health Associates and cofounder of the Coastal Plains Institute, a foundation that conducts environmental education projects in North Florida.

Barbara Braxton Wilks, Ed.D., MPH received her B.A. from the University of North Carolina, Chapel Hill; her M.A. from the University of Missouri; and her Ed.D. from the University of Georgia in 1974 where she is presently a faculty member. She did a postdoctoral Master of Public Health degree at Emory University School of Medicine. She is a nationally certified health education specialist (CHES), and has been active in the Association for the Advancement of Health Education, in the district and state level organizations. She holds membership in the American School Health Association and life membership in American Alliance of Health, Physical Education, Recreation, and Dance and the Georgia Federation of Professional Health Educators of which she is a charter member and Editor of the Catalyst. She teaches Health and Wellness, Issues in Consumer Health, Community Health, Methods, Curriculum courses, and supervises student teachers in Health Promotion and Education. She has published in *Health Education, Innovative Higher Education,* writes curriculum resource materials for the Georgia State Department of Education, and conducts in-service staff development workshops.

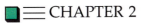

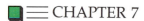

CHAPTER 6
Energy Balance and Weight Control   131

CHAPTER 7
Fitness   165

CHAPTER 8
Drugs as Medicines   201

CHAPTER 9
Drugs of Abuse   221

■≡ CHAPTER 20

The Consumer, Health Information, and the Health Care System 563

■≡ CHAPTER 21

The Environment and Personal Health 589

■≡ APPENDIXES

The U. S. Department of Health and Human Services completed a review of the health status of the population and established specific goals to be achieved by the year 2000. These goals express our nation's foremost health needs:

Infants. Reduce the incidence of low birthweight and birth defects.

Children. Improve health and development patterns, reduce childhood deaths from violence and other abusive behavior, accidents, environmental factors, and infectious disease. Reduce dental caries.

Young adults. Prevent accidents, suicide, and violent behavior. Prevent the use of tobacco, prevent the misuse of alcohol and other drugs, prevent unwanted pregnancies and sexually transmitted diseases including AIDS.

Adults. Reduce the incidence of HIV infection, stroke, heart attack, other coronary heart disease, diabetes, obesity, chronic obstructive pulmonary disease, and cancer. Reduce work-related injuries and deaths from work-related injuries and environmental causes. Reduce violent and abusive behavior.

Older adults. Increase independence; reduce the incidence of flu and pneumonia.*

We therefore adopted these objectives as missions of this book. We describe health promotion for infants and children in the chapters on emotional health, pregnancy, and parenting. To address young adults' major health threats, we devote a chapter each to cover topics of alcohol, other drugs, tobacco, sexually transmitted diseases, emotional health and problems, and contraception. As for the problems of adults, the book addresses the educational objectives the American Public Health Association identified. Chapters or parts of chapters are devoted to coronary heart diseases, diabetes, obesity, chronic obstructive pulmonary disease, cancer, and environmental risks. Hostility is covered with emotional problems; family violence is presented in an appendix. Accidents and injury prevention are also covered in an appendix.

This book is written for the individual: you. Thus each chapter contains not only basic information (*concepts*), but also the other two elements of our title: the options that the information gives people (*choices*) and applications (*strategies*). An objective for each chapter is not only to learn optimal health behavior, but also to learn the steps toward establishing that behavior as a routine. To that end, each chapter features a list of **Strategies** set apart from

*This list was adapted from the Public Health Service implementation plans for attaining the objectives for the nation, *Summary of Healthy People 2000,* national health promotion and disease prevention objectives for the year 2000, September 1990.

the text. Following each chapter is a **Spotlight** on information of special interest to students.

Clear defintions of terms ease the mastery of information, so we have made it a high priority to supply such definitions. To facilitate the reader's learning them, all key terms in the chapters are in boldface type and are defined nearby in the margins. **Miniglossaries,** presented at intervals throughout the chapters, contain groups of terms related to single concepts. The intent of the Miniglossaries is twofold: to ease study by presenting the information in small, manageable blocks; and to offer flexibility to the instructor who wants to assign some but not other sets of terms. The **Index** serves as an alphabetical list of all glossary terms: page numbers where definitions appear are in the index in boldface type.

The book addresses the reader as a consumer, not only of health products and services, but also of information. To guide the student through the process of evaluating health information, **Critical Thinking** sections appear throughout the book. The book cites its references following each chapter, modeling the characteristics of a reliable health information source.

A theme of the book is that a person's state of health is, to a great extent, that person's own responsibility. At the same time, it is important to acknowledge that not all of life's outcomes are chosen. Each chapter makes clear what people can control (their lifestyle habits) and what they cannot (their heredity, some of the circumstances of their lives, and chance events, including some accidents). Guidelines are offered, wherever relevant, to suggest when to get help with states of mind and body that are the subjects of the chapters that follow.

Another thing we emphasize is that someone else's choices are not a person's responsibility. From teaching, we know that students often ask what they can do to persuade friends and relatives to change their behavior. No matter how much a person may want to persuade Aunt Sally to give up smoking, or a sister to quit using pills, or a spouse to go jogging, one person cannot make the choice for another. The best bet is often to keep quiet about the choices others are making. We offer suggestions in the chapters about facilitating versus enabling behavior.

The book is positive. Its emphasis is on what *to* do, not on what *not* to do, to enhance the quality of life. Therefore, the chapters on diseases make it clear how different (and how preferable) *prevention* is in comparison with *cure.*

The chapters on nutrition encourage the reader, not to diet, but to eat well. The book suggests that people not only give up destructive habits, but that they find adaptive habits to replace negative ones.

The abundant thought we have put into the topics of this book has brought about changes in our own awareness and behavior. If reading the book has one-tenth of the impact on its users that writing it has had on us, it should help to bring about behavior changes that will enhance the quality of its readers' lives.

Lori W. Turner

Frances S. Sizer

Eleanor N. Whitney

Barbara B. Wilks

ACKNOWLEDGMENTS

We are grateful to Sharon Rolfes for writing Chapter 14 and for her availability and advice during the production of this book. We are also grateful to Linda DeBruyne for writing Chapter 11 and for her support throughout the preparation of this book. We thank Betty Hands and Bob Geltz for the data from which Appendix F was generated. We appreciate the artwork of John and Judy Waller, Cyndie Clark-Huegel, Wayne Clark, and Rolin Graphics, that graces the pages throughout. We thank our editors Mélina Brown, Peter Marshall, and Rebecca Tollerson for their many efforts in behalf of the book.

We are grateful to Sandra Woodruff for her preparation of the instructor's manual, test bank, and student activity manual for this text. We express our appreciation to Bill Beers, Sabrina McGriff, Teddy Benson, and Nancie Hopkins for their word processing assistance and helpful suggestions. We thank Linda Patton for her research assistance. Penelope Easton, Mike Khandijan, Linda Young, and Irwin Jahns have provided information and experience that now appear on the pages, and we thank them.

We are grateful to the outstanding Health Education faculty of Tallahassee Community College: Bob Bowers, Steve Owens, Roseann Poole, and Janella Silvey, for sharing their knowledge and experience. We are grateful to our students for their questioning minds and sharing of themselves that has inspired many of the words in this book and provided mutual learning as well as much fun.

We also appreciate the efforts of our reviewers:

Bill Beavers
Georgia Tech

Dave Buchanan
University of Massachusetts–Amherst

Mary Cessna
Indiana University of Pennsylvania

Suzanne Christopher
Portland Community College

Magsood Faguir
Palm Beach Community College

Barbara Greenberg
Nassau Community College

Joanna Hayden
William Paterson College

Dona Lange
Los Angeles Pierce College

Loretta Liptak
Youngstown State University

Henry Petraki
Palm Beach Community College

Grover Rusty Pippin
Baylor University

Nevin Posey
Kutztown University

Dale Wagoner
Chabot College.

CHAPTER 1

The Choice to Be Well

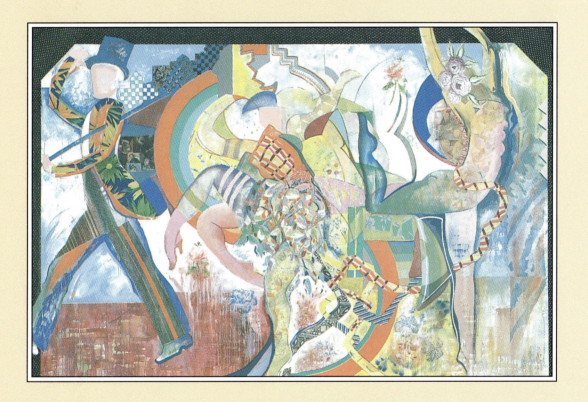

═══════════════════════════════════════

FACT OR FICTION

═══════════════════════════════════════

Just for fun, respond true or false to the following statements. If false, say what is true.

■ Being well is best defined as being free from disease. (Page 2)

■ The way adults contract most diseases today is by catching them from somebody else. (Page 3)

■ People can make themselves physically younger or older by the ways they choose to live. (Page 4)

■ Accidents are among the major causes of death for middle-aged to older adults. (Page 4)

■ A person who wants to change a harmful health habit, and knows how, will do so. (Page 6)

■ To help improve other people's health behavior, it is useful to offer constant reminders. (Page 18)

This book is about enjoying life. It challenges you to increase your knowledge, strengths, and skills in many areas—in self-awareness, emotional health, stress management, nutrition, fitness, intimate relationships, family planning, disease prevention, consumerism, and many others. It aims to enhance your ability to take action in all these areas with confidence and competence.

This is a tall order—especially since everyone already possesses vast experience in, and considerable knowledge about, these things. Why read a book about them? Oddly, the experience and knowledge people pick up about life always have gaps in them. Standard schooling, no matter where obtained, ensures that people learn the basics of language and mathematics, but the skills with which they are to manage their lives are taught only in bits and pieces. This book hopes to fill in some of the gaps for everyone who reads it.

How, then, can people maximally enjoy their lives? By feeling well, confident, and as much as possible, in control of their worlds. And what does it mean to be well? Traditional definitions of health define it as a state of complete physical, mental, and social well-being and not merely the absence of disease and infirmity.[1]* Other health educators claim that health should include even more than this.[2] They have expanded the term to **holistic health,** also called **wellness** or **high-level wellness.** These terms state that a person who has holistic health or high-level wellness functions well as a total person. These definitions suggest that a person's health should not be limited to physical, mental, and social components but should extend to include intellectual and spiritual dimensions. To say that a person has wellness, then, is to say that the person has reached the full potential possible for a human being. This book continues to use the term *wellness* to express that high ideal, but does not use the term *holistic health* again, for it has been abused by faddists and quack practitioners.

■ *FACT OR FICTION:* Being well is best defined as being free from disease. *False.* Wellness includes freedom from disease, but it also includes emotional, interpersonal, social, intellectual, and spiritual well-being.

health a state of complete physical, mental, and social well-being and not merely the absence of disease and infirmity.

holistic health (also called **wellness** or high-level wellness) maximal well-being, which includes physical, emotional, social, intellectual, and spiritual well-being. *Holistic health* refers to functioning well as a total person, achieving the full human potential.

---

*Reference notes are at the end of the chapter.

■≡ Wellness and Your Choices

You make choices that affect your wellness all the time. You choose your daily habits, such as how regularly you eat, what kinds of foods you eat, whether you smoke, and so forth. You choose your attitudes: when faced with a problem, for example, you choose whether to take it as bad luck or as a challenge. When a problem is medical, you choose whether to treat it yourself or to see a health care provider—and, if the latter, whom to see. You also make frequent choices as to what health claims to believe; you are bombarded with new information all the time in all forms from billboards to research studies.

This book focuses on those choices that are yours to make. You make dozens of such choices every day, and they determine your behaviors, set the probabilities of future events in your life, and affect the attitudes with which you meet those events. Your choices therefore influence your wellness profoundly, both now and in the future. A brief look at four categories of choices lays the groundwork for scrutiny of how you make them—how you choose to behave. The first category is the behaviors you choose to engage in.

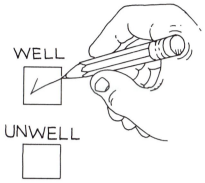

For most people, wellness throughout life is largely determined by the choices they make.

Lifestyle Choices

Your **lifestyle choices** are powerful in determining how well you are now, and how well you will be in the future. This assertion may seem overly optimistic at first glance, for there are many aspects of life over which people have no control. People cannot choose their heredity, for example, and many people inherit susceptibility to diseases through no fault of their own. Nor can people choose their environments, except in a limited way, and many people live in environments that present threats to their health.

In what sense, then, do people's lifestyle choices affect their wellness? They can choose behaviors that will influence the probabilities of negative or positive health outcomes. To give specific examples, a person cannot wish away susceptibility to an inherited disease, but can choose to learn about it and adopt behaviors that will postpone its arrival, reduce its severity, or maximize wellness within the limits the disease imposes. A person cannot choose to live completely free of polluted air, but can choose not to smoke. A person cannot choose to experience no health or accident risks, but can learn what risks are out there and choose behaviors to minimize them.

Even a single day's lifestyle choices either enhance or impair wellness a little. Repetitions over time compound the effects of these choices. A day's behaviors, repeated over a week, will have seven times the impact. Repeated every day for a year, they will have 365 times the impact. Over years, the effects accumulate still further, improving or damaging the quality of your life and even altering your statistical life expectancy.

For each poor choice, there is a positive alternative: people can choose not to smoke, not to abuse alcohol, to eat well, and to be physically active. These lifestyle choices are among the many that enhance wellness and maximize the probability of enjoying life into a healthy old age.

Researchers have provided a dramatic demonstration that lifestyle choices directly affect physical health. In a long-ago study, now viewed as classic,

lifestyle choices choices of daily behaviors such as eating habits, smoking, alcohol use, and level of physical activity.

■ *FACT OR FICTION:* Fact or Fiction: The way adults contract most diseases today is by catching them from somebody else. *False*. People don't "catch" most of today's major diseases; they "contract" many of them as a result of their own lifestyle choices.

chronological age   age as measured in years from date of birth.

physiological age   age as estimated from the body's health and probable life expectancy.

■ *FACT OR FICTION:* People can make themselves physically younger or older by the ways they choose to live. *True.*

■ *FACT OR FICTION:* Accidents are among the major causes of death for middle-aged to older adults. *False.* Accidents are among the major causes of death for younger adults.

infectious disease   a disease that can be passed from person to person and is caused by a specific disease-carrying agent. Also called *communicable disease.*

lifestyle diseases   diseases characterized by degeneration of body organs due to misuse and neglect, that cannot be passed from person to person but are influenced by personal lifestyle choices. Also called *degenerative diseases.* Examples are heart disease, cancer, and diabetes.

1890	1990
Tuberculosis	Heart disease
Digestive diseases	Cancer, Stroke
Pneumonia	Pneumonia
Flu, Bronchitis	Flu, Bronchitis
Stroke	Accidents
Scarlet fever	Suicide
Kidney disease	Diabetes
	Liver disease

The ten leading causes of death. Note that in the 1890s, most of them were infectious diseases. By the 1990s, most of the leading causes of death were primarily related to lifestyle.

they examined nearly 7,000 adults in California and noticed that some people seemed younger and others older than their **chronological age.** To find out what made the difference, the researchers focused on health habits and identified six factors that had maximum impact on **physiological age:** regular, adequate sleep; regular meals, including breakfast; regular physical activity; abstinence from smoking; abstinence from, or moderation in, alcohol use; and weight control. The effects of these factors were cumulative. That is, those who followed all six positive practices were in better health, even if older in calendar years, than people who failed to do so. In fact, the physical health of those who reported all positive health practices was consistently about the same as that of people *30 years younger* who followed few or none.[3] You have noticed this yourself, if you think about it: some older adults are extraordinarily healthy, and they invariably appear much younger than their peers. Have you noticed, too, that the most attractive people in a group are usually those who appear healthiest?

These research findings demonstrate that although you cannot alter the year of your birth, you can, in effect, make yourself younger or older by the way you choose to live. Try answering the questions in this chapter's Life Choice Inventory to see the effects of your lifestyle choices on the probable length of your life.

Middle-aged to older people served as subjects for the California study just described, and for these people, poor lifestyle choices were the most significant causes of loss of life and health. For younger people, accidents are another major cause of loss of life and health. The Life Choice Inventory includes prevention of driving accidents as one of the strategies most likely to promote physical health for adults, and Appendix E offers prevention and first aid strategies for common accidents.

This reality that lifestyle choices profoundly affect the quality of life differs from the reality of the past. Children and young adults, as well as older people, used to die helplessly of **infectious diseases,** such as smallpox, that raged out of control. Today, science has yielded so much knowledge about the causes of these diseases that over much of the world, control of many of them has made longer, higher-quality lives possible.

(One infectious disease, AIDS, is becoming a major killer of young people today, but not because its cause is unknown—it is known to be transmitted from person to person by sexual contact, blood transfusions, or injections using infected needles. AIDS is invariably fatal, but it is almost totally preventable, as Chapter 17 describes.)

Ironically, the control of yesterday's major infectious diseases has made possible a whole set of different diseases—those that develop in later life, due partly to people's making poor lifestyle choices over years of their lives. These **lifestyle diseases** are largely the result of people's abuse and neglect of their own bodies. Putting it negatively, the choice to smoke, for example, is a major cause of lung diseases; the choice to abuse alcohol is a major cause of accidents and liver disease; and poor choices in the realms of nutrition and physical activity can make heart disease and diabetes likely. The cartoon in the margin contrasts the major causes of death 100 years ago with those today, and shows that while people used to "catch" many diseases from disease agents ("germs"), they now are more likely to "contract" diseases by virtue of the ways they choose to live (also see Figure 1–1).

LIFE CHOICE INVENTORY

How long will you live? No one can answer this question for sure, of course. But you can lengthen or shorten the *probable* length of your life by a good many years depending on what choices you make. That is, your statistical *chances* of dying younger or older are affected by how you live.

The Longevity Game illustrates this principle. To play the game, start on the top line (age 74, the average life expectancy for adults in America today). Then answer the eleven questions that follow. For each question, add or subtract years as instructed. If a question doesn't apply, go on to the next one. If you are not sure of the exact number to add or subtract, make a guess. Don't take the score too seriously, but do pay attention to those areas where you lose years: they could point to choices you might want to change.

Start with: 74 years

1. Physical activity   _____
2. Relaxation   _____
3. Driving   _____
4. Blood pressure   _____
5. 65 and working   _____
6. Family history   _____
7. Smoking   _____
8. Drinking   _____
9. Gender   _____
10. Weight   _____
11. Age   _____

The probable length of your life: _____

1. *Physical activity.* If your work requires regular, vigorous activity or you work out each day, add 3 years. If you don't get much exercise at home, work, or play, subtract 3 years.
2. *Relaxation.* If you have a relaxed approach to life (you roll with the punches), add 3 years. If you're aggressive, ambitious, or nervous (you have sleepless nights, you bite your nails), subtract 3 years. If you consider yourself unhappy, subtract another year.
3. *Driving.* Drivers under 30 who have had traffic tickets in the last year or have been involved in an accident, subtract 4 years. Other violations, minus 1. If you always wear seatbelts, add 1.

4. *Blood pressure.* High blood pressure is a major cause of the most common killers—heart attacks and strokes—but most victims don't know they have it. If you know you have it, you are likely to do something about it. If you *know* your blood pressure, add 1 year.
5. *65 and working.* If you are 65 or older and still working, add 3 years.
6. *Family history.* If any grandparent has reached age 85, add 2 years; if all grandparents have reached age 80, add 6. If a parent died of a stroke or heart attack before age 50, minus 4. If a parent, brother, or sister has (or had) diabetes since childhood, minus 3.
7. *Smoking.* Cigarette smokers who finish:

   More than two packs a day, minus 8 years.

   One or two packs a day, minus 6.

   One-half to one pack day, minus 3.

8. *Drinking.* If you drink two cocktails (or beers or glasses of wine) a day on average, subtract 1 year. For each additional daily libation, subtract 2.
9. *Gender.* Women live longer than men. Females, add 3 years; males, subtract 3 years.
10. *Weight.* If you avoid eating fatty foods and don't add salt to your meals, your heart will be healthier, and you're entitled to add 2 years.

    Now, weigh in:

    Overweight by 50 pounds or more, minus 8 years.

    30 to 49 pounds, minus 4.

    10 to 29 pounds, minus 2.

11. *Age.* How long you have already lived can help predict how much longer you'll live. If you're under 30, the jury is still out. But if your age is:

    30 to 39, plus 2 years.

    40 to 49, plus 3.

    50 to 69, plus 4.

    70 or over, plus 5.

SOURCE: From "The Longevity Game" by Northwestern Mutual Life Insurance Company, with permission.

FIGURE 1–1 ■ **Lifestyle choices affect health.**

A few people are cut short by disease, even though they maintain excellent health habits. A few others have long lives and remain healthy even though they ignore all health warnings. The rest of us are affecting our health by the choices we make.

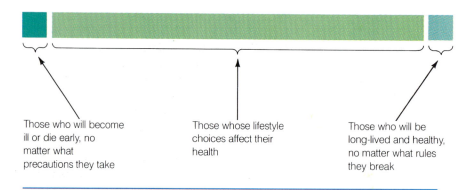

Those who will become ill or die early, no matter what precautions they take

Those whose lifestyle choices affect their health

Those who will be long-lived and healthy, no matter what rules they break

It should be emphasized that people who contract lung disease, liver disease, heart disease, or cancer are not always responsible for having done so, though. Heredity and environment clearly do contribute to the incidence of these diseases. Some people are simply susceptible to certain diseases, and sometimes they can do nothing to avoid them. And environmental factors other than infectious disease agents, such as pollution of air, water, and food, do influence people's susceptibility. Figure 1–2 shows how heredity, environment, and lifestyle choices all interact in the causation of disease. Still, the more you know, the better you can control the effects, even of hereditary and environmental influences. Knowledge of your

FIGURE 1–2 ■ **Heredity, environment, and lifestyle choices influence disease susceptibility.**

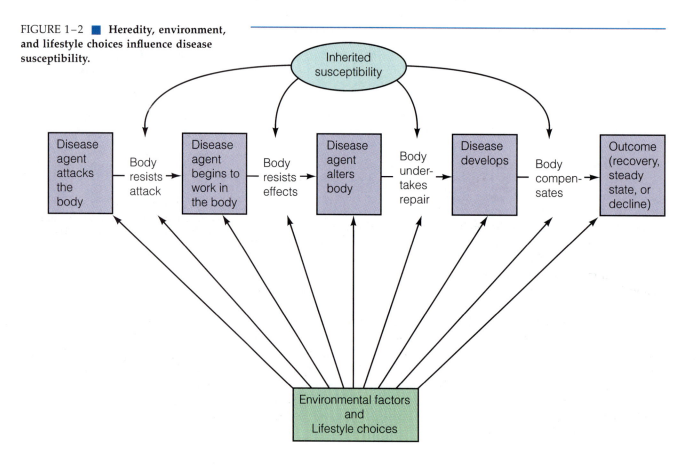

inherited risks can help you choose which lifestyle choices to emphasize in planning your disease-resistance strategy. And knowledge of the effects of your environment on your health can help you decide where to choose to live, what laws to vote for, and what causes to support.

In short, the more you learn, the more control you can gain. Figure 1–3 shows the probable course of a person who invests in learning about health and wellness. The investment leads to improved quality of life.

When people understand that they can exert some control over their health, they perceive that the **locus of control** is within themselves.[4] They realize that many of their actions and behaviors have an impact on their health; they see that for many aspects of their lives, they are not just helpless victims of external chance. It is vital to learn the difference between what can be controlled and what cannot be controlled, because when people realize that certain behaviors will make a difference, they are often most likely to take positive action.

This concept brings us to another related topic: personal responsibility. Since many facets of health can be influenced by personal choices and behaviors, to gain optimal wellness, people must take an active role in their health and assume responsibility. Figure 1–4 shows that personal responsibility is at the center of all components of health; responsibility is what makes the wheel turn.

■▶ *Lifestyle choices affect physiological age and life expectancy. Lifestyle diseases are also influenced by people's lifestyle choices. People who perceive the locus of control with respect to wellness as being internal actively take steps to stay healthy and well.*

The Choice of Attitude

Suppose a person chooses all the right behaviors, and still bad things happen. People cannot choose, after all, whether accidents will happen to them or not, and they certainly can't choose never to die. Can an accident victim be a well person? Can a dying person be well? Yes, in a sense, they can, because they can choose their own attitudes toward these circumstances.

Consider the contrast between two people—one, who is relatively untouched by life; the other, who has suffered many misfortunes but is cheerful and strong. The first has never been ill, never had an accident, and never suffered a loss. The second has gained strength and character from every tough experience life has presented. Of the two, the first is *healthy* and may, with luck, remain so throughout life, but it remains to be seen whether this person can face hardships and stay *well* through them. The second person is a well person, for whatever misfortunes have beset this person have not defeated him or her.

The quality the well person is demonstrating is **resiliency.** Resiliency is probably the most valuable trait that one can cultivate; it may be even more valuable in promoting wellness than the lifestyle behaviors described in the previous section. When adversity strikes, a person with resiliency uses it as an opportunity to practice coping skills and comes out stronger.[5] Such a person will die, in the end, of course, for everyone dies. But even then, this person will not be defeated, for he or she will choose to prepare for death so as to face it with clarity and dignity.

locus of control a person's perception of the impact that personal behaviors will have on some outcome, such as contracting a disease or achieving recovery. People who view the locus of control with respect to disease or health as external to themselves will perceive that their efforts have nothing or little to do with illness or recovery. In contrast, people who see the locus of control as internal or within themselves, perceive that their actions will have a strong impact on their health.

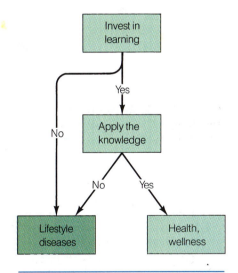

FIGURE 1–3 ■ **Invest in learning.**
For the majority of people, it pays to learn about health and apply the knowledge.

resiliency the ability to bounce back; in terms of emotional health, the quality of choosing to view each of life's hardships as a challenge, to learn from it, and as a result, to become stronger in the face of the next one.

5 stages to personal health

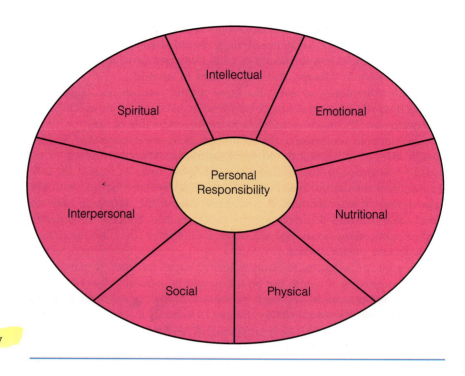

FIGURE 1–4 ■ **Personal responsibility and health.**

≣▶ *The choice of attitude is a key component of wellness. The person who takes hardships as challenges, and uses them as opportunities to practice coping skills, possesses resiliency and becomes stronger with each adverse experience.*

The Choice of Health Care Provider

The choice of a **health care provider** is mundane, compared with the choice of attitude, but it requires consideration at the start of this book.* It is important to choose one who is qualified to offer the medical and health care you need. Choose a physician (M.D., D.O.), a physician's assistant (P.A.), or a nurse practitioner (R.N.P.). These people all can provide care for ordinary medical problems; all can refer you to specialists for extra-ordinary problems. Physicians can write prescriptions for medicines not available over the drugstore counter; the other two work under physicians' auspices and can be authorized by their supervising physicians to write prescriptions.

Chapter 20 offers details on this and other health care options, but two other choices demand consideration here. One is the choice of how to relate to the health care provider. Since you are personally responsible for your wellness, it follows that you will not let someone else take this responsibility from you. You hire the health care provider to serve you. You are a **client,** the boss of the process, active in your own behalf. If you were a **patient,** on the other hand, the health care provider would be the active one and you

health care provider a person qualified to offer the following services:

- ■ Diagnosis and treatment of ordinary medical problems.
- ■ Referral to specialists when appropriate.
- ■ Preventive health care—that is, routine checkups at appropriate intervals and advice on preventive health behaviors.

client a person who actively pays another to perform a service.

patient a person who passively receives the benefit of a physician's services.

*As used in this book, the term *health care provider* refers to only three types of professionals: physicians (with the credential M.D., for *medical doctor,* or D.O., for *doctor of osteopathy*), physicians' assistants (abbreviated P.A.), or nurse practitioners (with the credential R.N.P., for *registered nurse practitioner*).

would be passive. Reflecting the view that people can guide their own health care, the term *client* is gradually replacing the term *patient* in health care circles, and the relationship between client and provider is becoming more equal than in the past.

The other choice that demands mention is the choice of when to attend to your own medical care needs, and when to go to a provider. The Spotlight at the end of this chapter shows that in some areas, you can perform your own health care: it is titled "Your Body—An Owner's Manual." It also shows how you can tell when you need professional medical attention.

≡▶ *Choose a qualified health care provider. Expect to work actively with, not to depend passively on, that person. Learn to distinguish between times when you can attend to your own health care, and times when you need to see your health care provider.*

The Choice of Whom to Believe

If you are responsible for your own wellness, it also follows that you will make your own choices of health and wellness products and services. This means, in turn, that you have to learn to see through health and wellness **fraud** or **quackery:** many salespeople are out there, competing for your dollars, and not all of them are honest. Figure 1–5 describes some of the tricks the dishonest ones use. To help enhance your skills in distinguishing fact from fraud, this book offers special Critical Thinking sections in every chapter; this chapter's version is on page 15.

≡▶ *Learn to distinguish valid from fraudulent health information. Health quackery is characterized by unidentified sources, emotional appeals, and the profit motive. Valid information reveals its sources, which are reputable, and it states scientifically derived findings.*

■≡ Health Behavior and Behavior Change

Health knowledge is hardly beneficial if it merely enables people to make A's on tests. It is valuable only if people use it to guide their behavior, a choice that depends first on motivation and commitment, then on action.

Motivation

The term **motivation** refers to the force that moves people to act. It may be either instinctive or learned. Instinctive motivation consists of **drives,** and is the strongest: hunger, thirst, fear, and tiredness propel people to take the actions necessary to meet their needs for food, water, safety, and sleep. Drives may also propel people to act in relation to others; the sex drive, protectiveness toward family members, and aggression are examples of drives. Learned motivation may also be powerful—consider the desire some people have for possessions, recognition, or achievement; or the desire others have to *relieve* themselves of possessions and lead a simpler life, or to work extremely hard for things they believe in. Powerful motivation virtually impels a person to act.

fraud conscious deceit, practiced for profit. Every chapter of this book deals with health and wellness information and misinformation, and Chapter 20 sums up ways to keep it all straight.

quackery another term for fraud. A *quack* is a person who practices health fraud. The word comes from an old word, *quacksalver*, which meant a person who boasts loudly about a medicine.

motivation the force that moves people to act.

drives instinctive motivation arising from sensations such as hunger, thirst, fear, and needs for sleep and sex.

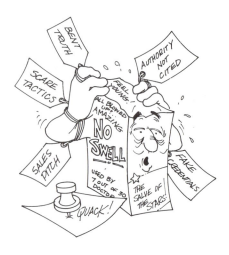

FIGURE 1–5 ■ **Identifying marks of health quackery.**

Becoming skillful at recognizing false, misleading, or unproven health and wellness information means learning the kinds of tricks that are used to mislead the unwary reader, viewer, or listener. One way to do this is to have a collection of "tags," like these, to identify these tricks. The more of these tags you can tie on a package of health information, the less likely it is to be valid.

In contrast, if a health claim has the following characteristics, it is likely to be valid:

■ It identifies its author, who is a recognized authority in the field—and the field is relevant to the health claim being made.
■ It is based on scientific findings published in reputable journals, and is interpreted correctly without bending or stretching the implications.
■ The source has no profit motive, but is merely communicating information.
■ The language is reasonable, not overly enthusiastic or optimistic. (For more on evaluating health claims, read Chapter 20.)

A psychologist explains motivation using the analogy of a black box with a reward inside. Suppose you were told, "If you'll put a dollar in the slot, you can take $1,000 out." Most people would not hesitate for a moment. They would drop their dollar in. But suppose you were told, "If you'll put a dollar in the slot today, you can take $1,000 out 20 years from now." Now you might think a minute. Today's dollar may mean more to you than the deferred gratification of many more dollars years away. Still, you might decide to drop your dollar in. Now suppose you were told, "If you put a dollar in, you may take $1,000 out—but when you touch the box, you'll get an electric shock." Most people want to know, "How much will it hurt?" Or suppose you were told, "If you put a dollar in, there's a 1 in 10 *chance* you can take $1,000 out." People are motivated to act in circumstances like these only if they perceive that the positives (rewards or benefits) outweigh the negatives (barriers, risks, and consequences).

Motivation can be viewed as being modified by three factors: the value of the reward (how big is the reward, and what does it cost?), its timing (how soon will the reward come, or how soon will the price have to be paid?), and its probability (how likely is the reward, and how certain is the price?).[6] The strength of a person's motivation depends on what weights the person assigns to these factors. Those weights, in turn, are modified by personal and social characteristics, such as age, gender, ethnic group, religion, personality, social class, and peer pressure.

Now contrast these situations:

■ Enjoy ice cream now (immediate reward); notice your weight gain tomorrow (pay later).
■ Forgo ice cream now; expect weight loss next week.
■ Smoke a cigarette (a certainty) now; pay with lung disease (a probability) in the future.
■ Give up smoking now; enjoy better health in the future.

No wonder it's difficult to motivate people to change their health habits!

Researchers have identified what motivates people to change their health behaviors. These payoffs seem to work best:

■ Cosmetic effect (you'll look better, younger, more attractive).
■ Employability (you'll compete better in the job market).
■ Sex relations (you'll get along better with the other gender).
■ Self-image (you'll be proud of yourself).
■ Reversal of any negative impressions other people have (people will be less put off by you).[7]

These motivators are at work in guiding behavior and in determining whether it will change.

≡▶ *Motivation is the force that moves people to act. It is influenced by the perception of the value and timing of rewards, and by the perception of the probability that consequences will result from the action.*

From Awareness to Action

How does health behavior change? This question is important, for many people *know* what to do to benefit their health, yet few actually *do* those things. The steps that lead to behavior change seem to group themselves into three phases—a contemplation period, in which no action is taking place; a period of action, in which progress is continually occurring; and a period of stability, in which the new behavior is cemented into place.[8]

During the contemplation period, these steps take place:

■ Awareness: "I could choose to change."
■ Cognition: "I know how to change."
■ Emotion: "I want to change."

Then, during the action period, the person commits to the change and starts making it:

■ Decision: "I will change."
■ Action: "I am changing."

While making the change, the person may shift back and forth from the old behavior pattern to the new; or may, in rare cases, exhibit only the new behavior. Finally, the person arrives at

■ Completed action: "I have changed."

When this achievement is realized, the person is at the point of feeling no inclination to revert to the old behavior, no matter what temptations may arise; and is confident of being able to resist relapse in all situations.

These steps don't always appear in the same order, but they always seem to appear. Nor do they appear in rapid succession; it may take months or even years for a person to go from one to the next.[9]

An example may help to show some of the dynamics of behavior change. Being overweight is a problem familiar to many people. (If you can't identify with this problem, substitute some other while reading this.) No doubt you know someone who wants to lose weight. He has taken the first two steps: he is *aware* of the need, and he *knows how*—at least, to some extent—yet still he is taking no action. Eating fattening foods brings him great pleasure, for one thing. For another, without being aware of it, he may receive some benefits from being fat. (He can develop friendships with women with fewer sexual implications, for example.) He may claim he wants to lose weight, and he may be chronically upset with himself for not getting thinner; yet deep inside he may not really *want* to change. Many people get stuck at this point.

Wanting is emotional—and when the emotions become positively involved, a rush of energy may enable a person to act. Still, even if the wanting is so strong that it brings tears of frustration or anger, emotion alone is not enough to change behavior. We all can name people who desperately want to lose weight, and yet still do nothing. The person has to make a decision not just for today, but for the long term, a step in which the will is involved. This is **commitment**.

At the point of deciding to commit to action, your friend who needs to lose weight says, "I'm going to eat wisely from now on," and does it. From that point on, possibly for months, he will stick to his plan faithfully. If he deviates, he will view the deviation as a momentary lapse, not as a relapse, will promptly return to his plan. (Chapter 6 describes the difference between lapses and relapse with respect to weight control.)

When the changed behavior holds up in the face of all temptations, your friend may seem to have become a completely different person. And in a sense, he is a different person. He has had to let go of his old habits. He has

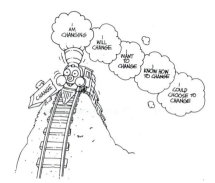

The elements of behavior change.

■ *FACT OR FICTION:* A person who wants to change a harmful health habit, and knows how, will do so. *False.* Wanting and knowing how to change a harmful health habit are not enough; a person also must have the will to change.

will a person's intent, which leads to action.

commitment a decision adhered to for the long term; a promise kept.

had to go through a grief experience—the loss of a cherished behavior with its rewards. His self-image has had to change. He *was* an overeater; he is now an *ex*-overeater. He *was* a person who avoided facing certain problems by overeating; he is now a person who owns those problems and deals with them constructively. He knows himself better, and he asserts himself more effectively.

In case you are reflecting on your own behavior and possible changes, it is as important to know when you are *not* ready as to know when you are. Much needless time and anxiety is wasted struggling with "I should; I ought to; I must" and struggling with shame and guilt over "I can't; I failed again." An important part of arriving at permanent desired behavior change is the awareness that success may require many practice runs. You should expect to stumble along the way; you don't have to succeed totally the first time.

≡▶   *People who successfully change their behaviors go through several steps from awareness to action. This process leads to commitment, a decision adhered to for the long term. Even people who are successful at changing their behaviors usually experience temporary setbacks.*

Behavior Modification

Suppose a person has firmly decided to make a change and is now about to begin. Many factors affect behavior and researchers have developed several theories to explain behavior in an attempt to help people make positive behavior changes. One popular theory states that people adopt health behaviors when they perceive they are susceptible to a condition, when they perceive the condition as severe, when they see great benefit in making a change, and when minimal barriers stand in their way.[10]* Another theory states that people adopt positive behaviors when they value health and are confident in their abilities to follow through with positive actions.[11]** So, valuing health and having self-confidence seem to be important parts of behavior change.

Another popular theory states that human behavior can be somewhat regulated by environmental factors. This is the theory of **behavior modification.†** In simple terms, this theory states that behavior can be seen as being sandwiched between two environmental conditions, those that precede it and those that follow it—the **antecedents** and the **consequences.** Because people can, themselves, use behavior modification techniques to change their own behavior, and because these techniques are recommended later in this book to help with weight control and fitness, they are described a little further here.

A (antecedents) → B (behavior) ←→ C (consequences)

According to the behavior modification theory, each behavior occurs in response to one or more cues (antecedents). The more intense the cues are, the more likely the behavior will occur. The behavior leads to positive or negative consequences, and the more intense these are, the more or less

behavior modification   the changing of behavior by manipulating the cues that trigger a behavior, the behavior itself, and the penalties or rewards attached to the behavior.

antecedents   cues, or environmental factors that trigger a behavior.

consequences   the penalties or rewards that follow a behavior.

---

*This is the Health Belief Model of behavior change.
**This is the Social Cognitive Theory of behavior change.
†Behavior modification strategies are derived from the theories of *operant conditioning*. (Operant behaviors are voluntary behaviors—those we can choose to do or not do; *conditioning* means learning; so the term *operant conditioning* means learning to change our choices.)

likely the behavior is to occur again. So to change behavior, the theory goes, you can adjust the cues and the consequences. By doing so, you can make desired behaviors occur more often and make unwanted behaviors occur less often or not at all.

Figure 1–6 illustrates behavior modification at work, showing the strategies in rectangular boxes and an example of each in ovals. The example is that of Chris, who needs to write a paper but lacks enough motivation to get started on it. Conditions are unfavorable: the TV is blaring, two friends have dropped in and are conversing, and there is no inviting place to settle down and work. Chris is tempted to procrastinate (unwanted behavior). Knowing the principles of behavior modification, though, Chris modifies the cues. Turning off the TV *eliminates* one cue to procrastination (strategy 1). Requesting that the friends come back later *suppresses* another cue to procrastination (strategy 2). Clearing off the table and turning up the lamp *strengthen* cues to studying (strategy 3). Once Chris begins to concentrate, the tendency to procrastinate fades, and the work begins to move forward (strategy 4). Now Chris indulges in self-congratulation (strategy 6).

A note about emphasizing negative consequences (strategy 5): if Chris had chosen to procrastinate, the result would have been work left undone—a negative consequence. But to pay much attention to this would be to reward it. Punishment is a form of attention—and attention is a reward. That is why unruly children, when they are punished, sometimes misbehave more. The most effective way to use strategy 5 is to ignore the unwanted behavior, not to call attention to it, and not to punish it.

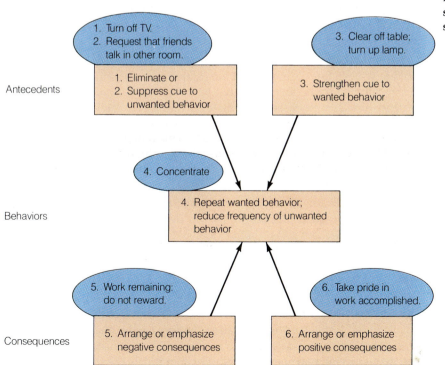

FIGURE 1–6 ■ **Behavior modification strategies used to facilitate effective studying.**

Behavior modification techniques equip people with a means of effectively changing their behavior if they want to. A particularly attractive feature of these strategies is that they don't involve blaming oneself or putting oneself down—a point of importance in fostering emotional wellness. The person who understands these techniques can say, "I know how to change—when I'm ready."

≡▶ *Some people use the theory of behavior modification to help themselves adopt positive lifestyle habits. Behavior modification strategies manipulate three things— the cues that trigger actions, the actions themselves, and the consequences of the actions—in the attempt to cement desired behaviors in place.*

From Action to Stability

Health behaviors usually don't change abruptly, nor, once changed, do they typically "stick" forever afterwards. Sometimes, even after what seems to be a firm commitment to changed behavior, a person slips back. Why? Once you have instituted a change in your life, you will maintain that change only for as long as you continue to feel rewarded by the change, or until it becomes a habit.

Let's switch our attention to a woman who smokes, to examine the broader application of behavior-change principles. She has decided to give up smoking, but after a day without cigarettes, she is a nervous wreck. After two days, she is experiencing extreme anxiety. At this time, the rewards of eventual respiratory health seem far away, and all that she is aware of is her desperate desire for a cigarette. This being the case, it is not surprising that she fails to give up smoking and returns to the habit within one or two days after making the initial effort.

To succeed, this person needed to have realistic expectations from the outset. She needed to know how difficult it would be and, especially, how long it would take before the pain would go away and the rewards would begin to come in. It would have helped her, too, to be alert to the immediate rewards—immediate, that is, in terms of days, not years. After a week, she could have been free of thoughts about cigarettes for several hours at a time, and in climbing stairs, she would not have become as winded as before. If she had tuned in to these immediate rewards, she might have made it through the hard part.

In resuming smoking, this person may have been unaware that the pain of withdrawal was about to diminish and that rewards were so soon to come. These awarenesses would have helped to cement the desired behavior change in place.

People need to know, too, that they can't undertake too large a change and expect to succeed. Suppose a person decides to give up cookies and cakes and candies and colas—in fact, to avoid all sugar—and not only to do that, but also to avoid all fatty foods—and not only that, but also to give up all alcoholic beverages—and to switch from whole milk to nonfat milk and never to use cream—and to give up salt—and to start jogging a mile every morning and do sit-ups every night—to go to church on Sundays—and to spend at least two added hours each day on homework. . . . That person may be in for a rude surprise. All these changes can be made, but not all at once. After only a few days, such a person will be exhausted and will give it all up, achieving none of the goals. We congratulate the person on having

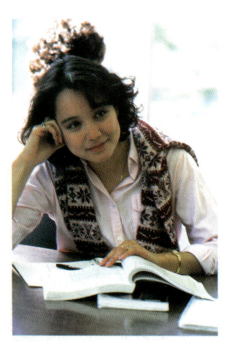

Once you are achieving the behavior you seek, congratulate yourself.

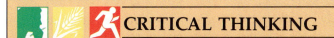 **CRITICAL THINKING**

The Miracle of Hard Work

Notice the attitude being demonstrated in the person switching from whole to nonfat milk. The person is making a behavior change for life. He isn't going "on a diet" that he plans to abandon later. He is cultivating a health habit that he is committed to maintaining. It may help him lose weight, yes, but it will also help him stay thin once he has reached his goal.

Notice, too, that he is willing to put in the necessary effort and practice for a permanent change. Now compare him with his roommate, who wants to get thin but *not* to change any of his habits permanently. The roommate has bought some diet pills to cut his appetite long enough to lose 20 pounds, but he has no plans to change any of his eating habits. You should have no trouble predicting which person will keep the weight off and which will regain it. Our nonfat milk–drinking friend will gradually lose weight and keep it off; his roommate will be a yo-yo.

The contrast is worth contemplating, because consumers are more susceptible to advertisements promising instant health gains without effort than to those suggesting they may have to work to get what they want. That's why diet pills and other quick fixes are advertised more often on TV than are permanent behavior changes that require hard work. But diet pills are precisely that—quick fixes, not permanent solutions. Permanent behavior changes, like switching to nonfat milk, are effective over the long term.

Permanent changes take work, not miracles.

identified many worthy goals. Now it's time to plan realistically. New behaviors require energy. They need to be taken up a few at a time—in fact, probably one by one.

For example, consider the effort needed just to switch from whole milk to nonfat milk. Registered dietitians sometimes use a "rule of three" to help people learn to like something new. Try nonfat milk once, and you may not like it; try it a second time, and you may say to yourself, "This isn't as good as whole milk, but I can drink it"; try it a third time, and you may say, "This is about the same as whole milk; I guess I don't prefer either one any more." Others say that it takes three weeks of conscious effort to set a new habit firmly in place. In any case, at some point, the habit of drinking nonfat milk becomes easy to maintain, because the preference for whole milk is gone. The new choice may even become the preferred choice.

This section has not identified all the many steps you can take to ensure that your behavior change efforts will be successful, but it has outlined some of the more important ones. A plan of action that incorporates these steps and others appears in Strategies: Changing Behavior.

Sometimes people comply with a suggested behavior only for a short time. When people revert to negative health habits, it is usually because they have forgotten the negative consequences associated with the old behaviors. For example, they failed to remember the time when they suffered

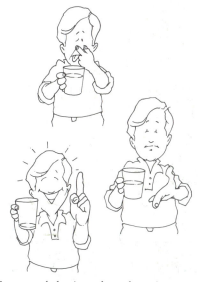

Try a new behavior at least three times to give it a real chance to stick.

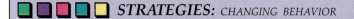

STRATEGIES: *CHANGING BEHAVIOR*

To make a behavior change:

1. Identify a goal. List the behaviors that will lead to the goal (desired behaviors) and the behaviors that will hinder progress toward the goal. List as many as you can.
2. For each behavior you have listed, identify the cues that prompt that behavior and the cues that tend to oppose the behavior.
3. Now set about changing the cues in all the ways you can to favor the desired behavior. Commit to changing. Plan. Dedicate the necessary time and money. Buy the equipment you need (owning a pair of jogging shoes gives you a boost toward being a jogger). Face what you'll have to give up or displace to give high priority to making the change. Mobilize the support of family and friends.
4. Envision your changed future self. Role-play the new you in your imagination.
5. Mark your progress in small, manageable portions. Break up your main goal into several small, achievable goals ("The next time, I'll take only one alcoholic drink on each weekend day"). Plan periodic rewards ("When I wake up feeling great, I'll go for a swim").
6. Start trying out the plan.
7. Modify the plan in ways that will succeed.
8. Try the modified plan.
9. Evaluate your progress often.
10. Savor your results, and value the benefits.

from shortness of breath; or weighed 250 pounds; or caught cold after cold; or were painfully paying, in whatever way, the price of the habit they might otherwise be tempted to resume. People who are totally, finally, absolutely committed to not slipping back have to make a conscious effort to remember the negative consequences of the old ways.

People who have long maintained a new way of life sometimes report episodes in which the old way springs back to consciousness, in dreams or unexpected memories. An ex-drug addict reports that she suddenly felt high again, and it scared her. A dieter dreams that he's been bingeing on chocolate. An ex-alcohol abuser awakens in a cold sweat from a nightmare in which she has vastly overindulged in alcohol. No one seems to know why these episodes occur, but they do serve a useful purpose: they bring back a vivid memory of the old behavior—and its price. Alcoholism counselors tell recovering addicts, "If you can't remember the last drink, then it wasn't your last." The maintenance of a new behavior sometimes depends on not forgetting that a return to the old behavior would be worse.

Finally, people changing their behavior have to realize that their self-images must change as well. Sometimes the self-image is slow to change, and the behavior slips back. People have to do some psychological work along with their physical work in order to change through and through. A person who gives up smoking has to learn to see herself as a confirmed ex-smoker. A person who takes up swimming every day has to own his new identity: "I am a swimmer."

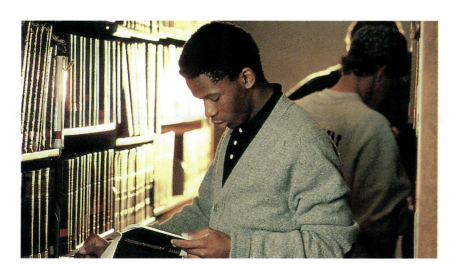

To help others effectively, make sure your information is accurate.

In summary, the maintenance of changed wellness-promoting behavior is facilitated by:

■ Continued motivation (remembering vividly the price of the old behavior and remaining aware of the benefits of the new).
■ A changed self-image.

One additional factor helps immensely if behavior change is to succeed, a factor that may be more important than any of those named above:

■ High self-esteem.

People who start out feeling worthwhile, who prize themselves enough to invest energy and effort in their own wellness, are most likely to maintain healthy behavior changes. The person who begins to succeed in changing behavior gains improved self-esteem from the effort and so wins an advantage for the efforts ahead.

≡▶ *Maintenance of improved health behavior depends on continued rewards, realistic expectations, and continued commitment. Remembering the negative consequences of old behaviors and improving self-image and self-esteem can help people maintain positive behavior changes.*

▣≡ Other People's Health Behavior

Perhaps you are concerned about someone else's behavior: "How can I get my father (mother, roommate, friend) to change?" These people's choices are *not* your responsibility. You can care about them and you can help them, but you can't change their behavior. No matter how much you may want them to do what you think is best, you cannot make the choice for them. In fact, your best bet is usually to say nothing and let the awareness of what they need to do come upon them from inside. Most important, make no negative judgments; these reduce the other person's self-esteem and make change less, not more, likely.

You can, however, facilitate the dawning of awareness. These strategies are especially effective:

- Give straightforward feedback.
- Set an example with your own behavior.
- Offer accurate information, or make sure it is available.

An example of the first strategy is offered by a student who baby-sat for a young mother who went out to parties several evenings a week. The student observed that the mother usually had two or three drinks before she went out and often came home dangerously drunk. All the student dared to say to the woman was, "Gee, every time I see you, you have a drink in your hand."

As it turned out, this was all she needed to say. The woman chose to seek treatment for alcoholism and later thanked the student for her help. "What did I do to help?" the student wanted to know. "You made me aware that I had a problem," the woman replied. "I hadn't realized how far I had gone until I saw myself as you saw me." The student had delivered straightforward feedback, as a mirror does, with no judgment implied.

The second strategy, setting an example, is also effective because it is nonjudgmental. No one likes to be told, "You really ought to quit doing this," or "You really ought to start doing that." In fact, people often do not even like to be reminded of resolutions they themselves have made: "Aren't you going to work out today?" If you change a health habit yourself, however, the person you are concerned about will surely notice and may begin thinking about doing the same thing. When ready, this person may ask you how you did it or ask to join you.

The third strategy, to supply accurate information, helps increase people's knowledge, so that when they become ready to make a change, they are equipped to do it. The information you offer may be statistics on the risks of having unprotected sex or "how-to" facts such as the meeting time and place for the next smoke-enders class. To be most helpful, don't push such information at others, but simply make sure it is available in case they want it.

If you try to influence someone and think you've failed, take comfort. The "failure" may be a success waiting to happen. Your feedback and information may not tip the scale right now, but together with other factors will weigh on the favorable side. It may take years before someone decides to make a lifestyle change for health's sake, but when the change happens, the person may well credit it to something someone said years earlier. Don't hesitate to care. Do what you can; then take satisfaction in having done your best, and let it go.

When someone does make the choice to change to a health-promoting behavior, you then have a further opportunity to help:

Offer positive reinforcement and support.

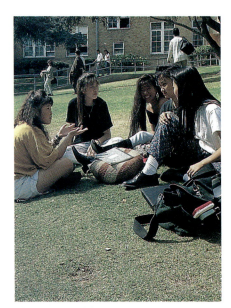

The support of friends strengthens motivation.

Keep the verbal praise moderate, however; some people don't like to have too much attention drawn to their first tentative efforts. Also, make sure the reinforcement you give is positive, not negative: "I'm glad to see you doing that," not "It's about time you did that" (which takes the credit from your friend). Also: "You look wonderful," not "You look better" (which implies that your friend looked awful before).

Much more is involved in promoting positive behaviors, but these ideas are enough for a start. Whether you keep your own life or other people's in mind as you read, we hope the chapters to come will bring you the information you need to facilitate informed health choices.

≡▶ *To help motivate other people to adopt desired health behaviors, offer feedback, provide examples, and supply accurate information. Don't push, and don't take responsibility for their choices. If they do change, offer congratulations and support.*

■≡ Portrait of a Well Person

The lists that follow itemize the elements of wellness, roughly in the order of the chapters to come. To cultivate mental, emotional, and spiritual wellness, a person:

■ Maintains high self-esteem; is willing to attempt new learning and behaviors, and is able to handle setbacks without loss of self-esteem.
■ Monitors emotions, managing and expressing them appropriately.
■ Recognizes potential emotional problems in self or others and seeks help with them when appropriate.
■ Feels that life has meaning; lives by cherished values.
■ Trusts and relies on a power greater than self; feels part of a beneficial process, not isolated.
■ Manages stress with skill and enjoyment, not letting it become overwhelming.

Chapters 2, 3, and 4 describe the strategies you can employ to pursue these goals.

To cultivate physical wellness, a person:

■ Obtains sufficient sleep to function well.
■ Enjoys food and uses it both for pleasure and to meet nutritional needs; maintains appropriate weight.
■ Cultivates physical fitness; enjoys outdoor play.
■ Uses over-the-counter drugs with respect, accurately matching each product to the need for it.
■ Uses prescription drugs with care, following directions fully.
■ Does not abuse any drugs. Uses no tobacco; uses alcohol in moderation, if at all.

The Spotlight following Chapter 4 explains the importance of sleep, and the series of chapters that follow address nutrition and fitness.

To cultivate interpersonal and social wellness, a person:

■ Develops supportive friendships; can socialize with others without the influence of alcohol or other drugs.
■ Can develop and maintain intimacy with another; can form a successful long-term partnership.
■ Understands and appreciates his or her sexuality; manages sexual relationships so as to enhance the quality of life.
■ Understands the principles of contraception, can communicate about it, and makes informed decisions about its use.

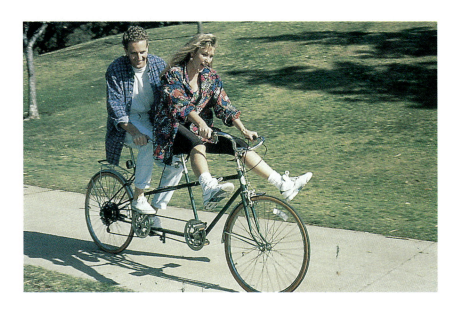

Well people enjoy outdoor play.

■ Continues growing, learning, and facing new challenges with advancing age.
■ Knows what is involved in facing death (one's own or someone else's) and faces grief with understanding of its stages.

Chapters 9 through 16 address these subjects.

Since life's events are at times outside an individual's control, a well person also has to be aware of the possibilities of accidents and diseases and be adequately defended against them. Thus a well person:

■ Is aware that accidents are a real possibility and takes appropriate preventive measures.
■ Is aware that infectious diseases (including sexually transmitted diseases such as acquired immune deficiency syndrome, or AIDS) are a real possibility and takes appropriate measures to prevent them.
■ Learns about his or her own risk factors for diseases and takes whatever measures are indicated to prevent them.
■ Knows how to evaluate health claims and products and successfully resists being victimized by misinformation and fraud.
■ When necessary, can use the health care system to advantage; when appropriate, can tend to his or her own medical needs.
■ Relates to the larger environment (home, community, world) and takes an appropriate share of the responsibility for it.

Chapters 17 through 21 and Appendix E address these subjects.

This long description not only defines wellness but implies actions to achieve it. It could be termed a list of **life management skills.** It feels good to be in control, to manage your own life. People who have already developed these skills to some extent, and who are actively moving forward along these lines, are maximizing their chances for enjoyment of life.

life management skills   the skills that help a person to realize his or her potential to be well and enjoy life; this book's strategies.

▶ *A person who chooses to cultivate wellness adopts many positive behaviors in all realms: mental, emotional, spiritual, physical, interpersonal, and social. These behaviors could be called life management skills.*

Your health now and in the future is largely influenced by your lifestyle choices. Heredity governs some aspects of health to some extent, and environmental factors put control of some aspects of health out of reach, but within these limits, your health is yours to enhance or impair. To enjoy youth and vitality throughout your entire life, learn and cultivate positive life choices.

For Review

1. Explain the differences in meaning between the terms *health* and *wellness*.
2. Identify the areas of life to which the terms *health* and *wellness* apply.
3. Describe the difference between chronological and physiological age.
4. Identify six factors shown by research to have maximum impact on the physiological age of adults and an additional factor that affects life expectancy in younger adults.
5. Contrast the lifestyle diseases and the infectious diseases. Explain how the nature of the lifestyle diseases places the locus of control for them within the individual.
6. List some factors that influence motivation.
7. List and describe the steps that lead to behavior change.
8. Describe ways in which people can manipulate antecedents, behaviors, and consequences to facilitate behavior change.
9. Identify some requirements for maintaining a changed behavior.
10. Describe a plan of action for ensuring successful behavior change.
11. Describe effective strategies for facilitating desirable health behavior change in other people.
12. Itemize life management skills to promote wellness in the following areas: (1) physical; (2) mental, emotional, and spiritual; (3) interpersonal and social; and (4) life events such as accidents and diseases.

Notes

1. World Health Organization: Constitution of the World Health Organization, *Chronical of the World Health Organization* 1 (1947): 29–43.
2. Joint Committee on Health Education Terminology, *Report of the 1990 Joint Committee on Health Education Terminology* 22 (1991): 173–184.
3. N. B. Belloc and L. Breslow, Relationship of physical health status and health practices, *Preventive Medicine* 1 (1972): 409–421.
4. D. S. Gochman, *Health Behavior* (New York: Plenum Publishing, 1988), pp. 43–63.

5. G. E. Richardson, B. L. Neiger, S. Jensen, and K. L. Kumpfer, The resiliency model, *Health Education,* November/December 1990, pp. 33–39.
6. We are indebted to Dr. Richard L. Hagen, associate professor of psychology at Florida State University, for sharing the analogy of the black box with us.
7. The art of counseling for weight reduction, *Nutrition and the MD,* July 1977.
8. J. O. Prochaska, Assessing how people change, *Cancer* 67 (1991): 805–807.

9. Prochaska, 1991.
10. D. S. Gochman, 1988, pp. 27–41.
11. I. M. Rosenstock, V. J. Strecher, and M. H. Becker, The role of self-efficacy in achieving health behavior change, *Health Education Quarterly* 15 (1988): 175–183.

SPOTLIGHT

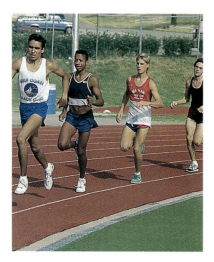

Your Body—An Owner's Manual

Advice about health care usually has more to say about curing illnesses than it does about staying healthy. But the most important aspect of health care most of the time is *self*-care. Doing a few simple things for your body can enable you to maintain it at least as lovingly as you would maintain a fine car. By attending to a few simple self-care techniques, you can spend less time trying to cure illnesses and more time doing the things you like doing. The trick is to adopt the necessary health habits—some daily, others only once a month or once a year.

That sounds like a worthwhile objective. I invite you to give me an owner's guide to the care of my whole body, starting with my bright smile.

A bright smile says something about its owner—that the person has high enough self-esteem to tend daily to tooth care. You probably already know how to brush your teeth, but you may not know that tooth decay can lead to major illness of the whole body. Even without decay, teeth that collect food particles and **dental plaque** create unpleasant mouth odor. (See the Miniglossary of Personal Health Terms for definitions of words in boldface type.)

The bacteria that live in plaque break down food particles and create acid. The plaque holds this acid like a sponge, and this dissolves away the tooth's outer layer, its **enamel.** The person may not feel a **cavity** forming in its early stages, but as the decay advances into the tooth's middle layer, its **dentin,** it eats into nerves, and the pain can be shocking. Should the decay infect the tooth's deepest layer, its **pulp cavity,** it may kill the tooth. If a cavity is discovered in the early stages, a dentist can drill away the damaged part of the tooth surface and replace it with a substance that seals and saves the tooth.

Brushing your teeth after each meal and flossing once each day, as shown in Figure S1–1, can remove particles and plaque—if, that is, you brush and floss correctly. Some people brush and floss wrong, every day, all their lives, and suffer tooth and gum disease despite their efforts. Dental plaque takes hold at the gum line and beneath it, and the gums themselves become diseased if plaque gets out of hand. Gum disease causes mouth odor and causes more tooth loss than tooth decay does. Ninety percent of all adults will develop gum disease; the early symptom is gums that bleed easily. But gum disease is a problem everyone can avoid.

In brushing, angle your brush so as to pull plaque out from below the gum line along the outside and inside surfaces of your teeth. Brush down on the upper teeth, up on the lower ones. In flossing, use the floss to pull the plaque up from below the gum line, *between* the teeth. If you do only this, only once a day, you will be doing more to protect your teeth and gums than you can by any amount of brushing of tooth surfaces.

By the way, you need not buy expensive toothpastes and mouthwashes for a clean mouth. They do taste good and freshen the breath for a few minutes, and some even provide a little fluoride, but this amount is not nearly so effective as the treatments given by dentists. For everyday cleaning, a toothbrush, clean water, and baking soda is all you need.

If I do all that, do I still have to visit the dentist?

Yes. A professional cleaning about once every six months and a full examination about once a year can go a long way toward helping you keep your teeth for life. Your dentist can advise you as to the intervals that are appropriate for you. And, of course, you are advised to obtain adequate fluoride and avoid sugary snacks.

Talk about my skin—I'm concerned about acne.

First, of course, daily washing of your skin is important. Millions of bacteria live on your skin, and this is normal, but if they are allowed to accumulate without removal, they may penetrate deeply into the skin and cause infections. Dirt may harbor disease-causing bacteria, too, as well as the normal ones. Wash with soap, not just water, for soap makes the bacteria slippery enough to be washed away.

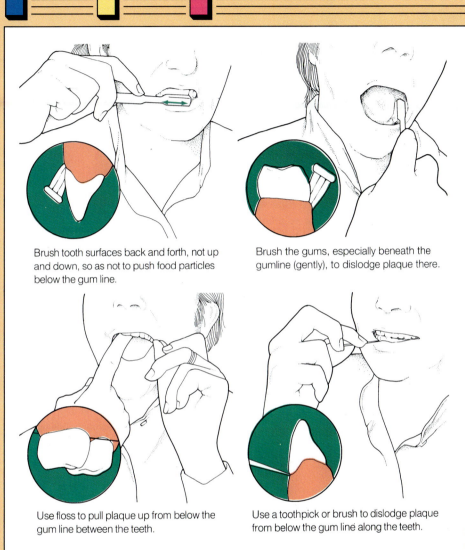

Brush tooth surfaces back and forth, not up and down, so as not to push food particles below the gum line.

Brush the gums, especially beneath the gumline (gently), to dislodge plaque there.

Use floss to pull plaque up from below the gum line between the teeth.

Use a toothpick or brush to dislodge plaque from below the gum line along the teeth.

FIGURE S1–1 ■ **Brushing and flossing the teeth and gums.**

As for **acne,** no one knows why some people get acne and others do not, but it is known to run in families. The hormones of adolescence also play a role by making the glands in the skin more active.

The skin's natural oil is **sebum.** Sebum is made continuously in deep glands and is supposed to flow continuously to the skin's surface through the tiny ducts around the hairs. Each duct has a lining that normally sheds by scaling and

flaking, and the oil, constantly being secreted, carries these scales and flakes to the surface of the skin. In acne, the oil is not brought to the surface of the skin; instead, skin-surface bacteria may find their way down into the ducts. The scales, instead of being carried out of the duct, stick together and form a plug, which weakens the duct so that oil and bacteria leak into the surrounding skin. The oil and bacteria irritate and cause redness, swelling, and **pus**

formation—the beginning of a **whitehead,** or pimple. A **cyst** may form—a sort of enlarged, deep pimple. Or the skin may open above the plug, revealing an accumulation of dark skin pigments just below the surface—a **blackhead.** These eruptions may cause permanent scarring.

Now, many people think skin bacteria cause acne, but they do not. Bacteria make it worse, once the process has begun. Also, the color of a blackhead is caused by pigments, not by dirt, so cleanliness alone isn't the answer. Squeezing or picking at the pimples to try to remove their contents does not help—it can cause more scars than the acne itself does.

How, then, can you treat acne?

Many remedies have been suggested: washing constantly, sunbathing, taking antibiotics, spreading vitamin A acid on the skin, avoiding certain foods and beverages, or obtaining relief from stress. Each of these has helped some people, but people respond differently to them. While science searches for future treatments, there is no surefire way of getting rid of acne.

Some products are worth a try. Among the over-the-counter (available without prescription) treatments are those that contain benzoyl peroxide. These have been proved safe and effective, although they can dry out and irritate the skin. Careful washing with mild soap helps remove skin-surface bacteria and oil and helps to keep the oil ducts open.

Other products and treatments are available by doctor's prescription. Among them are antibiotics to be either applied on the skin's surface or taken internally. Skin creams that contain an acid related to vitamin A are available: the acid loosens the plugs that form in the ducts, allowing the oil to flow again so that the ducts will not burst. But follow a physician's advice carefully in using the acid. It may burn the skin and even *cause* pimples to form, making the acne look worse at first.

Can acne be prevented?

Possibly—or at least its severity can perhaps be lessened. Many people think that certain foods and drinks

worsen their acne. Chocolate, cola beverages, fatty or greasy foods, nuts, sugar, and foods or salt containing iodine have all been blamed for worsening acne. Although it's not proved that these foods do worsen acne, if they do seem to affect your skin, there's no harm in avoiding them.

Stress clearly worsens acne, by way of the hormones that are secreted in response to it. Vacations from school or other pressures slow secretion of stress hormones and so help to bring relief. The sun, the beach, and swimming also help, because they are relaxing; the sun's rays also kill bacteria, and the swimming can help cleanse the skin. Beachgoers and other swimmers should exercise extreme caution, though. Too much sun can also bring on skin cancer, so steps to prevent sunburn are essential. Also, if you take antibiotics for acne, be aware that these can make the skin extra sensitive to the sun's rays—check with your physician before spending a day outdoors.

One remedy always works: time. While waiting for acne to clear up, keep the symptoms under control with treatments that work for you. Refrain from probing or picking at the skin to prevent scarring, and keep your eyes open for new developments.

What sorts of products should I use on my skin?

All you really need is soap and water. Companies that make other self-care products, of course, promote them as absolutely necessary to help you stay clean: vaginal sprays, douches, scented powders, and cologne. But the truth is that none of these products are needed for *health*. Most simply mask odors for a while.

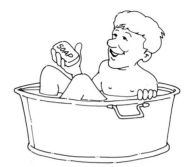

All you need is soap.

Body odor is caused by the action of normal skin bacteria on sweat and skin debris. While no threat to health, unpleasant odors may make others withdraw and damage a person's self-esteem. People may want to use an antiperspirant to reduce the sweat that feeds the bacteria that cause body odor. Also, a deodorant may help a little to mask any odor that may form during the day. Antiperspirants and deodorants are not substitutes for cleanliness, though, and even the most aromatic ones cannot totally mask the odor of unclean skin.

Hair gets dirty like the rest of the body, but you can use the same soap for the hair as for the body or you may choose a shampoo. If you have dandruff, most so-called dandruff shampoos do not actually cure dandruff. To find a truly effective dandruff treatment, ask a pharmacist for suggestions.

Many other products are on store shelves. Scented powders are nice, and they can relieve chafing and irritation, but unscented ones or plain cornstarch works just as well. As for cologne, if it boosts your self-image, it may be valuable. However, cologne is like many other products—unneeded for health. Don't be misled by sellers trying to force products on you.

What about care of the genitals?

For both males and females, a careful daily washing of the external genitals is all that is required to keep them free of infections and odors. Vaginal sprays and **douches** are not needed—a healthy vagina cleans itself all the time. An unpleasant discharge or bad odor may indicate an infection and should be checked by a physician. Not only are douches unnecessary, they can be downright dangerous. Douching interrupts the normal cleaning cycle and may wash bacteria up into the normally bacteria-free areas of the reproductive tract. Douching may even increase the risk of developing cancer of the reproductive system. And women should know that the vagina, usually clean and healthy, can easily become infected with bacteria from the stools. To prevent this, always wipe toilet paper from front to back, never from back to front.

What else should a body owner do by way of daily maintenance?

Consider your skeleton. Have you ever wondered why it is that some people seem to radiate energy, have a bounce in their step, and seem to be a picture of high self-esteem? One of the best things good posture does is to give a person that energetic look. By the same token, a person who slumps or sways appears tired, bored, or negative. Since you have to stand, sit, walk, and lie down anyway, why not align your body for its best posture?

The way you walk, sit, and sleep affects your skeleton profoundly over the years. The bones and disks of your spine are of particular interest, and if you have had even a twinge of back pain, you will know why. Think

of your spine as a set of 26 delicate hollow bones (**vertebrae**) stacked upon one another like doughnuts with pads between them (the disks). Think of your spinal cord running right up through the holes in the doughnuts.* (A difference from doughnuts is that the holes in the vertebrae are near their edges, not at the center; see Figure S1–2.) Major nerves exit and enter at every level between the vertebrae—and if the bones or disks are damaged, they can bulge out and pinch those nerves. The result: stabbing pain, like an electric shock, torturing the muscles of the neck, shoulders, back or legs. This may sound like something that will never happen to you, but if you learn the statistics, you can figure the odds: during their adult lives, eight out of ten people have back pain severe enough to warrant a visit to the doctor.[1]*

That's still not likely to happen to me. I don't do strenuous work that involves my back.

You might be surprised to learn that people in the sedentary (sitting) occupations are most susceptible. If they don't exercise, their back and abdominal muscles become weak, and their spines tend to become less and less well supported. Poor posture combined with weakened muscles provides a virtual guarantee of major back trouble.

What do the abdominal muscles have to do with it? Are you telling me I should exercise my stomach to protect my back?

*Counting the "tailbones," there are 33 vertebrae in most people's spines; some have 34.

*Reference notes are at the end of the Spotlight.

Yes. Most people know that walking, bicycling, swimming, or other regular exercise that works the long muscles of the back is protective, but they do not know that they need strong abdominal muscles, too. Overly strong back muscles can bend your spine backward unless you have strong abdominal muscles to work against them.[2] Abdominal crunches or modified sit-ups (see Chapter 7) are therefore important. And how you sit, stand, and walk also matter. The image to keep in mind is of that stack of doughnuts. Keep it in its normal S curve so that it will not topple; so that it will hold your heavy head up by balancing, not by straining; and so that the nerves will run straight through it unimpeded.

You mentioned how I sleep as being important, too.

Yes. You spend a third of your life sleeping—8 hours out of every 24. By the time you have lived 75 years, you will have spent a quarter of a century lying down. Whatever position you choose to lie in for 25 solid years is bound to affect the shape of your skeleton permanently.

I hope you're not going to tell me to change the position I sleep in. I doubt I could learn to sleep in any other position.

No one position is right for sleeping, but there are some to avoid. Figure S1–3 shows the principles. In general, the idea is to keep your spine in its normal curve while sleeping, just as you would try to do while awake. If you sleep on your back, support your knees, so as not to develop a swayback, and do not use too high a pillow under your head. If you sleep on your side, use a

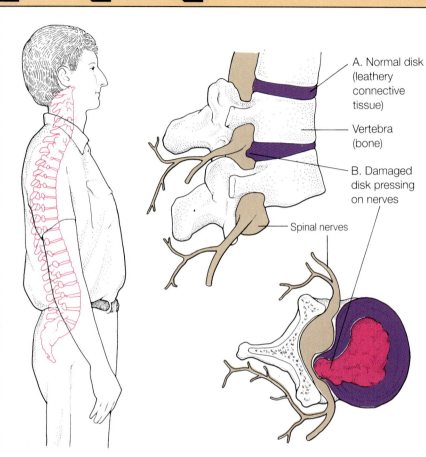

A. Normal disk (leathery connective tissue)

Vertebra (bone)

B. Damaged disk pressing on nerves

Spinal nerves

Normal curve of the spine. When the bones are stacked this way the discs bear the weight evenly, and the nerves feel the least pressure.

FIGURE S1–2 ■ The spinal column.

The spinal cord runs through the hollow part of the bones of the spine. Branches of nerves leave the main trunk at each level to carry messages to and from the body parts. Disks provide padding between the bones. Disk A is normal and protects the nearby nerves from being pinched. Disk B has bulged out of shape and is pinching the nearby nerves. Depending on how high in the spine this defect is, the result will be pain in the neck, shoulder, lower back, or legs. Other common back damage causing pain includes flattened disks, bone spurs, worn-out vertebral joints, or degeneration of the vertebrae themselves (osteoporosis).

pillow just high enough to keep your neck straight. Do not sleep on your stomach; this stresses the back. Figure S1–3 shows how to sit, stand, and walk, too.

That sounds like good advice. Any other daily habits I should be conscious of?

None we haven't covered elsewhere. We stress nutrition; fitness; and alcohol, drug, and tobacco use in later chapters.

You mentioned monthly and yearly chores, though. What did you have in mind?

Breast and testicular self-examinations fall into the monthly category. Chapter 19 shows how to do them, but knowing how is not enough. You also have to *remember* to do the examinations every month. Some people keep a reminder with the monthly bills.

As for yearly health care duties, a woman needs a Pap smear every year, but neither women nor men need complete physical examinations every year. Once every five years is frequent enough for young people, and for older ones, schedules are available that will help catch the

major diseases of later life in time to treat them (ask your health care provider).

What can I do to protect my hearing and vision?

For hearing—don't listen to loud music through earphones, and don't attend loud concerts without earplugs. If you use guns, use ear-protecting muffs along with them. For vision—watch television from 6 feet or more away and with lights on in the room. Don't stare into the television from up close, especially in a dark room. Don't expose your eyes to

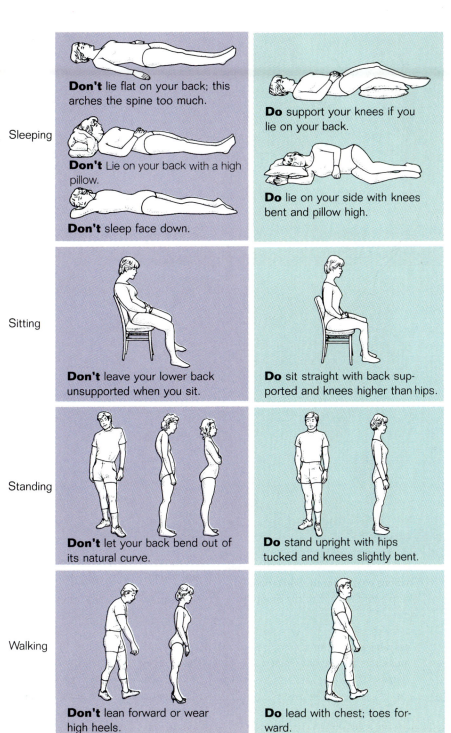

Sleeping

Don't lie flat on your back; this arches the spine too much.

Don't Lie on your back with a high pillow.

Don't sleep face down.

Do support your knees if you lie on your back.

Do lie on your side with knees bent and pillow high.

Sitting

Don't leave your lower back unsupported when you sit.

Do sit straight with back supported and knees higher than hips.

Standing

Don't let your back bend out of its natural curve.

Do stand upright with hips tucked and knees slightly bent.

Walking

Don't lean forward or wear high heels.

Do lead with chest; toes forward.

FIGURE S1–3 ■ **Care of the spine.**

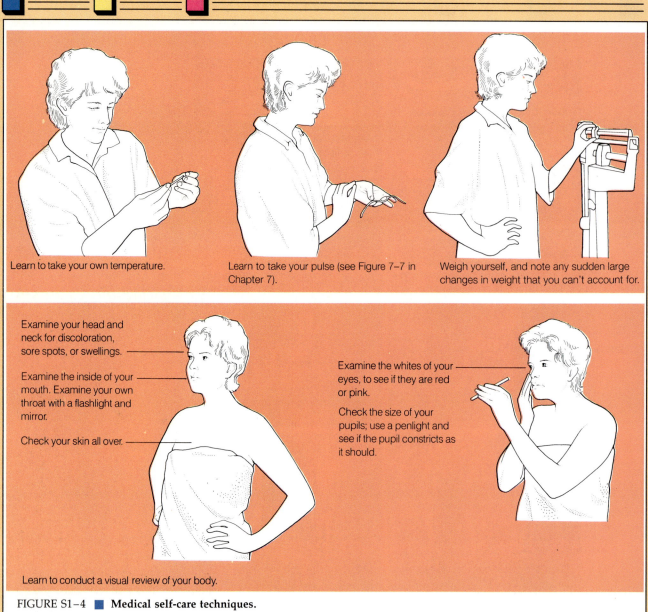

Learn to take your own temperature.

Learn to take your pulse (see Figure 7–7 in Chapter 7).

Weigh yourself, and note any sudden large changes in weight that you can't account for.

Examine your head and neck for discoloration, sore spots, or swellings.

Examine the inside of your mouth. Examine your own throat with a flashlight and mirror.

Check your skin all over.

Examine the whites of your eyes, to see if they are red or pink.

Check the size of your pupils; use a penlight and see if the pupil constricts as it should.

Learn to conduct a visual review of your body.

FIGURE S1–4 ■ **Medical self-care techniques.**

These are observations you can make, yourself, before visiting a health care professional. The keener your self-awareness, the better you can take care of yourself, and the better you can cooperate with medical personnel when necessary.

any kind of radiation other than ordinary light, and never stare at the sun or at an ultraviolet light.

That about takes care of all the maintenance activities you need to engage in to keep your body in smooth

running order—other than to seek medical help when necessary, of course.

What signs should send me running for medical care?

People could save themselves a lot of time, money, and needless worry if

they knew when *not* to visit a health care provider, as well as when *to* see on. One time not to go is when you have an ordinary cold, as explained in Chapter 8. You also need not go if you have:

■ A mild rash without other symptoms.

■ A single episode of vomiting or diarrhea without abdominal pain.

■ A fever of less than 102 degrees Fahrenheit (39 degrees centigrade).

You do need to go for periodic checkups and immunizations; your provider can give you a schedule for these. And you should make a special visit if you have any of the symptoms listed in the box ''When to Obtain Medical Help,'' in Appendix E.

Those are useful lists. Now, all I need to know is how to take my temperature and how to take my pulse, and I'll be all set.

Figure S1–4 offers these and a few other techniques everyone can learn to use. To learn more of the same, you may want to purchase a self-care book such as the American Medical Association's *Family Medical Guide.**

You should also learn and practice the basics of accident prevention, and take a course in first aid, to be maximally responsible for your own health care. And if you have a chronic condition (such as hypertension, diabetes, arthritis, or kidney disease), there are many ways in which you can learn to monitor and regulate it yourself. Self-care initiatives do not replace professional health care, but they certainly complement it nicely, and they give you the sense, which is appropriate, that your health care is your own responsibility.

*Other good references: D. W. Kemper, K. E. McIntosh, and T. M. Roberts, *Healthwise Handbook: The Practical Family-Based Guide to Care* (Boise, Idaho: Healthwise, 1991); D. M. Vickery and J. F. Fries, *Take Care of Yourself: The Consumer's Guide to Medical Care* (Reading, Mass.: Addison-Wesley, 1990); Better Homes and Gardens's *Family Medical Guide;* Consumer Guide's *Family Medical and Health Guide;* or Good Housekeeping's *Family Health and Medical Guide.* Look for the latest edition.

■ MINIGLOSSARY
of Personal Health Terms

acne a continuing condition of inflamed skin ducts and glands, with a buildup of oils under the skin forming pimples.

blackhead an open acne pimple with a buildup of dark skin pigment (not dirt) in its opening.

cavity a hole in a tooth caused by decay. (Tooth decay is also called dental *caries*.)

cyst (SIST) an enlarged, deep pimple.

dental plaque (PLACK) a buildup of material on the surfaces of the teeth.

dentin a tooth's softer middle layer.

douches fluids, supposedly sold to cleanse the vagina; actually, vaginas clean themselves constantly with no help, and douching can wash dangerous bacteria into the reproductive tract.

enamel a tooth's tough outer layer.

pulp cavity a tooth's deepest chamber that houses its blood vessels and nerves.

pus A mixture of fluids and white blood cells that collects around infected areas.

sebum (SEE-bum) the skin's natural oil, actually a mixture of oil and waxes, that helps keep the skin and hair moist.

vertebrae (singular, **vertebra**) the bones of the spine—26 above the point of attachment to the pelvis, 7 or 8 below it.

whitehead a pimple filled with pus, caused by the plugging of oil-gland ducts with shed material from the duct lining.

■≡ Spotlight Notes

1. T. Nordstrom, Steps to a healthy back, *Healthline,* May 1985, pp. 14–16.

2. J. Willis, Back pain: Ubiquitous, controversial, *FDA Consumer,* November 1983, pp. 5–7.

CHAPTER 2

Emotional Health

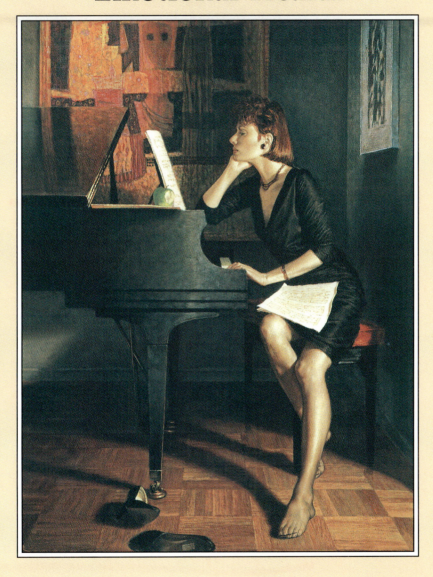

Becoming Emotionally Healthy
Developing Self-esteem
Relating to Others

Finding a Place in Society
■ **SPOTLIGHT** Spiritual Health

FACT OR FICTION

Just for fun respond true or false to the following statements. If false, say what is true.

■ Emotional health is not related to physical health. (Page 32) F

■ The most important relationship in life is the relationship with your lifemate. (Page 33) T

■ It is best to reject illogical or unpleasant feelings. (Page 35) T

■ If you sometimes feel like a child when you are sad, you are emotionally immature, and you need to grow up. (Page 37) F

■ Since one cannot change the past, it is a waste of time to examine childhood experiences. (Page 38) F

■ People with high self-esteem focus on their positive qualities and do not see their negative attributes. (Page 41) T

Emotional health is a key part of total wellness. Most emotionally healthy people take care of themselves physically—they eat well, exercise, and get enough rest. They work to develop supportive personal relationships and are often well developed spiritually. Thus emotional health benefits overall wellness and all areas of life.

In contrast, many people who are emotionally unhealthy are self-destructive. For example, emotionally unhealthy people often abuse alcohol, nicotine, or other drugs; they often overeat or overwork. These self-destructive behaviors can lead to drug addictions, cancer, obesity with its associated risks, heart disease, and other ills.

The idea that emotional health and physical health are closely intertwined has received national attention. Many people claim that our emotional health is so important that it "affects what we do, who we meet, who we marry, how we look, how we feel, the course of our lives, and even how long we live."[1]*

How can you know if you are emotionally healthy? What can you do to improve your emotional health? This chapter attempts to help you answer these questions. It begins by exploring the most important relationship in your life—the relationship with yourself.

■≡ Becoming Emotionally Healthy

To become emotionally healthy, you must function well in three spheres—in relation to yourself, to others, and to society. To obtain a preview of what is involved, try the Life Choice Inventory on page 48.

In becoming emotionally healthy, you first need to know yourself. You need to examine your thoughts, needs, values, and feelings. You also need to discover the various aspects of your personality and to recognize the stages of life that await you. The relationship with self is the most important and must be positive before the relationships with others and society can be truly rewarding.

■ **FACT OR FICTION:** Emotional health is not related to physical health. *False.* Emotional health is a key part of overall wellness.

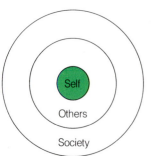

The emotionally healthy person functions well in three spheres—in relation to self, to others, and to society.

*Reference notes are at the end of the chapter.

Self-knowledge is not given at birth. Human beings normally are conscious of only a small part of themselves, and to discover more takes learning and practice that, ideally, continue for a lifetime.

Self-knowledge begins when you ask yourself, "Who am I?" You may answer this question by just saying your name: "I am Leslie Owens." You may add that you are a man or woman, an important aspect of yourself. Then you may go on to describe other observable traits, such as your height, weight, age, occupation, and race. Beneath these surface traits, though, who are you, really? What are your intimate, secret thoughts, needs, values, and feelings?

Thoughts, Needs, and Values

Your **thoughts** take place in the outermost layer of your brain. They are conscious; you are always aware of them. Your thought processes assist you in integrating information about yourself.

Your thoughts shape your life. If you think distorted, negative thoughts, you probably will feel unhappy. Norman Vincent Peale claims in his successful book, *The Power of Positive Thinking*, that you can have peace of mind, improved health, and a never-ceasing flow of energy through learning to think positively.[2]

Training your mind to think positively is a challenging discipline and requires persistent practice—but the rewards are well worth the work. Recent research shows that such training can protect people from illness, even better than the positive health practices mentioned in Chapter 1.[3] Through positive thought processes you can also begin to work on the next task in becoming emotionally healthy—identifying your **needs**.

Some people don't even know they have needs, but everyone does, and recognizing them and learning how to meet them fosters emotional health. The psychologist Abraham Maslow has described a hierarchy of needs that provides an excellent start. According to Maslow, people will struggle to meet their basic needs before they can begin to think about "higher" things.[4] Hunger is such a need. People who are hungry may not be able to think about their need for love. Once the basic need for food is met, however, other needs naturally arise. In other words, needs form a hierarchy, and when you have met the most basic ones, you become more aware of, and can strive to meet, the "higher" ones (see Figure 2–1).

Most primitive are needs related to survival—needs for food, clothing, and shelter (physiological needs). Next are the needs to feel physically safe and secure (safety needs). If safe and secure, people are free to notice their needs to be loved, to feel emotionally secure (love needs). If those needs are met, they can be in touch with their needs for respect and esteem; and given that, they can seek to achieve the ultimate—self-actualization, or the realization of their full potential. Only a few people, perhaps 1 to 2 percent, ever evolve that far.

Becoming aware of your needs is an important step in getting to know yourself. As you continue to learn about yourself, you will identify more specific needs, and you will seek ways to meet them. Through this process, you will become aware of another important component of yourself—your values. Exploring your values also increases self-knowledge.

Your **values** are your rules for behavior—more simply, what you view as right and wrong. You learned the first ones from your family and society,

thoughts those mental processes of which a person is always conscious.

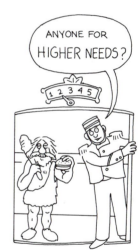

Once basic needs are met, a person can aspire to meet higher needs.

needs elements that are essential for health and wellness.

self-actualization the final step in Maslow's hierarchy of needs, the realization of a person's full potential.

values a person's set of rules for behavior.

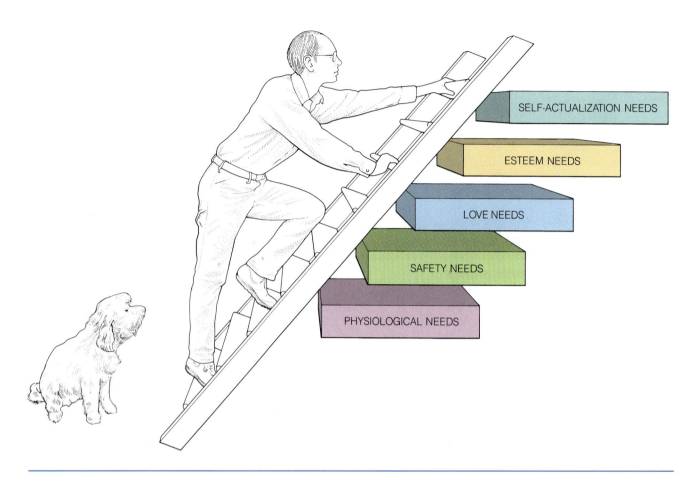

SELF-ACTUALIZATION NEEDS

ESTEEM NEEDS

LOVE NEEDS

SAFETY NEEDS

PHYSIOLOGICAL NEEDS

FIGURE 2–1 ■ **Maslow's hierarchy of needs.**

and later you continued working them out for yourself. Values assign positive and negative weights to things and lead to decisions.

Values are both conscious and unconscious; sometimes you can state them in words, but sometimes they influence your behavior without your awareness. People who are well acquainted with themselves are keenly aware of their values, and that helps them to choose their behaviors without confusion. For example, a student who values honesty and is conscious of this value probably will choose without hesitation not to cheat on exams.

You can discover your values by stating your beliefs. Then, to discover how strong your values are, you can ask some questions about them.[5] For each value that you state, ask the questions in the margin.

Values often arouse strong emotions (feelings) within a person. A student who values honesty, yet cheats on an exam, is likely to feel guilty. Being able to identify and find the source of a feeling is a key step in emotional development. People who are emotionally healthy are able not only to recognize, but also to deal with, their emotions, often by expressing them, and sometimes by taking action.

≡▶ *Knowing your thoughts, needs, and values is a key part of self-knowledge. Learning to manage your thoughts, meet your needs, and live by your values is an important part of emotional health.*

To discover how strong your values are, ask:

■ Would I be willing to affirm this value publicly?
■ How faithfully will I stand by this value when it is challenged, or when the acts it implies bring negative consequences?
■ Do I act consistently and repeatedly in line with this value?[6]

Emotions

An **emotion** is defined as a felt tendency to move toward something assessed as good or favorable or away from something assessed as bad or unfavorable. The terms *emotions* and *feelings* are often used interchangeably. A sampling of emotions and their extremes appears in the margin.

The emotions that arise in response to events often depend on prior experiences with events of that kind. The experience of hearing a twig crack in the woods, for example, may arouse the emotion of fear or joy or interest, depending on what you are expecting. The experience of being frustrated in your attempt to reach a goal may arouse a mixture of emotions including impatience, anger, and irritation. Losing a loved one (the experience of grief) evokes a series of emotions including both anger and sorrow.

Sometimes a person has a feeling and cannot pinpoint its cause. When this happens, often the person will discount the feeling as illogical. But even when feelings seem unreasonable, they are not "wrong"; they are as natural as the wind. Feelings are acceptable and healthy—all of them.

The cartoon in the margin shows a person shouting. The person is angry but won't admit it. Anger is not accepted in many social settings, so people often deny it. Other emotions people often deny are hurt, loneliness, and the like—feelings that reveal weakness and vulnerability.

Some feelings are labeled acceptable for women, but not for men—for example, feeling sad and crying. Women in our society are "allowed" to cry, but men are viewed as weak if they cry. A message that boys hear early on is, "Big boys don't cry." Some men carry this unhealthy message into their adulthood and do not learn to express sadness.

It is acceptable to feel anything. It may not be acceptable to act on all feelings, but you must deal with them somehow; and often your mind has to decide how to handle them. It may be necessary to suppress an emotion momentarily (for example, if fear would be incapacitating, and action is needed). It is fine to do so (and necessary for survival in some instances), but it is best to face the feeling as soon as possible. Repressed emotions can accumulate and ultimately make it difficult for a person to function either emotionally or physically. (More about the negative consequences of "stuffing feelings" will follow in the next chapter.)

Some people are closely in touch with their feelings and easily express them. Others find it hard to express their feelings or even to know what these feelings are. Generally, people who are aware of their feelings and who express them appropriately are more emotionally healthy than people who ignore them.

The first step in dealing with your emotions is to recognize them when they occur. If your heart is pounding, your knees are shaking, and your palms are sweating, you are feeling fear. Other steps follow, not necessarily in the order presented here, but all are essential to emotional health.

An important part of dealing with emotions is to accept them. People often have a hard time accepting some feelings, especially unpleasant ones such as hurt; they may feel overwhelmed by the intensity, and they may fear that the pain will not pass. Feelings are like waves, and if you ride them out, they pass and leave you peaceful. Only if you fight them do they keep on coming back.

Another reason people may resist their feelings is that the actions contemplated in response to the feelings may be unacceptable. It helps to keep

emotion   a felt tendency to move toward something assessed as good or favorable or away from something assessed as bad or unfavorable. Also called a *feeling*.

A sampling of emotions and their extremes:

Affection—love.

Anger—rage.

Desire—lust.

Dislike—revulsion.

Distress—anguish.

Excitement—frenzy.

Fear—terror.

Happiness—ecstasy.

Interest—fascination.

Possessiveness—jealousy.

Shame—humiliation.

Sorrow—agony.

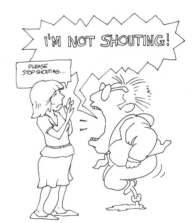

People deny anger because, in our society, it seems unacceptable or inappropriate.

■ *FACT OR FICTION:* It is best to reject illogical or unpleasant feelings. *False.* It is best to face and deal with all feelings as promptly as possible, even those that seem illogical or unpleasant, although it is not always best to act on them.

To verbalize your feelings, name them:

I'm angry.

I'm upset.

I'm hurt.

I'm sad.

I'm excited.

I'm resentful.

I'm envious.

I'm anxious.

I'm frustrated.

I'm afraid.

I'm thrilled.

I'm stressed.

I'm uneasy.

I'm touched.

I'm nervous.

I'm lonely.

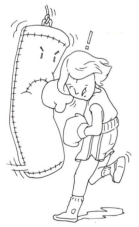

Express anger physically in order to become able to relax enough to consider the situation rationally.

in mind the distinction between feelings and actions. Some actions are not acceptable, of course, but impulses toward them are OK. A young mother, listening to her baby crying, may have a sudden impulse to hit the baby; that is natural, and all mothers have such impulses. A person who feels sexual desire may imagine having sex with a stranger; the impulse is natural. A rejected lover, in a flood of self-pity, may feel like committing suicide; that feeling, too, is natural. When you can recognize, own, and express in acceptable ways even negative feelings, you have grown emotionally.

The next step in dealing with feelings is to express them appropriately. That means doing something physical—speaking, writing, crying, shouting, laughing, or otherwise acting out emotions. Let's take the first alternative: speaking. How often in the last two or three weeks have you made any of the statements listed in the margin, either to yourself or to someone else? Knowing that you have these feelings is helpful in dealing with them.

Expressing feelings is sometimes best done physically. Calmly saying, "I'm angry," for example, doesn't fully express the feeling. It releases more of the emotion to speak angrily (you can do this in a room by yourself), or even to beat on a punching bag (you can do this in private, too). It is not acceptable to knock down another person with a blow to the jaw just to express your anger, but doing nothing at all can be harmful to you. Once you have let off steam by yelling, crying, running, dancing, or whatever, then you can relax again and calmly reassess the situation that triggered the emotion in the first place.

In some instances, you may find that expressing the feeling is all you need to do to cope with it. But other times negative emotions return over and over again. If they do, they are a signal that you need to assess the situation. You may need to act, to change something. You may need to confront another person.

For example, someone we know was furious at his lifemate. In addition to recognizing the anger, owning it, and verbalizing it, this person expressed it physically in a socially acceptable way every day after work—by digging a hole in the backyard. After a year the hole was big enough for a swimming pool, and our friend was a superb physical specimen—but still an angry person. He had to reassess the situation; it was time for a change; and a confrontation became necessary. How to express grievances is described later in this chapter: see ''Relating to Others.'' (Dealing with resentment is discussed in the next chapter, and working through conflict is described in Chapter 12.)

So far, this section has presented ways of identifying needs, exploring values, and expressing emotions. The accompanying Strategies sum up the steps in dealing with emotions just described. Now, to help you develop a

Emotions are expressed physically.

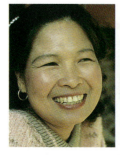
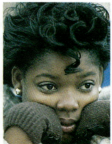
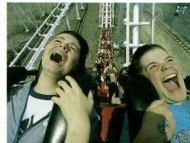

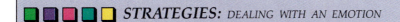

STRATEGIES: *DEALING WITH AN EMOTION*

To deal with an emotion, you must:

1. Recognize it.
2. Own it: accept that you feel it.
3. Verbalize it: express it in words to yourself or someone else.
4. Express it: take physical action.
5. If a negative emotion persists or returns, reassess the situation. A confrontation may be necessary.

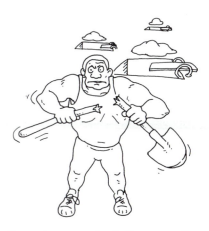

Expressing anger physically may produce fitness but no resolution. Either action or acceptance is needed.

fuller understanding of your emotions and yourself, the discussion turns to meeting the personalities within.

≡▶ *Recognizing, accepting, and expressing feelings are important facets of emotional health. Feelings sometimes need physical expression and sometimes indicate other needs for action.*

The Personalities Within

Many people have learned much about their emotions and themselves through the theory of **transactional analysis (T.A.)**. This theory holds that everyone's personality is made up of a cluster of selves that develop during the early years: the Child, the Parent, and the Adult.[7] The Child is the little person characterized by spontaneity and curiosity. The Child in you experiences many of your feelings. This is why you may often feel like a child when you are very angry or sad. The Parent is composed of all the people who wielded parental authority over you in the past; this figure exemplifies your values. The Adult is the reasoning person who collects information, weighs facts, and makes meaning of them. The Adult is like the character Mr. Spock from the science fiction adventures of "Star Trek"—emotionless, dull, measured, and factual. Table 2–1 lists the traits of the Parent, Adult, and Child; corresponding examples are in the margin.

The figures we carry within us exert a major influence on our emotional health. Take the Parent figure, for example. Parents (simply stated) can be

transactional analysis (T.A.) the theory that everyone's personality includes Parent, Child, and Adult figures.

■ *FACT OR FICTION:* If you sometimes feel like a child when you are sad, you are emotionally immature, and you need to grow up. *False.* It is normal to feel like a child when you are sad.

TABLE 2–1 ■ **Traits of the Parent, Adult, and Child in Transactional Analysis**

Parent	Adult	Child
Nurturing	Information giving	Loving
Tender	Fact finding	Impulsive
Helpful	Reality testing	Curious
Judgment making	Intelligent	Playful
Value conveying	Objective	Exuberant
Tradition transmitting	Able to estimate probabilities	Spontaneous
Critical	Able to compute dispassionately	Irresponsible
		Selfish
		Manipulative

Examples of T.A. personalities:

On seeing an older child wildly pushing a baby in a park swing:
PARENT: Oh, dear, she'd better stop that before someone gets hurt.
ADULT: The baby seems to be enjoying the ride, the swing is sturdy, and it looks as though he's buckled in pretty well.
CHILD: Whee! That looks like fun! Me next!

On seeing a row of tulips in early spring:
PARENT: Mustn't touch!
ADULT: I wonder how a person goes about growing such lovely flowers.
CHILD: I want to pick them all for myself!

On waking up in the morning feeling extra sleepy:
PARENT: Stay in bed, Honey; you need your rest.
ADULT: If I stay in bed, I could catch up on rest, but I stand a chance of missing something important today.
CHILD: Zzzzzz . . .

■ *FACT OR FICTION:* Since one cannot change the past, it is a waste of time to examine childhood experiences. *False.* It is important to examine childhood experiences, because the messages received in childhood influence emotional health today.

either of two kinds: critical or nurturing. The critical Parent reacts to the child in a predominantly negative, judgmental way. A person raised in this type of atmosphere can develop a negative self-concept that interferes with emotional growth. A person who heard condemning messages throughout childhood about being unwanted, in the way, no good, sloppy, or lazy usually adopts a critical Parent as a permanent part of the personality. Naturally, such a person continues in adult life to hear negative judgments from within.

In contrast, the nurturing Parent reacts to the child positively as being cute, funny, industrious, achieving, and the like. The child then, on becoming an adult, carries a more self-approving Parent inside, and the accepting messages heard during childhood are repeated throughout adult life. These statements are confirming and support emotional health.

Part of becoming emotionally healthy is learning to adopt a nurturing parental attitude toward yourself. Those who received criticism and negative judgments during childhood must work hard to change the negative internal messages into positive ones, so as to foster emotional well-being.

Exploring the personalities within requires that you examine your childhood experiences and how they affected you. This can help you grow toward emotional maturity. You can also gain insight by looking forward, so as to know what changes life may bring you. Psychologists study the stages of life to acquire insight into the dynamics of individuals.

≡▶ *The theory of transactional analysis holds that everyone's personality includes Child, Adult, and Parent components. Being a nurturing Parent to your one's internal Child, and using one's internal Adult to make realistic judgments, fosters emotional health.*

The Stages of Life

Several theorists have studied the patterns of change that take place during adult life. When people see the patterns of their lives, they can assume some control and make conscious choices that would not be possible otherwise.

According to the psychoanalyst Erik Erikson (see Table 2–2), the first two decades of adult life are spent working on the issue of intimacy versus isolation. In this stage, the person works out the details of relationships with others and society. The person also learns to balance healthy self-centeredness with unselfishness, avoiding both extremes. The person, by age 30, ideally has a strong sense of self and direction.

Sometime around age 30 the so-called midlife crisis may strike. People may painfully come to fear that their dreams may not be fully realized. With full adulthood (often around age 40), the person is established and self-accepting. At 60 or so, the shift into old age begins; Erikson sees it as a challenge to maintain the sense of personal worth during retirement, when the self may begin to seem less important.

Another thinker, Gail Sheehy, has described the pattern of life in slightly different terms—as a series of crucial turning points, or crises. A person who is going through one of these crises may be comforted to know that it is a normal part of life. Sheehy's predictable crises of adult life are shown in Table 2–3.

It takes years to develop emotional health; in fact, the process never ends. No one ever becomes perfect; one just keeps on becoming. But to provide a

---

TABLE 2–2 ■ **Eight Stages of Life According to Erikson**

Stage and Age	Developmental Task
Infancy (0 to 1)	To learn **trust** as opposed to distrust. The infant receives affection and learns that needs will be met. (If neglected, abused, or deprived of love, the individual may go through life mistrusting the world.)
Toddler stage (1 to 2)	To learn **autonomy** as opposed to shame and self-doubt. The toddler, even though dependent on parents, learns to be a separate person with self-will. (If thwarted in this development, the toddler learns to feel inadequate and ashamed. As an adult this person may remain dependent and have feelings of inadequacy.)
Preschool age (3 to 5)	To learn **initiative** versus guilt. The child explores the world with eager curiosity and an active imagination. (If discouraged in this development, the child will feel guilt at natural impulses and as an adult may hesitate to display initiative or take risks.)
School age (6 to 12)	To develop **industriousness** as opposed to inferiority. Having built on the three previous stages, the child now has the confidence to pursue self-chosen goals at play and at school with vigor. The child works well and functions well socially. (If this development fails, the adult will lack confidence and will perform poorly.)
Adolescence (13 to 20)	To develop an **identity** as opposed to suffering role confusion. The adolescent develops a strong sense of self, goals, and timing; becomes busy learning how to fit in the social circle—as leader, follower, female, male. The adolescent picks out role models to emulate and grows in confidence and self-definition. (The failure of this development produces a confused young person without a secure time sense or sense of direction.)
Young adulthood (21 to 40)	To develop **intimacy** versus isolation. The well-developed young adult can commit to love, to work, and to a social group or community. (The failure of this development leads to avoidance of intimacy, sexual promiscuity, isolation, and destructiveness.)
Adulthood (41 to 60)	To develop **generativity** versus stagnation. The mature adult moves through life with confidence, taking pride in others' accomplishments (especially those of children or young people). (The negative side of this development is self-involvement and failure to encourage others.)
Older adulthood (61 and older)	To retain **ego integrity** as opposed to falling into despair. The person feels fulfilled and faces death with serenity. (The adult who has not enjoyed the positive sides of each of these developmental stages experiences increasing isolation and despair and fears death.)

---

sense of the goals, Table 2–4 presents a description of the ideal end result and sets the stage for the next chapter's discussion of emotional problems.

Notice that the first attribute mentioned in Table 2–4 is self-esteem. This quality is the most crucial part of all in becoming emotionally healthy, so the next section is devoted entirely to it.

TABLE 2–3 ■ **Predictable Crises of Adult Life According to Sheehy**	
Age	**Crisis**
18–22	"Pulling up roots"—breaking free from family.
22–29	"Trying Twenties"—getting started on life, locating peer group, gender role, occupation, philosophy of living.
30–34	"Catch 30"—making new choices, developing more realistic goals.
35–45	"Deadline Decade"—reevaluating of accomplishment, discovering of autonomy.
mid-40's	"Renewal or Resignation"—developing a hardened, stale attitude or revitalizing warmth and mellowing.

≡▶ *To cultivate emotional health means to keep on growing, to continue to deal with the psychological changes life brings. Many of the changes are predictable, and it helps to know what they may be.*

TABLE 2–4 ■ **Characteristics of Emotionally Healthy People**
Emotionally healthy people:

Have high self-esteem.

Are confident that their behavior is normal.

Are honest.

Accept themselves.

Can have fun.

Don't take themselves too seriously.

Recognize that other people can enhance their lives but are not the sole source of their happiness.

Can have intimate relationships.

Do not try to control things they cannot control.

Do not constantly seek approval and affirmation from others.

Do not manipulate others or get their way by underhanded means.

Usually feel they are similar to other people.

Take responsibility appropriately, but do not take too much responsibility for others.

Give loyalty when it is appropriate and deserved.

Consider consequences before acting.

Deal with emotional pain by feeling and expressing it appropriately.

Are able to grieve when they suffer losses.

Continue to mature mentally, emotionally, and spiritually throughout their lives.

Live with balance, not extremes.

Validate and acknowledge their observations, feelings, and reactions.

Creatively express themselves, if inclined, by dancing, painting, writing, singing, acting, or other artistic activities.

Attend to their physical and psychological needs.

Disclose family problems when appropriate.

Refuse to tolerate inappropriate behavior.

Are not prone to stress-related illnesses.

SOURCE: J. G. Woititz, *Adult Children of Alcoholics* (Pompano Beach, Fla.: Health Communications, 1983); R. Hemfelt, F. Minirth, and P. Meier, *Love Is a Choice* (Nashville: Thomas Nelson, 1989), pp. 9–16.; Artistic expression may boost physical and mental health, *University of Texas Lifetime Health Letter*, July 1991, p. 7.

▣≡ Developing Self-esteem

How many people do you know who really believe in and respect themselves? Do you? People who are emotionally healthy have high self-esteem: they know and like themselves. People with high self-esteem do not think they are perfect; in fact, they know they are not, but like themselves anyway. They not only cherish their positive qualities; but have learned to accept the negative, even though they may be trying to improve. In contrast, a person who claims to be perfect probably has low self-esteem; that's why the person denies having imperfections.

Self-esteem is so crucial for emotional health that some psychologists use attitudes toward the self as criteria for evaluating mental health.[8] Self-esteem is valued as so important to individuals and society that the state of California has formed a task force to promote self-esteem and personal and social responsibility in its young people.* The rationale is that poor self-esteem is closely linked with alcoholism, drug abuse, crime and violence, child abuse, teenage pregnancy, prostitution, chronic welfare dependency, and failure of children to learn. The need for people to develop stronger self-esteem is evident from the millions of people with alcoholism and the huge illicit drug trade, which cost millions of dollars in medical expenses, lost productivity, law enforcement, and corrections every year. Poor self-esteem diminishes not only the individual, but also society.

High self-esteem facilitates emotional growth. If you know you are a worthwhile person, then you will take care of your total health. Some unhealthy people claim that so much attention to self is indulgent and selfish, but as it happens, those who take care of themselves actually have more to offer their families, friends, and society.

You can enhance your self-esteem in two ways: one, by fostering a positive view of your inner self; the other, by developing a healthy relationship with your outer self, your body.

A Positive View of the Inner Self

A technique for viewing the inner self positively is to practice making affirmative statements.[9] These statements, called **affirmations**, can be ones perceived as true now or statements to be made true by means of practice. Affirmations **empower** people—that is, they make people feel effective. Affirmative ideas replace defeating messages.

To practice making affirmations, repeat positive messages so often that they embed themselves in your subconscious mind and manifest themselves in your life. Affirmations should all be "I" statements, phrased positively: "I can relax when under stress"; "I can be alone without being lonely"; "I deserve success"; "I accept myself as I am." Also helpful is to visualize yourself succeeding at a task or developing a quality you desire. Visualizing success helps people build self-esteem, improve their school performance,[10] battle disease, win athletic contests, and overcome emotional problems.

self-esteem belief in oneself; self-respect and self-liking.

■ *FACT OR FICTION:* People with high self-esteem focus on their positive qualities and do not see their negative attributes. *False.* People with high self-esteem have learned to accept the positive and negative sides of themselves.

affirmations positive statements about one's self, often used to increase self-esteem.

empower to give ability to, to make effective or powerful.

*Most U.S. public school health education curricula are built on improving self-esteem.

As well as thinking positively, you can take actions:[11]

■ Write out your affirmations.
■ Pursue activities (occupational and recreational) that reflect your skills and interests.
■ Be grateful; appreciate what you have.
■ Attend support groups.
■ Read meditation books and concentrate on uplifting thoughts.
■ Read positive literature and watch movies with positive themes.
■ Listen to self-help audiotapes.
■ Attend seminars, lectures, and workshops.
■ Surround yourself with friends who believe in you.
■ Affirm others—believing in, supporting, and empowering others affirms ourselves.
■ Relax.
■ Have fun.
■ Celebrate your successes.
■ Exercise and nourish your body.
■ Obtain therapeutic massage.
■ Give and receive affection (hugs, for example).

Another suggestion for making desired affirmations become reality is "acting as if" you already have the quality you are seeking. This is often called "fake it 'til you make it." This technique is not only useful for personal growth, but also for teaching salespeople how to sell products successfully.

Still another way some people empower their inner selves is through cultivating spiritual health—through a relationship with their **higher power**. These people enjoy a sense of peace, because they feel in touch with a force greater than themselves and greater than human limitations. Spiritually healthy people feel loved by their higher power, and this facilitates self-acceptance. People who have a relationship with a higher power have a sense of purpose, not just a meaningless day-to-day existence. They feel significant, part of a big plan on a large scale. This chapter's Spotlight further explores the concept of spiritual health.

Finally, a way to foster a positive view of your inner self is to appreciate your own uniqueness. Too many unhappy people compare themselves to others and strive to be like those around them. Knowing that you are special in your uniqueness and that no one else can be you can improve your self-esteem.

Part of developing self-esteem is to like yourself for who you *are*, not for what you *do*. Society's focus on achievement can result in overvaluing externals such as how much money you make, the car you drive, or the position you hold. This subtly erodes self-esteem and creates a frenzy of striving to achieve according to society's standards. Then when people fail, they think this, too, reflects on them: when they make mistakes, they become their mistakes. The mistake actually is what a person does, not who the person is. Knowing that you are unique and worthwhile aside from your achievements and accomplishments, and in spite of your failures and mistakes, supports your self-esteem.

higher power   a power greater than the individual human self. Some people refer to their higher power as God.

≡▶   *Self-esteem is central to emotional health. To foster self-esteem, affirm your positive qualities, and develop those you desire. Act as if qualities you wish for were already yours. Discover your relationship with a higher power.*

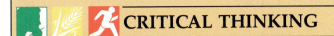

CRITICAL THINKING

Marketing Tricks

People who try to sell products to improve your outward appearance are motivated to benefit themselves, not you. To benefit themselves, they have to extract money from you. If you are satisfied with yourself as you are, they lose; they have nothing you'll be willing to buy. So their marketing strategy is to promote your self-dissatisfaction, to convince you that your appearance is not acceptable. They want you to believe that you have a problem and that they have the solution. A person with low self-esteem is practically defenseless against these tricks; in fact, low self-esteem is one of the marks of a person who is vulnerable to quackery. The higher your self-esteem, the easier it is to see through these tricks, the more confidently you develop your own image, and the less you will feel compelled to bend yourself out of shape to fit into other people's molds.

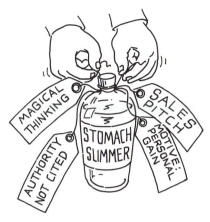

Low self-esteem benefits image sellers; high self-esteem benefits you.

A Positive Body Image

The second part of self-esteem is a positive body image. Poor body image is prevalent in our society, partly because people have accepted emaciated fashion models as models not for clothes, but for body size. Poor body image causes adolescent depression and poor self-esteem, particularly among females.[12] Each year, millions of people try to change the way they look. Half a million undergo cosmetic surgery; 40 million go on diets; and multitudes try contact lenses, facials, and new cosmetics in hopes of becoming more attractive.[13] People feel that they must be sexually attractive, and our society has high standards for sexual attractiveness. As you might guess, the intense desire for a sexier appearance makes us sitting ducks for quacks (see Critical Thinking: Marketing Tricks).

Improving your body's appearance is a worthwhile goal, though, if you do it by means of good nutrition and physical activity, so that it benefits your physical health as well. Chapters 5, 6, and 7 offer many tips on how to develop nutritional health and fitness. Once you've attained a healthy body, though, let that be enough. Don't compare your body with society's unrealistic, unhealthy standards for sexual attractiveness. Be content with being healthy and fit; don't try to get thin at the expense of your wellness.

≡▶ *A positive body image can contribute to self-esteem, but society's goals for body image are unrealistic. Learn to see through sales pitches that insult people; aim for health and fitness, not for emaciation.*

We've said that the emotionally healthy person functions well in three spheres—in relation to self, to others, and to society. So far, this chapter has been devoted primarily to the most important relationship in anyone's life—the relationship with self. Now, what about relationships with others?

■≡ Relating to Others

As individuals, we need relationships with other people—it is normal and healthy to turn to relationships to meet some of our needs. However, a vast difference exists between meeting normal needs in relationships and becoming dependent and overly needy. An emotionally healthy person develops a balanced give-and-take with others.

Relationships are varied. Relationships you have with your parents are different from those you have with your siblings or your friends. Friendships can vary tremendously. Your intimate love is different from any other relationship. All of these connections with others form a web that helps define who you are.

People who value themselves cultivate a strong **support system**; this may consist of family; neighbors; friends; people at work, school, or church; a mentor or adviser; and a therapy or self-help group. Of course, the person participating in such friendships and social groups stands ready to give, as well as to receive, and so does not need to be embarrassed about asking for support sometimes.

Most people derive their first support from the family, and it is from the family that they learn how to interact with others. Those who have positive, nurturing family experiences are most likely to have positive relationships in their adult lives. An emotionally healthy family provides an environment conducive to healthy emotional development. (The emotionally unhealthy family is discussed in the next chapter.)

People also develop friendships for support. Friends are a vital aspect of a healthy and fulfilling life, and studies show those with social ties are physically healthier than those who are isolated.[14] Many people are afraid to cultivate friendships at first, often because they are shy. *Why Am I Afraid to Tell You Who I Am?* is a book written to help shy people overcome their fears about relationships.[15] Its title reveals the primary problem shy people have: fear—specifically, fear of being rejected. In one survey of 120 college students taking a personal health course, 80 percent of those who heavily

---

support system a network of individuals or groups with which one identifies and exchanges emotional support.

The emotionally healthy person maintains strong relationships with others.

A support group lends security to its members.

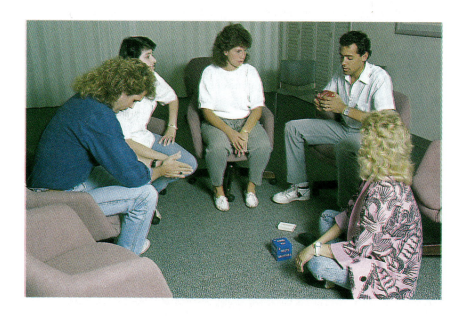

drank alcoholic beverages stated they did so because they were shy and needed extra courage to socialize. Table 2–5 lists tips for overcoming shyness.

Reaching out to other people usually does not lead to rejection, but to get started, you have to be willing to risk rejection and to handle it if it occurs. It helps to keep two things in mind: first, "If I'm rejected, I won't be any worse off than I am now"; second, "If it doesn't work out, it's no reflection on me; I tried. The other person had other needs." More often, when you reach out, you find that the other person is pleased to be approached. At least you have the benefit of some contact; at best, a rewarding relationship has a chance to form.

Multitudes of people who know this can't act on it, though, because they don't know how. A few specific suggestions can help. Each can be practiced in isolation, in front of a mirror, or with one close friend you already trust. One authority recommends remembering these suggestions by thinking of the word *soften* (see margin)[16]. To these, we'd add:

■ Disclose your own feelings (people always find feelings interesting).
■ Ask questions about the other person's feelings (people like you to be interested in them).
■ Listen attentively (people love to be listened to).

■ S Smile.
■ O Open posture.
■ F Forward lean.
■ T Touch.
■ E Eye contact.
■ N Nod.

TABLE 2–5 ■ Tips for Overcoming Shyness

For 2 million American adults, shyness is a serious problem that inhibits their social and professional growth. If you are shy, there is hope; shyness experts say you can conquer your fears. The following guidelines are from psychologists who treat shyness:

■ Build your self-esteem by focusing on your strong points and praising yourself for good deeds or a good performance. Don't put yourself down. Focus only on the positive. Do not dwell on what you or others perceive as failures or weak points. Concentrate on turning stumbling blocks into stepping stones.
■ Practice talking to people. First, write down what you want to say and rehearse in front of a mirror. Then, progress to a good friend or relative; then try it with acquaintances; and finally with new acquaintances.
■ Work to improve your speaking voice and volume by talking into a tape recorder.
■ Observe and copy the behavior patterns of people who are assertive, who can get what they want without being obnoxious or aggressive.
■ Learn to laugh at yourself when things go wrong, rather than launching into a self-depreciating tirade.
■ Remember that you are not alone. At least two out of every five people are probably as uncomfortable as you are in the same situation.
■ Do not try to hide your "true self." Accept who you are. Think of your peculiarities as traits that make you distinctive, rather than odd.
■ When with other people, focus your attention on them and what they are saying. Do not focus on your own words, actions, and appearance.
■ Before you enter a social setting, vividly imagine yourself succeeding in it.
■ Practice relaxation techniques (see Chapter 4).
■ Avoid using alcohol or other drugs to relax. Although you may feel inhibited without them, using them will not teach you the social skills you desire. Also, using them can increase the chance that you will make a fool of yourself.

SOURCE: J. E. Brody, You can kick the queasy feeling, 30 November, 1989. *New York Times*

assertive expressing wants and needs appropriately; expressing desires in a way that is respectful toward others; direct, healthy communication.

aggressive insulting others or otherwise being disrespectful; an inappropriate and ineffective way of expressing wants and needs.

To form successful relationships, you must express wants and needs in a way that is respectful toward others. To find the happy compromise between the extremes of timidity and assault is to be **assertive rather than aggressive**. There is usually a gap, sometimes large, sometimes small, between what you want or need and what you are receiving in every setting—school, job, home, friendships, dealings with storekeepers or creditors, and more. To close the gap, you need to express your wants and needs appropriately and, at the same time, remain mindful of other people's feelings so that you do not wound them unnecessarily.

To be assertive is to say what you mean, not to tiptoe around dropping hints and not to attack the other person. This does not come naturally to many people and has to be learned and practiced. In each of the following situations, a person is behaving nonassertively; see if you can decide what the person really means. (Assertive responses are given in the accompanying box.)

SITUATION	NONASSERTIVE BEHAVIOR
A person steps in front of Ms. A, who has been standing in line for an hour.	MS. A.: Says nothing aloud; mutters, "Some people. . . ."
Mr. B comes home, gets a drink, sits down, and starts reading the paper.	MS. B (from the kitchen): "I sure wish I could rest like that at the end of the day. But no, I have to cook dinner, bathe the baby, wash up. . . I'm so tired, too."
Mr. C notices that Child C hasn't cleaned up her room even though he told her to do so earlier.	MR. C: "Child, I told you to clean up your room. What's the matter with you? You're the laziest child I ever saw."

In the first example, Ms. A is not assertive at all; she simply does not speak up for herself. In the second, Ms. B makes it clear to her husband that she feels overworked, tired, and grumpy, but she doesn't tell him what she wants him to do about it. In the third example, Mr. C tells his child what to do, which is assertive, but then goes on to insult the child, which is aggressive.

Ms. B and Mr. C share a problem common to people who have trouble being assertive. They have let their resentments build up for so long that when they do speak, they express not a simple wish of the moment but an age-old gripe. Ms. B does it slow-burn style; Mr. C does it by way of a loud explosion. Both are painful to express and painful to witness. By contrast, notice how the appropriate responses differ in tone and content: they each express a single, specific, concrete request of the moment. Assertive statements are like that: "Please wash the dishes." "Please pay me the five dollars you owe me." Also, they speak of the action they want, not of the person. The responder knows exactly what to do and does not have to feel attacked.

To make your wishes known assertively but not aggressively:

■ Isolate the incident. Don't discuss everything that has been bothering you for months.

■ Be specific and positive. Describe the behavior you want.

Assertive Behaviors for Ms. A, Ms. B, Mr. C.

Ms. A: "Excuse me, I was here first. The end of the line is back there." (Points.)

Ms. B: "Would you please cook dinner while I bathe the baby?"

Mr. C: "I told you to clean up your room. Now do it." (And he sees that she does.)

A way to choose what to mention is to ask yourself, "Does this bother me every time it happens, or is it an isolated incident?" If it happens often, mention it. If not, handle it yourself by walking it off or waiting it out.

If a major grievance has built up, don't just casually mention it the next time the occasion arises. Here are pointers for expressing major grievances:

- Pick a time to express them; don't just burst forth with them.
- Pair a resentment with an appreciation: "I appreciate [this] but resent [that]."
- Make feeling statements about yourself ("It hurts my feelings when you . . ."), not judgment statements about the other person ("You are insensitive").

Assertiveness is the key to obtaining cooperation: it makes you easier, not harder, to get along with. It is worth practicing for the person who wants to achieve harmonious relationships with others. Chapter 12 develops this theme further with respect to intimate relationships.

Relationships with others can be the most difficult, yet the most rewarding, part of our lives; they are a challenge in emotional growth. Equally challenging is the development of a relationship with society.

≡▶ *Relationships with others are vital to emotional health. Many kinds of relationships contribute to a person's support system. To develop relationships, people need, among other things, to learn to overcome shyness and to assert themselves.*

■≡ Finding a Place in Society

Another way people can grow toward emotional health is by finding a place in society that suits them. Each person needs to establish some relationship with the larger world. One person may choose to live a relatively isolated life, pursuing goals of personal value. Another may choose to become one of a large group of people pursuing society's main goals. Still another may choose to associate with a subgroup in society whose values differ from the majority's values. The Spotlight following Chapter 9 revisits the topic of social health and examines it from several angles.

An important component for many people in establishing a place in society is finding a job or career.[17] If you are a college student, you are probably preparing yourself for some line of work. The better you know yourself, the better you can choose, and succeed at, a job or career. To be satisfying, a job ideally meets several of a person's needs, including the needs for

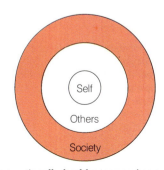

The emotionally healthy person has a strong relationship with society.

LIFE CHOICE INVENTORY

Do you cultivate emotional wellbeing? Try answering these questions to get an idea. Don't take your score too seriously; this is just for fun.

1. I spend time doing work that I enjoy.
   a. almost always
   b. sometimes
   c. almost never

2. I find it easy to relax.
   a. almost always
   b. sometimes
   c. almost never

3. In my spare time, I participate in activities that I enjoy.
   a. almost always
   b. sometimes
   c. almost never

4. When I am about to be in a stressful situation, I realize it ahead of time, and I prepare for it.
   a. almost always
   b. sometimes
   c. almost never

5. I handle anger:
   a. by expressing it in ways that hurt neither myself nor other people
   b. by bottling it up so that no one knows I'm angry
   c. I never am angry, or I express anger aggressively

6. I participate with group organizations such as school, sports, church, or community activities.
   a. quite often
   b. very seldom
   c. never

7. I find it easy to express my feelings.
   a. almost always
   b. sometimes
   c. almost never

8. I can talk to close friends, relatives, or others about personal matters.
   a. almost always
   b. sometimes
   c. almost never

9. When I need help with personal matters, I seek it out.
   a. almost always
   b. sometimes
   c. almost never

10. When I am under stress, I make extra sure to exercise regularly, to work off my tension.
   a. almost always
   b. sometimes
   c. almost never

For each *a* answer, give yourself 2 points; for each *b* answer, give yourself 1 point; for each *c* answer, give yourself 0 points. A score of 18 to 20 is excellent; 16 or 17 is very good; 14 or 15 is good; and 13 or below means that you need improvement.

SOURCE: Adapted from U.S. Department of Health and Human Services, *Health Style*, HHS publication no. (PHS) 81-50155, 1981 (a self-test distributed by National Health Information Clearinghouse).

Three levels of work:

■ Job—meets basic needs for survival and physical security.
■ Career—can help meet needs for other people's esteem and respect, for a position in life.
■ Life's work—helps meet needs for self-actualization.

security, for a feeling of competence, for autonomy, for creativity, for variety, and for the sense that one is performing worthwhile work.[18] Your work may be school or homemaking right now; it is still a job, in a sense. Ask yourself how many of your needs are met by your work.

Some claim that having rewarding work is the single most important determinant of well-being in the adult.[19] Those who have satisfying jobs, then, have a built-in life advantage. Those who do not may find that they can enhance their emotional well-being by seeking satisfying work outside of their jobs. Many people, for example, obtain satisfaction through activities such as hobbies or volunteer work.

This chapter has touched on each of the three major realms of emotional health: relationships with self, others, and society. Unfortunately, not everyone is given an easy path to developing the qualities described in this chapter. Most people become sidetracked by obstacles that can hinder healthy emotional development. The next chapter explores these obstacles and how people can overcome them.

■≡ For Review

1. Describe the importance of emotional health to physical health.
2. Explain ways to gain self-knowledge and why it is important.
3. Describe thoughts, needs, and values and how they are important in emotional health.
4. List three feelings, and describe acceptable ways to express them.
5. List traits of the three personalities within according to transactional analysis.
6. List the stages of life according to Erikson.
7. List characteristics of an emotionally healthy person.
8. Describe a person with self-esteem. Discuss why self-esteem is important.
9. List ways to go about improving self-esteem.
10. Compare and contrast assertive and aggressive behavior.
11. Describe some possible sources for a support system.

■≡ Notes

1. M. Beattie, *Beyond Codependency* (New York: Harper and Row, 1989), pp. 125–137.
2. Norman Vincent Peale, *The Power of Positive Thinking* (New York: Prentice-Hall, 1955).
3. G. E. Richardson, B. L. Neiger, S. Jensen, and K. L. Kumpfer, The resiliency model, *Health Education,* November/December 1990, pp. 33–39.
4. A. Maslow, *Toward a Psychology of Being* (Princeton, N.J.: Van Nostrand, 1968).
5. L. Raths, H. Merrill, and S. Sidney, *Values and Teaching* (Columbus, Ohio: Merrill, 1966), as cited in S. B. Simon, L. W. Howe, and H. Kirschenbaum, *Values Clarification: A Handbook of Practical Strategies for Teachers and Students*, rev. ed. (New York: Hart, 1978), p. 19.
6. H. Kirschenbaum, as cited in Simon, Howe, and Kirschenbaum, p. 20.

7. A classic transactional analysis reference is E. Berne, *Games People Play: The Psychology of Human Relationships* (New York: Grove, 1964).
8. M. Jahoda, *Current Concepts of Positive Mental Health* (New York: Basic Books, 1958), pp. 22–80.
9. D. McGonigle, Making self-talk positive, *American Journal of Nursing* 88 (1988): 725.
10. B. J. Mushinski-Fulk, Training positive attitudes: "I tried hard and did well," *Intervention in School and Clinic* 26 (1990): 79–83. (abstract), cited in *Journal of School Health,* March 1991, pp. 141–142.
11. Beattie, 1989, pp. 125–137.
12. *Journal of Abnormal Psychology* as quoted in Great bodies come in many shapes, *University of California Berkeley Wellness Letter,* February 1991, pp. 1–2.
13. How your looks shape your life, *Parade*, 4 July 1982, pp. 11–13.

14. Social ties: Friendships Are important to your health, *University of Texas Lifetime Health Letter*, April 1990, p. 7.
15. J. Powell, *Why Am I Afraid to Tell You Who I Am?* (Chicago, Argus Communications, 1969).
16. A. C. Wassmer, *Making Contact* (New York: Dial, 1978), as cited in A. F. Grasha and D. S. Kirschenbaum, *Psychology of Adjustment and Competence* (Cambridge, Mass.: Winthrop, 1980), p. 349.
17. G. Brim, Losing and winning, *Psychology Today*, September 1988, p. 48.
18. T. J. DeLong, Re-examining the career anchor model, *Journal of the American Dietetic Association* 81 (1981): 365.
19. H. Selye, as cited in Your job—Love it or leave it, *Executive Fitness Newsletter*, 30 December 1978, p. 1.

SPOTLIGHT

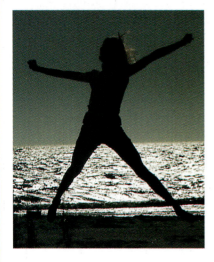

Spiritual Health

People have always contemplated the reason for their existence. Imagine, for a minute, someone standing alone on the globe, looking out into the deep, dark recesses of space, asking, "Why am I here?" "What purpose do I serve?" "What is the reason for my existence?" Whenever people clear their minds of all other thoughts and look inside themselves and to the world to ask these questions, they are expressing a need for spiritual health.

Questions regarding the ultimate purpose of human life can be traced from humankind's earliest beginnings.[1*] At times, almost all people experience a sense of temporary futility in life's events and feel a need for a greater purpose—something to anchor their lives to. People have a basic need for direction, mission, or duty. People need a larger goal.

*Reference notes are at the end of the Spotlight.

I haven't heard much talk about the value of a spiritual life. It seems that our society focuses instead on making a lot of money.

Unfortunately, this is true. Recently displayed on a car bumper was a sticker that read, "He who dies with the most toys wins." This way of life equates value with material possessions and is pleasure centered. People who seek happiness through ownership and acquiring things are locked into continually seeking *more* material things. Because possessions only bring fleeting pleasures, such people never have enough. Ultimately, materialism brings boredom and emptiness.

A story is told of a wealthy man who heard his servant exclaim, "Oh, if I only had $5!" Thinking that was little enough to ask for, he gave the servant a five-dollar bill. Moments later, when he was almost out of earshot, he heard the servant complaining to himself, "Oh, why didn't I say $10?" That is the cry of a person who never will find satisfaction, and in fact who is looking for it in the wrong place. People also search for comfort from alcohol, other drugs, or sex. These bring temporary pleasure, but not permanent peace, contentment, and satisfaction. One writer claims that people have a hunger in their hearts, a vacuum that can only be filled with spirituality.[2] A person who tries to fill this emptiness with possessions or worldly pleasures stays empty.

Many people seem to equate spirituality with formal religions and with rules like the Ten Commandments. Is this what spirituality is?

Some people find spirituality through organized religion, but living by a set of rules is not what spirituality is about. It is not measured by how often people attend church. Optimal spiritual health expresses itself as the ability to reach one's highest potential. This includes discovering and acting on a higher purpose in life; learning "how to give and receive love, joy, and peace; to pursue a fulfilling life; and to contribute to the improvement of the spiritual health of others."[3] It means having a connectedness to a larger meaning or purpose,[4] or a personal relationship with a higher power.

How can you tell if someone is spiritual?

Those who are satisfied with life regardless of their circumstances are often spiritual. These peoples' degree of satisfaction with life does not depend on their age, gender, life circumstances, income, or even health.[5]

Regardless of religious affiliation, people with spirituality seem to share a faith that consists of certain beliefs:

■ They believe that a power greater than themselves exists.
■ They believe that this power is in control of the universe and of their lives (is all powerful).
■ They believe that this power is good, cares for and loves them, and controls and guides their lives according to their best interest.

Spirituality is tested at times of crisis, which present opportunities to develop maturity and character.[6] The spiritual person goes through trials with grace and peace and trusts that whatever is happening is happening for a good reason. Those without spirituality take hardships with bitterness.

One spiritual author, the Apostle Paul, writes: "I know what it is to be in need, and I know what it is to have plenty. I have learned the secret of being content in any and every situation, whether well fed or hungry, whether living in plenty or in want."[7]

That serenity sounds like something to strive for. Are there other benefits of spiritual health?

Yes, there are many. Besides enhancing the quality of life, it improves physical well-being and aids in physical healing. Many people with chronic illness live longer than medically expected due to their spirituality. One study showed that faith and hope added to the amounts of pain-killing hormones (endorphins) secreted by the brain, which enhance the physical feeling of well-being, even in extremely stressful situations.[8]

Spiritual health also helps heal emotional injuries. Spirituality is the foundation of addiction recovery programs of all kinds.[9] For depression and grief, spirituality helps provide comfort. For anxiety and stress, spirituality can provide a sense of peace.[10] For problems with guilt and resentment, it offers forgiveness and enables people to forgive others.

Spiritual health helps meet emotional needs, too. Remember Maslow's hierarchy of needs mentioned in the chapter? Through spiritual development, the needs for esteem, love, and self-actualization can be met.

The person with spiritual health relates well to self, others, and society, and acts as part of the environment rather than in opposition to it (see Chapter 21). Spiritual health provides a sense of belonging and of connectedness, which gives a person a sensitivity and respect for all things. Spiritual people are good stewards of the earth.

How does lack of spiritual health affect people?

People who lack spiritual health feel disconnected and lonely, and their lives lack meaning and purpose. These feelings are known to harm people's health.[11] Too little interest in spiritual health can contribute to apathy, dissatisfaction, and wasted human potential.[12]

continued on next page

TABLE S2–1 ■ **How's Your Spiritual Health?**

When was the last time you:	Score[a]
1. Shared ten minutes with a child and talked about a common interest?	
2. Spent a half hour listening intently to someone different from yourself in age, culture, social class, philosophy, or other major factor?	
3. Went to a church, synagogue, or religious service?	
4. Helped someone who is less fortunate (in your opinion) than you?	
5. Took a walk in the park or woods with someone you love?	
6. Prayed for someone?	
7. Watched the sun come up (or go down) while at a lake, in the mountains, in the woods, or at home, or wherever you might be?	
8. Read inspirational or devotional materials?	
9. Spent 15 to 30 minutes meditating, praying, pondering, or reflecting on your purpose in life?	
10. Attended an art exhibition, a theater or dance performance, or a concert of high spiritual quality?	
TOTAL SCORE	

SCORING: Give yourself 6 points for each activity that you did yesterday or today, 5 points for each done in the last week, 4 for each done in the last month, and 3 for each done in the last year.

ANALYSIS

After totaling your score, take a look at the general guidelines for interpreting results below.

Score	Interpretation
40–60	You are enjoying all the benefits of a spiritually rich life.
30–39	You emphasize spiritual values in your life.
20–29	Spiritual concerns are a part of your life, but you may want to spend more time concentrating on them.
0–19	Your spiritual life is underdeveloped. Try to bring these values into the limelight, even if it takes some extra effort on your part.

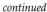

continued

Atheistic philosophers believe that the universe is impersonal, and that life's events are a product of blind chance. This view holds that since there is no higher power, life has no ultimate meaning. Therefore life is absurd and futile, and people are miserable because they feel uncertain and insignificant. A life without spirituality is cynical and pessimistic; a spiritual life is optimistic.

How can I develop spiritual health?

You may get some hints from Table S2–1, How's Your Spiritual Health? Here are some more. There are as many different ways to go about developing spirituality as there are spiritual and religious traditions:

■ Keep a journal of events, thoughts, feelings, prayers, and dreams.
■ Pray and meditate on a regular basis.
■ Read books suggested by your church or friends.
■ Stay open and receptive to messages about how to live your life.
■ Apply spiritual principles in your life. Review your behavior periodically in light of these principles and keep trying to improve.
■ Think of others as spiritual seekers, too. Cultivate humility and your sense of oneness with others.

The benefits of spiritual health are many. Human beings can reach their full potential only if they develop the spiritual side of themselves. Life is hardly worth living without joy, faith, and love. Spiritual health brings peace that surpasses all understanding.

■ ≡ Spotlight Notes

1. V. Frankel, *Man's Search for Meaning* (New York: Simon and Schuster, 1963).
2. J. R. W. Scott, *Basic Christianity* (Downers Grove, Ill.: Inter-Varsity Press, March 1978).
3. L. S. Chapman, Developing a useful perspective on spiritual health: Love, joy, peace and fulfillment, *American Journal of Health Promotion,* Fall 1987, pp. 12–17.
4. R. Bellingham and coauthors, Connectedness: Some skills for spiritual health, ed. L. S. Chapman, *American Journal of Health Promotion,* September/October 1989, pp. 18–32.

5. G. Brim, Losing and winning, *Psychology Today,* September 1988, p. 48.
6. M. Khandijan, Wildwood Presbyterian Church, personal communication, 1990.
7. Philippians 4:12, in *The NIV Study Bible,* New International Version, ed. Kenneth Barker (Grand Rapids: Zondervan, 1985), p. 1809.
8. J. Folkenberg, Hope: Is it a hidden health factor? *Journal of the American Dietetic Association* 85 (1985): 357.

9. C. Whitfield, Stress management and spirituality during recovery: A transpersonal approach, Part I: Becoming, *Alcoholism Treatment Quarterly,* Spring 1984, pp. 3–54.
10. Chapman, 1987, pp. 31–39.
11. Bellingham and coauthors, 1989, pp. 18–32.
12. L. S. Chapman, Spiritual health: A component missing from health promotion, *American Journal of Health Promotion,* Summer 1986, pp. 38–41.

CHAPTER 3

Emotional Problems

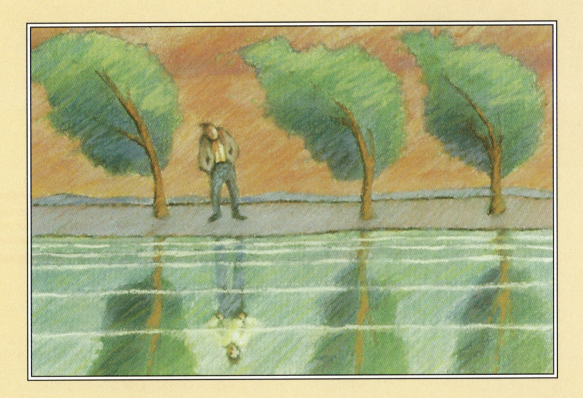

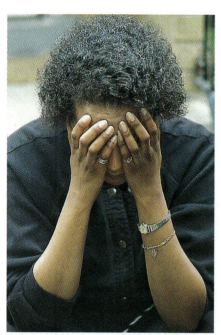

A person who feels troubled emotionally may feel alone, but comfort can come easily.

FACT OR FICTION

Just for fun, respond true or false to the following statements. If false, say what is true.

■ People who are emotionally healthy never need psychological help. (Page 54)
■ A person who can carry another's share of responsibility is emotionally strong, but the dependent one has emotional problems. (Page 62)
■ People who engage in regular physical activity experience less depression and anxiety than people who do not. (Page 62)
■ Anxiety can be beneficial. (Page 65)

■ To express resentment only provokes conflict; it is best to deal with resentment in private. (Page 67)
■ To deal with an emotional problem, one first needs to discover who is at fault. (Page 72)
■ If a person is self-destructive, the best way to help is to keep the person from getting into trouble. (Page 73)

■ *FACT OR FICTION:* People who are emotionally healthy never need psychological help. *False.* Even emotionally stable people may benefit from such help.

emotional problems   behavioral or psychological patterns that are abnormal enough so that a person may feel significant emotional pain or be unable to function in one of three important areas:

1. Social or family relations.
2. Occupation (including school).
3. Use of leisure time.

Emotional problems are a normal part of everyone's life. A person who feels troubled emotionally may feel alone and ashamed, but comfort can come easily. The hardest part of dealing with an emotional problem is facing the fact that you have it; once that's done, you quickly discover that you are not alone and need not feel ashamed. No matter how extreme a problem may seem to its possessor, it is not unique: others have suffered with it, and ways of dealing with it have been worked out and are available.

People are more aware of, and better informed about, emotional problems than they used to be, and they value psychological help from counseling and support groups more than in the past. Most people realize now that counseling is not an ordeal, and not just for people who are seriously mentally ill, but a path toward wellness. For people who are already very healthy, counseling and support groups can be enjoyable explorations of the self. Psychological help can provide support through crises, solve problems in relationships, provide insights into behaviors, build self-esteem, and assist in making important decisions.

The choice of exactly when to obtain help varies with the individual. Many people seek outside help immediately for even mild problems, while some wait until problems become so overwhelming that they can hardly function. Yet, some people *never* obtain outside help even for serious emotional problems. Many therapists claim that the people who most need professional help often are least likely to seek it.

This chapter uses the term **emotional problems** to describe behavioral or psychological patterns in a person that are abnormal enough so that the person may feel significant emotional pain or be unable to function in one of three important areas—social or family relations, occupation (including school performance), or use of leisure time.[1]* According to this definition, emotional problems range from common, temporary mild depression or anxiety to severe problems, such as those characterized by a loss of the sense of reality. The emotionally healthy person is compared with the emotionally unhealthy person in Table 3–1.

*Reference notes are at the end of the chapter.

TABLE 3–1 ■ **Characteristics of Emotionally Healthy People versus Emotionally Unhealthy People**

Emotionally Healthy People	Emotionally Unhealthy People
Have high self-esteem.	Have low self-esteem.
Are confident that their behavior is normal.	Guess at what normal behavior is.
Are honest.	Often lie when it would be just as easy to tell the truth.
Accept themselves.	Judge themselves without mercy.
Can have fun.	Have difficulty having fun.
Don't take themselves too seriously.	Take themselves very seriously.
Recognize that other people can enhance their lives but are not the sole source of their happiness.	Are certain their happiness hinges on others.
Can have intimate relationships.	Have unusual difficulty with intimate relationships.
Do not try to control things beyond their control.	Try to control things they cannot control.
Are able to affirm themselves.	Constantly seek approval and affirmation from others.
Communicate openly and assertively about their needs and wants.	Communicate indirectly and try to meet their needs using aggressiveness or manipulation.
Usually feel they are similar to other people.	Usually feel they are different from other people.
Take responsibility appropriately, but do not take too much responsibility for others.	Are super-responsible or super-irresponsible.
Give loyalty when it is appropriate and deserved.	Are extremely loyal, even when loyalty is undeserved.
Consider consequences before acting.	Act impulsively without considering consequences.
Deal with emotional pain by feeling it and expressing it.	Deal with emotional pain by resorting to addictions and compulsive behaviors.
Continue to mature mentally, emotionally, and spiritually throughout their lives.	Tend to remain immature; their mental, emotional, and spiritual growth is blocked.
Live with balance, not extremes.	Live lives that are punctuated by extremes.
Validate and acknowledge their observations, feelings, and reactions.	Invalidate and repress their observations, feelings, and reactions.
Attend to their physical and psychological needs.	Neglect their needs.
Disclose family problems when appropriate.	Hide family or other secrets.
Refuse to tolerate inappropriate behavior.	Have a high tolerance for inappropriate behavior.
Feel emotional pain; are able to grieve when they suffer losses.	Are unable to grieve losses to completion.
Cope with stress in positive ways, so are not prone to stress-related illnesses.	Are prone to stress-related illnesses.

SOURCES: Adapted from J. G. Woititz, *Adult Children of Alcoholics* (Deerfield Beach, Fla.: Health Communications, 1983); R. Hemfelt, F. Minirth, and P. Meier, *Love Is a Choice* (Nashville, Tenn.: Thomas Nelson, 1989), pp. 9–16.

This chapter is devoted mostly to common emotional problems. The emphasis is practical: how to recognize them, understand them, and deal with them. First, though, how do they develop?

■ The Mingled Causes of Emotional Problems

For many emotional problems, it is impossible for anyone but an expert to pinpoint an exact cause. Many different causes can produce symptoms that, on the surface, may appear quite similar. A person who feels too apathetic to study for a test may think the cause is psychological when in reality it is physical—a new carpet, for example, can give off fumes that make a person feel sick. Some severe emotional problems are caused by brain damage from drugs, injuries, or diseases such as AIDS and syphilis.

People should not attempt to diagnose their own or their friends' emotional problems.

Some nutrient deficiencies can cause an impressive list of symptoms that mimic emotional problems: apathy, irritability, restlessness, confusion, insomnia, hysteria, hostility, depression, lack of appetite, headaches, and loss of memory.[2] If a vitamin or mineral deficiency causes symptoms, repeated doses of the nutrient that is lacking will clear them up[3]; but if a deficiency is not at fault, then taking nutrient supplements will only delay correct diagnosis and treatment. Lack of exercise or sleep can also bring on symptoms of emotional problems as can alcohol or other drug abuse. It is important to obtain an accurate diagnosis before undergoing treatment. People should not attempt to diagnose their own or their friends' problems. Only a mental health professional can provide a correct diagnosis.

Some emotional problems tend to occur in certain families. This suggests that they may be inherited and/or learned. Some people may be genetically predisposed to certain emotional problems. Others may develop problems by learning destructive thought patterns or behaviors from their environments.

The disorder known as manic depression* is an example of a genetically inherited emotional problem. It is caused by an abnormality in a gene located in a narrow band on the chromosome known as "number 11." The major mental disorder schizophrenia is another example of a disease with a strong genetic component.

People may inherit diseases like manic depression or schizophrenia, or they may inherit the potential for developing them.[4] For example, if one identical twin develops schizophrenia, then the other twin has a 46 percent chance of developing it, too.[5] You might think that this proves conclusively that schizophrenia is hereditary, but environmental and hereditary influences often cannot be disentangled from each other. Many cases show that people who develop schizophrenia were exposed to disturbed family environments including violence or sexual abuse.[6] In addition, alcohol and other drug abuse often pervade the environments in which people with schizophrenia grow up.

Childhood trauma does not always leave people emotionally crippled, though. Why some people who were abused as children remain apparently functional is a mystery. Perhaps healthy heredity can endow people with exceptionally strong resilience.

Whatever the role of heredity, some environmental conditions clearly foster the development of emotional problems. One environmental condition is chemical dependency. Chemical dependencies can intensify or even cause emotional problems. Foremost among these are alcohol abuse and the abuse of illegal drugs, which together account for close to half of the hundreds of billions of dollars' worth of each year's treatment costs for mental illness.[7]

Another environmental trigger of emotional problems may be societal pressures. Each child arrives in this world with certain inborn characteristics: some are physically active, some artistic, some sensitive, and so forth. Yet parents and society may want children to conform to certain molds. A parent who wants a child to play sports is a familiar example; the child may not be inclined that way. This puts the child in a bind between the wishes of the parent and inner guidance. Such pressure can precipitate an emotional problem.

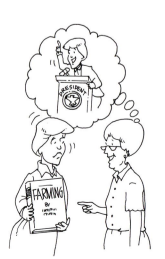

Society's ideals don't always fit individuals.

*Terms referring to major emotional problems appear in Appendix C.

A person who tries to measure up to parental or societal ideals may fall short, and this may diminish self-esteem. In severe cases, it can precipitate emotional problems. The student who is expected to perform beyond inner ability or motivation may turn to alcohol or drugs for escape and so develop an **addiction**. The young person attempting to achieve the ideal of slimness may first try to starve, then eat out of control, and then vomit in an attempt to undo the damage—an eating disorder (see the Spotlight following Chapter 6). Something is wrong with the society that puts such pressure on people, but unfortunately it is the individuals who suffer and who require treatment.

We said earlier that some emotional problems run in families, partly because families provide the environments in which people grow up. As a result, most emotional problems appear in childhood and adolescence.[8] Studies of dysfunctional family dynamics offer hope in the search for prevention and treatment of emotional problems.

addiction being dependent on a substance or strong habit or behavior.

≡▶ *Emotional problems cause pain and impair functioning socially, on the job, and in leisure time. Inheritance has a strong influence, making some people prone, and some resistant, to emotional problems, but environmental contributors are also important.*

■≡ Dysfunctional Family Dynamics

As described in Chapter 2, an emotionally healthy family supports emotionally healthy development.[9] Conversely, a **dysfunctional family** may lay the foundations for problem thought patterns and behaviors. A dysfunctional family is one with abnormal, impaired, or incomplete functioning that impairs the emotional health and self-esteem of the family members.

dysfunctional family a family with abnormal, impaired, or incomplete functioning that impairs the emotional health and self-esteem of the family members.

All families express some degree of dysfunction, at least at times. Families are neither perfectly healthy nor totally unhealthy. Healthy families may behave in unhealthy ways during times of crisis. However, healthy families do not remain dysfunctional; they return to a normal, healthy state. Dysfunctional families tend to grow increasingly dysfunctional; the unhealthy interactions grow more frequent and more severe.

Dysfunctional family dynamics both cause and result from several conditions:

■ Alcoholism and other chemical addictions, chronic mental illnesses, or disabling physical illnesses.
■ Dependence on, or obsession with, people who have such conditions (codependency, described later).
■ Active physical or sexual child abuse.
■ Passive child abuse, such as withholding of affection and physical neglect.[10]

When these conditions are present, parents do not meet their children's emotional needs consistently.[11] Addictions, particularly, consume parental energy and focus, leaving children to fend for themselves. Parenting may be inconsistent, unpredictable, arbitrary, and chaotic—sometimes loving, warm, caring, interested, and involved; and other times unloving, cold, unavailable, and preoccupied. The more severe the family dysfunction, the more emotional damage to the children.

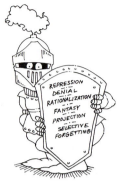

Defense mechanisms: forms of mental avoidance.

People from dysfunctional families bear a painful legacy of confusion, fear, anger, and hurt. Then, because they instinctively seek what is familiar even if it is unpleasant, they tend to repeat the patterns they have learned. In making relationships, they choose people who will interact with them in the same distorted ways that their families of origin did.[12] Each person from a dysfunctional family is at high risk of marrying someone with alcoholism (or another such condition), repeating a life of addictions, or both.[13]

A dysfunctional family is characterized by family secrets (such as alcoholism or other drug problems), seriousness (no sense of humor), lack of cohesiveness or unity, and rigid rules. The most damaging of the rules are understood by all but never spoken:

■ Don't talk—do not discuss problems or unpleasant feelings.
■ Don't feel—do not admit feelings, particularly unpleasant feelings such as sadness and anger.
■ Don't trust—because you cannot discuss problems or admit feelings to those who care for you.[14]

In contrast, the functional family is characterized by sharing and acceptance of feelings—a sense of caring, support and trust.[15] Functional and dysfunctional families are compared in Table 3–2.

The "don't talk" and "don't feel" rules of dysfunctional families force family members to repress pain and other unpleasant feelings. Rather than dealing with them in healthy ways, as described in the last chapter, they use **defense mechanisms** such as repression to survive in their dysfunctional homes. Defense mechanisms are useful for dealing with the first, shocking impact of major life problems but are destructive when used over prolonged periods. These behaviors interfere with people's emotional health and with the development of positive relationships in adult life. Rather than defense mechanisms, people should turn to **coping devices** (see the two miniglossaries that contrast these two sets of responses).

defense mechanisms inappropriate automatic and often unconscious forms of emotional avoidance in reaction to emotional injury.

coping devices appropriate behaviors used to deal with unpleasant or painful situations.

TABLE 3–2 ■ **Characteristics of a Functional versus a Dysfunctional Family**

Functional Family	Dysfunctional Family
Establishes rules for the sake of functioning cooperatively, which are appropriate, consistent, and reasonably flexible.	Establishes rules for control's sake, which are rigid and arbitrary.
Encourages its members to develop well-rounded personalities with many facets.	Establishes rigid roles for each member: for example, one is always the scapegoat, one is unnoticed, one is overly responsible, and one is the family clown.
Accepts its problems and treats them as factual.	Has deep, dark secrets that no one may ever disclose (alcoholism, infidelity, or other).
Welcomes outsiders into the system.	Resists allowing outsiders to enter the system.
Typically has members who are relaxed and have a sense of humor.	Has members who are usually serious and tense.
Permits members the right to personal privacy, so that they can develop a sense of self.	Permits members no personal privacy, so that they have difficulty defining themselves as individuals.
Fosters a spontaneous "sense of family," so that members feel free to leave and reenter the system.	Enforces loyalty to the family; members must always act as part of the system.
Allows and resolves conflict between members.	Denies and ignores conflict between members.
Continually changes.	Resists change.
Has spontaneous loyalty and a sense of wholeness.	Has no real unity; is fragmented.

■ MINIGLOSSARY
of Defense Mechanisms

denial the refusal to admit that something unpleasant or painful has occurred: "No, I don't believe it."

fantasy delusion, in the face of a painful or unpleasant situation, that something positive has happened instead: "He hasn't really left me. He's gone to buy me a present."

oral behavior ingesting substances such as drugs, alcohol, or unneeded food.

projection the conviction, in the face of an unpleasant or painful situation you have caused, that it is the other person's fault: "The teacher asked the wrong questions on the exam."

rationalization the justification of an unreasonable action or attitude by manufacturing reasons for it: "I couldn't prevent the accident because I had to pay attention to something else."

regression reversion to inappropriate childish ways of coping with painful realities, such as chronic crying or whining.

repression the refusal to acknowledge an unpleasant or painful event or piece of news: not hearing it.

selective forgetting memory lapse concerning an experience or piece of news too painful to bear: not remembering it.

withdrawal disengaging from people and activities to avoid pain. Examples: engaging in extended periods of fantasy (daydreaming), refusing to talk with anyone, or sleeping excessively.

■ MINIGLOSSARY
of Coping Devices

displacement channeling the energy of suffering into something else—for example, using the emotional energy churned up by grief for work or recreation.

ventilation the act of verbally venting one's feelings; letting off steam by talking, crying, swearing, or laughing.

To make matters worse, when children express their needs to their parents, the parents may respond that having and expressing needs is wrong. Children may feel ashamed, and so respond by ignoring their needs and themselves; they may focus on the family problem instead. They interpret the signals they receive as meaning that they are unimportant; thus begins a loss of sense of self that defines these family systems. They enter adulthood focusing on the needs of others, unable to take care of themselves.

In families with dysfunctional interactions, the parents are not to be blamed; the problem is with the family system. Most parents truly love their children and genuinely try to benefit them; they repeat the dysfunctional interactions for two reasons:

■ The parents were emotionally impoverished; they grew up with unmet emotional needs.
■ The parents learned dysfunctional behavior patterns as children and never learned to replace them with other patterns.

Without realizing it, the parents in dysfunctional families may unconsciously turn to their children to meet their emotional needs. To do so, they draw from their children what little love they can offer, leaving the children drained of emotional energy. The children grow up with an enormous hunger for love that they carry into adulthood. Lonely as adults, they unsuccessfully seek to fill the void with alcohol, other drugs, money, possessions, sex, prestige, power, other people, food, or compulsive behaviors. Then they pass the same family dynamics to their children. Thus addictive behaviors and dysfunctional family dynamics are handed down from generation to generation. All of these conditions have recently received a great deal of media attention. Public figures such as comedian Louis Anderson and actress Suzanne Somers have spoken out about how growing up in dysfunctional homes has complicated their adult lives.

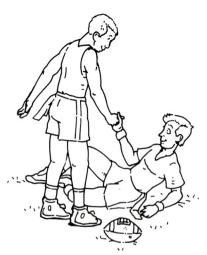

In an unhealthy relationship, one is dependent, the other codependent.

codependency a pattern of helping others; a system of learned behaviors, beliefs, and feelings that lead to obsession with people and things outside the self, along with neglect of the self to the point of having little self-identity.

Codependency

Suppose that you live with (or were raised with) someone who suffers from an addiction or other problem. Can you remain emotionally healthy? A healthy adjustment to such a situation is rare. More commonly, the person who is close to someone with a dependency develops codependency—meaning literally, "with a dependent person." Codependency inflates the giver and diminishes the receiver so that neither is appreciated, loved, or supported on his or her own merits.

If you are concerned about a parent's or another relative's drinking, drug use, or other compulsive behavior, or if you grew up in a dysfunctional family, you may find it helpful to answer the questions in Table 3–3. This survey can provide you with useful information about yourself. It can give you clues to decide if you may be caught in codependency.

People with codependency become so focused upon, or preoccupied with, important others in their lives that they neglect themselves and their own needs. Remember from Chapter 2 that a basic component of emotional health is self-knowledge. People with codependency have focused on helping others for so long that they do not know themselves. If asked, "How do you feel?" people with codependency will often respond by saying how other significant people in their lives feel, or by interpreting the look on *your* face. People with codependency can be pictured going through life with a bright spotlight shining outward. They vividly illuminate people and things outside of themselves but leave themselves and their own needs in the dark.

Codependent people are certain their happiness depends almost totally on what others do and think. Members of couples who suffer from codependency say things like, "If only he would listen to me, I could be happy." "If she would only change, I would be happy." Many single people with codependency feel that perfect mates would make them happy. Actually, the only thing that can make a person happy is self-acceptance and self-esteem.

Correcting problems of codependency can improve self-esteem and the quality of life. Also, correcting these problems can break the pattern so that it will not be passed on to the next generation. This chapter's Spotlight describes the healing of emotional problems.

SOURCES: Adapted from Codependency, *Wellness Letter*, October 1990, p. 7; S. S. Mull, Help for the children of alcoholics, *Health Education*, September/October 1990, p. 42; R. Hemfelt, F. Minirth, and P. Meier, *Love Is a Choice* (Nashville, Tenn.: Thomas Nelson, 1989), pp. 9–16.

Understanding reasons for childhood emotional deprivation and abuse is important, but does not reverse the damage or heal the victims. To restore their emotional health, people who were abused as children must know that they are entitled to their feelings about the mistreatment. They need to express those feelings and resolve them. This chapter's Spotlight, "Emotional Healing," describes the pathway back to wholeness and emotional health.

One major form of dysfunctional behavior is an unhealthy reaction to people with addictions, known as **codependency**. The person with the ad-

---

TABLE 3–3 ■ **Family Function Survey**

The following questions refer to a family situation in which the irresponsible behaviors of a person with an addiction are causing overly-responsible behaviors of codependency in other family members. Answer the following questions about a family member's addictive behavior to see if you may be caught up in such a situation. Remember, addictive behaviors include: alcohol or other drug abuse, excessive gambling, compulsive spending, overworking, fanatical religious behavior, excessive exercising, and the like.

1. Does the person often undergo extreme personality changes?
2. Do you feel that the person's behavior or belief system is more important to the person than you are?
3. Do you feel sorry for yourself and frequently indulge in self-pity because of what you feel this behavior is doing to your family?
4. Has the person's behavior ruined special family occasions?
5. Do you find yourself covering up, or feeling apologetic for, the consequences of the person's behavior?
6. Does the person's behavior make you feel depressed or angry?
7. Is your family having financial difficulties because of this person's behavior?
8. Have you ever tried to prevent this person's behavior by hiding the car keys, pouring liquor down the drain, etc.?
9. Are holidays more a nightmare than a celebration because of the person's behavior?
10. Do you find it necessary to lie to employers, relatives, or friends in order to hide the person's behavior?
11. Does the person's behavior cause you to fear for your own safety or for the safety of other members of your family?
12. Have you ever threatened to leave home or to leave this person because of the behavior?
13. Did the person ever make promises and then break them because of the behavior?
14. Did you ever wish that you could talk to someone who could understand and help with the problems of this family member?
15. Have you ever felt sick, cried, or had a knot in your stomach after worrying about this family member's behavior?

If you answered yes to any two of the above questions, there is a good possibility that your family may be dysfunctional.

If you answered yes to four or more of the above questions, you might benefit from a professional evaluation of your family's functioning and your own possible codependency. Besides reading this chapter and the Spotlight, you can call Alanon for help with problems like this. Look up "Alcoholism" in the yellow pages and call Alcoholics Anonymous. (They help with codependency problems too, even if they are not alcohol- or even drug-related.) Or call 1-800-356-9996 for a brochure on all services.

SOURCE: Inspired by C. L. Whitfield, *Healing the Child Within* (Deerfield Beach, Fla.: Health Communications, 1987), pp. 25–53.

diction becomes dependent; the other becomes overly responsible; and this is damaging for both people. For whenever one person carries another's share of responsibility, both are unhealthy. The discovery that traits people thought of as signs of strength may actually be signs of an emotional problem may be a surprise—but a welcome one, for it will be a relief to let those traits go. The accompanying box, "Codependency," describes the person with these traits.

■ *FACT OR FICTION:* A person who can carry another's share of responsibility is emotionally strong, but the dependent one has emotional problems. *False.* Both are unhealthy. One is codependent; the other is dependent.

≡▶ *One reason emotional illness runs in families is that learned dysfunctional patterns of behavior are passed from parents to children. Abused or neglected children often become parents who abuse or neglect their children. Those who go out of their way to care for emotionally ill (dependent) family members can become ill themselves (codependent), by failing to meet their own needs.*

■≡ Common Emotional Problems

Whether or not they grew up in dysfunctional families, all people experience negative feelings from time to time that may become problems if they go unresolved. Foremost among those feelings are depression, grief, anxiety, guilt, and resentment. Normally, people can deal with these feelings and resolve them relatively quickly. However, a person with unresolved issues left over from childhood may experience these feelings chronically and deeply, and be unable to resolve them without outside help. For each feeling, the ordinary, transient version and the extreme, prolonged, or unresolved problem are described in the following sections.

Prolonged Depression

If you have never felt "down," you are a most unusual person. Described as the common cold of emotional health, **depression** drives more people to seek counseling than does any other emotional problem. Most likely, you know exactly what depression feels like, because you have been there: taking no joy in life, looking forward to nothing, wanting to withdraw from people and activities. Being extremely tired can make you feel this way, but in the case of depression, it doesn't go away, even after a good night's sleep.

depression   an emotional condition of varying duration and severity in which the person feels apathetic, hopeless, and withdrawn from others. A *clinical depression* is one that lasts for more than two weeks. A *major depression* is an emotionally crippling depressed state; at the extreme, a suicidal state.

Sometimes a depression is the warning sign of a disease. Depressed mood is one of the early symptoms of the sexually transmitted disease AIDS, for example (see Chapter 17). A major depression can, at least sometimes, be due to biochemical abnormalities in the brain. It is important, therefore, to go for a physical checkup if a depression sets in for no known reason and refuses to go away.

Sometimes a mild depression goes away by itself, but often you can hasten its departure. People can learn how to recognize the signs of impending depression and how best to prevent or relieve it. The accompanying Strategies review ways of coping with depression.

People who engage in regular physical activity experience less depression and anxiety than people who do not. Running has been shown to be useful, even in place of psychotherapy, to treat mild depression. Physical activity alters mood and attitude for the better in heart disease, alcoholism, and other conditions. Both running and weight-lifting routines have been demonstrated to improve mood.

■ *FACT OR FICTION:* People who engage in regular physical activity experience less depression and anxiety than people who do not. *True.*

Persistent depression, whatever the cause, can be terrifying. Some people who have experienced it say that they would rather have any kind of physical pain than the mental anguish of total hopelessness and helplessness. A person in a prolonged depression (more than two weeks) needs a skilled diagnosis, for if unrelieved, depression can lead to suicide. The signs of a prolonged depression or impending suicide appear later (see Table 3–4 in "Suicide" Section).

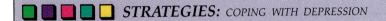

STRATEGIES: COPING WITH DEPRESSION

To ease the passing of a mild depression:

1. Identify the cause.
2. Take action. Make a change in your life; renegotiate the terms of a negative relationship; stop wishing for something or someone you can't have; renew self-care activities you have been neglecting (bathe, wash your hair).
3. Force yourself to do something different, something fun (the first move in this direction is the hardest).
4. Do something physically active.
5. Take a nap.
6. If possible, avoid unpleasant tasks.
7. Find reasons to laugh; time off from self-pity may end a depression.
8. Go outdoors; the green color of living plants in the sun has a known therapeutic effect on the viewer.
9. If you feel stuck, get help.

Depressed people, by their very behavior, repel others as if they were saying, "Leave me alone." Too often, they get what they seem to be asking for. It takes a discerning friend or family member to recognize such unattractive behavior as a call for help. (See the later section, "Suicide," for more information.)

≡▶ *Depression can be mild and short-lived or severe and long-lasting. People can often pull themselves out of mild depressions by changing their routines. If a depression lasts longer than two weeks professional attention is needed.*

Unresolved Grief

Depression at a time of loss is natural and even desirable, for it is one of the stages of grief. All losses evoke what therapists call the **grief process**. To maintain emotional health after a loss, it is beneficial to allow yourself to feel the pain and share your sadness with safe and supportive others. This permits completion of the grieving process and enables you to become free of it. Grief heals, given time, and the greater the loss, the greater the time required. Unfortunately, some people have not learned how to complete the grief process, and therefore they accumulate lifetimes of unresolved grief.

Education about the grief process can help people cope during times of loss. For those who normally express their feelings easily, it helps to know what feelings to expect. For those who avoid feeling pain, it helps to know that once they allow themselves to experience it fully, it will pass—not all at once, but it will pass.

A person faced with a loss typically goes through a series of stages of grief. These stages were first described by Elizabeth Kubler-Ross, who spent many hours with dying persons during the 1960s. She wrote specifically about the anticipation of death, but the same stages occur in reaction to losses of all types: the loss of a loved one, a pet, a job, a possession, money, a belief, a habit, or anything a person cherishes. Adverse external circumstances can cause grief, too: a prolonged drought on the farm, a long spell

grief process the series of feelings that follow a loss: denial, anger, bargaining, depression, acceptance.

of rain during a vacation, the threat and fear of war, or widespread financial disaster. The stages of grief are:

- Denial—"No, it can't be!"
- Anger—"Why me? I don't deserve this!"
- Bargaining—"I'll do anything; just let this not happen."
- Depression—withdrawal, loss of hope.
- Acceptance—"It's all right. I can move on now."

The grief process, or doing "grief work," is different for everyone. People do not necessarily go through the stages in the sequence described. Most people move back and forth from stage to stage or experience more than one at a time. For example, you may feel angry and depressed at the same time. Those who repress such feelings associated with losses carry a heavy load of unresolved, lifelong grief in the form of chronic anxiety, tension, fear, nervousness, anger, resentment, sadness, emptiness, unfulfillment, confusion, or shame. This often results in difficulty sleeping; body aches and pains; or full-blown emotional or physical illness.

chronic shock a condition that arises when people repeatedly suppress (usually painful) feelings; commonly seen in people who have experienced emotional or physical injury or abuse.

Those who grew up in troubled families may not have been allowed to grieve childhood losses when they occurred. As adults, many developed feelings of numbness or "no feelings at all" that therapists call **chronic shock**. For example, during moments of extreme stress, combat soldiers are often required to act, regardless of how they feel. Their survival depends upon their ability to suspend feelings in favor of taking steps to ensure their safety. Unfortunately, the resulting "split" between one's self and one's experience does not heal by itself, even with the passage of time. Until active healing takes place, the individual continues to feel numb and loses the ability to recognize which feelings are present.

post-traumatic stress disorder a reaction to psychological stress such as wartime trauma or rape, arising after the event is over.

trauma = wound

These soldiers, as well as other people who have been through stressful experiences such as episodes of abuse, bombings, rape, floods, torture, kidnapping, or hurricanes, often suffer long afterwards from feelings of extreme anxiety known as **post-traumatic stress disorder**. They may have disturbed sleep and impaired memories (especially with respect to the stressful time).[16] For example, many women, after being raped, show signs of distress months or years after the actual incident. The person may repeatedly relive the experience and may be unable to concentrate or focus on present responsibilities, sometimes acting unresponsive to other people and sometimes overreacting to minor disturbances.

The time to recovery from post-traumatic stress disorders may be as long as 15 to 20 years or even longer. For example, many of the veterans who fought in Vietnam during the 1960s were just beginning to come to terms with their experiences in the 1980s and finally resolved their pain during the Persian Gulf war of 1991.

Growing up or living in a severely abusive or dysfunctional family often brings about post-traumatic stress disorders.[17] Such disorders are most likely to appear if the following conditions are present:

- The trauma occurs over a prolonged time (longer than six months).
- The trauma is of human origin.
- Those around the affected person deny the existence of the emotional injury.

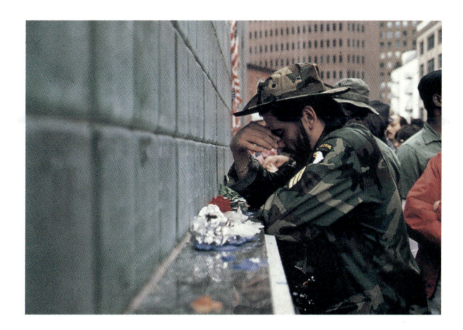

To become free of pain, one must go through it.

All three conditions are usually present in actively alcoholic and similarly troubled families.

≡▶ *Depression is natural at a time of loss; it is one of the stages of grief. Others are denial, anger, bargaining, and acceptance. Grief resolves with full experience of the associated pain. Those who suppress the pain (unresolved grief) may still suffer numbness and post-traumatic stress disorders years later.*

Extreme Anxiety

Like depression and grief, **anxiety** is familiar to everyone. And like depression, anxiety is a normal state, some of the time. However, while depression is a low-energy state, anxiety is characterized by high energy and therefore can be beneficial on occasion. A small dose of anxiety can spur a student to tackle a test with intense concentration, but excessive test anxiety can also freeze the test taker's mind. Too much anxiety is disabling.

The body's reaction to anxiety is the stress response: rapid heartbeat and respiration, extreme alertness, and the other aspects of readiness needed in an emergency. Chapter 4 deals with the stress response and shows how to manage stress.

An **anxiety attack** is a sudden, extreme, and incapacitating attack of panic that comes on for no apparent reason. You may have experienced an anxiety attack at some time in your life: you felt suddenly panicky, your heart started hammering uncontrollably, you felt dizzy, and you broke out in a sweat. Such an episode lasts only a few minutes but renders you helpless to cope with anything for as long as it is going on. An occasional attack of anxiety can hit anyone—in fact, an overdose of caffeine (six to eight cups of coffee in as many hours) can bring one on—but some people have such attacks frequently and never know when to expect them. This makes them

anxiety an emotional state characterized by high energy; the body's reaction to it is the stress response (see Chapter 4).

■ *FACT OR FICTION:* Anxiety can be beneficial. *True.*

anxiety attack a sudden, unexpected episode of severe anxiety with symptoms such as rapid heartbeat, sweating, dizziness, and nausea.

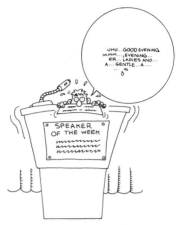

A little anxiety heightens performance, but too much anxiety can be debilitating.

constantly fearful and is a chronic handicap. The post-traumatic stress disorder described earlier is a chronic anxiety state of this kind.

If you find yourself in an anxious state, it is wise to:

■ Identify the cause. What do you fear? State it in words.
■ Face it. Can you change it? How? Do it.
■ If you can't change it, let it go. Worry is not helpful, and it wastes energy. Substitute concentration, meditation, or prayer, where useful.
■ Visualize a positive outcome, and work toward that. Live in the solution, not in the problem.
■ Use any accumulated energy in some physical way: be active. People who are regularly active experience less anxiety than people who are not.[18] Lack of physical activity aggravates, and can even cause, anxiety.
■ Practice relaxation techniques (see Chapter 4 for details).

Prolonged or intense anxiety out of proportion to any real danger or threat is a signal that a situation may be becoming unmanageable. Signs of extreme anxiety are the same as those of extreme stress (see Table 4–3 in Chapter 4). If these symptoms persist, it is time to get help.

■▶ *Small doses of anxiety can propel a person to meet challenges. The emotionally healthy person uses slight anxiety to advantage, and copes with extreme anxiety by finding relief for it.*

Inappropriate Guilt and Shame

guilt the awareness of having acted inconsistently with one's own values (having done "wrong").

Ordinary **guilt**, like ordinary anxiety, is desirable up to a point. A guilty feeling says that you have crossed a line your values dictate you should not cross; it is a reminder from your conscience to act consistently with your values.[19] Appropriate guilt can be useful to keep your ethics and conscience functioning.

shame the feeling of being at fault; the sense of being blameworthy; the identification of guilt with self.

The extreme version of guilt is **shame**. Also, while guilt arises from within, shame is imposed from outside as a form of control—a tool used by parents and societies probably since the beginning of time. Shame is communicated with a look, a tone of voice, or with words such as "Shame on you!" In contrast to guilt, shame can handicap a person's functioning and destroy self-esteem.[20]

Another difference between appropriate guilt and shame is that guilt separates the behavior from the person; shame equates the behavior with the person. Guilt says, "What you did was bad, but you are acceptable." Shame says, "What you did is bad, you are bad, and nothing you do will change that."[21]

An example may help to show the difference between appropriate guilt and shame. A student parties, rather than studying, then fails an exam, and feels guilty: "I guess next time I'd better go to the library, and save my partying for Saturday night." This is appropriate guilt, and leads to a desirable correction in the student's behavior. Notice, though, that the student doesn't lose self-respect or self-esteem. The idea is, "I'm OK, but my behavior on that occasion was not OK."

Now contrast the student who does the same thing, but then is disabled by shame: "What a stupid jerk I am. What a worthless, dumb failure." This person has not distinguished the mistake from self, but "is" the mistake.

Shame for behavior becomes shame for being. This erodes self-esteem and destroys emotional health. To become emotionally healthy, the student will need to learn to stay tuned into guilt when appropriate, but reject shame-casting and nurture self-esteem.

≡▶   *The emotionally healthy person tunes in to appropriate guilt to stay in touch with values, but rejects shame as destructive to self-esteem.*

Unexpressed Anger, Resentment, and Hostility

Some people, who feel **hurt** easily, say they seldom feel **anger**. Others, who deny that they are ever hurt, often become angry. Actually, though, hurt underlies anger. Both feelings are provoked by an offense—either physical injury or emotional assault. When injured or offended, you feel pain (hurt); then you feel the impulse to protect yourself by lashing out against the offender (anger).

Hurt and anger are among the hardest of all emotions to deal with because our society frowns on the qualities they seem to reflect. To say "I feel hurt" is to admit that you are vulnerable, and our society tends to label vulnerability, especially in men, as a sign of weakness. To say "I am angry" is to admit that you are experiencing an aggressive impulse, and our society deems aggression unacceptable, especially in women.

Remember, though, that all feelings are OK. Feeling hurt is OK; and feeling angry is OK (although aggressive *acts* usually are not). The ability to simply say "I am hurt" or "I am angry" is a hallmark of strong emotional health. Having expressed themselves, people can resolve the conflict that evoked the pain. Real peacefulness can follow. Rather than pretending to be serene (suppressing anger), a person can actually become serene.

A person who feels hurt or anger and is afraid or unable to express it, suppresses it and builds **resentment** instead. It is unhealthy to be consumed inwardly by resentment. Suppose your roommate entertains friends in your crowded quarters when you would rather be alone. You have only two alternatives—to express anger, or to suppress it and feel resentful. Suppose that, to avoid conflict, you suppress your anger and burn inwardly. You pay a price when you stuff (swallow) feelings: your relationship with your roommate will be impaired until you express your resentment and both of you resolve it. This chapter's Life Choice Inventory asks how well you express resentment.

As offenses accumulate and a person repeatedly represses anger and resentment, internal pain builds up, causing a smoldering rage or **hostility**. Having not worked through this accumulated pain, a hostile person is similar to a time-bomb easily able to explode at even minor irritations or annoyances. A hostile person will snap at, cut off, withdraw from, and insult others in ways that bewilder them, because the displayed rage is inappropriate for the present situation. What people do not know is that the hostile person is responding not to the present situation, but to a lifetime of accumulated, unresolved pain and anger.

Hostility makes people tense and anxious. Carried over years, it imposes stress on the body that causes physical illnesses of all kinds, including heart disease, which is a major killer of adults in our society. That is one reason why stress management strategies are important in disease prevention, and why this book devotes a whole chapter to them (Chapter 4).

hurt   the feeling of pain.

anger   a protective response to being hurt; the impulse of wanting to lash out in defense.

resentment   repressed anger.

■ *FACT OR FICTION:* To express resentment only provokes conflict; it is best to deal with resentment in private. *False.* To express resentment helps resolve conflict; to keep it private can harm a relationship.

hostility   chronic unexpressed resentment usually displayed as rage.

LIFE CHOICE INVENTORY

How well do you express resentments? This is a measure of how assertive or aggressive you are. (Some items may not apply to you. Try to imagine that they do.)

1. Your mother has emphasized that she wants you with the family at six o'clock today. At five o'clock, a friend invites you to a get-together you can't refuse. You:
   a. Go with your friend, stay through six, and explain to your mother later.
   b. Call your mother and tell her that you will be going with your friend.
   c. Complain to your mother that she is too demanding, but stay home.
   d. Tell your friend you can't go, and say nothing to your mother.

2. Several of your friends and you studied together for a test. All of your friends got good grades. You wrote the same kinds of answers on the test but got a low grade. You think your work was just as good as theirs. You:
   a. Write an anonymous note to the instructor's supervisor saying that the test grades are obviously unfair.
   b. Take your test to the instructor and ask why your grade was low.
   c. Complain to all your friends, and say nothing to the instructor.
   d. Keep your mouth shut so that the instructor won't be even more unfair to you the next time.

3. You have just cleaned up the kitchen area. The next person puts a greasy frying pan on the countertop and starts to leave. You:
   a. Wait until you are alone, and then put the greasy frying pan between the bedsheets, where the person will be sure to find it.

b. Tell the person, "Please wash your frying pan before you leave."
   c. Make a general remark about inconsiderate people who leave dirty dishes for others to clean up.
   d. Say nothing, and wash it yourself later.

4. You are on your first date with someone you have admired from a distance for a long time. At the end of the evening, the other person gets much more sexual than you want to be. You:
   a. Back off, and leave as quickly as you can without saying anything.
   b. Tell the other person that things are going too far for you.
   c. Keep pulling away, and let the other person guess the message.
   d. Say nothing and go along, because you want to date the person again.

5. You get home with a newly bought bag of groceries, only to find that the chicken you bought is already spoiled in the package. You:
   a. Storm back into the store and make a scene, so that all the other customers will know you were sold some rotten chicken.
   b. Go back to the store, ask to see the manager, and explain that the chicken you just bought is spoiled.
   c. Never shop in that store again.
   d. Do nothing.

6. You are in your room, studying for a big exam. Your neighbor is playing the stereo loudly. You:
   a. Knock on your neighbor's door, walk in, and switch off the stereo.
   b. Ask your neighbor to turn down the volume, and explain why.

c. Go someplace else to study, and never speak to your neighbor again.

d. Give up and stop trying to study.

7. Your friends like horror movies, but you don't enjoy them at all. Your friends are making plans to see the latest horror movie this Saturday night. You:

a. Tell them you think horror movies are for mental midgets, and you're not going.

b. Tell them you don't enjoy horror movies and ask if they'd consider another movie.

c. Go to the movie and afterward make some humorous negative remarks about it, hoping they will get the message.

d. Stay home Saturday night.

8. You occasionally babysit for Mrs. Harper's three children. Lately she has been making excuses when it comes time to pay you. You:

a. Tell her that you're fed up and that you won't babysit for her anymore.

b. Tell her that it's inconvenient for you to be paid late.

c. Decide you won't work for her again.

d. Say nothing.

9. You and your friend are in a record store together, and you see your friend slip a cassette into a coat pocket. You:

a. Grab the cassette, put it back on the shelf, and threaten to turn your friend in.

b. Tell your friend how you feel about shoplifting and recommend replacing the cassette.

c. Say nothing, but resolve never to go shopping with your friend again.

d. Act as if nothing has happened.

10. Your parents have given you some money to spend on clothes, and they have told you exactly what they want you to buy. You need clothes, but you disagree with the style they are urging on you. You:

a. Buy what you want, and tell them they are way out of touch with today's styles.

b. Tell them how you'd rather spend the money and why it's important to you.

c. Buy what they want you to have, and try to trade it for something else later.

d. Buy what they want you to have, wear it, and thank them for it.

Scores: Give yourself 10 points for each *a* answer, 8 for each *b*, 6 for each *c*, and 4 for each *d*. Add them up. If you scored:

85 to 100—You have no trouble asserting yourself, but your behavior borders on aggressiveness. You know what you want, but you have to give more thought to how you go about getting it.

70 to 84— You have a good sense of what you want, and you speak your mind. You are assertive.

45 to 69— You need to practice voicing your opinions and speaking up for your rights.

Below 45—You almost never voice an opinion. You may be building up some resentments. Start practicing assertiveness—be honest with yourself and direct with others.

SOURCE: Adapted from S. Schlatner, Get smart, *Coed*, March 1981, p. 36b.

≡▶ *Anger is a natural response to hurt, and should be expressed in appropriate ways. Appropriately expressed, anger resolves into serenity. Unexpressed anger becomes resentment, and chronic resentment (hostility) can cause disease.*

■≡ Suicide

During one day in the United States, about 20 young people end their own lives. In the same day, 1,000 attempt to do so but fail. According to the experts, suicide in young people is an epidemic problem.[22] Suicide attempts suggest that people may want to die. However, except for a tiny percentage, those who attempt suicide actually want to live. Thus it should be possible to prevent suicides from occurring. The signs of prolonged depression, which may signal the threat of an impending suicide, are shown in Table 3–4.

People who attempt suicide usually believe that they are not loved or accepted. A suicide attempt is really a cry for help; it says, "Look at me, help me, save me!" The person wants desperately to know that someone cares. The ambivalence of some victims' intentions is obvious: some are found dead while still holding the telephone, others call the police to say they plan to overdose, and the majority of attempts are made in such a way that someone will be sure to save them.

Most people who commit suicide suffer from deep despair, loneliness, and hopelessness. They feel that their lives are completely out of their control, and that the only way they can regain control is to take their lives. Other reasons young people attempt suicide:

■ They may have become involved with alcohol or other drugs to an extent that impairs their mental health.
■ They may be trying to impress another person with the urgency of their feelings.
■ They may have an unrealistic, romantic view of death.
■ They may be under too much parental pressure to succeed.
■ They may not be able to express anger or pain.

TABLE 3–4 ■ Signs of Depression That May Warn of Impending Suicide

These signs, especially if many appear at once and if they are prolonged, may warn of an impending suicide:
■ Withdrawal from friends; cessation of hobbies and activities.
■ Slackening of interest in schoolwork and decline in grades.
■ Not caring what happens, good or bad; passive behaviors.
■ Feeling bad about oneself, pessimistic, and helpless.
■ Ceasing to groom oneself or care for one's room, possessions, or clothes.
■ Ceasing to meet responsibilities (pay bills, return calls, or answer the phone).
■ Changes in eating or sleeping habits, alcohol or drug use.
■ Abrupt changes in personality; aggressive, hostile behavior; impulsiveness; sudden mood swings.
■ Anxiety at times of separation.
■ Inability to concentrate.
■ Refusal to leave the room or the bed.
■ Obsession with death; a death wish.

■ They may feel rootless, without the anchor of a strong parent-child relationship.

■ They may not have firm values or rules on which to base life decisions.

■ They may have suffered a loss and see no end to their unbearable grief.

■ They may have a parent or friend who committed suicide, making the act seem feasible.[23]

■ They may believe there is no other solution to a problem.

■ They may want to reunite with a deceased loved one.

To help someone, if you suspect an oncoming suicide attempt, take the person seriously and get involved. Don't wait to see what develops, because tomorrow may be too late. Ask outright if the person is planning suicide; do not be afraid that you'll plant the idea. Chances are, your friend already has it in mind, and could benefit by talking about it with a clear-headed person.

Be careful not to deny the seriousness of the intent. If you imply that your friend doesn't mean it, you may unintentionally convey a dare. At the same time as you show your concern, try to convey that you know the crisis is major, but offer reassurance that it is temporary. If the person seems on the verge of making a suicide attempt, the two most important things to do are these:

■ Phone a suicide hotline or crisis intervention center immediately. Dial 911, the operator, or the police.

■ Stay with the person until help arrives.

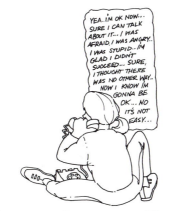

Ask someone to listen to you; you'll be glad you did.

If you fail to prevent a suicide, you can expect to feel the loss deeply. Emotional support is available for survivors,* and learning about the process of grief can help you work it through.

If you sometimes feel like ending your own life, you aren't alone. Almost everyone feels that way, sometimes. Things can seem very bad, but they always get better, given time. You can talk to someone during the bad times without saying who you are: call the helping hotline in your area. Or ask someone you trust to listen to your thoughts; you'll both be glad you did.

▶ *Take suicide signs seriously; never make light of suicidal talk. Offer a listening ear and some clear-headed perspective; obtain help if indicated. Suicidal thoughts and attempts will pass, given time.*

■ About Getting Help

If you have any questions about your own state of well-being, you are not alone. Whatever you fear, others have feared it too—and have conquered it or come to terms with it. Emotional problems are treatable. It is the responsibility of the person with an emotional problem to acknowledge it and to seek the help necessary to cope with it. Assigning blame is not useful; in fact, the concept of blame for an emotional problem and the question of whose "fault" it is are out of date, irrelevant, and destructive. Rather, the

---

*A reference we recommend is Iris Bolton's *My Son . . . My Son . . . A Guide to Healing after a Suicide in the Family,* 4th ed. (Atlanta: Bolton Press, 1985).

■ *FACT OR FICTION:* To deal with an emotional problem, one first needs to discover who is at fault. *False.* Assigning blame is not useful and is destructive.

question to ask is: How can I most efficiently recover? The choice to get help is a choice that the emotionally healthy person can make.

The exact moment when a person decides to get help is often the moment when that person starts to get better. Having felt helpless, the person is now taking charge, regaining a sense of control.

How to Help Yourself

If you have concluded that you might benefit from having psychological help, be selective. First and foremost, don't try to buy your way out of an emotional problem with a quick fix. This chapter's Critical Thinking section shows how extensively health fraud permeates the mental health field.

Having faced down the wish for a magical cure, you can turn to the search for appropriate help. Be choosy, because not all "therapists" are well qualified. Try the following possibilities:

■ Call or go to the campus counseling center.
■ If you are reading this book as the text for a course, check with the instructor.
■ Call the college psychology department.
■ Look in your telephone book for a telephone counseling service; call; ask what to do. You don't have to give your name if you don't want to.
■ Look up "Mental Health," "Health," "Social Services," "Drugs," "Alcohol," "Family Services," "Suicide Prevention," or "Counseling" in the telephone book; call; ask what to do. Again, you can choose whether to say who you are.
■ Call a hospital or any physician and ask for advice.
■ Ask your mentor whom to see. Call or ask around for a member of the clergy who is known to be helpful.

Persist. The first source you try may not work out well, but there *is* someone out there for you to talk to. Often, several referrals will take place before a problem is resolved. You might start by seeing a counselor for anxiety but end up getting help by learning from an accountant how to balance your checkbook—and that might solve the anxiety problem. Often a single clear-headed discussion will lead to a simple solution. People may hesitate to consult professional helpers for fear of what they may be forced to discover about themselves. Yet the most earth-shaking discovery people are likely to make is that they are not alone—that other people have the same problem, and that, with help, they can deal with it.

≡▶ *Seeking professional help for an emotional problem is a sign of growth toward wellness. Choose therapists carefully based on good advice and credentials. For more about helping yourself, see this chapter's Spotlight.*

How to Help Another Person

It is sometimes possible to help another person who has an emotional problem. Simply caring and offering support is often beneficial. Listening is therapeutic, too. Often a person can work out problems, given sufficient opportunities to discuss them.

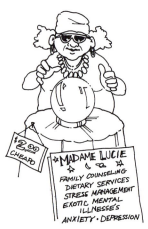

It's dangerous to go to the wrong person for therapy.

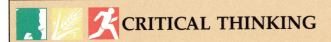 **CRITICAL THINKING**

Substitutes for Coping

"Are you tired, run-down? You may be deficient in Vitamin Z." "Do you suffer from insomnia? Use our soothing little E-Z-Sleep caplets and enjoy a sound snooze." "Do you freak out easily? Drink Sister Sybil's Syrup and slide smoothly back to spiritual serenity."

If only emotional problems could be solved so easily! Unfortunately, what they usually require is honest hard work. But ads like these can easily take people in, for three reasons. First, occasionally a symptom like tiredness, insomnia, or anxiety does reflect a simple physical problem such as a vitamin deficiency; Chapter 5 describes a case of this kind. Second, symptoms of emotional illness are often vague, and suggestible people may be led to believe they have them when they don't ("Yes, now that you mention it, I haven't been sleeping well lately.") And third, people often don't want to face and work on stressful emotional issues, and would rather believe that taking a little blue pill will make their problems go away. So hucksters lead people to focus on their symptoms, convince them that a nutrient or medicine will cure them, and encourage people to postpone dealing with their real problems.

Often, though, tiredness, insomnia, and anxiety are signs that you need to work through some emotional issue in your life. If that is the case, the sooner you face and deal with it, the less stress it will ultimately cause. And the work of resolving a problem is almost invariably less than the work it takes to keep avoiding it. As the last chapter said in other words, if you feel pain and try to push it back, it will push back at you. If you face it and ride it out, it will resolve into serenity.

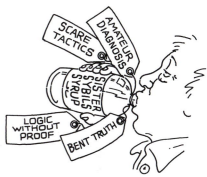

There's no sure way out of an emotional problem but through it.

Not many people, however, are professionally qualified to help others. The untrained person can often do more harm than good by saying or suggesting the wrong things. Sometimes, too, a person may actually harm someone by allowing a troubled person to evade feelings that should be confronted and resolved. This misguided attempt to help is what people with codependency do; it is termed **enabling**. Enablers, with the best intentions in the world, actually prolong other people's drinking, gambling, or other self-destructive behaviors by rescuing them from the consequences of their own actions (see Chapter 10). It is the *least* helpful thing they can do except in life-or-death situations.

A person may help another for the wrong reasons. Helping others may be a way of avoiding facing one's own problems. It provides an excuse: "I couldn't go to class because I was helping Jane." People who focus on other people's problems to this extent are often codependent and need help for themselves.

When helping others, be sure to protect yourself. For your emotional well-being, it is important to be aware of the limits of your ability to give support. A depressed person can be a sort of emotional sink into which you pour your energy without getting anything back. Such a relationship drains you, to no useful purpose.

enabling misguided "helping." An enabler is a person who actually does harm by supporting a troubled person's continued indulgence in a self-destructive attitude or behavior.

■ *FACT OR FICTION:* If a person is self-destructive, the best way to help is to keep the person from getting into trouble. *False.* Rescuing a person from the consequences of self-destructive behavior promotes a repeat performance.

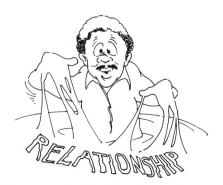

If you are mired in a dependency relationship, you may need help getting out of it.

If such a situation drags on for very long, wisdom dictates that it is best for you and the other person if you extricate yourself from it. Your continued listening may be postponing a solution. Put the person in touch with expert help and bow out. Make it clear that you are taking this action to obtain truly effective help for your friend and peace of mind for yourself. In a life-or-death situation, when you have to help, you need a special set of strategies. You may have to break out of ordinary social norms. If a person is clearly irrational and in danger, you may have to risk the friendship in order to benefit the person. To tell when to take this risk, ask yourself:

■ Do I perceive that the person's life or health is in serious danger?
■ Is the person threatening someone else's life or health?
■ If I fail to intervene, will the situation become dangerous?

If so, intervene. It is a risk, but the risk of not intervening is worse. Your judgment may not be perfect, but it is the best you have available, so use it.

A crisis requires professional help, and the person who needs help should be the one to call. Mental health agencies will not step in unless the person with the problem initiates the request. If your friend is resistant, place the call yourself, but then persuade your friend to talk to a helping person on the other end of the line. If that fails, or in the case of a very sick, weak, or debilitated friend, call the police or an ambulance. The move may be awkward, but its urgency justifies it.

Continue helping until you are satisfied that you have done what you can. Then let go. Should the outcome disappoint you, remember, you did your best.

≡▶   *Offering emotional help to others is beneficial only if the help does not undermine their independence or prevent their recovery. When a person becomes overly dependent, it is best to establish a link to professional help, and bow out. In a life-or-death situation, obtain professional help promptly.*

More people have emotional problems than not. In fact, those with emotional problems who have faced them often develop more character and depth than those who never had to face such challenges. And as Chapters 1 and 2 have both emphasized, people who gain practice and skill dealing with life's problems often win even better health, both mentally and physically, than those who have few problems to begin with.

The next chapter describes many ways of dealing with stress—a sort of catch-all term for all the problems discussed so far, as well as other problems. Before it begins, though, the Spotlight shows how emotional healing takes place.

■≡ For Review

1. Define emotional problems.
2. Identify and contrast several causes of emotional problems.
3. List characteristics of dysfunctional families.
4. Define codependency, and describe how it can impair emotional development.
5. List and describe common emotional problems.
6. Identify some strategies for coping with depression.
7. List and describe the stages of grief.
8. Describe the differences between normal anxiety and extreme, disabling anxiety.
9. Compare and contrast guilt and shame.
10. Explain how the feelings of hurt and anger are related.
11. Define resentment, and describe how it can be harmful.
12. List signs indicating that a depressed person needs help.
13. Describe how to find help for emotional problems.
14. Describe how to intervene in a life-or-death emergency.

■≡ Notes

1. *Diagnostic and Statistical Manual of Mental Disorders,* 3d ed. (Washington, D.C.: American Psychiatric Association, 1980), p. 8; often referred to as *DSM III*.

2. E. M. N. Hamilton, E. N. Whitney, and F. S. Sizer, Behavior, nutrient deficiencies, and sugar, in *Nutrition: Concepts and Controversies,* 3d ed. (St. Paul, Minn.: West, 1983), pp. 438–443.

3. D. Lonsdale and R. J. Shamberger, Red cell transketolase as an indicator of nutritional deficiency, *American Journal of Clinical Nutrition* 33 (1980): 205–211.

4. D. Coon, *Introduction to Psychology,* 4th ed. (St. Paul, Minn.: West, 1986), pp. 504–527.

5. S. E. Nicol and I. I. Gottesman, Clues to the genetics and neurobiology of schizophrenia, *American Scientist* 71 (1983): 398–404.

6. D. Rosenthal and O. W. Quinn, Quadruplet hallucinations: Phenotypic variations of a schizophrenic genotype, *Archives of General Psychiatry* 34 (1977): 817–827.

7. Alcohol, drug, mental illness costs put at $273 billion, *The Nation's Health,* April 1991.

8. Peak ages for developing mental illness are childhood, adolescence, *The Nation's Health,* November 1990.

9. S. S. Mull, Help for the children of alcoholics, *Health Education,* September/October 1990, p. 42.

10. C. L. Whitfield, *Healing the Child Within* (Deerfield Beach, Fla.: Health Communications, 1987), pp. 25–53.

11. Mull, 1990, p. 42.

12. E. Taylor, Taking care of herself, *Time,* 10 December 1990, pp. 106–107.

13. W. Kritsberg, *The Adult Children of Alcoholics Syndrome* (New York: Bantam, 1988), outside back cover.

14. C. Black, *It Will Never Happen to Me* (New York: Ballantine, 1981), pp. 24–48; also cited in Mull, 1990, p. 42.

15. G. S. Belkin, *Introduction to Counseling* (Dubuque: Wm. C. Brown, 1988), as cited in Mull, 1990, p. 42.

16. D. Gelman, Treating war's psychic wounds, *Newsweek,* August 1988, pp. 62–64, as cited in Mull, 1990, p. 42.

17. T. L. Cermak, Children of alcoholics and the case for a new diagnostic category of co-dependency, in *Growing up in the Shadow,* ed. R. Ackerman (Pompano Beach, Fla.: Health Communications, 1986), pp. 23–32, as cited in Mull, 1990, p. 42.

18. K. T. Francis and R. Carter, Psychological characteristics of joggers, *Journal of Sports Medicine* 22 (1982): 386–390.

19. Hilda Fried, ed., *Plain Talk about Feelings of Guilt,* National Institute of Mental Health, Division of Scientific and Public Information, Plain Talk Series, (Washington, D.C.: Government Printing Office, 1989).

20. M. Beattie, *Beyond Codependency* (New York: Harper and Row, 1989), pp. 101–112.

21. Beattie, 1989.

22. Much of this information is from M. Giffin and C. Felsenthal, *A Cry for Help* (Garden City, N.Y.: Doubleday, 1983).

23. Many of these items are from Giffin and Felsenthal, 1983.

SPOTLIGHT

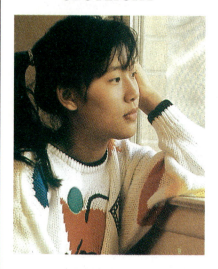

Emotional Healing

Chapter 3 described emotional problems that need healing. To see whether you tend to have such problems in relationships with self and others, answer the questions in Table S3–1. This survey reflects not only your present emotional health, but also your need for emotional healing.

Now that I've completed the survey, I think I probably could benefit from emotional healing. Where do I start?

First, you need to learn what sorts of therapeutic activities are available and which may be appropriate for you.

What do you mean by therapeutic activity?

Any activity that has a healing or health-promoting effect is a form of *therapy*. For one person, going out for the softball team after work may be therapeutic. For another, it may be

therapeutic to get out of the noise, clamor, and exertion; go home to a quiet kitchen; listen to music; and cut up fresh vegetables for a gourmet dinner. Painting, lovemaking, writing, walking on the beach or in the mountains—all these can be therapeutic activities.

A person with an emotional problem can also benefit from the help of another person or persons to achieve healing. This can take the form of *psychotherapy* (which means, literally, therapy for the spirit). Psychotherapy is offered in many different places, in several formats, by many types of therapists. Among places to go for therapy in most urban locations are:

- ■ Counseling centers at schools or colleges.
- ■ The community mental health center.
- ■ The offices of psychiatrists, psychoanalysts, and psychiatric nurses.
- ■ Private counseling centers and psychological clinics.
- ■ Employee assistance programs.
- ■ Crisis centers (drug crisis, spouse abuse, and others).
- ■ Alcohol and drug abuse programs.
- ■ Self-help groups.
- ■ Telephone counseling.

How can I find the right therapy program?

One way you can tell if a program is right for you is to ask yourself if you

---

TABLE S3–1 ■ **Recovery Potential Survey**

Answer the following questions with words such as "Never," "Seldom," "Occasionally," "Often," or "Always."
1. Do you seek approval and affirmation?
2. Do you fail to recognize your accomplishments?
3. Do you fear criticism?
4. Do you overextend yourself?
5. Have you had problems with your own compulsive behavior?
6. Do you have a need for perfection?
7. Are you uneasy when your life is going smoothly? Do you continually anticipate problems?
8. Do you feel most alive in the midst of a crisis?
9. Do you care for others easily, yet find it difficult to care for yourself?
10. Do you isolate yourself from other people?
11. Do you respond with anxiety to authority figures and angry people?
12. Do you feel that individuals and society in general are taking advantage of you?
13. Do you have trouble with intimate relationships?
14. Do you attract and seek people who tend to be compulsive?
15. Do you cling to relationships because you are afraid of being alone?
16. Do you often mistrust your own feelings and the feelings expressed by others?
17. Do you find it difficult to express your emotions?
Every honest person would answer "occasionally," "often," or "usually" to some of these questions. Those to which you gave positive answers indicate areas in your life that you might want to explore.

SOURCE: If you answered "occasionally," "often," or "usually" to any of these questions, you may find it useful to read the book *Healing the Child Within* by C. L. Whitfield (Deerfield Beach, Fla.: Health Communications, 1987), pp. 2–3.

feel comfortable with the counselor. The outcome depends more on that than on anything else.

Effective therapy always contains three ingredients:

1. A warm or mutually respectful and trusting relationship between the therapist and the client.
2. The exploration of the present problem's causes, effects, or both.
3. The exploration of new, more adaptive ways of dealing with the problem (attitudes or behaviors). Short glossaries for types of therapists and the therapies they offer appear in Appendix C.

In addition to formal therapies, there are many "Anonymous" groups: Alcoholics Anonymous (AA), Overeaters Anonymous (OA), Narcotics Anonymous (NA), Gamblers Anonymous (GA), and others like them. These are self-help groups run by and for people with compulsions and addictions. Their services are free; members support them voluntarily. Most make use of a "12-step" program that progresses from admitting the problem, through dealing with it, to helping others deal with it. (Spotlight 10 lists the 12 steps.) Members assist one another in working their recovery programs.

What does it mean to work a recovery program?

The work of recovery involves these steps:

1. Feeling the pain associated with not getting your original needs met in the past.
2. Expressing and resolving that pain so that it no longer interferes with your living a contented and peaceful life.
3. Learning to interact with people in healthy ways, as would have

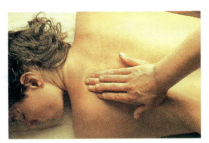

A therapeutic touch can hasten healing.

happened naturally if your original needs had been met.

For many people, the most efficient way to accomplish these tasks is to engage in formal therapy, although healing can occur without it. The many self-affirming activities listed in Chapter 2 facilitate recovery. Also helpful is to connect with other recovering people and to keep a journal or diary.

What can I expect to experience during recovery?

During recovery, you will experience growing awareness of your feelings, acceptance of your past, and changes in your attitudes and behaviors. The process occurs in stages, all of which are necessary for healing to take place. People can recover without knowing they are passing through these stages, or may recognize them only in retrospect. This is one reason why it is helpful for a person to have a sponsor, guide, counselor, or therapist during recovery.

Before recovery, a person denies any problem and uses defense mechanisms (described in Chapter 3) to survive. In this stage, people do not realize that their behaviors are self-defeating. Then, as recovery begins, the person recognizes these behaviors as destructive, and begins to uncover underlying problem thoughts, which

are described by therapists as *core issues*. Some of these problems are described in Table S3–2 along with the transformations that occur in recovery. Finally, healing becomes complete, not in the sense that the person becomes perfect, but in the sense that all the parts—new behaviors, attitudes, and feelings—come together and work together without awkwardness. The recovery work is used, applied, and integrated into the person's life. The new, positive behaviors become automatic; the learned actions occur almost as though by reflex.

How would you go about uncovering an underlying problem? What types of underlying problems could people have?

An example of a typical situation may help illustrate this process. Michelle began a recovery program when she sought help through counseling for depression and anxiety. She reported that, in spite of her outward accomplishments, she felt empty and sad and had low self-esteem. She commented that her friends would be surprised if they knew how she felt about herself. Michelle's friends and acquaintances viewed Michelle as successful and happy: in fact, they were even envious of her. She was attractive and well-groomed. She exercised faithfully. Her career achievements were remarkable.

In counseling, Michelle revealed that, as a child, she had been an excellent student and a class leader. Her teachers had always described her as more responsible, organized, and mature than most children her age. Being the oldest in her family, Michelle had an overdeveloped sense of responsibility. She remembered that during her childhood, her father had been actively alcoholic, and her mother had spent most of her energy trying to control his drinking. Michelle had prepared the meals, cleaned the house, and taken care of the other children. In taking responsibility for running the family, she thwarted her own normal developmental need to spend time playing. As a result, she emerged as an outwardly successful adult, but she could never take satisfaction in her achievements. She had become a "workaholic," and was never able to enjoy feeling satisfied with herself. She also found herself inappropriately helping (enabling) other people and neglecting herself.

In counseling she identified her underlying problems as being overly responsible for others and neglecting her own needs. Through therapy she identified her problem behaviors and corrected them. She learned to take care of herself, to assert her valid needs to her close friends, and to play and enjoy herself. This raised her self-esteem and relieved her depression and anxiety.

This recovery process sounds wonderful, but isn't it an overwhelming task? How long does it take?

For a person who has unresolved childhood issues, it may take three to five years or even longer to arrive at the stage of final healing; people progress at different individual rates. Recovery may feel overwhelming at times, and it is natural and healthy to take time off at such times.

Recovery is individual. At the beginning, it may take weeks, months, or even years before people become able to talk about and express their feelings around their wounds.

TABLE S3–2 ■ Core Issues Transformed by Recovery	
Core Issue	**Recovery Transforms This Issue into**
Trying to control other people or external circumstances	Learning responsibility, while letting go of trying to control other people and/or circumstances
Being overly responsible for others	Being responsible for self; letting others take responsibility for themselves
Neglecting needs of self	Meeting needs of self in a healthy way
Tolerating inappropriate behavior	Learning what is appropriate; not tolerating inappropriate behavior
Having difficulty identifying and expressing feelings	Developing ease in identifying and expressing feelings; using feelings to help guide behavior
Grieving past and current losses	Grieving current losses
Fearing abandonment	Having freedom from fear of abandonment
Having difficulty resolving conflict	Resolving conflict with ease

SOURCE: Adapted from C. L. Whitfield, *Healing the Child Within* (Deerfield Beach, Fla.: Health Communications, 1987), p. 108.

Then it may take even more time to practice new behaviors, and more time still for those behaviors to become automatic.

Is it really worth it for people to go through all that work?

The rewards of recovery are tremendous. People emerge with high self-esteem. They have confidence in their problem-solving skills. The negative messages from the past never completely disappear, but through therapy people develop keen ears for identifying these messages and learn to quickly combat them with positive self-talk. Relationships with self, friends, family, and a higher power improve. True intimacy becomes a possibility. Serenity, once unknown, becomes the rule.

What does a person's relationship with a higher power have to do with recovery?

A relationship with a higher power—spirituality—is a vast area in recovery that is crucial to emotional healing. Spirituality pervades all experiences, including suffering, healing, and serenity. Spirituality is a heightened awareness of the relationships with self, others, and the universe.

Spirituality is necessary to heal completely, for people who have been through emotional trauma must forgive those who caused the pain. "Turning it over" is a phrase used in recovery programs that means to turn the upset or resentment over to a higher power in order to be free of the pain.

In emotional healing, people identify past traumas, experience them, let go of them, and become well. Emotional healing finally leads to taking care of the self and enjoying a richer, fuller, happier life. The process continues throughout life.

CHAPTER 4

Stress and Stress Management

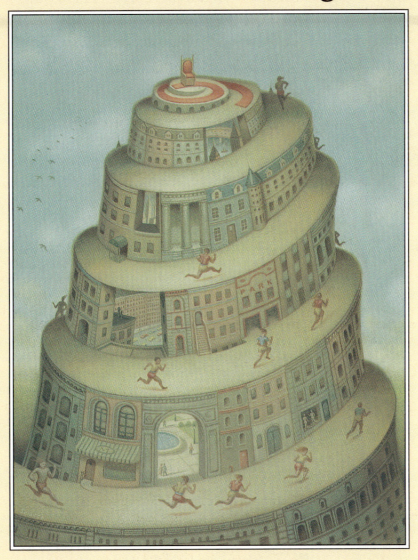

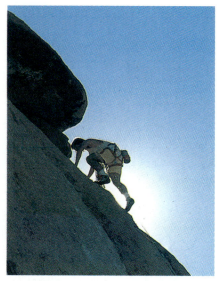

Challenges can be stressful—and beneficial.

stress   the effect of demands (stressors) on a person. Stress that is perceived as a welcome challenge is *eustress* (YOU-stress); stress that is perceived as negative is *distress*. This term encompasses both stressors and the body's response to them.

   eu = good, beneficial

   dis = bad, negative

stressor   a demand placed on the body to adapt.

FACT OR FICTION

Just for fun, respond true or false to the following statements. If false, say what is true.

■ Some stress is beneficial. (Page 80)
■ Prolonged stress can make a person vulnerable to disease. (Page 85)
■ The fight-or-flight reaction was experienced by our distant ancestors, but people today do not experience it. (Page 85)

■ Whether an event is stressful depends more on the person experiencing it than on the event itself. (Page 87)
■ Machines can help you learn to relax. (Page 94)

The word *stress* is widely used today. The experience has been known since prehistoric times, but the term as applied to modern society was not used until the physiologist Hans Selye (pronounced SELL-yeh) examined stress scientifically earlier in this century.[1]* Now the word is so widely used that it seems to apply to every life situation. When a person says, "I am under stress," he may mean that he is ill, that his love life has gone awry, that he is under financial pressure, or any of a hundred other things.

In contrast, another person who says she is under stress may mean that she is thriving. Stress can be a threat to wellness, or it can be the fuel for progress and achievement. For some, it almost borders on inspiration.

Many young adults have yet to learn to deal with stress, for their role models may not have done so successfully. Life in today's urban world can be so demanding that people respond by overloading themselves. They drive cars and talk on their phones at the same time. They study on the way to school and eat on the run between classes. Even when on vacation, people supposedly at leisure cover 15 countries in two weeks. Unfortunately, many people have not learned how to relax on their own, so they turn to alcohol or other drugs for help.

The college years are stressful, for they represent a period of transition requiring students to adapt to many life changes. This chapter shows how people respond to stress and how you can deal with your own stress.

■☰ Stressors and Stress

To say that a person is under **stress** means that the person is responding to **stressors** in a characteristic way. A stressor is anything that requires you to cope with or adapt to a situation. Physical stressors include all environmental stimuli. Psychosocial stressors include life-changing events, both desirable and undesirable (see Tables 4–1 and 4–2).

*Reference notes are at the end of the chapter.

TABLE 4–1 ■ **Physical Stressors**

The Greater the Intensity the Greater the Stress

Light and changes in light
Heat/cold and changes in temperature
Sound and changes in sound level
Touch/pressure and changes in touch stimuli
Airborne chemical stimuli (odors, smoke, smog, air pollution)
Waterborne chemical stimuli
Drugs/medicines/alcohol
Foodborne chemicals and contaminants
Bacteria/viruses/other infective agents/allergens
Injury, including surgery
Exertion, work
X rays/radioactive rays/other forms of radiation

TABLE 4–2 ■ **Psychosocial Stressors for College Students**

Life Event	Stress Points	Life Event	Stress Points
Death of spouse	100	Son or daughter leaving home	29
Divorce	73	Trouble with in-laws [trouble with parents]	29
Marital separation [breakup with boyfriend/girlfriend]	65	Outstanding personal achievement	28
Jail term	63	Spouse beginning or stopping work	26
Death of close family member (except spouse)	63	School beginning or ending [final exams]	26
Major personal injury or illness	53	Change in living conditions	25
Marriage	50	Revision of personal habits (self or family)	24
Being fired from a job [expulsion from school]	47	Trouble with boss [trouble with professor]	23
Marital reconciliation	45	Change in work [or school] hours or conditions	20
Retirement	45	Change in residence [moving to school, moving home]	20
Change in health of a family member (not self)	44	Change in schools	20
Pregnancy	40	Change in recreation	19
Sex difficulties	39	Change in church activities	19
Gain of new family member [change of roommate]	39	Change in social activities [joining new group]	18
Business readjustment	39	Taking on small mortgage or loan	17
Change in financial state	38	Change in sleeping habits	16
Death of close friend	37	Change in number of family get-togethers	15
Change to different line of work [change of major]	36	Change in eating habits	13
Change in number of arguments with spouse	35	Vacation	13
Taking on a large mortgage [financial aid]	31	Major holidays like Christmas and Thanksgiving	12
Foreclosure of mortgage or loan	30	Minor violations of the law	11
Change in responsibilities at work [change in course demands]	29		

Check the list and identify the events that have happened to you in the past year or that you expect within the next year. Use the number system to determine how many stress points you are experiencing in this period of your life. Then score yourself as follows: over 200—urgent need of intelligent stress management; 150–199—careful stress management indicated; 100–149—stressful life, keep tabs on your mental health; under 100—no present cause for concern about stress.

SOURCE: Adapted from Lifescore: Holmes scale, *Family Health*, January 1979, p. 32.

College students experience a variety of stressors. Some authorities believe that the college years may be the most stressful in one's life.[2] The most common kinds of stressors experienced by students include:

■ Pressure to achieve. Students may create their own pressure, if they have high internal standards. Or parents and teachers may create pressure by holding up high expectations.

■ Financial burdens. Many students have to work while earning their degrees. These students have to balance employers' expectations with academic goals. For those with families to support, the stress is even more intense.

■ Living adjustments. Many students are living away from home, usually for the first time, and have not established a network of social support, which is crucial for coping.

■ Social pressure. Students are confronted with choices regarding alcohol, drug use, and sexuality.[3] The current epidemic of sexually transmitted diseases adds even more pressure.

Figure 4–1 illustrates these and other stressors. Although some stress can be beneficial, unmanaged stressful demands can arouse anxiety, which in turn often causes mental and physical harm, as the next sections describe.

FIGURE 4–1 ■ **Stressors in the lives of students.**

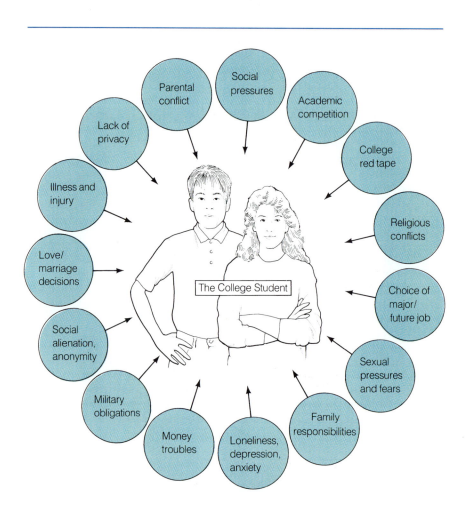

≡▶ *A stressor is anything that requires you to cope with or adapt to a situation. College students face many stressors.*

■≡ Stress and the Body's Systems

What can a stressor such as exercising, taking an exam, or buying a new car do to your body? You may say it is "scary" or "exciting" (as opposed to "relaxing"), but what does that mean, physically? It means, among other things, that your heart beats faster and that you breathe faster than normal, signifying that your body is getting ready to exert itself physically. All external changes stimulate you this way to some extent, requiring you to change internally in some physical way—that is, to adapt. All environmental changes—changes in the temperature, the noise level around you, what is touching you, and countless others—require such adaptation. So do all psychological events, both desirable and undesirable.

All of the body's systems are affected by stress, but of particular importance are the **nervous system**, the **hormonal system**, and the **immune system**. Figures 4–2 and 4–3 show the anatomy and describe the workings of the hormonal and nervous systems. As for the immune system, the parts are so widespread in the body that to show them in a figure would require a picture of almost every organ and tissue. Included in the immune system are **white blood cells** made in the bone marrow and incubated in other

nervous system the system of nerves, organized into the brain, spinal cord, and peripheral nerves that send and receive messages and integrate the body's activities.

hormonal system the system of glands, organs that send and receive blood-borne chemical messages that integrate body functions in cooperation with the nervous system.

immune system the cells, tissues, and organs that protect the body from disease; it is composed of the white blood cells, bone marrow, thymus gland, spleen, and other parts.

white blood cells the blood cells responsible for the immune response (as opposed to the red blood cells, which carry oxygen).

FIGURE 4–2 ■ **The hormonal system.**

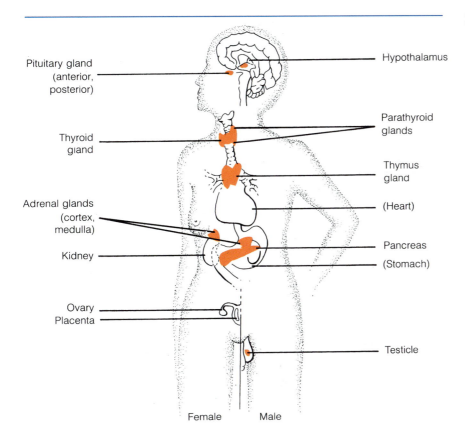

Pituitary gland (anterior, posterior)

Hypothalamus

Parathyroid glands

Thyroid gland

Thymus gland

(Heart)

Adrenal glands (cortex, medulla)

Kidney

Pancreas

(Stomach)

Ovary
Placenta

Testicle

Female   Male

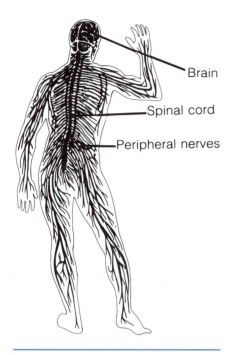

FIGURE 4–3 ■ The organization of the nervous system.

antibodies   large protein molecules produced to fight foreign tissue.

immunity   the body's capacity for identifying, destroying, and disposing of disease-causing agents.

homeostasis   (HO-me-oh-STAY-sis)   the maintenance of relatively constant internal conditions by corrective responses to forces that would otherwise cause life-threatening changes in those conditions. A homeostatic system is not static. It is constantly changing, but within tolerable limits.

stress hormones   epinephrine and norepinephrine, hormones with many roles, one of which is to help modulate the reaction of the nervous system to stress.

epinephrine   (EP-ih-NEFF-rin), norepinephrine (NOR-ep-ih-NEFF-rin)   two hormones of the adrenal gland, sometimes called the stress hormones, although they are not the only hormones modulating the stress response. (The adrenal gland nestles in the surface of the kidney.)

glands, and **antibodies** made by white blood cells. These other tissues all work together to confer **immunity** on the body. These systems connect all the body's parts so that they act as a unit.

Whether a particular stressful event presents a mental challenge such as an exam, or a physical one such as a fistfight, the responses always have the same effect: to restore balance. If unmet, the challenge would upset the body's balance, but the body adjusts to meet it. The efficient functioning that results from the body's adjustments to changing conditions is **homeostasis**.

The stress of cold weather can serve as an example to show how the nervous system in particular works to maintain homeostasis. (Remember, all stressors call forth similar balance-restoring efforts from the body, so even if you never experience cold weather, you do perform adjustments of the same general kind.) When you go outside in cold weather, your skin's temperature receptors send "cold" messages to the spinal cord and brain. Your nervous system reacts to these messages and signals your skin-surface capillaries to shut down so that your blood will circulate deeper in your tissues, where it will not lose heat. The system also signals involuntary contractions of the small muscles just under the skin surface: goose bumps with their by-product, heat. If these measures do not raise your body temperature enough, the nerves signal your large muscle groups to shiver. The contractions of these large muscles produce still more heat. All of this activity adds up to a set of adjustments that maintains your homeostasis (a constant temperature, in this case) under conditions of external extremes (cold).

Let's say you now come in and sit by a fire and drink hot cocoa. You are warm, and you no longer need the body's heat-producing activity. At this point, the nervous system signals your skin-surface capillaries to open up again, your goose bumps to subside, and your muscles to relax. Your body has maintained homeostasis throughout the cold time with extra effort; now it can relax and maintain homeostasis without extra effort.

Now imagine that the system is constantly under stress—having to work to stay warm, to repair injuries, and to deal with fears and anxieties. Without periods of relaxation between times, in which to recover, these constant demands would wear the body down.

This example described only the nervous system's role in managing a brief period of stress, but all the body's parts act smoothly together. Like the nervous system, the hormonal system is busy during times of stress, sending messages from one body part to another to maintain order. Among the hormones that mediate the stress response, collectively called the **stress hormones**, are **epinephrine** and **norepinephrine**, secreted by the adrenal gland.

The immune system is suppressed during the stress response, but rebounds between times. With small amounts of stress, that alternate with times of relief from stress, the immune system maintains optimal health, but prolonged stress can impair immunity and make a person unusually vulnerable to disease.

The immune system, after all, is crucial in defenses against infectious disease agents, which are always present in all environments: agents that cause colds, flu, measles, tuberculosis, pneumonia, and hundreds of other diseases. The immune system also helps defend against cancer. Cancer cells grow from a person's own body tissues, but the immune system can often recognize them as abnormal cells and fight them off. Anything that impairs the immune system threatens life; anything that strengthens the system supports health.

≡▶ *The nervous, hormonal, and immune systems cooperate to maintain balance during stress. During the stress response, the nervous and hormonal systems are activated, and the immune system is suppressed. Prolonged stress can impair immunity and make a person unusually vulnerable to disease.*

■≡ Stress and Too Much Stress

A little stress can be beneficial, but too much stress, unrelieved, can be exhausting and debilitating. Consider what stress, whether it is physical, psychological, or both, does to you. Whatever stressor you encounter, the **stress response** has three phases, but the third phase is not always the same. The three phases may be either **alarm**, **resistance**, and **recovery** or alarm, resistance, and **exhaustion** (see Figure 4–4).

Alarm occurs when you perceive that you are facing a challenge. Stress hormone secretion increases, activating all systems to achieve resistance. Resistance is a state of speeded-up functioning in which enhanced stress hormone secretion continues, favoring muscular activity over other body functions (we'll describe this unbalanced state in more detail shortly). During the resistance phase, your resources are mobilized just as a nation mobilizes its manpower to fight a battle. In the case of your body, the resources are your attention, strength, fuels, and others, but the principle is the same. You can use these resources for emergency purposes for a while, but only for a while. Just as the fighters must return to farm their fields, your resources must return to support your normal body functions.

Hopefully, before your resources run out, the stressor leaves you and a recovery period arrives. You relax and recuperate. Enhanced stress hormone secretion ceases, all systems slow down, normal functioning resumes, needed repairs take place, fuel stores are refilled, and you become ready for the next round of excitement. It is because of the need for recovery between times of stress that the military provides "R and R" (rest and recreation) times for its personnel. If you have to stay in overdrive (resistance) for too long, however, your resources become depleted, and recovery is delayed or becomes impossible. This is exhaustion.

In learning to manage stress so as to protect yourself from becoming exhausted, you need to appreciate its physical nature. The stress response evolved eons ago to permit our ancestors to react appropriately to *physical* danger, not to psychological threats.

Consider how physical the response is. It is often called the **fight-or-flight reaction,** because when someone is faced with a physical threat, the two major alternatives are to fight or run away. Every organ responds to the alarm and readies itself to take action. The heart rate and respiration rate speed up. The pupils of the eyes widen so that you can see better. The muscles tense up so that you can jump, run, or struggle with maximum strength. Circulation to the skin diminishes (to protect against blood loss from surface injury); circulation to the digestive system and internal organs (which can wait) also diminishes. Circulation to the muscles and nerves (which are needed now) increases. The kidneys retain water (in case you

■ *FACT OR FICTION:* Prolonged stress can make a person vulnerable to disease. *True.*

stress response The response to a demand or stressor, brought about by the nervous and hormonal systems, also called the *general adaptation syndrome*. It has three phases: alarm, resistance, and recovery or exhaustion.

alarm the first phase of the stress response, in which the person perceives a stressor.

resistance the second phase of the stress response, in which the body mobilizes its resources to withstand the stressor's effects.

recovery the third phase of the stress response, in the case in which the stressor is withdrawn and the body returns to its normal state of balance.

exhaustion the third phase of the stress response, in the case in which the stressor continues to act beyond the body's ability to resist; breakdown with harmful effects.

fight-or-flight reaction the response to immediate physical danger; the stress response.

■ *FACT OR FICTION:* The fight-or-flight reaction was experienced by our distant ancestors, but people today do not experience it. *False.* People today experience the fight-or-flight reaction just as our ancestors did.

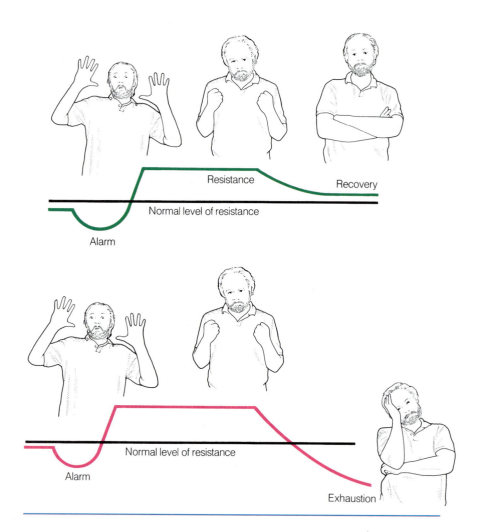

FIGURE 4–4 ■ **The stress response and its ending in recovery or exhaustion.**

should lose fluid by bleeding). The immune system temporarily shuts down (the body needs to cope with external threats).

While the nerves bring about some of these effects, the hormones go to work, too. The brain initiates a hormone cascade that calls gland after gland into play and affects every organ in the body.

Today, the same stress response occurs, even though the stressors people face are often psychological, not physical. Our Stone Age ancestors had to cope with fierce tigers and spear-wielding foes, not with bouncing checks or final exams. But bouncing checks and final exams evoke fear, just as tigers and foes do, and fear evokes the same response in you today that it did in your Stone Age ancestors. The stress response serves you well when physical action is called for, but it can actually handicap you when you have to contain your fear and take no physical action.

Consider what happens if you experience alarm (anxiety, fear), and you *don't* fight or flee—that is, your body takes no physical action. The body gets *ready* to exercise, and mobilizes its resources, but doesn't use them. Now your muscles are tense and can't relax; your blood is rich with fuels that will tend to accumulate and damage your heart; you are in a state of heightened anxiety with no relief in sight. This state of chronic arousal drains your reserves, exhausts you psychologically, and renders you vulnerable to diseases of all kinds, especially heart disease. (Chapter 18 shows the links between unused fuels and heart diseases.)

The state of stress resistance is an unbalanced state. It is a state in which muscular activity is favored over other necessary body functions such as digestion and immune defenses. The stress response represents the body's effort to deal with an emergency to preserve life so as to get back to the normal desirable state as quickly as possible; the digestion and normal immune defenses can then resume. Both states are important—normal functioning to keep you running smoothly during peaceful times, and stress resistance to get you through times of change and back to normal functioning.

If a round of stress leads to recovery, then it has benefited you. It may even strengthen your ability to adapt to the next round. On the other hand, if it leaves you drained, it may have harmed you. You may be *less* able to adapt the next time. How can you make sure to obtain benefit, rather than harm, from your stressful experiences? The next section provides some insight.

≡▶ *The stress response (fight-or-flight reaction) is a physical reaction, even if the stressor is psychological. The phases are alarm, resistance, and recovery or exhaustion. If the reaction ends in recovery, it can benefit you. If it ends in exhaustion, it may harm you.*

■≡ Stress Management Strategies

People who are educated about stress management strategies are better able to cope than those who are not.[4] This section describes those strategies, beginning with personal health habits.

People who maintain strong programs of personal wellness during ordinary life are best able to withstand crises when they arrive. Eating well, sleeping well, being physically active, cultivating daily joy and laughter, and acting on your spiritual values can help you lead a serene and largely stress-free life. To determine how well you protect yourself from stress during ordinary life, complete the first 20 questions of this chapter's Life Choice Inventory. Answer the last 5 questions to see how well you manage especially stressful times.

Physical activity is especially beneficial as a stress reducer: it works your tense muscles so they can relax again. It burns the fuels in your blood, preventing their accumulation. It resolves your anxiety and brings relief.

In addition to maintaining a program of personal wellness, you can improve your reaction to stress by bolstering your self-esteem. People with high self-esteem learn to view challenges as positive and therefore experience less stress than those with low self-esteem. For example, a person with low self-esteem might fear meeting new people as a threat, whereas a person with high self-esteem would enjoy it. Whether an event is stressful depends more on the person experiencing it than on the event itself.

You can change the way you react to events so that the events aren't so stressful. An example is public speaking. The stress response can help you get "up for it." Some excitement and anticipation ahead of the event, with the associated rapid heartbeat and breathing, will give you the physical

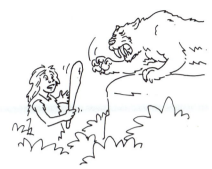

The threats your ancestors faced were physical, and the reaction was to fight or flee.

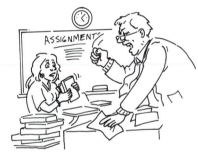

The threats you face today are seldom physical, but your reaction is still the same.

This chapter's Spotlight describes what sleep does for the body.

■ *FACT OR FICTION:* Whether an event is stressful depends more on the person experiencing it than on the event itself. *True.*

See Chapter 2 for suggestions about improving self-esteem.

LIFE CHOICE INVENTORY

How vulnerable are you to stress? To determine how likely you are to be affected by stressors, answer the following questions. Beside each question, fill in the number corresponding to how much of the time each statement applies to you: 4: always.   3: almost always.   2: most of the time.   1: some of the time.   0: never.

Part 1. During ordinary life I: Score

1. Eat at least one hot, balanced meal a day. _____
2. Get seven to eight hours' sleep at least four nights a week. _____
3. Give and receive affection regularly. _____
4. Have at least one relative within 50 miles on whom I can rely. _____
5. Exercise to the point of perspiration at least twice a week. _____
6. Do not smoke or use smokeless tobacco. _____
7. Take fewer than five alcoholic drinks a week. _____
8. Am the appropriate weight for my height. _____
9. Have an income adequate to meet basic expenses. _____
10. Get strength from my spiritual beliefs. _____
11. Regularly attend club or social activities. _____
12. Have a network of friends and acquaintances. _____
13. Have one or more friends to confide in about personal matters. _____
14. Am in good physical health (including eyesight, hearing, and teeth). _____
15. Am able to speak openly about my feelings when angry or worried. _____
16. Have regular conversations with the people I live with about domestic problems (e.g., chores, money, and daily living issues). _____
17. Do something for fun at least once a week. _____
18. Am able to organize my time effectively. _____
19. Drink fewer than three cups of caffeinated beverages (coffee, tea, or cola drinks) a day. _____
20. Take quiet time for myself during the day. _____

Part 1 score _____

Scoring for Part 1:

61 to 80:   Congratulations. Your defenses against daily stresses are strong.

41 to 60:   You are well-defended against stress, but you could still improve your defenses.

0 to 40:   You are too vulnerable to stress; try to improve.

Part 2. During highly stressful times I:

1. Prioritize my responsibilities and meet the most important ones first. _____
2. Refuse assertively to take on too many responsibilities. _____
3. Ventilate my feelings at intervals. _____
4. Use willed relaxation techniques at intervals. _____
5. Seek outside help as needed. _____

Part 2 score _____

Scoring for Part 2:

15 to 20:   You handle highly stressful times very well.

10 to 15:   You handle highly stressful times well.

0 to 9:   You need to learn to handle stressful times better.

energy to turn out a spectacular performance. You are at your most attractive when you are aroused and alert. But too much nervous energy is debilitating. If you allow yourself to think about what a catastrophe it will be if you do less than a perfect job, you will be trembling visibly, your teeth will be chattering, and your knees will be knocking together. In such a state, you

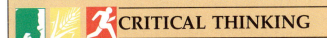

CRITICAL THINKING

Use Skills, Not Pills, to Manage Stress

Some people want to reduce their stress so much that they are willing to pay large sums of money to do so. People spend hundreds of dollars needlessly on "stress vitamins," tranquilizing pills, sleeping pills, and many more products, in hopes of eliminating the harmful effects of stress on their health. Beware of any product or service that takes your money, and promises you something great for little effort.

A program suggesting that you practice a discipline such as maintaining a routine of regular, strenuous physical activity is one that asks you to work. On the other hand, a pill or potion that promises to make you feel better instantly, without any effort on your part, is one that suggests magic. The first will be effective, the second will not.

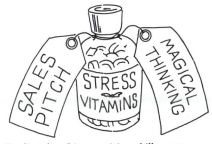

Be disciplined in practicing skills, not deceived into buying pills.

can hardly reach your audience at all, and you will be unduly exhausted afterward. It is to your advantage to learn to *perceive* the event as not so stressful and to relax before and after it.

This example illustrates another strategy: use the stress response to your advantage. Direct and control the energy it gives you. It is a magnificent response to challenges, after all. It's only when the energy is scattered and wasted that it drains you without giving you anything in return. (In other words, it's OK to have butterflies in your stomach as long as they're all flying in formation.)

Notice that every strategy suggested here is a skill you can learn. Practicing these skills improves your personal competence; you assume control. Developing these skills requires discipline which is more demanding than buying gimmicks that promise stress relief without effort. This chapter's Critical Thinking section develops this thought.

Wise time management can also help you to minimize stress. Time is similar to a regular income: you receive 24 hours of it each day. It is like money, too, in that you have three ways in which to spend it. You can save ahead (do tasks now so you won't have to do them later); you can spend as you go; or you can borrow from the future (have fun now and hope you will find the time later to do things you have to do). If you manage time wisely, you can gain the two advantages that wise money management also gives you—security for the future and enjoyment of the present. It takes skill to treat yourself to enough luxuries so that you enjoy your present life, while saving enough so that you will have time available when you need it. When your friends call on a Sunday to invite you out, you don't want to be caught with no money on hand, no clean clothes, and no studying done for the big exam on Monday. That is an avoidable stress, and planning ahead circumvents it. Make a time budget. If this sounds boring, remember, you have to do it only once, and an hour of time spent in organizing buys many hours of time doing what you choose.

Several planning techniques can help you get the most out of your day while keeping tabs on long-term time needs. One such technique is to make two records—one, a weekly time schedule, and the other, a list of things to do (see Figure 4–5). To make the time schedule, set up a grid that lists the days of the week across the top, and lists blocks of time (such as each hour from waking to bedtime) down the left-hand side. Fill in your set obligations, such as class meetings, in the appropriate spaces. Then add study time, travel time, and mealtimes. Allot a space each day to exercise. In the time remaining, decide when to take care of your regular weekly obligations, such as laundry, bill paying, or grocery shopping. Attend to your nutrition, your bathing and grooming, your sleep needs, and your need for play and relaxation.

Now make a list of things you have to do, and prepare to assign tasks from this list to the empty spaces in your days. Decide how urgent each one is ("This I can postpone; this I have to do today"). Enter the most urgent items into today's schedule, carry it with you, and check off each item when you have completed it. At the end of the day, return uncompleted tasks to the list of things to do.

To schedule a long-term assignment, such as a term paper, first identify every task you must do to complete the project. Then, working backward from the due date, schedule the tasks. For example, if it will take you six hours to type the paper, schedule those six hours on a grid that you have started for the due-date week. Back up and schedule time before that to write the final draft, and allot time still earlier for the research and first

FIGURE 4–5 ■ **Time management.**

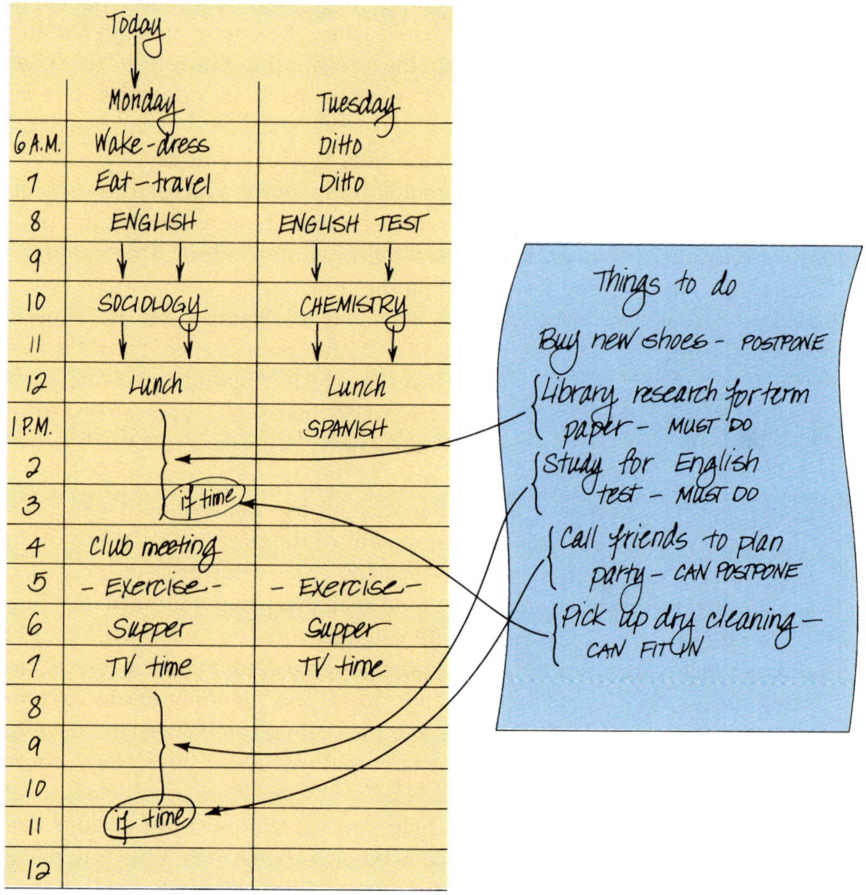

drafts. If you have been realistic about the time each step will take, you will not be caught short at the end.

A part of wise time management is knowing your limits so you don't take on more tasks than you can handle. If you spread yourself too thin, you may have difficulty giving any of your activities the concentration and energy they require.

After identifying your limits, maintain them. For some people, staying within their limits requires learning assertiveness so that they can say no when others ask for their involvement in projects and activities. (Assertiveness was covered in Chapter 2.)

Another stress management strategy is to monitor your body sensitively. Too many people believe they have to wait until they are suffering before they take steps to reduce their stress. That's not true. At each step along the way, you can monitor your body for the early warning signals of too much stress. If you are alert to their appearance, you can initiate preventive action before exhaustion sets in and does damage. Cold hands and feet are among the first signs; Table 4–3 itemizes others. When you see these signs, seek relief; don't let the situation get worse.

TABLE 4–3 ■ **Signs of Stress**

Physical Signs	Psychological Signs
Pounding of the heart; rapid heart rate.	Irritability, tension, or depression.
Rapid, shallow breathing.	Impulsive behavior and emotional instability; the overpowering urge to cry or to run and hide.
Dryness of the throat and mouth.	Lowered self-esteem; thoughts related to failure.
Raised body temperature.	Excessive worry; insecurity; concern about other people's opinions; self-deprecation in conversation.
Decreased sexual appetite or activity.	Reduced ability to communicate with others.
Feelings of weakness, light-headedness, dizziness, or faintness.	Increased awkwardness in social situations.
Trembling; nervous tics; twitches; shaking hands and fingers.	Excessive boredom; unexplained dissatisfaction with job or other normal conditions.
Tendency to be easily startled (by small sounds and the like).	Increased procrastination.
High-pitched, nervous laughter.	Feelings of isolation.
Stuttering and other speech difficulties.	Avoidance of specific situations or activities.
Insomnia—that is, difficulty in getting to sleep, or a tendency to wake up during the night.	Irrational fears (phobias) about specific things.
Grinding of the teeth during sleep.	Irrational thoughts; forgetting things more often than usual; mental "blocks"; missing of planned events.
Restlessness, an inability to keep still.	Guilt about neglecting family or friends; inner confusion about duties and roles.
Sweating (not necessarily noticeably); clammy hands; cold hands and feet; cold chills.	Excessive work; omission of play.
Blushing; hot face.	Unresponsiveness and preoccupation.
The need to urinate frequently.	Inability to organize oneself; tendency to get distraught over minor matters.
Diarrhea; indigestion; upset stomach, nausea.	Inability to reach decisions; erratic, unpredictable judgment making.
Migraine or other headaches; frequent unexplained earaches or toothaches.	Decreased ability to perform different tasks.
Premenstrual tension or missed menstrual periods.	Inability to concentrate.
More body aches and pains than usual, such as pain in the neck or lower back; or any localized muscle tension.	General ("floating") anxiety; feelings of unreality.
Loss of appetite; unintended weight loss; excessive appetite; sudden weight gain.	A tendency to become fatigued; loss of energy; loss of spontaneous joy.
Sudden change in appearance.	Nightmares.
Increased use of substances (tobacco, legally prescribed drugs such as tranquilizers or amphetamines, alcohol, other drugs).	Feelings of powerlessness; mistrust of others.
Accident proneness.	Neurotic behavior; psychosis.
Frequent illnesses.	

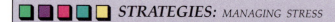

STRATEGIES: *MANAGING STRESS*

To manage stress:

1. During ordinary times, maintain a program of strong personal wellness.
2. Be sure to include regular physical activity.
3. Develop high self-esteem.
4. Maintain a positive attitude toward stressors—view them as opportunities for growth.
5. Manage time wisely.
6. Take on tasks within your limits.
7. Practice assertiveness to maintain your limits.
8. Monitor your body for the early warning signs of too much stress.
9. Release tension by crying, laughing, talking with friends, or willing yourself to relax.
10. When stress begins to intensify, identify which stressors you can control. Put the others out of your mind. Prioritize and take action by focusing your attention on immediate tasks.
11. If stress becomes unmanageable, seek outside help.

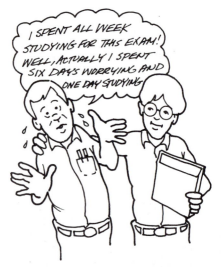

It only slows you down to worry about things you have to do.

Sometimes stress becomes really severe, in spite of all your efforts. Then even small details become overwhelming. Example: a student who is breaking up with his girlfriend, moving out of his home, and changing schools all at the same time is trying to get his belongings packed. He picks up a paper clip and can't decide what packing box to put it in. He starts to sob; he can't cope.

There's nothing wrong with crying at such a time; it is a form of ventilation, and it will help to relieve tension. Once relaxed, though, our student still has a problem to solve. He needs to ask himself which elements of the situation he can control, and pay strict attention only to those. The breakup, the move, and the change of schools are beyond his control right now. The packing is not. He can go on with it, or stop. He may need to take a break—for food, sleep, exercise, or willed relaxation (see later section). He may need to tap a friendship—to get help moving boxes or just to talk to someone. If his friend can help him laugh, so much the better, for laughter works as crying does, to relieve tension. And being able to talk to close friends about personal matters helps people manage stress.

If you find yourself chronically unable to function because stress is so overwhelming, it may be time to seek outside help. (Chapter 3 provided information about getting help.) The Strategies above sum up this section's pointers on stress management.

≡▶ *Learning and practicing stress management strategies can improve your life and your wellness.*

■≡ Willed Relaxation

relaxation response the opposite of the stress response; the normal state of the body.

The exact opposite of the stress response is the **relaxation response**. This response reduces blood pressure, slows the pulse, quells anxiety, and releases tension (see Table 4–4). Relaxation permits your body to recover from

---

TABLE 4–4 ■ The Stress Response and the Relaxation Response

Stress Response	Relaxation Response
Rapid metabolism	Normal metabolism
Fast heart rate	Normal heart rate
Raised blood pressure	Normal blood pressure
Rapid respiration	Normal respiration
Muscles tense	Muscles relaxed
Blood supply to digestive organs and skin diverted to muscles	Normal blood circulation restored
Water retained in body	Normal water balance restored
Immune resistance lowered	Immune resistance restored

---

the effects of stress, and you can will it to happen, even in the midst of a stressful situation.[5]

You can relax anywhere, any time. You can simply tune into a tranquilizing thought or word, and relax. For most people, though, relaxation is first learned through a formal exercise, as described here.

Willed relaxation always has these components: a comfortable position, a noninvasive (noninterrupting) environment, and a passive attitude toward intervening thoughts. The following paragraphs describe various methods of achieving this response.

"Relax!" When someone tells you this, can you do it? How do you know when you've succeeded? Many clinics use a **biofeedback** technique to teach people how to monitor their own physical condition. One such technique uses a machine (the electromyograph, or EMG) that can measure muscle tension. Harmless electronic sensors are fastened to the forehead, neck, jaw, or anywhere muscles may be tense. A tone tells the person when the muscle tension changes, by changing pitch. The pitch drops lower and lower as the person relaxes, and so the person learns what to do to become fully relaxed.

biofeedback a clinical technique used to help a person learn to relax by reflecting muscle tension, heart rate, brainwave activity, or other body activities.

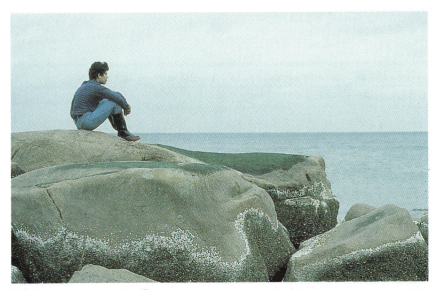

Relaxation can occur naturally . . .

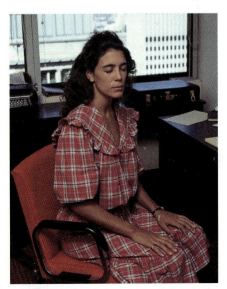

. . . but you can also learn to relax at will.

Another biofeedback tool, the pulse monitor, can make the heartbeat audible, so that the person can learn how to slow it down, thus achieving the same thing—relaxation. Still another biofeedback machine (an electroencephalograph, or EEG) can be used to monitor brainwave activity. The EEG is wired to pads attached painlessly to the outside of the head. It displays patterns that reflect the person's brainwaves on a monitor. By watching the monitor, the person can note which brainwaves are associated with tension and which with relaxation. The person feels different sensations occurring along with these brain states, and can learn to bring on the states voluntarily.

A way to achieve the same result without machines is **progressive muscle relaxation**. The technique involves lying flat and relaxing the muscles all over the body, beginning with the toes. The goal is to locate and erase tension wherever it is occurring in the body. People who have never tried this are astonished to discover the number of different muscles involved in creating tension, especially in the belly, the upper back and neck, and the face. Fifteen different sets of muscles in the face alone can become tense—those involved in smiling, in squinting the eyes, in frowning, in operating the jaw—and each of these must relax. Some people learn that the only thing preventing them from relaxing is that the tongue is held too tightly against the roof of the mouth; others find that they clench their jaws; others, that they are squinting their eyes in a forced smile.

With practice, you can learn to relax your muscles whenever you think of it—not only when you have time to keep still for 30 minutes. Professional mountain climbers train themselves to do it while climbing—the so-called mountain rest step. Any time you take a step, you have to tense one leg—but why tense the other one? At each step, relax the unused leg and let the tension go. That way, you're resting throughout the climb, and you don't have to be exhausted when you get to the top. Students don't have physical mountains to climb, but they do have intellectual ones. If your shoulders (for example) are tense while you are reading, what good does that do you? Relax them.

The benefits of systematic relaxation are so great that many cultures have developed forms of discipline to promote it. One such discipline is **meditation**. Meditation usually involves sitting erect, closing the eyes, breathing deeply, and relaxing the muscles. Table 4–5 presents one sum-

■ *FACT OR FICTION:* Machines can help you learn to relax. *True.*

progressive muscle relaxation a technique of learning to relax by focusing on, and relaxing, each of the body's muscle groups in turn.

meditation a method of relaxing that involves closing the eyes, breathing deeply, and relaxing the muscles.

TABLE 4–5 ■ **Steps to Relaxation**

To relax at will:

1. Assume a comfortable sitting position.
2. When you are ready, close your eyes.
3. Become aware of your breathing. Breathe in deeply, hold it, then breathe out. Each time you breathe out, say the word *one* silently to yourself.
4. Allow each of your muscles to relax deeply, one after another. Imagine that you are floating, drifting, or gliding.
5. Maintain a passive attitude and permit relaxation to occur at its own pace. (Any way that you are proceeding is correct.) Thoughts will pass through your mind; allow them to come and go without resistance.
6. Continue for 20 minutes. You may open your eyes to check the time, but do not use an alarm. When you finish, sit quietly for several minutes, and open your eyes when you are ready.

mary of the steps that might be used, although many variations are possible, and a complete set of instructions would provide many more details. If you practice meditation as described here once or twice daily, after a while, the relaxation response will come with little effort. Practicing it before meals is better than after, since the digestive processes seem to interfere with the response.

To practice relaxation at intervals is to assume control of the body's responses, and it offers a benefit beyond the simple pleasure it brings. Just as stress leads to disease, stress management helps prevent it.

≡▶ *People who learn to will themselves to relax can enjoy the benefits of the relaxation response regardless of their circumstances and surroundings.*

The joy of life is in meeting its challenges, developing new ways of dealing with them, and engaging in experiences that will facilitate new learning. The next chapter explains how to obtain adequate nutrition to enhance physical health and well-being.

■≡ For Review

1. Define stress.
2. Distinguish between eustress and distress.
3. Show how the nervous and hormonal systems regulate the body's functioning during times of stress and between those times.

4. Describe the harmful side effects of prolonged stress on the body's systems.
5. Describe an effective time management strategy.
6. Enumerate some of the physical

and psychological signs of stress.
7. Summarize stress management strategies.
8. Describe the relaxation response and several different means of achieving it.

■≡ Notes

1. The story of Dr. Selye's research into the nature of stress is told in (among others) H. Selye, *The Stress of Life* (New York: McGraw-Hill, 1956; rev. ed. 1976).
2. S. A. Ramsey, J. S. Greenberg, and S. F. Hale, Evaluation of a self-instructional program in stress management for college students,

Health Education, February/March 1989, pp. 8–13.
3. J. S. Greenberg, A study of stressors in the college student population, *Health Education* 12 (1981): 8–12.
4. G. E. Richardson, S. Beall, and G. T. Jessup, The efficacy of a three week stress management unit for high

school students, *Health Education* 14 (1983): 12–15; R. G. LaCivita, Stress-management programming and the college student: A report, *Journal of American College Health* 30 (1982): 237–239.
5. H. Benson, *The Relaxation Response* (New York: Morrow, 1975).

SPOTLIGHT

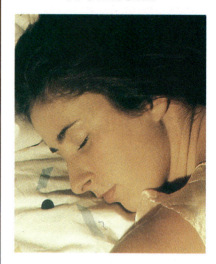

Sleep and Dreams

As mentioned in the chapter, part of managing stress is getting enough sleep. Sleep is indispensable to health. During sleep, people recover from physical and emotional stresses and injuries; they also dream. Chapter 1 cited statistics showing that people who regularly slept about eight hours a night were physiologically younger than people who did not. This Spotlight explores the importance of sleep and dreams and reveals what is known about their effects on health.

I've always wondered what goes on during sleep. What exactly does sleep do for me?

Oddly enough, this is the one question that may be the hardest to answer about sleep. Even though people spend a third of their lives sleeping, no one seems to know for sure what goes on during all that time. However, we do know some of the things that happen physiologically: the blood pressure falls, breathing and heartbeat slow down, the muscles relax, and the body temperature falls. Perhaps most significantly, a hormone known as growth hormone is secreted during sleep almost exclusively—and growth hormone provides for growth and regeneration of body cells. It is probably growth hormone that accounts for the physical renewal that sleep brings.

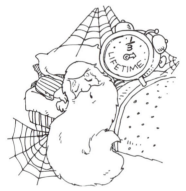

People spend a third of their lifetimes sleeping.

What happens to a person who doesn't get enough sleep?

All body systems work less efficiently. People become irritable, can't concentrate, think slowly, and lose coordination. If deprived of sleep long enough, people may start feeling confused, having hallucinations, or even feeling that they are going insane—a finding used to torture people under oppressive regimes. Irregular sleep or chronic sleep deprivation over years can shorten life. Other problems with too little sleep include fatigue, reduced productivity, and increased risks of heart disease and digestive disorders.[1]* Drivers who fall asleep at the wheel cause 6,000 auto-related deaths a years.[2] Even without having accidents, people have died from getting too little sleep.[3]

Does everybody need eight hours of sleep a night?

People's sleep needs vary. About 2 percent of adults habitually sleep 10 hours a night, and some even more. Most adults need about 6 to 7 hours.

Is there such a thing as beauty sleep? I've heard that an hour of sleep before midnight is worth two afterward.

There's nothing special about the hour of midnight, but it is true that early hours of sleep are "deeper" and more beneficial (more efficient, you might say) than others. You cycle repeatedly through several stages during sleep. Some of these stages seem to be essential to a person's well-being. People deprived of sleep become hostile, irritable, and anxious, or depressed and apathetic. When uninterrupted sleep is again possible, people will experience longer periods of the type of sleep they've missed, to "make up" for it. This is one reason why sleeping pills may actually harm people; many of them suppress important phases of sleep.[4]

What is the function of dreams?

There have been many theories, but the emerging view seems to be that dreams are "the royal road to the unconscious mind."[5] Researchers who earlier dismissed dreaming as irrelevant or random have revised their

*Reference notes are at the end of the Spotlight.

views and now acknowledge the deep psychological significance of dreams. Some have thought that people dreamed to forget—that is, to discharge images and impressions for which they had no further use. But these researchers have revised their theory; they now ascribe considerable importance to dream narratives.

As for the symbols in human dreams, which many people think are "weird," many have universal meaning and appear in all people's dreams—father figures, the cross (symbol of wholeness), the fish (symbol of self), and the like. The appearance of these symbols in our dreams may seem bizarre occasionally, but this does not make the dreams trivial.

Should I try to remember my dreams?

Some people who do, and who learn to interpret them, say their dreams provide profound insights that help them to guide their lives.[6] But dreams will work for you anyway; they help people integrate their experiences in a useful fashion even if they don't become aware of them.[7]

I often have difficulty sleeping. Are you saying that I shouldn't take sleeping pills?

Millions of people in the United States have difficulty sleeping (insomnia) and spend tens of millions of dollars on medications to relieve it.[8] But drugs may actually cause more sleeping problems than they solve, since they create a dependence in the user, as well as interfering with normal sleep patterns. The combination can leave a person exhausted and hooked, afraid to stop taking the pills and sleeping poorly because of

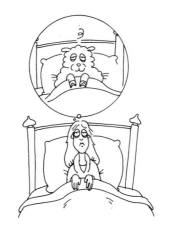

Millions of people suffer from insomnia.

them. A lot of sleep aids are quack devices, too: watch out for them.

I hate being tired. What should I do?

Investigate, perhaps with your health care provider's help, the possible causes of your insomnia. Most common is pain or discomfort. A simple change of position or bedding may be enough to remedy that. Another common cause is anxiety, including anxiety over your sleeplessness. In such cases, you need to deal with your problems (as discussed in Chapters 2 and 3).

A change of surroundings may also affect your ability to sleep. You hear strange noises in a new place, and you don't feel completely secure at first. But these problems should pass quickly—one way to help is to make your environment safe (install safe locks). A change in schedule may also affect your sleep cycle. Most stressful is a constantly changing schedule, such as shift work. The need for repeated readjustment to rotating shifts deprives workers of many hours of sleep after each changeover.

If you can't find the cause of your

insomnia, try using the relaxation exercises described at the end of the chapter. Make sure you can move easily and are not too hot or too cold. If small noises nearby are bothering you, mask them with some "white noise"—a fan, an air conditioner, or a radio or TV tuned to produce a continuous fuzzy sound (not words that might keep you interested). And of course, make sure you don't drink too much coffee, tea, or cola late in the day, because caffeine can interfere with your night's sleep (the Spotlight following Chapter 8 is devoted to caffeine).

Smoking cigarettes, especially in the evening, will probably keep you awake, because nicotine is a stimulant. People who quit smoking say living a smoke-free life helps them sleep better.[9]

Check your daytime schedule for exercise, too. Exercise promotes relaxation, and regular exercise promotes regular sleep. If possible, exercise early in the day, not just before bedtime, because it takes a while to calm down after exercising. Exercising outdoors may be beneficial; it is recommended to get exposure to the natural light each day.

Develop a bedtime ritual.[10] Some activities will make you sleepy. About an hour before bedtime, begin clearing your mind; set worries aside. Read a boring book. Listen to quiet music. Have a light snack. Take a warm bath. Count backward slowly from 1,000 to 0 (don't try to stay awake until you finish). One therapist tells clients with insomnia, "Promise that if you awaken tonight, you will do a job you hate (example: clean the oven)." He finds that they unconsciously "choose" to stay asleep rather than face the unpleasant task.

Finally, sleep clinics that employ hypnosis and other techniques can help. Inquire about their credibility, though; like all such services, some are rip-offs and some are real. You can write for evaluations of such services.*

Once you're sleeping successfully, stay on the schedule that works best for you. Go to sleep and get up at the same times each day—regularity facilitates easy sleeping.[11]

*Write to the American Sleep Disorders Association, 604 Second St., S.W., Rochester, MN 44902.

What do you think of the "nightcap" idea—an alcoholic beverage at bedtime?

Nightcaps can cause dangerous sleep abnormalities. Researchers studied 20 young men of normal sleeping habits and found that after drinking a single nightcap of vodka and orange juice, 18 of the 20 experienced "abnormal respiratory events"—stoppage of breathing for long periods, followed by gasping without waking up.[12] Alcohol and many drugs cause nightmares, and their withdrawal causes nightmares, too.

Is it OK to sleep during the day?

Some. Whatever pattern keeps you refreshed and vigorous is fine. Some people choose to work at night, and they find that an afternoon nap can allow them that privilege. Winston Churchill wrote that napping was essential for anyone who wanted to get the last scrap of energy out of the human structure. Many people famous for their personal energy have made similar statements. Some people passively accept sleep whenever it comes, but others take charge of their sleep and use it to great advantage.

■≡ Spotlight Notes

1. Creatures of the light, *University of California, Berkeley, Wellness Letter,* February 1991, p. 7.
2. Sleep: A little extra can boost alertness, improve mood, *University of Texas Lifetime Health Letter,* December 1990, pp. 3–6.
3. E. Weck, Why aren't you asleep yet? A bedtime story, *FDA Consumer,* October 1989, pp. 13–15.
4. When you can't sleep, *Consumer Reports Health Letter,* July 1990, p. 49.

5. J. Winson, The meaning of dreams, *Scientific American,* November 1990, pp. 86–96.
6. G. M. V. Delaney, *Living Your Dreams* (San Francisco: Harper and Row, 1979).
7. Winson, 1990.
8. J. C. Gillin, The long and short of sleeping pills, *New England Journal of Medicine* 324 (1991): 1735–1737.
9. Eight hours a night and other myths, *University of California,*

Berkeley, Wellness Letter, April 1989, pp. 4–5.
10. Sleep: A little extra can boost alertness, 1990.
11. P. Goldberg and D. Kaufman, *Everybody's Guide to Natural Sleep* (New York: St. Martin's, 1990), pp. 151–153.
12. P. Gunby, A drink a night keeps good slumber at bay (Medical News), *Journal of the American Medical Association* 246 (1981): 589.

CHAPTER 5

Nutrition

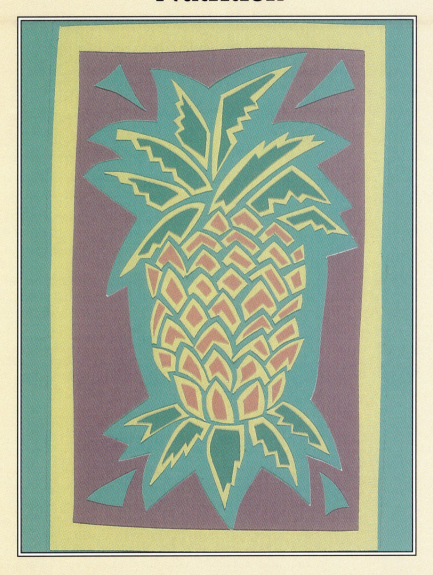

Just for fun, respond true or false to the following statements. If false, say what is true.

■ You can rely on your appetite to tell you when you are hungry. (Page 101)

■ Too much protein can make you fat. (Page 103)

■ It is virtually impossible to eat a diet too high in fiber. (Page 106)

■ Honey and sugar are the same, as far as the body is concerned. (Page 108)

■ Of all the things in foods that cause diseases, sugar is probably the biggest culprit. (Page 112)

■ The more vitamins you consume, the better it is for your health. (Page 115)

■ Fast foods can be nutritious. (Page 125)

Y ou choose to eat a meal about 1,000 times a year. Eating is so habitual that people hardly give it any thought, yet it is a voluntary activity. You choose when to eat, what to eat, and how much to eat—70,000 times in a lifetime.

Each day's intakes of nutrients may affect body organs and their functions only slightly, but over years and decades the effects of those intakes are cumulative. Chapter 1 said that your lifestyle choices can add years to, or subtract years from, your physiological age, and your nutrition choices are among the most influential in this regard.[1]* By age 65, or even earlier, your choices will have affected your physiological age for better or worse by 15 to 30 years.[2] Sound nutrition cannot alone ensure a long and healthy life, but it weighs things in your favor.

■≡ Benefits of Nutrition

Your body renews its structures continuously: each day it replaces some old muscle, bone, skin, and blood with new tissues. In this way some of the food you eat today becomes part of your body tomorrow. The best food for you, then, is the kind that supports today's growth and maintenance of strong muscles, sound bones, healthy skin, and sufficient blood to cleanse and nourish all parts of your body.

Further, the best food minimizes your risks of developing ill health, for your food choices weave together with other choices in a pattern that raises or lowers your chances of contracting diseases later. Obesity, a topic of the next chapter, can result from overeating, and is a pivotal condition that compounds the risks of developing many other diseases. The choice to eat high-fat foods not only renders obesity likely but also increases risks of contracting cancer, high blood pressure, diabetes, heart disease, and chronic intestinal disorders.

In short, good nutrition both promotes health and helps prevent disease. But to manage your nutrition in your own best interest, you have to learn

*Reference notes are at the end of the chapter.

what foods to eat, for not all foods are equally nutritious. Some people, especially those with low incomes, do not obtain sufficient nutrients from their foods. Pregnant women are especially vulnerable to nutrient deficiencies, and deficiencies can retard the growth of developing infants, both before and after birth. Among migratory workers and certain rural populations, more than 1 in every 10 children suffers stunted growth caused by a poor diet.[3] Iron deficiencies affect one to five percent of people severely enough to cause the deficiency symptom of anemia. These are forms of **undernutrition.**

At the same time, **overnutrition** also threatens people's health. About 30 percent of men and 40 percent of women are overweight.[4] Many people's average daily intakes of salt, fat, cholesterol, and alcohol are too high for the health of their hearts. Others eat too few vegetables and too much meat, choices linked to high incidences of several degenerative diseases.[5] Even vitamins and minerals can be toxic if they are consumed in excess. Table 5–1 summarizes some guidelines presented to the U.S. population intended to promote health and help prevent disease. Most nations have similar sets of recommendations.

≡▶ *Good nutrition promotes health and helps prevent diseases. Both undernutrition and overnutrition threaten health.*

■≡ Food Choices

Because your accumulated food choices profoundly influence your health, it is worth questioning why you eat when you do, why you choose the foods you do—and, most importantly, whether they supply the nutrients you need.

To the question of what prompts you to eat, you may reply that it is **hunger.** That is often true, but hunger, the physiological need for food, is not the only stimulus that triggers eating behavior. Another cue is **appetite,** the psychological desire for food, which may arise in response to the sight, smell, or thought of food even when you do not need to eat. You may have an appetite when you are not hungry—or the reverse. Hunger, appetite, obesity, and underweight are the subjects of the next chapter.

As for the question of why you choose the particular foods you do, several answers come to mind:

■ Personal preference (you like them).
■ Habit or ethnic tradition (they are familiar; you always eat them).
■ Social pressure (they are offered; you feel you can't refuse).
■ Availability (they are there and ready to eat).
■ Convenience (you are too rushed to prepare anything else).
■ Economy (you can afford them).
■ Emotional needs (foods can make you feel better for a while).
■ Values or beliefs (they fit your religious tradition, square with your political views, or honor the environmental ethic).
■ Nutritional value (you think they are good for you).

All but one of these reasons are psychological and social reasons; only the last one reflects that you are conscious of nutrition's importance to your wellness. But this is not to say that your other reasons for choosing foods are

undernutrition   underconsumption of food energy or nutrients severe enough to cause disease or increased susceptibility to disease; a form of malnutrition.

overnutrition   overconsumption of food energy or nutrients sufficient to cause disease or susceptibility to disease; a form of malnutrition.

Chapters 18 and 19 provide more details of the links between food and diseases.

hunger   the physiological need to eat; a negative, unpleasant sensation.

appetite   the psychological desire to eat, which normally accompanies hunger; by itself a pleasant sensation.

■ *FACT OR FICTION:* You can rely on your appetite to tell you when you are hungry. *False.* You may have an appetite when you are not hungry.

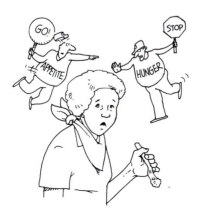

You may have an appetite when you are not hungry—or the reverse.

TABLE 5-1 ■ **Dietary Guidelines for Americans/Nutrition and Your Health**

---

1. *Eat a variety of foods daily.* Include these foods every day: fruits and vegetables; whole-grain and enriched breads, cereals, and other products made from grains; milk and milk products; meats, fish, poultry, and eggs; and dried peas and beans.

2. *Maintain healthy weight.* To increase calorie expenditures, increase physical activity. To decrease calorie intake, control overeating by eating slowly, taking smaller portions, and avoiding second helpings; eat fewer fatty foods and sweets and less sugar, drink fewer alcoholic beverages, and eat more foods that are low in calories and high in nutrients.

3. *Choose a diet low in fat, saturated fat, and cholesterol.* Choose low-fat protein sources such as lean meats, fish, poultry, and dry peas and beans; use eggs and organ meats in moderation; limit intake of fats on and in foods; trim fats from meats; broil, bake, or boil—don't fry; limit breaded and deep-fried foods; read food labels for fat contents.

4. *Choose a diet with plenty of vegetables, fruits, and grain products.* Substitute starchy foods for foods high in fats and sugars; select whole-grain breads and cereals, fruits and vegetables, and dried beans and peas, to increase fiber and starch intake.

5. *Use sugars only in moderation.* Use less sugar, syrup, and honey; reduce intakes of concentrated sweets like candy, soft drinks, cookies, and the like; select fresh fruit or fruits canned in light syrup or their own juices; read food labels—sucrose, glucose, dextrose, maltose, lactose, fructose, syrups, and honey are all sugars; eat sugar less often to reduce dental caries.

6. *Use salt and sodium only in moderation.* Learn to enjoy the flavors of unsalted foods; flavor foods with herbs, spices, and lemon juice; reduce salt in cooking; add little or no salt at the table; limit salty foods like potato chips, pretzels, salted nuts, popcorn, condiments (soy sauce, steak sauce, and garlic salt), some cheese, pickled foods and cured meats, and some canned vegetables and soups; read food labels for sodium or salt contents, especially in processed and snack foods; use lower-sodium products when available.

7. *If you drink alcoholic beverages, do so in moderation.* For individuals who drink, limit all alcoholic beverages (including wine, beer, liquors, and so on) to one (for women) or two (for men) drinks per day. "One drink" means 12 oz of beer, 3 oz of wine, or 1½ oz of distilled spirits.[a] People who should *not* drink alcohol include pregnant women,[b] those who must drive, those taking medication, those who have trouble limiting alcohol intakes,[c] and children and adolescents.

---

[a]For an expanded discussion of what constitutes "a drink," see Chapter 10.
[b]For a discussion of the risks of drinking during pregnancy, see Chapter 14.
[c]For discussions of driving and alcohol, as well as of alcohol addiction, see Chapter 10.
SOURCE: U.S. Department of Agriculture, U.S. Department of Health and Human Services, *Nutrition and Your Health: Dietary Guidelines for Americans*, 3d ed. (Washington, D.C.: Government Printing Office, 1990).

■ MINIGLOSSARY
of Nutrient Terms

---

nutrients   substances obtained from food and used in the body to promote growth, maintenance, and repair. The *essential nutrients* are those the body cannot make for itself in sufficient quantity to meet physiological need, and which, therefore, must be obtained from food.

carbohydrates   nutrients, most of which yield energy the human body can use. The *complex carbohydrates* include starch (energy-yielding) and some fibers (primarily not energy-yielding); the *simple carbohydrates* are the sugars.

fats (technically, lipids)   energy-yielding nutrients that include fats and oils, cholesterol, and other compounds.

protein   a type of nutrient that can serve as working parts of cells, or can yield energy.

vitamins   essential nutrients synthesized by living things, required in minute amounts to help do the body's work (not energy-yielding).

minerals   the earth's basic elements, some of which are essential nutrients required in small amounts to help do the body's work (not energy-yielding).

water   a substance necessary for life that provides a medium for, participates in, and results as a waste product from, life processes.

fiber   indigestible carbohydrates and other compounds in food that provide bulk in the digestive tract.

---

invalid or will necessarily damage your health. After all, food nourishes not only the body but the mind and spirit, too. Still, when you learn about nutrition, you are in a position to design a diet that meets your body's needs while honoring your preferences, social values, and other individual needs.

≡▶ *People eat in response to hunger or appetite. The choice of which food to eat is influenced by preference, economy, and many other factors.*

Foods, Nutrients, and Fiber

Food supplies **nutrients, fiber,** and other materials. The nutrients fall into six classes: the **carbohydrates,** the **fats, protein, vitamins, minerals,** and **water** (see accompanying Miniglossary of Nutrient Terms). Fibers are mostly carbohydrates and are discussed in their section of this chapter.

Three classes of nutrients provide **energy** the body can use: carbohydrate, fat, and protein. The body uses energy from these nutrients to do its work and to generate heat. Carbohydrate supplies the body with one of its two major fuels, the sugar **glucose;** the brain and nervous system can normally use only this fuel as their energy source. Fat supplies the body's other major fuel, **fatty acids;** the muscles, including the heart muscle, rely heavily on this fuel. Protein is the major structural and working material of cells, but it, too, can be broken down (to **amino acids**) and used for energy to some extent. In adverse conditions such as undernutrition or severe stress, body protein may become a major fuel.

The units used to measure energy are **calories,** familiar to everyone as a reflection of how "fattening" a food is. (Indeed, both protein and carbohydrate as well as fat, if taken in excess of need, are converted to body fat and stored, so the calorie count of a food does reflect its fattening power.) One other compound people ingest provides energy: the alcohol of alcoholic beverages. Alcohol is not a nutrient, because it does not promote growth, maintenance, or repair of the body; but it has to be counted as an energy source.

An important point is apparent here. People tend to think of carbohydrate as "fattening," but this reputation is undeserved. Peddlers of dangerous low-carbohydrate diets would like you to believe that carbohydrate causes weight gain, but carbohydrate is not especially fattening. On the other hand, protein is thought of as promoting thinness, but excess protein loads you down with calories that are stored as fat. Also, protein often goes hand in hand with large amounts of fat in foods; for example, meats and cheeses are high in both protein and fat, so they are high in calories. Carbohydrate, on the other hand, rarely comes packaged by nature with large amounts of fat. Gram for gram, the calories in fat are more than double those of carbohydrate or protein; thus any food that provides much fat provides calories in abundance.

The other nutrients, vitamins and minerals, do not provide energy themselves, but help both to regulate energy's release and to mediate other body activities. As for water, it is the medium in which all of the body's processes take place. Probably about 60 percent of your body's weight is water, which transports materials to and from cells, and provides the environment in which these cells live. When fuel nutrients break down to release energy, they break down to water and other simple compounds. Since you lose water from your body daily, you must replace it daily. To this end, adults need to drink about eight glasses of fluid a day. Second only to oxygen, water is the most vital nutrient; you can live only a few days without it.

Nutrients fall into six classes. Among these, carbohydrates, fats, and protein yield energy the body can use. Vitamins and minerals assist the body in energy release and regulate its functions. Water provides the medium in which all these processes take place.

energy the capacity to do work or produce heat.

glucose one of the body's two major energy fuels; derived from carbohydrate.

fatty acids simple forms of fat that supply energy fuel for most of the body's cells.

amino acids building blocks of protein.

Energy-yielding nutrients:

Carbohydrate—provides energy as glucose.

Lipid—provides energy as fatty acids.

Protein—provides amino acids that can be made into working cell proteins, or that can be transformed into glucose or fatty acids under some conditions.

calories units used to measure energy; determined from the heat food releases when burned. Calories reflect the extent to which a food's energy can be stored in body fat.

■ *FACT OR FICTION:* Too much protein can make you fat. *True.*

Vitamins—play regulatory roles.

Minerals—play regulatory roles.

Water—provides the medium for life processes.

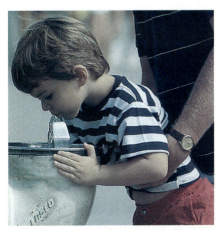

Water is the most vital nutrient of all.

Liver glycogen is for the whole body's use. Muscle glycogen is used within the muscles only. See Chapter 7 and its Spotlight.

hypothalamus (high-po-THALL-uh-mus) a brain regulatory center.

glycogen the form in which the body stores glucose.

balanced meal a meal containing sufficient, but not excessive, amounts of foods from each food group and therefore sufficient, but not excessive, carbohydrate, fat, protein, vitamins, and minerals.

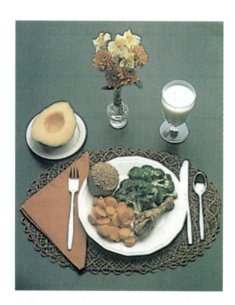

FIGURE 5–1 ■ **A balanced meal.**

This meal supplies foods from every food group, as well as a recommended balance of energy sources: less than 30 percent of its calories are from fat, and about 60 percent are from carbohydrate (the rest are from protein). Note the moderate meat portion and the generous portions of vegetables and fruit. The bread is without butter, and the beverage is nonfat milk. Total calories: about 500.

A mistake people commonly make is to think that if fat should contribute 30 percent of the calories, then it should take up a third of the plate. On the contrary: fat is much more calorie-dense than the other constituents of food, and much of it is invisible. In this 500-calorie meal, the only visible fat is in the chicken skin, and yet fat contributes almost 30 percent of the calories.

Energy from Food

The body derives its energy chiefly from two fuels: glucose and fatty acids. The supply of glucose is temporary, and you must eat to maintain it. The brain's **hypothalamus** sends out a hunger signal when blood glucose gets too low. If you don't eat, the body turns to its four or so hours' worth of liver **glycogen** (a concentrated storage form of glucose in your liver) to generate glucose. And if you still do not eat after most of the liver's glycogen has been used, then lean body tissues including the liver itself and the muscles begin to break down, releasing amino acids. Some amino acids are converted to glucose, and others can be used for fuel in its place. (Amino acids from lean tissue must step in to play the role of glucose, because although the muscles and other organs can use fat as fuel, the brain ordinarily cannot. The brain needs a steady and large glucose supply, which the body's abundant fat cannot supply.) But the wise eater obtains food before incurring tissue protein losses. Why dismantle your house for firewood when the woodpile is nearby?

When you eat, you replenish your fuels. Within seconds when you eat carbohydrate, your blood glucose rises. Your liver and muscle cells store some extra glucose as glycogen, and the fat cells store much more as fat.* Thus your body creates reserve supplies of both fuels to draw on the next time you have to postpone eating.

When you get hungry, what should you eat? The obvious choice might seem to be a candy bar ''for quick energy,'' and it is true that the body can quickly raise its blood glucose from a concentrated sugar source such as candy. The only trouble is that a dose of sugar by itself lasts only a short time; you'll soon be hungry again, and possibly shaky besides. You may remember how cranky and irritable you became as a child when you were hungry; a candy bar seemed to help for a while but may have made you feel worse in the end.

A better choice than pure sugar is a **balanced meal**—that is, a meal that contains several different kinds of food that offer protein, fat, and carbohydrate all together. Here's why a balanced meal is better:

■ The carbohydrate in the meal provides an immediate source of glucose energy.
■ The fat in the meal slows down the digestive system so that the glucose is absorbed gradually. It also provides fatty acids that cells can use for energy.
■ The protein in the meal prompts the body to regulate its use of the glucose, keeping it available in the bloodstream longer.

Figure 5–1 provides an example of a balanced meal, and Figure 5–2 shows how the energy-yielding nutrients are distributed among servings of foods.

The body stores energy nutrients as glycogen or fat. When starved for glucose, the body breaks down its own lean tissues for the raw materials with which to make glucose. The best source of energy for the body is a balanced meal.

_____

*The liver cells convert excess glucose to fat and release it; the fat cells pick it up and store it.

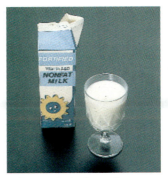

Milk = carbohydrate plus protein (plus vitamins, minerals, and water).

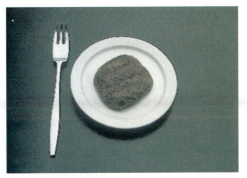

Meat = protein plus fat (plus vitamins, minerals, and water).

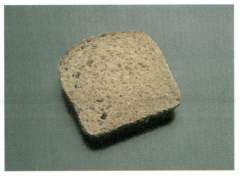

Bread (and starchy vegetables) = carbohydrate (plus protein, vitamins, and minerals).

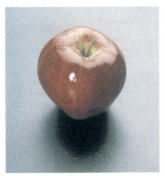

Fruit = carbohydrate (plus vitamins, minerals, and water).

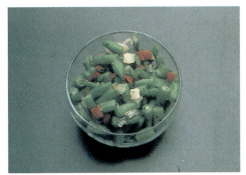

Vegetable (except starchy vegetables) = carbohydrate plus protein (plus vitamins, minerals, and water).

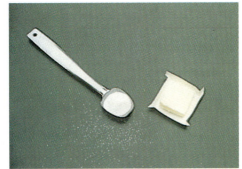

Pure fat = fat only. Pure sugar equals carbohydrate only.

FIGURE 5–2 ■ Foods and the energy-yielding nutrients in them.

Five categories of foods contain vitamins, minerals, and energy. The sixth contains essentially pure energy. These portion sizes are useful for diet planning. The meat portion is moderate (3 ounces) and the vegetable portion, ample (1 cup), consistent with recommended guidelines.

The Carbohydrates

The terms *complex carbohydrate* and *simple carbohydrate* refer to an important distinction among carbohydrates—simply stated, the distinction between starch and fiber versus sugars. Another important distinction among the simple carbohydrates (sugars) is that they come in both natural (dilute) and processed (concentrated) form—simply stated, fruit versus candy.

The complex carbohydrates are composed of long chains of glucose units. (The complex carbohydrate glycogen has already been mentioned as the form in which glucose is stored in the human liver and muscle cells.) **Starch,** the principal complex carbohydrate in grains and vegetables, is the chief energy source for human beings throughout the world and it is highly desirable in the human diet. Starch provides the body with the glucose it needs in a form it uses best. And if the starchy foods you eat are such wholesome foods as whole-grain breads (not refined white bread), potatoes (not potato chips), or whole-grain cereals (not the sugary vitamin-enriched kind) then your body obtains many of the *other* nutrients it needs, along with a steady supply of glucose. Most people would do well to boost their intakes of such starch foods, and the Spotlight that follows Chapter 7 shows how important a diet high in such foods can be to athletic performance.

starch a complex carbohydrate, the predominant food energy source for human beings.

Complex carbohydrates (long chains of glucose):

Glycogen—the body's storage form of glucose.

Starch—people's main food energy source.

Fibers—indigestible carbohydrates.

■ *FACT OR FICTION:* It is virtually impossible to eat a diet too high in fiber. *False.* Too much fiber can be as harmful as too little.

sugars   simple carbohydrates; examples are glucose, fructose, sucrose, and lactose.

The four sugars important in nutrition:

Glucose.

Fructose.

Sucrose.

Lactose.

empty calories   a popular term referring to foods that contribute energy but negligible nutrients.

Other complex carbohydrates in foods—fibers—are mostly indigestible by human beings and so yield no calories, but they help to maintain the health of the digestive tract.

Most fibers in foods move through the digestive tract essentially unchanged. They hold water and so provide bulk inside the intestines, enabling the muscles of the digestive tract walls to push their contents along (see Figure 5–3). Foods high in fibers also make softer stools. The subject may be unglamorous, but it intensely interests anyone who suffers from the consequences of a lack of fiber: constipation (hard, sluggish stools), hemorrhoids (swollen, painful rectal veins that bulge out from straining to pass hard stools), or a host of other intestinal ills.

Because fiber keeps the intestinal contents moving, it helps to prevent infection of the appendix (appendicitis). Additionally, fiber helps to control the blood cholesterol level, a risk factor for heart disease. (Certain fibers bind cholesterol and keep it from being absorbed into the body; it is excreted with the feces instead.) Fiber also helps control the blood glucose concentration and so helps to prevent diabetes. Some fibers bind cancer-causing agents in the digestive tract and keep them from being absorbed or from touching the intestinal walls.

Fiber may also help to prevent obesity. The person who eats fiber-rich foods chews longer and fills up sooner on fewer calories. Consistently, foods that are high in fiber are low in calories and vice versa, so it is hard to eat a diet high in fiber and also gain weight.

Clearly, fiber is beneficial, but is there such a thing as too much fiber? There certainly is. Some years ago, many college students overdid the high-fiber diet, much to their intestinal distress. They suffered diarrhea, prolonged and severe enough to cause dangerous dehydration. More recently, a man hoping to ward off diseases courted disaster instead when he wolfed down a half dozen oat bran muffins. He required emergency surgery to remove a blockage of bran lodged in his intestine. Too much of anything, in nutrition as in all areas of life, is as harmful as too little.

Plant foods—particularly those with their skins and seeds intact—are high in fiber. Fiber breaks down when foods are refined or cooked. Apples have more fiber than applesauce; apple juice has none. Baked potatoes with the skins have more fiber than mashed potatoes; potato chips have almost none. If you want to eat a diet high enough in fiber to benefit your health, choose whole grains, whole fruits, and whole vegetables most of the time. Cook these foods sparingly, and eat some raw.

The simple carbohydrates are the **sugars.** All sugars are chemically similar to glucose and can be converted into glucose in the body. All their names end in *ose*, which makes them easy to recognize as carbohydrates. The four sugars most important in human nutrition are glucose (the body's fuel), fructose (the sweet sugar of fruits, honey, and maple syrup), sucrose (table sugar), and lactose (milk sugar). Simple carbohydrates come mostly from fruits and milk or in concentrated form as sugar, honey, and other sweets.

Nutritionists recommend that you consume abundant quantities of fruits and vegetables that contain sugars, but they urge you in the same breath to "avoid consuming too much sugar." What's the difference?

Part of the answer lies in the phrase **empty calories.** When you eat an apple, you receive about 100 calories from the sugars in it, together with a little vitamin A, a bit of thiamin, some vitamin C, a moderate dose of fiber,

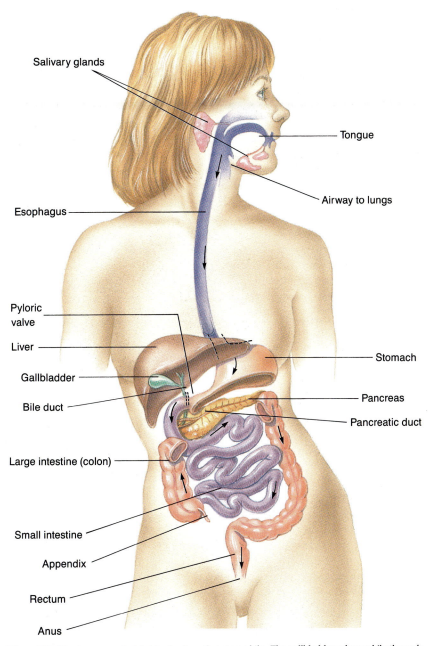

Salivary glands

Tongue

Esophagus

Airway to lungs

Pyloric valve

Liver

Gallbladder

Bile duct

Stomach

Pancreas

Pancreatic duct

Large intestine (colon)

Small intestine

Appendix

Rectum

Anus

FIGURE 5–3 ■ **The digestive system.**

Mouth:
  Chews and mixes food with saliva
  Donates mainly starch-digesting enzymes

Esophagus:
  Passes food to stomach

Stomach:
  Adds acid, enzymes, and fluid
  Churns, mixes, and grinds food to a liquid mass

Small intestine:
  Secretes enzymes that digest all food to small nutrient particles
  Cells of wall absorb nutrients into blood and lymph

Liver:
  Manufactures bile, a detergentlike substance, to help digest fats

Gall bladder[a]
  Stores bile until needed

Bile duct:
  Conducts bile into small intestine

Pancreas:
  Manufactures enzymes to digest food and bicarbonate to neutralize stomach acid

Pancreatic duct:[b]
  Conducts pancreatic juice into small intestine

Large intestine (colon):
  Reabsorbs water and minerals
  Passes undigested waste (fiber, bacteria, and some water) to rectum

Rectum:
  Stores waste prior to elimination

Anus:
  Holds rectum closed
  Opens to allow elimination

[a]The gallbladder is a sac embedded in the liver that stores bile. The gallbladder releases bile through a duct into the small intestine whenever fat is present there.
[b]In some people, the pancreatic duct merges with the bile duct before they open into the small intestine. The common portion is called the *common bile duct.*

a healthy bit of potassium, and several dozen other nutrients. By contrast, a 12-ounce cola beverage gives you about 150 calories from sugar without any nutrients. In fact, it creates a sort of debt, for to avoid overconsuming calories, you now have to derive the nutrients you need in a day from food

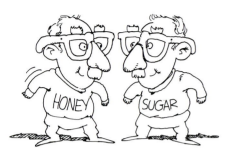

In terms of nutrition, there's no significant difference between honey and sugar.

Snacks dentists recommend:

Milk, cheese, and yogurt (not fruit and flavored yogurts, though, which are as sugary as ice cream).

Fresh fruits (not dried fruits, jams, and jellies).

Vegetables (but not candied or glazed).

Grains (but not granola bars, which are as sticky as candy bars).

CRITICAL THINKING

Honey versus Sugar

Some people believe honey to be the ideal substitute for sugar because, they say, it offers nutrients with its sweetness, rather than just empty calories. True, honey does contain traces of a few vitamins and minerals, but relative to a person's daily need, these nutrients don't add up to much. A tablespoon of honey (65 calories) offers one-tenth of a milligram of iron, for example, but an adult's daily need for iron can be as high as 15 milligrams or more. Consequently, to meet the need for iron, an adult would need 150 tablespoons in a day—almost 10,000 calories of honey! (Most people can eat only 2,000 to 3,000 calories a day without getting fat.) The nutrients in honey just do not add up as fast as the calories do, so honey, like sugar, is a relatively empty-calorie food. Honey is almost identical to sugar chemically, too. And spoon for spoon, sugar contains *fewer* calories than honey, because the sugar crystals take up more space.

containing 150 fewer calories. The same criticism applies to both honey and sugar (see this chapter's Critical Thinking section).

Also, the bacteria that cause dental caries (cavities) thrive on sugar. They can double their numbers when carbohydrate sticks to tooth surfaces for 20 minutes or more at a time—and sugar tends to stick. Caries form when three factors are present: a susceptible tooth, a carbohydrate supply, and bacteria to consume the carbohydrate and produce acid from it that decays the tooth enamel. A few people are born with decay-resistant teeth, but most people need to protect their teeth to prevent decay. Two obvious preventive measures are, first, to avoid exposing the teeth to carbohydrate for long periods; and second, after exposure, to brush and floss them promptly. If you drink a cola beverage, finish it quickly and follow with a vigorous water rinse.

To get around the problems sugars present while still enjoying the pleasures they offer, people often turn to alternative sweeteners. For a view of their pro's and con's, see the accompanying box, Sugar Substitutes.

≡▶ *Complex carbohydrates (starches and fiber) benefit the body in many ways. Simple carbohydrates (sugars) may benefit nutrition when they are dilute, as they occur in fruits, but may be deleterious to nutrition when overconsumed in the form of concentrated sweets.*

The Fats

Nearly all the body's tissues (except the brain and nervous system) can use fat as an energy source. It is the major fuel for muscles, as long as they have enough oxygen to break it down.

Fat is stored in a layer of cells beneath the skin and also in many pads surrounding and underlying vital organs. As well as providing an energy

Sugar Substitutes

People dream of calorie-less doughnuts, calorie-free candy, and ice cream with the calories of skim milk. At the same time, consumers insist that no risks to health must accompany calorie savings. The desire of most people to control body weight while eating as they like pushes many people to use sugar substitutes.

Such people may choose from two sets of substitutes. One set is the sugar alcohols, which are energy-yielding sweeteners (sometimes referred to as *nutritive* sweeteners); the other is the artificial sweeteners, which provide virtually no energy (also referred to as *nonnutritive* sweeteners).

The sugar alcohols are familiar to people who use special dietary products. (Among them are *maltitol, mannitol, sorbitol,* and *xylitol.*) A benefit of sugar alcohols is that ordinary mouth bacteria cannot metabolize them as rapidly as they metabolize sugar, so sugar alcohols do not contribute as much to dental caries. All the sugar alcohols provide as many calories as table sugar (sucrose), though.

The person who wishes to reduce energy intake should be aware that the sugar alcohols *do* provide as much energy per gram as sucrose. In spite of this, products that contain them are labeled "sugar-free." The person who is limiting calorie intake must limit sugar alcohols just as carefully as sugars. For this person, artificial sweeteners may offer a preferable alternative.

Like the sugar alcohols, artificial sweeteners make foods taste sweet without promoting dental decay. Unlike sugar alcohols, they have the added attraction of being calorie-free. The big three synthetic sweeteners are *saccharin, cyclamate,* and *aspartame,* and a fourth that is seeking acceptance is *acesulfame potassium* or *acesulfame K.*

Saccharin is used primarily in soft drinks, and as a tabletop sweetener. Due to questions about its safety, products containing saccharin must carry on their labels the warning that "use of this product may be hazardous to your health. This product contains saccharin, which has been determined to cause cancer in laboratory animals." However, although studies have shown an increase in bladder tumors in animals fed saccharin, these tumors may not have been cancerous. In any case, the risks of saccharin's causing cancer are low compared to other risks.

Cyclamate has had a shorter life than saccharin, dominating the artificial sweetener market for only 20 years. The 1970 ban on its use in the United States, although repeatedly appealed, has been continued, even though, like saccharin, cyclamate has never been conclusively proven guilty of causing cancer in human beings. Both saccharin and cyclamate have been handicapped by another disadvantage, though: they do not taste exactly like sugar.

As for aspartame, within only a few years, it received the approval of the Food and Drug Administration (FDA). Thereafter, it appeared in dozens of food products. Worldwide, people gratefully accepted aspartame as NutraSweet in diet drinks, chewing gum, presweetened cereal, gelatins, and pudding and as Equal, a powder to

(continued on next page)

(continued)
use at home in place of sugar. Aspartame sales have far surpassed the sales of saccharin and are also encroaching on sugar sales in some markets.

This amazing popularity is mostly due to aspartame's flavor, which is almost identical to that of sugar. Another lure drawing people to aspartame is the hope that it may be completely harmless, unlike the other sweeteners, whose laboratory records are tarnished. Furthermore, aspartame is touted as safe for children, so families wishing to limit their children's sugar intakes are turning to it. Aspartame appears to be safe for all people except those with the rare inherited disorder known as phenylketonuria (PKU). Product labels offer a special warning for people with PKU.

Some 500 individual complaints were received after aspartame's approval by the Centers for Disease Control. The researchers investigating these claims concluded that some individuals may exhibit vague but not dangerous symptoms due to unusual sensitivity to aspartame but that the product is generally safe. Aspartame seems to have only one drawback: it breaks down when heated.

The FDA has recently approved the artificial sweetener acesulfame K, which has been used without reported health problems in several other countries. Marketed under the trade name Sunette, this sweetener is about as sweet as aspartame and has been approved for use in chewing gum, beverages, instant coffee and tea, gelatins, and puddings. Unlike aspartame, acesulfame K holds up during cooking, and it is safe for people with PKU. Like its predecessors, however, acesulfame K is being challenged by consumer groups concerned about its safety. Further research and consumer acceptance will determine its place on the grocery shelves.

As a sweet-toothed, overweight population, many people perceive sugar substitutes as the only way to cheat the scales. Current evidence seems to suggest that artificial sweeteners, used in moderation as part of a well-balanced, nutritious diet, pose no health risks. The question remains whether they serve their intended purpose, though. People who use artificial sweeteners may ingest just as many calories as always, but from different foods than they ate before.

SOURCES: L. D. Stegink, The aspartame story: A model for the clinical testing of a food additive, *American Journal of Clinical Nutrition* 46 (1987): 204–215; H. Carlson and J. Shah, Aspartame and its constituent amino acids: Effects on prolactin, cortisol, growth hormone, insulin, and glucose in normal humans, *American Journal of Clinical Nutrition* 49 (1989): 427–432; Position of the American Dietetic Association: Appropriate use of nutritive and non-nutritive sweeteners, *Journal of the American Dietetic Association* 87 (1987): 1689–1690.

reserve, it helps to insulate the body from the cold, from changes in temperature, and from mechanical shock. Whenever you eat, you store some fat, and within a few hours after a meal, you start taking it out of storage and using it for energy until the next meal. Thus both glucose and fat are stored after meals, and both are released later when needed as fuel for the cells' work.

The body has scanty reserves of carbohydrate and not much protein to spare, but it can store fat in practically unlimited amounts. A pound of body fat is worth 3,500 calories, and a person's body can easily carry 30 to 50 pounds of fat without looking fat at all. In fact, a man of normal weight might have about 15 percent, and a woman about 20 percent, of the body weight as fat.

Fat comes in different forms. In foods, most of it comes as fats and oils, and it is stored in the body's fat cells relatively unchanged. The fats you eat come in two forms—**saturated** and **unsaturated** (including **polyunsaturated**). People who are at risk for heart and artery disease are encouraged to reduce their total fat, and especially their saturated fat, intakes. Saturated fats come primarily from animal-derived foods such as meats, butter, and cream. They are identifiable by certain physical characteristics: they are firm at room temperature, they melt at high temperature, and they are not easily broken or changed by oxygen. Unsaturated fats come primarily from vegetable oils, including olive oil, corn oil, and canola oil. They are liquid or soft at room temperature, they melt at low temperature, and they are vulnerable to attack by oxygen.

Another form of fat is **cholesterol.** Some cholesterol is made from other fats in the body, and it is an important material for proper cell functioning. However, in excess it is associated with heart and artery disease. Cholesterol forms a major part of the deposits that accumulate along arteries and increase the risk of heart attacks and strokes. For people trying to lower blood cholesterol, it is *not* effective to limit only cholesterol intake; it is necessary to limit total fat intake, including both saturated fat and cholesterol.

Reducing fat intake offers a fringe benefit to people who wish to cut calories. A spoonful of fat contains more than twice as many calories as a spoonful of sugar or pure protein. By removing the fat from a food, you can drastically reduce the calorie count. Figure 5–4 shows that the single most

saturated pertaining to fatty acids, those with carbon chains filled to capacity with hydrogen atoms.

unsaturated pertaining to fatty acids, those whose carbon chains have hydrogen atoms missing at one or more points.

polyunsaturated fatty acids with hydrogens missing at two or more points along their carbon chains.

cholesterol a type of fat made by the body; and a minor constituent of fat in foods.

Details concerning dietary fats and blood cholesterol are provided in Chapter 18.

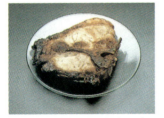

Small pork chop with ½ inch border of fat (25 grams fat) = 275 cal.

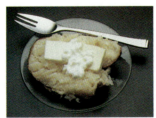

Large potato with 1 tbsp butter and 1 tbsp sour cream (14 grams fat) = 350 cal.

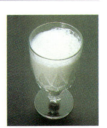

Whole milk, 1 c (8 grams fat) = 150 cal.

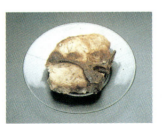

Small pork chop with fat trimmed off (13 grams fat) = 165 cal.

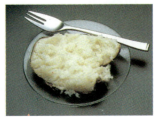

Plain large potato (less than 1 gram fat) = 220 cal.

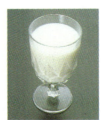

Nonfat milk, 1 c (less than 1 gram fat) = 90 cal.

FIGURE 5–4 ■ Fat and calories.
Fat hides calories in food. When you trim fat, you trim calories.

effective step you can take to reduce the energy value of a food is to eat it with less fat.

Of all the dietary factors related to diseases prevalent in developed countries, high fat intake is by far the most significant. Heart disease and many forms of cancer are linked to a high fat intake; probably many other diseases are, too, including arthritis, gallbladder disease, diabetes, and all diseases aggravated by obesity. The most important dietary steps you can take to prevent these diseases are to control your fat intake and to control your weight.

Because controlling fat intake is so important to everyone's health, food manufacturers have come up with some noncaloric fat substitutes. The accompanying box introduces them.

≡▶ *Fat is the body's major energy fuel and the body stores a generous supply. Food fat comes in saturated and unsaturated forms. Saturated fat and cholesterol in the diet both contribute to cholesterol in the body that damages the heart and arteries.*

Protein

Protein is well known as the body-building nutrient, the material of strong muscles—and rightly so. No new living tissue can be built without it, for protein is part of every cell, every bone, the blood, and every other tissue.

■ *FACT OR FICTION:* Of all the things in foods that cause diseases, sugar is probably the biggest culprit. *False.* Of all the things in foods that cause diseases, fat is by far the biggest culprit.

Fat Substitutes

Heart disease and obesity, two major health problems, are both linked to dietary fat, so artificial fats offer hope for their prevention and treatment. Food chemists have been working on artificial fats since the 1960s, and recently two products have received a great deal of attention. These artificial fats are not the same as granules that mimic the flavors of butter, cheese, or sour cream. Although such flavors have been available for years and they replicate the *taste* of fats, they lack the feeling of richness provided by the fatty foods themselves. Artificial fats are designed to provide the entire experience of eating fat—the creaminess as well as the taste—but without the calories.

One product is a calorie-free fat replacement formerly known as *sucrose polyester (SPE)*, now known by its generic name *olestra*. Olestra is a synthetic combination of sucrose and fatty acids, but unlike either, it is indigestible. Because the body cannot digest it, olestra passes through the digestive tract unabsorbed. An added advantage: its presence in the digestive tract reduces blood cholesterol concentrations by interfering with cholesterol's absorption.

Olestra looks, feels, and tastes like dietary fat, and can substitute for fats and oils in products such as shortenings, oils, margarines, snacks, ice creams, and other desserts. Scientific research on animals and human beings seems to support olestra's safety in general, although it does reduce vitamin E absorption somewhat. One proposed solution to this problem is to supplement olestra products with vitamin E.

The other fat substitute is made from protein, and its trade name is *Simplesse.* The FDA has approved it

Proteins constitute the cells' machinery—they do the cells' work. The energy to fuel that work comes from carbohydrate and fat as they break down.

Among the cells' working parts are a multitude of proteins called **enzymes.** Each enzyme performs a specific chemical reaction in the building or break-down of cellular materials. A single human cell may contain several thousand kinds of enzymes, each promoting a different chemical reaction.

Cells inherit their instructions on how to make proteins. When geneticists talk about hereditary differences among people, they are really talking about differences in the codes people inherit for their proteins, most of which are enzymes. Among proteins that confer individuality on people are the anti-bodies, which confer resistance to disease and facilitate the body's rejection of foreign materials.

Proteins are made of building blocks, the amino acids. A set of 20 distinct amino acids form proteins (much as letters form sentences), but your body can make only 11 of them. The nine amino acids the body cannot make are the **essential amino acids,** which you obtain from food.

Your body loses protein every day. Digestive tract cells wear out and are excreted in the feces. Skin cells flake off or are rubbed off. Hair and nails (made of protein) grow longer daily and are shed or cut away. An adult loses about 1/4 cup of pure protein a day. People need to eat protein-containing foods every day to replace the protein they lose.

enzymes proteins that facilitate chemical reactions without being changed, them-selves, in the process.

essential amino acids a group of nine amino acids that cannot be made by the body and thus must be obtained in food.

for use in certain products, such as frozen desserts, mayonnaise, and salad dressings. Simplesse is fabri-cated in a process that heats and blends proteins from egg whites or milk into tiny round particles which the tongue perceives to be as creamy as fat.

In the body, Simplesse is digested and absorbed, contributing to energy intake, while olestra passes through essentially unchanged. Simplesse provides 1 1/3 calories per gram—a substantial reduction from fat's 9 calories per gram, but more than olestra's zero calories. In the kitchen, Simplesse is unsuitable for frying or baking, because it becomes jelly-like when heated. Olestra can, however, partially replace cooking fats.

Artificial fats are taking their places on grocers' shelves and may become as commonplace as arti-ficial sweeteners. But do they really better people's nutrition? No one knows for sure. On the one hand, these products may help to increase the nutrient density of the diet, but on the other hand, their availability may encourage the consumption of more nutrient-poor foods. One thing is known, though: because they are so new to the market and are patented, artificial fats are costly and drive up the prices of foods that are made with them.

Ironically, the very existence of these products may make their use unnecessary. Food companies have responded to these new products by devising many other creative ways to reduce fats in their foods—for example, by substituting egg whites or skim milk particles for fat. These methods skirt the need to add expensive artificial fats to foods, and thus keep food prices down while providing no-fat and low-fat products to meet consumer needs.

SOURCES: M. Kroger, Can we have our cake and eat it too? *Priorities,* Winter 1989, pp. 37–39; No regulatory clearance needed for NutriFat (abstract), *Journal of the American Dietetic Association* 89 (1989): 426; L. McBean, Fat/cholesterol: An update, *Dairy Council Digest* 60 (1989): 7–12.

You know you are eating protein when you eat meats, fish, poultry, eggs, cheese, and milk. Plant foods such as grains, legumes (black beans, soybeans, blackeyed peas, lima beans, and the like), and other vegetables eaten in quantity also provide protein. In fact, an adult can obtain enough protein from one egg, two cups of milk, and an assortment of grains and vegetables—without a single serving of meat. Yet many people eat two or three eggs for breakfast, hamburgers for lunch, and 12-ounce steaks for dinner.

Protein-rich foods from animal sources are often high in fat and calories, and all are low in fiber, so in excess, they can pose a triple threat to health. It is beneficial to health for people to obtain at least half of their protein from plants, and it is possible to get enough protein from plant foods alone, as **vegetarians** do. Figure 5–5 gives examples of some high-protein vegetarian dishes.

Thus far, this chapter has dealt with the energy-yielding nutrients—carbohydrate, fat, and protein. The next section deals with the nutrients everyone thinks of when they think about nutrition—the vitamins and minerals.

vegetarians   people who omit meat, fish, and poultry from their diets. *Lacto-ovo vegetarians* use milk and milk products and eggs as well as plant foods; *strict vegetarians* eat only plant foods.

≡▶   *Protein is made of amino acids and serves as the building materials for many body structures and machinery. The essential amino acids must be obtained from food each day.*

FIGURE 5–5 ■ **Vegetarian protein choices.**

Choose from two or more of these columns to obtain balanced assortments of amino acids for the human body's use.

Grains	Legumes	Seeds and Nuts	Vegetables
Barley	Dried beans	Cashews	Broccoli
Bulgur	Dried lentils	Nut butters	Leafy greens
Cornmeal	Dried peas	Other nuts	Others
Oats	Peanuts	Sesame seeds	
Pasta	Soy products	Sunflower seeds	
Rice		Walnuts	
Whole-grain breads			

Examples:

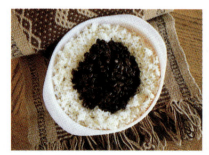

Beans and rice.

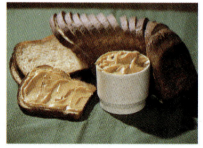

Peanut butter and bread.

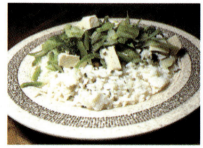

Soybean curd (tofu) and rice.

Vitamins and Minerals

Vitamins and minerals occur in foods in much smaller quantities than do the energy-yielding nutrients, and they make no contribution of energy themselves. Nor do they contribute building material, except for the minerals of bone. Instead they serve mostly as helpers, or facilitators, of body processes. They are, nonetheless, a powerful group of substances, as their absence attests. A vitamin A deficiency can cause blindness; a lack of niacin causes mental illness; a lack of vitamin D causes growth retardation; a lack of iron causes anemia. The consequences of deficiencies are so dire and the effects of restoring the needed nutrients so dramatic that they make wonderful stories for faddists to tell: Are you bald? Impotent? Do you have pimples? Are you nearsighted? The right vitamin will cure whatever ails you, they say.

Actually, a vitamin or mineral can cure only the disease caused by a deficiency of that vitamin or mineral. Also, an overdose of any vitamin or mineral can make people as sick as a deficiency can, and it can even cause death. A balanced diet of ordinary foods supplies enough, but not too much, of each of the vitamins and minerals.

The vitamins and minerals are listed along with some of their more important roles in the body, in Table 5–2. This section discusses only a few vitamins and minerals that exemplify the importance of meeting your body's needs for all of them. It refers frequently to foods, and the end of the chapter puts the foods together into an eating plan that can meet all needs for all nutrients.

■ *FACT OR FICTION:* The more vitamins you consume, the better it is for your health. *False.* All of the vitamins (and minerals) can be toxic when taken in large amounts.

THIAMIN. Thiamin is a typical vitamin in that its presence is not felt, but its absence makes itself known all over the body. A severe thiamin deficiency causes a paralysis that begins at the fingers and toes and works its way inward toward the spine, with extreme wasting and loss of muscle tissue, swelling all over the body, and enlargement of the heart and irregular heartbeat. Ultimately, the victim dies from heart failure. Few have ever witnessed such an extreme deficiency, but consider how a mild lack manifests its presence: stomachaches, headaches, fatigue, restlessness, disturbances of sleep, chest pains, fevers, personality changes (aggressiveness and hostility), and a whole string of symptoms often classed as neurosis. Mild thiamin deficiencies are likely to be seen in consumers of "junk" diets—that is, diets that emphasize foods low in nutrients and high in calories, sugar, fat, and salt.

Proof that thiamin was deficient in some people who snacked heavily on empty-calorie foods came from research that showed below-normal activity of a thiamin-containing enzyme in their blood.[6] They also had the symptoms of neurosis just mentioned. When they took thiamin supplements for a month or more, the symptoms disappeared as the blood enzyme activity returned to normal.

On hearing stories like this, people tend to want to rush out to the drugstore and buy bottles of vitamin pills. There's a problem, though. Although you might get the amount of thiamin you need this way, more than 40 other essential nutrients are all equally vital to your well-being. Nutritious foods are far more effective than pills in supplying the assortment of nutrients you

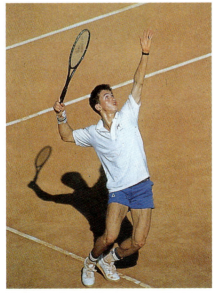

For perfect functioning, every nutrient is needed.

TABLE 5–2 ■ Major Roles of the Vitamins and Minerals

Fat-Soluble Vitamins[a]

Vitamin A	A pigment of the eye important in vision, especially night vision.
	A participant in the modeling of bones during growth and in the mending of breaks.
	A helper in maintaining the body's many surfaces (skin and linings of lungs, digestive tract, urinary tract, vagina, and eyelids).
	A participant in the repair of genetic damage that could otherwise lead to cancer.
	A factor in production of sperm and maintenance of pregnancy.
Vitamin D	A regulator of the calcium concentration in the blood.
Vitamin E	A protector of compounds that are susceptible to destruction by oxidation; important in protecting red blood cells from bursting as they pass through the lungs.
Vitamin K	A factor necessary for the clotting of blood.

Water-Soluble Vitamins[a]

Thiamin **Riboflavin** **Niacin**	Factors that help enzymes to facilitate the release of energy from nutrients, needed in every cell of the body.
Vitamin B$_b$	A factor necessary for the metabolism of protein.
Vitamin B$_{12}$ **Folate**	Factors that help cells to divide, especially blood cells and cells of the intestinal lining.
Biotin **Pantothenic acid**	Other B vitamins; seldom found deficient in human beings but known to be needed in the diets of experimental animals.
Vitamin C	A factor that maintains the body's connective tissue. Important to the healing of wounds. Part of the "glue" that holds cells together.

Major Minerals

Calcium **Phosphorus**	The principal minerals of bones and teeth. Calcium is involved with muscle contraction, nerve transmission, immune function, and blood clotting. Phosphorus is important in the genetic material and in energy transfer.
Magnesium	Another factor involved in bone mineralization, protein synthesis, muscular contraction, and transmission of nerve impulses.
Sodium **Chlorine** **Potassium**	Electrolytes that maintain fluid balances and the balance of acids and bases inside and outside cells. Chlorine is also part of the hydrochloric acid of the stomach, necessary for digestion. Potassium also facilitates protein synthesis and the maintenance of nerves and muscles.
Sulfur	A component of certain amino acids. Part of the vitamins biotin and thiamin and the hormone insulin.

TABLE 5–2 ■ continued

Trace Minerals

Iodine	A component of thyroid hormone, which helps to regulate growth, development, and metabolic rate in the body.
Fluoride	An element involved in the formation of bones and teeth; helps to make them resistant to loss of their minerals.
Selenium	A factor that, with vitamin E, protects body compounds from oxidation.
Iron	Part of the red blood cell protein hemoglobin, which carries oxygen from place to place in the body, and of the muscle protein myoglobin, which makes oxygen available for muscle work.
	A factor necessary for the use of energy in every cell.
Zinc	A working part of many enzymes and of the hormone insulin.
	A factor involved in the making of genetic material and proteins, immune reactions, transport of vitamin A, taste perception, wound healing, the making of sperm, and the development of the fetus.
Copper	A factor necessary for the absorption and use of iron in the formation of hemoglobin.
	Part of several enzymes.
	A factor that helps to form the protective covering of nerves.
Cobalt	Part of vitamin B_{12} and therefore involved in cell division.
Chromium	A factor associated with insulin and required for the use of glucose.
Molybdenum **Manganese**	Facilitators, with enzymes, of many cell processes.
Vanadium, Tin, Nickel, Silicon, Others[b]	Factors necessary for many biological functions in animals

NOTE: The vitamin names given here are the official names as of 1990. Other names still commonly used and seen on labels are *alpha-tocopherol* for vitamin E, *vitamin B_1* for thiamin, *vitamin B_2* for riboflavin, *pyridoxine* for vitamin B_6, *folic acid* or *folacin* for folate, and *ascorbic acid* for vitamin C.

[a]The fat-soluble and water-soluble vitamins were originally separated on the basis of their solubility. The fat-soluble vitamins tend to be stored in the body and so can be eaten in large quantities at intervals, whereas the water-soluble vitamins tend to be excreted daily in urine and not to accumulate, and so ideally are eaten daily.
[b]Specific human requirements remain undetermined.

need, because they contain rich mixtures of nutrients in forms the body is adapted to use.

What foods in particular supply thiamin, then? Almost no one food you can eat will supply your daily need in a single serving. In fact, thiamin is delivered in adequate amounts only to people who eat *ten or more servings of nutritious foods each day,* as the Daily Food Choices pattern describes (see Figure 5–6, later in this chapter).

FOLATE. Folate deficiency is probably more widespread than most people realize. It distorts the red blood cells and impairs their ability to carry sufficient oxygen to all the body's other cells, causing a kind of **anemia.** Folate deficiency causes a generalized misery with many symptoms, including fatigue, diarrhea, irritability, forgetfulness, lack of appetite, headache, and many more.

anemia   reduced size or number or altered shape of the red blood cells; a symptom of any of a number of different disease conditions, including several nutrient deficiencies.

The term *anemia*, which means literally "without blood," refers to a symptom, not a disease. Many nutrient deficiencies and diseases can cause it.

Why is folate deficiency so widespread? For one thing, the vitamin is predominantly found in *fresh* foods, the kind that do not store well, primarily vegetables. Folate is easily destroyed when foods are canned, dehydrated, or otherwise processed, or even when foods are overcooked. Finally, some people need more folate than others. For example, anyone who is growing new cells needs extra folate: children, pregnant women, and people recovering from illness or surgery.

VITAMIN B$_6$. Vitamin B$_6$, too, is an indispensable cog in the body's machinery, and the price of a deficiency is a multitude of symptoms. Vitamin B$_6$ illustrates another nutrition principle—excesses are also toxic. Whenever people start overusing a nutrient, no matter how nontoxic the nutrient may seem at first, it is only a matter of time before toxic effects appear. This happened in the 1970s with vitamin C after the publication of the popular book *Vitamin C and the Common Cold.*[7] In the 1980s, it happened with vitamin B$_6$. People were "diagnosing" vitamin B$_6$ deficiencies on grossly inadequate evidence and "prescribing" large doses.

The first major report of toxic effects of high doses of vitamin B$_6$ described people who had numb feet, then lost sensation in their hands, then became unable to work. Later, their mouths became numb.[8] Since then, other reports have followed, showing nervous system damage from more moderate doses of vitamin B$_6$.[9]

Not everyone is likely to suffer toxicity symptoms with high doses of vitamin B$_6$. Because it is easily excreted in the urine, vitamin B$_6$ is a relatively nontoxic nutrient, but individual tolerances vary, and we cannot say that supplements are "safe" for anyone. The same fact holds true for every vitamin, and every mineral, too.

osteoporosis   a disease characterized by progressively reduced density of the bones, which can cripple people in later life.

CALCIUM. Calcium bears the distinction of being the most abundant mineral in the human body. It is the major mineral of bones and teeth, and everyone is aware that children therefore need milk daily to support their growth. Calcium is not abundant in foods, however, and low intakes are common. A deficit of calcium during childhood and especially in young adulthood threatens the integrity of the bones and contributes to gradual bone loss, **osteoporosis,** that can totally cripple a person in later life. Chapter 15 tells more about who is at risk for osteoporosis, and what is known about its prevention and treatment.

For people who can tolerate milk and milk products, the obvious way to meet calcium needs is to include them in the diet daily, because they are almost the only foods that contain much calcium per serving. Table 5–3 shows the amounts of milk recommended for children and adults. People who cannot tolerate fresh milk can try cheese or fermented dairy products as substitutes for fluid milk. A few plant foods make significant contributions to those who plan their diets carefully: selected nuts; green vegetables

TABLE 5–3 ■ Recommended Fluid Milk Intakes	
Children under 9	2 to 3 c
Children 9 to 12	3+ c
Teenagers	4+ c
Adults	2 c
Pregnant women	3+ c
Lactating women	4+ c
Older women	3 to 5 c

such as some leafy greens and broccoli; and legumes. Calcium-fortified beverages and calcium supplements may be of some value.

IRON. Iron's presence in every living cell testifies to its enormous importance in the body. Iron is part of the protein **hemoglobin,** the body's oxygen carrier. Bound into hemoglobin in the red blood cells, iron enables them to ferry oxygen from lungs to tissues, thus permitting the release of energy from fuels to do the cells' work. Iron-deficiency anemia is characterized by weakness, tiredness, apathy, headaches, and a paleness that reflects a reduction in number and size of red blood cells. (In dark-skinned people, this paleness can be seen in the corner of the eye.) A person with this anemia can do very little muscular work without experiencing disabling fatigue, but will feel more energetic after a few weeks of eating the needed iron-rich foods.

Women may often have their blood iron levels pronounced normal, and yet they may still need iron because their body stores may be depleted. This condition is not detected by standard tests. Because most women eat less food than do men, their iron intakes are lower. And because women menstruate, their iron losses are greater. These two factors predispose women to iron deficiencies.

Iron is one of the **trace minerals,** so called because only tiny amounts are needed in the diet. Despite this, iron deficiency occurs in as many as half of all persons even in developed countries—most predictably, in inner-city and rural families of limited means. People begin to lose energy long before they are diagnosed as having iron-deficiency anemia. With no obvious disease, they still appear unmotivated and apathetic, they work and play less, and they are less physically fit. Incidence rates for iron-deficiency anemia in developed countries range from 10 to 20 percent; rates are higher in the developing countries. Therefore, the incidence of iron deficiency not severe enough to cause anemia may be higher still.[10] If this one worldwide malnutrition problem could be alleviated, millions of people's lives would brighten.

The cause of iron deficiency is usually poor nutrition—that is, inadequate intake, either from sheer lack of food or from high consumption of iron-poor foods. Among non-nutritional causes, blood loss, usually caused by infection, is the primary one. Meats, fish, poultry, and legumes are iron-rich foods, and an easy way to obtain the needed iron is to eat them regularly. But foods that are rich in iron are poor in calcium and vice versa. Thus plans for a balanced diet emphasize the importance of both.

SODIUM. Some minerals serve as **electrolytes,** dissolved substances in blood and body fluid that carry electrical charges. Fluids and electrolytes provide the environment in which the cells' work takes place—work such as nerve-to-nerve communication, heartbeats, contraction of muscles, and so forth. When people lose fluid—whether it is sweat, blood, or urine—they also lose electrolytes. When too much body fluid is lost, as in heat stroke, diarrhea, or injury, its replacement is essential and may require medical assistance.

Sodium is one of the electrolytes. It is best known as part of sodium chloride, ordinary table **salt,** a highly prized food seasoning and preservative. Because sodium is so abundant in the diet, people easily meet their

hemoglobin the oxygen-carrying protein of the red blood cells.

trace minerals minerals essential in nutrition, needed in small quantities (traces) daily. Iron and zinc are examples.

electrolytes minerals that carry electrical charges when dissolved in fluid.

Fluid replacement for sweat losses in heavy exercise or work is discussed in the Spotlight following Chapter 7.

salt a compound that, in water, separates into electrolytes.

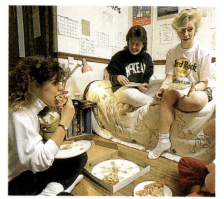

Your food choices may be better than you realize.

hypertension   high blood pressure.

Diet planning principles:

Adequacy—enough of each type of food.

Balance—not too much of any type of food.

Calorie control—not too many calories.

Economy—not too expensive.

Moderation—not too much fat, salt, or sugar.

Variety—as many different foods as possible.

Four Food Group Plan   the original and widely taught eating plan, developed to ensure dietary adequacy. (It calls for a minimum of 2 servings a day of milk/milk products, 2 of meat/meat alternates, 4 of vegetables and fruits, and 4 of breads and cereals.)

Daily Food Choices pattern   a modern plan for ensuring dietary adequacy that offers five categories of foods to choose from. (It treats vegetables and fruits separately; for recommended servings see Figure 5–6.)

need from food. This same abundance, however, means that some people must try consciously to control sodium excesses to avoid aggravating high blood pressure (**hypertension**). Foods high in salt are not always easy to recognize, so people wishing to avoid salt must be alert to the words *salt* and *sodium* on food labels.

ZINC. Zinc plays roles of major importance in association with the cellular machinery in every body organ. It is lost from the body daily, in much the same way as protein is, and so it must be replenished daily to ward off deficiencies. Zinc is highest in foods of high protein content, such as shellfish, meats, and liver.

At one time, zinc deficiencies were unheard of, but they are now known to be present in many of the world's people. In the Middle East, for example, zinc deficiencies have caused severe growth retardation and arrested sexual maturation in adolescent boys. In the United States and Canada, zinc deficiencies occur in the most vulnerable population groups—pregnant women, children, the elderly, and people with low incomes.

So far, we have introduced all of the classes of nutrients and given thumbnail sketches of a few of them. The last section of the chapter shows you how to arrange foods into patterns that provide the full spectrum of nutrients you need. However, some people are still not sure of meeting their nutrient needs using foods alone, and think they should take supplements. The Spotlight at the end of this chapter offers pointers to help make an informed decision on supplement use.

≡▶   *Vitamins and minerals are needed by the body in particular amounts; both too little and too much of a vitamin or mineral can be harmful. Each plays distinct roles in the body, and no one can replace the others.*

How to Choose Nutritious Foods

Altogether, people need about 40 vitamins and minerals. How can they meet their needs for all of these nutrients?

Each nutrient has its own unique pattern of distribution in foods. It might seem quite a tricky business, then, to work them all into the meals you eat, and yet you probably do well, as far as vitamins and minerals go, without even trying. People all over the world obtain these nutrients from an astonishing variety of diets.

Eating wisely doesn't require giving up favorite foods and all the pleasures they provide, although it may require moderation in their consumption. More often it just means fine-tuning your current diet a little. Eat this food more often, and eat that food a little less often; that's all. For many people, whether they know it or not, food plans such as the **Four Food Group Plan** they learned in school, or the new **Daily Food Choices pattern** serve as the basis for planning adequate, balanced diets.

Figure 5–6 shows the Daily Food Choices pattern. Adults need to choose a number of servings daily from each group that falls within the ranges shown. The pattern can help a diet planner design an adequate and balanced diet.

Milk and Milk Products

(These foods supply calcium, riboflavin, protein, and other nutrients.)
2 servings
Serving = 1 c milk or yogurt; ¼ c Parmesan cheese or process cheese spread; 2 c cottage cheese; 1½ c ice cream or ice milk; 2 oz process cheese food; 1⅓ oz cheese.

■ Nonfat milk, buttermilk, low-fat milk, plain yogurt.
■ Whole milk, cheese, fruit-flavored yogurt, cottage cheese.
■ Custard, milk shakes, pudding, ice cream.

Breads and Cereals

(These foods supply riboflavin, thiamin, niacin, iron, and other nutrients.)
6 to 11 servings per day.
Serving = 1 slice bread; ½ to ¾ c cooked cereals, rice, or pastas; 1 oz ready-to-eat cereals.

■ Whole grains (wheat, oats, barley, millet, rye, bulgur), enriched breads, rolls, tortillas.
■ Rice, cereals, pastas (macaroni, spaghetti), bagels.
■ Pancakes, muffins, cornbread, biscuits, presweetened cereals.

Vegetables

(These foods supply vitamin A, folate, and other nutrients.)
3 to 5 servings
Serving = ½ c or typical portion (1 medium artichoke, 1 wedge lettuce).

■ Bean sprouts, broccoli, brussels sprouts, cabbage, carrots, cauliflower, cucumbers, green beans, green peas, leafy greens (spinach, mustard, collard), lettuce, mushrooms, tomatoes, winter squash.
■ Corn, potatoes.
■ Avocados, sweet potatoes.

Fruits

(These foods supply vitamin C, vitamin A, potassium, and other nutrients.)
2 to 4 servings
Serving = ½ c or typical portion (1 medium apple, ½ grapefruit).

■ Apricots, cantaloupe, grapefruit, oranges, orange juice, peaches, watermelon, strawberries.
■ Apples, bananas, canned fruit, pears.
■ Dried fruit.

Meat and Meat Alternates

(These foods supply protein, iron, niacin, folate, zinc, and other nutrients.)
2 servings per day for adults, children, teenagers.
3 servings per day for pregnant/lactating women/teenagers.
Serving = 2 to 3 oz lean, cooked meat, poultry, or fish.
Note: 1 oz. meat, poultry, or fish = 1 egg, ½ to ¾ c legumes, 2 tbsp peanut butter, ¼ to ½ c nuts or seeds.

■ Poultry, fish, lean meat (beef, lamb, pork), dried peas and beans, eggs.
■ Beef, lamb, pork, refried beans.
■ Hot dogs, luncheon meats, peanut butter, nuts.

Miscellaneous Group

No serving sizes are provided because servings of these foods are not recommended. They provide few nutrients.

■ Miscellaneous foods, not high in calories, include spices, herbs, coffee, tea, and diet soft drinks.
■ Foods high in fat include margarine, salad dressing, oils, mayonnaise, cream, cream cheese, butter, gravy, and sauces.
■ Foods high in salt include potato chips, corn chips, pretzels, pickles, olives, bouillon, prepared mustard, soy sauce, steak sauce, salt, and seasoned salt.
■ Foods high in sugar include cake, pie, cookies, doughnuts, sweet rolls, candy, soft drinks, fruit drinks, jelly, syrup, gelatin desserts, sugar, and honey.
■ Alcoholic beverages include wine, beer, and liquor.

FIGURE 5–6 ■ Daily food choices pattern.

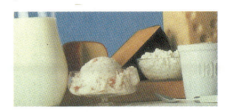

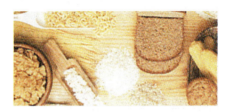

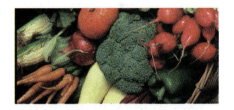

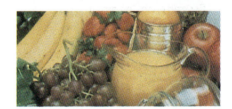

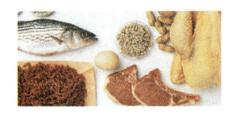

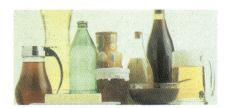

Key:

■ Foods generally highest in nutrient density.
■ Foods moderate in nutrient density.
■ Foods generally lowest in nutrient density.

LIFE CHOICE INVENTORY

How well do you eat? Answer these questions to find out.

Part I

Do you eat nutritious foods from all of these categories? Answer yes or no. For each "yes" answer, give yourself 2 points. Total possible points = 10.

                                        Score

1. I have two or more cups of milk or the equivalent in milk products every day. _____
2. I have two or more servings of meat or meat alternates every day. _____
3. On some days I eat dried peas or beans instead of meat. _____
4. I generally have at least six servings of grain products (breads, cereals, rice, and the like) each day. _____
5. I have at least three servings of vegetables and two servings of fruits every day. _____

                       Total for Part I _____

Part II

Do you maintain appropriate weight? If yes, give yourself 20 points, skip Part III, and go on to Part IV. If you are more than 10 pounds *over* your appropriate body weight, complete Part IIIa; if you are more than 10 pounds *below* your appropriate body weight, complete part IIIb.

I eat just enough food to stay within 5 to 10 pounds of the weight considered appropriate for my height. (20 points) _____

                       Total for Part II _____

Part IIIa

Do you choose a diet low in fat, saturated fat, and cholesterol? For each "yes" answer, give yourself 1 point. Total possible points = 10.

1. My milk and milk-product choices are mostly nonfat or low in fat (nonfat or low-fat milk rather than whole milk; ice cream or ice milk two or three times a week or less). _____
2. I seldom have more than about three teaspoons of margarine or butter per day. _____
3. My meat, fish, poultry, or egg choices usually amount to two moderate servings a day or less. _____
4. In choosing meats, I eat chicken and fish more often than beef, ham, lamb, or pork. _____
5. I remove fat or ask that fat be trimmed from meat before cooking. _____
6. In preparing meat, I usually broil, boil, bake, or roast it; I usually don't fry it. _____
7. On some days I eat dried peas or beans instead of meat. (This is the same as Part I question 3—it counts under both Part I and Part III.) _____
8. In choosing or preparing vegetables, I use little or no fat; if I use butter or margarine I add it after cooking. _____
9. The grain products I use have little or no fat added. _____
10. In buying foods, I read labels for fat contents and choose mostly foods with less than 3 grams fat per 100 calories. _____

                       Total for Part IIIa _____

Part IIIb

Do you have the characteristics of a person with an eating disorder? For each "no" answer, give yourself 2 points. Total possible points = 10.

1. Do you view yourself as overweight? _____
2. Are you presently on a weight-loss diet? _____
3. Do you engage in bingeing and vomiting? _____
4. Does your weight fluctuate over a range of more than 10 pounds? _____
5. Are you trying to lose weight? _____

                       Total for Part IIIb _____

A person can control calories while using this pattern. The foods color-coded with green boxes are the lowest in calories within each group; those with yellow boxes are intermediate; and those with red boxes are highest in calories. A person who chooses the smallest recommended number of serv-

Part IV

Do you get plenty of starch and fiber daily? For each "yes" answer, give yourself 2 points. Total possible points = 10.

1. When I am hungry, I choose starchy foods rather than fatty foods. _____
2. The grain products I use are mostly whole grains (whole-wheat bread, whole-grain cereals, brown rice, and the like). _____
3. I eat abundant fruits and vegetables (this resembles Part I question 5 above; you get added points for these as high-fiber foods). _____
4. I eat salads or raw vegetables (such as carrots and celery) at least every other day. _____
5. I eat dried beans or peas at least once a week (again, you receive credit for legumes as a high-fiber food). _____

Total for Part IV _____

Part V

Do you eat reasonable quantities of sugar, honey, and other concentrated sweets? For each "yes" answer, give yourself 2 points. Total possible points = 6.

1. I eat sweets (candy bars, etc.), if at all, in addition to, not in place of, the nutritious foods I need for a balanced diet, and only within the limits my weight allows. _____
2. I drink cola beverages, if at all, in addition to, not in place of, the milk and fruit products I need for a balanced diet, and only within the limits my weight and caffeine tolerance allows. _____
3. I don't let sweets and sugary drinks harm my dental health; I rinse or brush my teeth after eating and drinking them. _____

Total for Part V _____

Part VI

Do you use salt in moderation? For each "yes" answer, take 2 points. Total possible points = 4.

1. I generally choose foods salted lightly or not salted at all. _____
2. I add little or no salt to food after preparation. _____

Total for Part VI _____

Part VII

Do you drink alcohol, if at all, in moderation? For each "yes" response, give yourself 5 points. Total possible points = 10.

1. I drink no more than two drinks of alcoholic beverages in any one day (see Chapter 10 for the definition of "a drink"). _____
2. I drink no more than four drinks of alcoholic beverages in any one day. (If you answered "yes" to question 1, just before this, you should of course answer "yes" to this question, too, and take the full 10 points' credit for this section.) _____

SCORE:

I	_____
II or III	_____
IV	_____
V	_____
VI	_____
VII	_____
Total	_____ (out of 60)

RATING:

60	Incredible.
50–59	Excellent.
40–49	Your diet has room for improvement.
30–39	Not so good. Work on your weakest areas.
Below 30	Poor. Make major efforts to improve.

ings, all from the green-coded foods, will obtain the needed nutrients and only about 1,200 calories. A person choosing the highest number of servings, also from the green-coded foods, raises the calorie level to about 2,000 calories. Beyond this, a person who needs more food energy, say to support

The New Food Labels

Food labels still state what ingredients are in the package, just as they always have done. When they state what nutrients are in the food, though, they're beginning to do that in a new way. For the last 25 years, nutrient contents of foods have been expressed in terms of the U.S. RDA, a set of standard values that are intended to represent the nutrient needs of the consumer. Now the nutrients in foods are expressed on labels in terms of **Daily Values**.

The Daily Values provide consumers with two kinds of information—first, about essential nutrients that are known to be indispensable to health (protein, vitamins, and minerals); and second, about all other nutrients, such as fat and fiber, that have important relationships with health.[a] For many of the former group, the consumer wants to obtain *at least* the Daily Value each day. For the latter group (except fiber), the consumer wants to obtain *no more than* the Daily Value each day.

By presenting nutrient information in a standard format and as percentages of Daily Values, labels give consumers the opportunity to judge the contributions of individual foods to their daily diets and health goals. Daily Values also provide an easy way to compare the nutrition virtues of different foods.

[a]The Daily Values were established by the Food and Drug Administration (FDA) in 1990–1991. They use two sets of standards. For protein, vitamins, and minerals, they use Reference Daily Intakes (RDI), which are based on long–established recommended intakes for these nutrients. For nutrients and food components such as fat and fiber that do not have such long-established recommended intakes, but that do have important relationships with health, they use Daily Reference Values (DRV) based on scientific evidence and consensus.

Daily Values   reference values used on food labels as a standard with which to compare a food's nutrient contents. (For example, a food may state on its label that a serving provides "25% of the Daily Value for vitamin A.")

The more nutrients and the fewer calories a food offers relative to a person's needs, the greater that food's **nutrient density.**

nutrient density   the amount of nutrients a food contains relative to the calories it contains. The higher the nutrients and lower the calories, the more nutrient dense the food.

weight gain, may substitute some of the higher-calorie selections suggested by the pattern—that is, yellow and red-coded foods.

The beauty of the Daily Food Choice pattern lies in its simplicity and ease in learning. It is not rigid; it can be used with great flexibility. For example, cheese can be substituted for milk because both supply the same nutrients (protein, calcium, and riboflavin) in about the same amounts (although cheese is generally a much higher-fat choice than milk). Legumes and nuts are alternatives for meats. The pattern can also be adapted to casseroles and other mixed dishes and to different national and cultural cuisines. A study of the pattern and some thought about the questions asked in this chapter's Life Choice Inventory should provide the information you need to obtain a virtual guarantee of diet adequacy.

Three other dietary ideals as important as adequacy are variety, moderation, and calorie control. The strategies that follow can guide you in implementing them, but before you do so, realize that your body is unique. It responds to food in its own characteristic ways according to its genetic inheritance and its current needs. No doubt you already know its tendencies. For example, a sedentary young woman who tends to gain weight may need to take steps to reduce her intake of fat, but an active young man who tends to stay thin might be better off ignoring at least some such sugges-

STRATEGIES: *SELECTING NUTRITIOUS FOODS*

To select nutritious foods:

1. Given the choice between whole foods and refined, processed foods, choose the former (apples rather than apple pie; potatoes rather than potato chips). Fewer nutrients have been refined out of the whole foods; less fat, salt, and sugar have been added.
2. When choosing meats, choose the lean ones. Select fish or poultry often, beef seldom. Ask for broiled, not fried, to control your fat intake.
3. Use both raw and cooked vegetables and fruits. Raw foods offer more fiber and vitamins such as folate and thiamin that are destroyed by cooking. Cooking foods frees other vitamins and minerals for absorption.
4. Include milk, milk products, or other calcium sources for the calcium you need. Use low-fat or nonfat items to reduce fat and calories.
5. Learn to use margarine, butter, and oils sparingly; only a little gives flavor; a lot overloads you with fat and calories.
6. Vary your choices. Eat broccoli today, carrots tomorrow, and corn the next day. Eat Chinese today, Italian tomorrow, and hot dogs and beans on Saturday.
7. Load your plate with vegetables and unrefined starchy foods. A small portion of meat or cheese is all you need for protein.
8. When choosing breads and cereals, choose the whole-grain varieties.

To select nutritious fast foods:

9. Choose the broiled sandwich with lettuce, tomatoes, and other goodies—and hold the mayo—rather than the fish or chicken patties coated with breadcrumbs and cooked in fat.
10. Select a salad—and use more plain vegetables than those mixed with oily or mayonnaise-based dressings.
11. Order chili with more beans than meat. Choose a soft bean burrito over tacos with fried shells.
12. Drink low-fat milk rather than a cola beverage.

When choosing from a vending machine:

13. Choose cracker sandwiches over chips and pork rinds (virtually pure fat). Choose peanuts, pretzels, and popcorn over cookies and candy.
14. Choose milk and juices over cola beverages, or choose diet beverages over sugary ones to avoid empty calories.

■ *FACT OR FICTION:* Fast foods can be nutritious. *True.*

tions. She needs to avoid storing excess calories from fat; he needs them to add body weight. The point here is to think carefully about your own body and its needs before taking any action where your diet is concerned. The strategies listed here serve the needs of most people.

Good nutrition starts with wise food purchasing. Learn to identify the more nutritious foods. The box entitled The New Food Labels and the Miniglossary of Terms on Food Labels show how you can use food labels to make informed choices.

■ MINIGLOSSARY
of Terms on Food Labels

free "nutritionally trivial" and unlikely to have a physiological consequence.

high 20 percent or more of the Daily Value for a given nutrient.

less at least 25 percent less of a given nutrient than the comparison food.

low an amount that would allow frequent consumption of a food without exceeding the dietary guidelines. A food that is naturally low in a nutrient may make such a claim, but only as it applies to all similar foods (for example, "fresh cauliflower, a low-sodium food").

more at least 10 percent more of a given nutrient than the comparison food.

reduced must identify the comparison food, the percentage of reduction, and the amount in the comparison food.

source of 10 to 19 percent of the Daily Value.

Note: Foods containing more than 11.5 grams total fat or per 100 grams must indicate those contents immediately after a cholesterol claim. As you will see, all cholesterol claims are prohibited when the food contains more than 2 grams saturated fat per serving.

cholesterol-free less than 2 milligrams cholesterol per serving and 2 grams or less saturated fat per serving.

low in cholesterol 20 milligrams or less per serving and per 100 grams of food,
and 2 grams or less of saturated fat per serving.

less cholesterol 25 percent or less cholesterol than the comparison food (reflecting a reduction of at least 20 milligrams per serving), and 2 grams or less saturated fat per serving.

reduced cholesterol 50 percent or less cholesterol per serving than the comparison food (reflecting a reduction of at least 20 milligrams per serving), and 2 grams or less saturated fat per serving.

kCalorie free fewer than 5 kcalories per serving.

light one-third fewer kcalories than the comparison food. Any other use of the term must specify what it is referring to (for example, "light in color" or "light in texture").

low kcalorie less than 40 kcalories per serving and per 100 grams of food.

reduced kcalorie at least one-third fewer kcalories than the comparison.

fat free less than 0.5 grams of fat per serving (and no added fat or oil).

less fat 25 percent or less fat than the comparison food.

less saturated fat 25 percent or less saturated fat than the comparison food.

low fat 3 grams or less fat per serving and per 100 grams of food.

low saturated fat 1 gram or less saturated fat per serving, and not more than 15 percent of kcalories from saturated fat.

percent fat free may be used only if product meets definition of *low fat*.

reduced fat 50 percent or less of the fat in the comparison food *and* reduced by more than 3 grams fat per serving (for example, "reduced fat, 50 percent less fat than our regular cookies, reduced from 10 grams to 5 grams per serving").

reduced saturated fat 50 percent or less of the saturated fat in the comparison food *and* reduced by more than 1 gram.

high fiber 20 percent or more of the Daily Value for fiber; a high-fiber claim made on a food that contains more than 3 grams fat per serving and per 100 grams of food must also declare total fat.

sodium free and salt free less than 5 milligrams of sodium per serving.

low sodium less than 140 milligrams per serving and per 100 grams of food.

reduced sodium no more than 50 percent of the sodium of the comparison food.

very low sodium less than 35 milligrams per serving and per 100 grams of food.

sugar free less than 0.5 grams per serving.

SOURCE: E. N. Whitney and S. R. Rolfes, *Understanding Nutrition*, 6th ed., in preparation.

FIGURE 5–7 ■ **How to read a food label.**

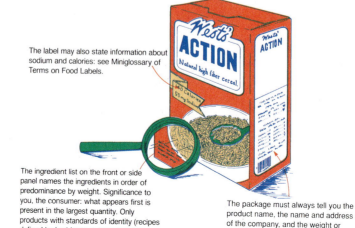

The label may also state information about sodium and calories: see Miniglossary of Terms on Food Labels.

The ingredient list on the front or side panel names the ingredients in order of predominance by weight. Significance to you, the consumer: what appears first is present in the largest quantity. Only products with standards of identity (recipes defined by law) have no ingredient list.

The package must always tell you the product name, the name and address of the company, and the weight or measure; and it may list the ingredients

≡▶ *Diet planning ideals include adequacy, balance, calorie control, economy, moderation, and variety. The Daily Food Choices pattern serves as a basis for planning adequate, balanced diets. To achieve the other ideals requires attending to individual food choices within the plan.*

No doubt you can create many ideas from the facts in this chapter. Apply them. And keep on learning about nutrition; it is worth a lot to your wellness. The next chapter takes you further in your pursuit of nutritional health by discussing weight control.

■≡ For Review

1. Explain the health risks associated with both undernutrition and overnutrition.
2. Describe some differences between hunger and appetite.
3. Describe what is meant by a *balanced meal*.
4. Explain why, although starch and sugar are both carbohydrates, starchy foods confer greater benefits on the body.
5. Identify foods high in fiber.
6. Identify some symptoms of deficiencies of several vitamins and minerals.
7. Outline the major principles of wise diet planning.
8. Describe strategies for putting diet-planning principles into practice.

■≡ Notes

1. *The Surgeon General's Report on Nutrition and Health: Summary and Recommendations,* DHHS (PHS) publication no. 88−50211 (Washington, D.C.: Government Printing Office, 1988).
2. N. B. Belloc and L. Breslow, Relationship of physical health status and health practices, *Preventive Medicine* 1 (1972): 409−421.
3. Improved nutrition, *Public Health Reports Supplement,* September/October 1983, p. 132.
4. T. B. Van Itallie, Health implications of overweight and obesity in the United States, *Annals of Internal Medicine* 103 (1985): 983−988, as cited in M. R. C. Greenwood and V. A. Pittman-Waller, Weight control: A complex, various, and controversial problem, in *Obesity and Weight Control: The Health Professional's Guide to Understanding and Treatment,* eds. R. T. Frankle and M. U. Yang (Rockville, Md.: Aspen Publications, 1988), pp. 3−15.
5. U.S. Department of Health and Human Services, Public Health Service, *Promoting Health, Preventing Disease: Objectives for the Nation* (Washington, D.C.: Government Printing Office, 1980), as cited in M. Nestle, Promoting health and preventing disease: National nutrition objectives for 1990 and 2000, *Nutrition Today,* June 1988, pp. 26−30.
6. D. Lonsdale and R. J. Shamberger, Red cell transketolase as an indicator of nutritional deficiency, *American Journal of Clinical Nutrition* 33 (1980): 205−211.
7. L. C. Pauling, *Vitamin C and the Common Cold* (San Francisco: W. H. Freeman, 1970).
8. H. Schaumberg and coauthors, Sensory neuropathy from pyridoxine abuse, *New England Journal of Medicine* 309 (1983): 445−448.
9. More B_6 toxicity reported, *Nutrition Forum,* November 1985, p. 84.
10. N. S. Scrimshaw, Functional consequences of iron deficiency in human populations, *Journal of Nutrition Science and Vitaminology* 30 (1984): 47−63.

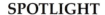

SPOTLIGHT

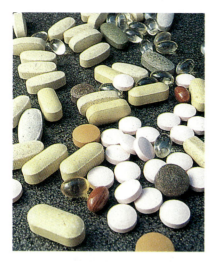

Vitamin-Mineral Supplements

Billions of dollars are spent on "vitamin pills" (actually, vitamin-mineral supplements) in the United States each year. Two-thirds of our citizens use them. You may be one of these users. Perhaps, after studying nutrition, you are wondering if you really need a supplement. This discussion is intended to help you make that decision.

A lot of people have the impression that they can't get the nutrients they need from food alone.

People who haven't learned enough about nutrition think they need supplements as insurance against their own poor food choices. Indeed, their food choices may be poor, but taking supplements is no guarantee that they will get the particular nutrients they need. It's just as likely that they'll get a duplication of the nutrients their food is supplying and still lack the ones they need. The only way to be sure to get the needed assortment of nutrients is to construct a balanced diet from a variety of foods. Besides, no supplement supplies all the nutrients you can get from food.

Even if you could get all your vitamins and trace minerals from a supplement, there is no way you can package the bulk nutrients you need—protein, fiber, carbohydrate, calcium, and others—because you need such large amounts. No one supplement can match a balanced diet, and no combination of supplements can, either. No one knows enough, yet, to construct a synthetic substitute for food. Even in the hospital, where the most advanced technology provides "complete" synthetic formulas for clients for months, the most these formulas can do is to enable clients to survive. They won't thrive until they are back on food.

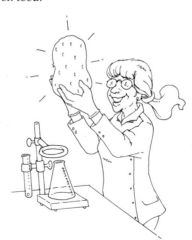

When science concocts the ideal supplement, it will probably turn out to be identical to food.

Nutrient supplements are useful at times. A person may need a specific nutrient to counteract a specific deficiency—iron for iron-deficiency anemia, for example. But it takes medical training and tests to make a correct diagnosis; people can't diagnose their own deficiencies, and they would be foolish to try.

Do people ever have unusually high nutrition needs that justify their taking supplements?

No two people have exactly the same nutrient needs, but people's requirements differ, at the most, only twofold or threefold. An ordinary diet of mixed foods can easily meet the highest of those needs. And the argument still holds that you can't tell, just by guessing, which nutrients you need more of. One shouldn't self-prescribe nutrients based on speculations about having unusually high nutrient needs.

In rare instances, genetic defects may alter nutrient needs considerably, but only one person in 10,000 has such a defect. That person needs a diagnosis and treatment by a qualified health care provider.

What about high nutrient needs induced by different lifestyles? I've seen vitamins advertised for people under stress, alcohol users, cigarette smokers, athletes—things like that.

Yes, the purveyors of supplements like to make the claim that ordinary people need their products—of course, because they can sell more products that way. The claim works; lots of people buy nutrient supplements because they identify with the ads. Stresses, including smoking and moderate alcohol use, do deplete people's nutrient stores somewhat, but the composition of the supplements for those people is just guesswork on the part of the manufacturers. The way to counteract nutrient losses is still to eat well, not to take supplements.

People who drink to excess have major nutrition problems and need to stop drinking, of course, not to take supplements. As for athletes, they need supplements *less* than other people, because they are able to eat more food. Chapter 7 and its Spotlight offer more nutrition information for these people.

Are there any times when I should be taking a vitamin pill?

Yes, when a health care provider recommends it, and yes, in at least two other instances:

☐ When your energy intake is below about 1,500 calories, so that you can't eat enough food to meet your vitamin needs. (People who can't exercise have this problem.)
☐ When you know that, for whatever reason, you are going to be eating irregularly for a limited time.

Remember that if vitamins are needed, minerals are needed, too, and a vitamin pill is not enough. A vitamin-mineral supplement is called for.

When I do need a vitamin-mineral supplement, what kind should I take? I've heard the organic, natural ones are preferable to the synthetic ones.

Organic and *natural* are terms that have no meaning in relation to the contents of vitamin-mineral supplements. All vitamins are organic, no matter where they come from. *Natural* has no legal meaning at all. These terms mean only that the product will be expensive. Don't let them fool you. Read the ingredient lists, and

buy the product that contains the nutrients you are looking for, at the lowest price.

Whenever a health care provider recommends a supplement, carefully follow directions as to the type and dose to take. When you are selecting one yourself, a single, balanced vitamin-mineral supplement should suffice. Look for one in which the nutrient levels are at or slightly below

the RDA (Appendix B), and avoid preparations that exceed the upper limits listed in Table S5–1. Remember, you will still be getting some nutrients from foods.

What about taking supplements as a preventive measure? I've heard that certain vitamins prevent cancer.

Good nutrition certainly helps protect you. Diets that are *deficient* in

TABLE S5–1 ■ Safe Doses for Vitamin and Mineral Supplements

Substance	Amount Recommended for Prevention[a]
Vitamins	
Vitamin A (IU)	250 to 2,500
Vitamin D (IU)	400 (up to age 18)
	200 (adults)
Vitamin E (IU)	6 to 30
Thiamin (mg)	1 to 2
Riboflavin (mg)	1 to 2
Niacin (as niacinamide, mg)	10 to 20
Vitamin B_6 (mg)	1.5 to 2.5
Folate (mg)	0.1 to 0.4
Vitamin B_{12} (µg)	3 to 10
Pantothenic acid (mg)[b]	5 to 20
Biotin (mg)	Not recommended in supplement form
Vitamin C (mg)	50 to 100
Minerals	
Calcium (mg)	400 to 800
Phosphorus (mg)	No need to supplement
Magnesium (mg)	No need to supplement
Iron (mg)	10 to 30 (women)
	30 to 60
Zinc (mg)	10 to 25 (adults)
	25
Iodine (mg)	Not recommended in supplement form

[a]The FDA and the Committee on RDA do not recommend that these nutrients be used to attempt to correct deficiencies, because deficiencies often arise from nonnutritional causes such as disease or interference by drugs. In these cases the underlying causes of the deficiencies must be correctly diagnosed and treated; supplements may mask, but will not correct, the problems.
[b]Use only in multivitamin form.

SOURCE: Parts adapted from The American Medical Association's Council on Scientific Affairs, Vitamin preparations as dietary supplements and as therapeutic agents, *Journal of the American Medical Association* 257 (1987): 1929–1936; A. Hecht, Vitamins over the counter: Take only when needed, *FDA Consumer,* April 1979, pp. 17–19; Food and Nutrition Board, *Recommended Dietary Allowances,* 10th ed. (Washington, D.C.: National Academy of Sciences, 1989).

nutrients render you defenseless against cancer and many other ills. But to say that a pill containing specific nutrients will protect you is to drastically oversimplify the case. You need foods, with all the multitude of nutrients and related compounds they contain, if you really want protection.

Suppose I just want to take a vitamin-mineral supplement as insurance against slight deficiencies. There's no harm in that, is there?

Perhaps not—but keep the dose low; vitamins in excess are toxic. All of them, not only the well-known vitamins A and D, but also the B vitamins and vitamin C, have been shown to have toxic effects, at least in some people, in large doses. And while overdosing with vitamins is risky, overdosing with minerals is still riskier. Excess minerals can be toxic—often in quantities not far above normal intakes.

A friend of mine routinely takes a pile of nutrient supplements. I am worried that some of her practices are dangerous. What should I tell her?

What supplements does she take?

Before breakfast, she takes 500 milligrams of vitamin C, 1,000 units of vitamin E, several tablespoons of nutritional yeast, some kelp tablets, a capsule of vitamins A and D, a spirulina tablet, some green pills, and other pills containing trace minerals. Then she sprinkles desiccated liver, powdered bone, bone meal, and wheat germ on her granola, and pours on some reconstituted powdered nonfat milk. Then for lunch . . .

Never mind what she takes for lunch. You have good reason to worry about her using such a huge stockpile of nutrient preparations. The potent supplements of vitamins A and D and the minerals are especially dangerous.

Not all her choices are dangerous, though. The wheat germ and powdered nonfat milk are nutritious and reasonable in cost. The other choices are more nearly neutral. Your best bet in advising your friend (if she wants your advice) is to suggest she consult a qualified professional such as a registered dietitian (R.D.) for nutrition advice. Congratulate her, because she cares about her health. Reinforce her use of the nutrient-dense foods; the nonfat milk and wheat germ. Then single out for attention her most dangerous practices, the overdoses of toxic vitamins and minerals. As for the others, keep your own counsel about them unless she asks you. That way you probably won't lose a friend, and you may provide a substantial boost to exactly what she treasures most—her good health.

CHAPTER 6

Energy Balance and Weight Control

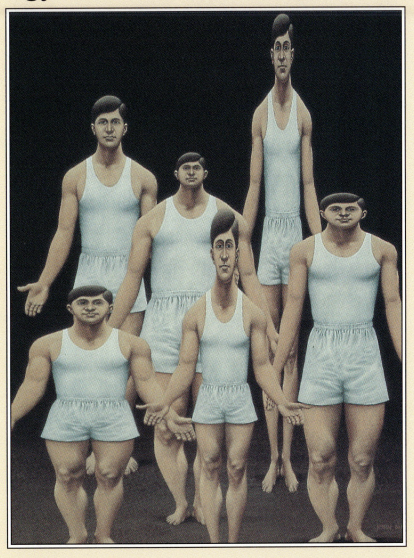

════════ ▗▄▄▄▄▄▄▄▄▄▄▄▄▄▄▄▄▄▄▄▖ ════════
          FACT OR FICTION
════════ ▝▀▀▀▀▀▀▀▀▀▀▀▀▀▀▀▀▀▀▘ ════════

Just for fun, respond true or false to the following statements. If false, say what is true.

■ Excess fat around the abdomen presents a greater risk to health than excess fat elsewhere on the body. (Page 133)

■ The dieter who sees a large weight loss on the scale can take this as a sign of success. (Page 141)

■ When you eat excess calories of fat or carbohydrate, you store them in fat; when you eat excess calories of protein, you store them in muscle. (Page 144)

■ To succeed in losing weight, you have to stop eating carbohydrate. (Page 144)

■ The fastest way to lose body fat is to stop eating altogether. (Page 144)

■ If an inactive person takes up a daily hour of exercise, the person will end up spending more calories all day, even during sleep. (Page 150)

■ It is harder to lose a pound than to gain one. (Page 153)

A re you pleased with your body weight? If you answered yes, you are a rare individual. Nearly all people in our society think they should weigh more or less (mostly less) than they do. Usually their primary reason is appearance, but they often perceive, correctly, that physical health depends on weight, too.

People also think of their weight as something they should control. They are right, but a pair of misconceptions makes their task difficult. The first is to focus on *weight*; the second is to focus on *controlling* weight. To put it simply, it isn't your weight you need to control; it's the fat in your body in proportion to the lean. And it isn't possible to control either one, directly; it is possible only to control your *behavior*. Thus this chapter presents weight control concepts in relation to the behaviors that promote weight change. People also need to maintain a new weight once they've achieved it, so the last section gives tips for holding body weight steady over the years. First, some links between body weight and health are of interest.

■≡ Underweight, Overweight, and Health

Both deficient and excessive body weight present health risks. It has long been known that thin people will die first during a siege or in a famine. A fact not always recognized, even by health care providers, is that overly thin people are also at a disadvantage in the hospital, where they may have to go for days without food so that they can undergo tests or surgery. Underweight also increases risks for any person fighting an infection or other wasting disease. In fact, people with cancer often die from starvation, not from the cancer itself. Thus underweight people are urged to gain body fat as an energy reserve and to acquire protective amounts of all the nutrients that can be stored.

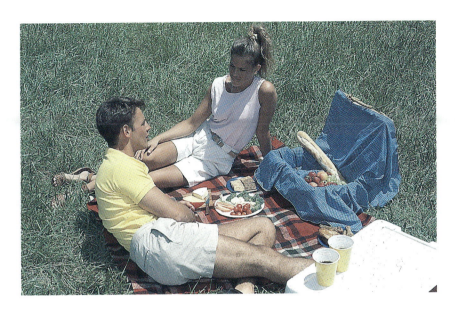

To control weight successfully, people must control their eating behaviors.

The health risks of overfatness are so many that it has been declared a disease: **obesity.**[1]* Obesity worsens hypertension, thereby increasing the risk of stroke; it precipitates diabetes in genetically susceptible people; it increases the risk of heart disease. Other conditions associated with overfatness include abdominal hernias, some cancers, varicose veins, gout, gallbladder disease, arthritis, respiratory problems, liver malfunction, complications in pregnancy and surgery, flat feet, and even a high accident rate.

One of the most serious consequences of obesity is heart disease, and even mild or moderate overweight can elevate the risk.[2] Overweight demands that the heart work extra hard to pump blood through miles of extra capillaries that feed excess fat tissue. Too, fatty deposits within the arteries restrict blood flow to the heart's pumping muscles, depriving them of nutrients and oxygen. This deprivation combined with the heart's extra work load can permanently damage the muscle tissue.

Especially dangerous is fat that collects around a person's middle—**central obesity.** A person with central obesity is fattest around the waist and belly, whereas other obese people's weight collects around their hips and thighs. A quirk of human anatomy may be partly to blame for the greater heart disease risk of people with central obesity. Veins in the abdominal area drain blood, along with a load of fat from the fat tissue, directly to the liver, where the fat is processed and packaged with cholesterol in a form easily deposited in the body's arteries. The fat packages then move into the bloodstream, where they release their fat and cholesterol to stick to the inner linings of the artery walls. When these lipids adhere to the delicate walls of the tiny arteries of the heart, they interfere with the free flow of blood that feeds and cleanses the heart's tissues, leading to that form of heart disease known as atherosclerosis. Veins in the hip area, on the other hand, bypass the liver and drain blood directly back into the heart's pumping chambers to be sent along to, and used or stored by, other body parts.

obesity overfatness with adverse health effects.

central obesity excess fat on the abdomen and around the trunk.

■ *FACT OR FICTION:* Excess fat around the abdomen presents a greater risk to health than excess fat elsewhere on the body. *True.*

*Reference notes are at the end of the chapter.

Some obese people can escape at least some of the health problems mentioned, even heart disease, but no one who is fat in our society quite escapes the social and economic handicaps. Fat people are less sought after for romance, less often hired for jobs, and less often admitted to college. They pay higher insurance premiums, and they pay more for clothing. Psychologically, too, a body size that embarrasses a person diminishes self-esteem. People who are severely obese often are required to pay for two seats on a bus or an airplane. People who are obese are urged to reduce their weight. Their health risks are expected to normalize as they do.

A warning about weight reduction is in order, though: some people are able to lose weight, but few are able to maintain the new desirable weight. Repeated cycles of weight loss and weight regain are common and can be more hazardous to health than obesity itself.[3] Weight maintenance, the steady state in which weight varies little over the years, is as important to health as weight loss.

Both underweight and obesity present risks to health. Underweight people are poorly defended against body fat loss, infections, and wasting diseases. Overweight people are susceptible to heart disease and social and other handicaps.

■ Definition of Appropriate Weight

Body *weight* roughly corresponds to body fatness, so weight on the scale is often used as an indicator of body fatness. A more accurate indicator would be a direct measure of body fatness, but this is hard to obtain.

The traditional way of assigning desirable weights to people is to use one of the insurance-company tables of weights for height, which used to be called the "ideal weight tables." You find your height in the table; decide whether you have a small, medium, or large frame; and then find your weight range. (Height and weight and frame size tables are inside the back cover, on page X.) That weight range is consistent with good health for most people, and you can narrow it down further, based on your own personal preferences. Traditionally, a weight 20 percent or more above the table weight defines obesity—that is, too much body fat for health; a weight 10 percent or more below the table weight defines **underweight** (too little body fat for health).

The use of body weight as an indicator of overfatness is unsatisfactory for some purposes. For one thing, weight and fatness do not always coincide: a healthy person with dense bones and muscles may seem overweight on the scale, while a person whose scale weight seems reasonable may have too much body fat (too little lean tissue) for health. For another thing, frame size measures are not valid. No matter what bone is chosen for use as an indicator of a person's frame size, it only roughly reflects the bulk of the person's bones and muscles.[4] Health care providers find it frustrating to have to use the available frame size measures.

Health care professionals would prefer to have some direct measure of body fatness, but it is hard to measure fat directly. Most resort to a **fatfold test,** using a fatfold caliper—a pinching device that measures the thickness of a fold of fat on the back of the arm, below the shoulder blade, on the side of the waist, or elsewhere. About 50 percent of the body's fat lies beneath

More on heart disease, atherosclerosis, and fat in Chapter 18.

underweight   a body weight so low as to have adverse health effects, generally defined as a weight 10 percent below standard.

Height and weight and frame size tables are inside the back cover on page X.

fatfold test   a clinical test of body fatness in which the thickness of a fold of skin on the back of the arm (triceps), below the shoulder blade (subscapular), or in other places is measured with an instrument called a caliper. The older, now outdated, term for this is *skinfold test.*

Quick Ways to Assess Body Fatness

These ways to answer the question "What is an appropriate weight for you?" are just for fun:

■ A crude measure of body fatness is the "pinch test" (this is a fatfold measure without the equipment to make it accurate). Pick up the skin and fat at the back of either arm with the thumb and forefinger of the other hand. Keep your fingers still, so as not to lose the "measurement" when you pull them away from your arm. Measure the thickness on a ruler. A fatfold over an inch thick reflects obesity.

■ Another shortcut method is to measure your waist compared with your chest (not bust). Every inch by which your waist measurement exceeds your chest measurement is said to take two years off your life.

■ Another crude measure: lie down, relax, and place a ruler across your abdomen from one hipbone to the other. If it doesn't easily touch both bones while you're relaxing, you're too fat.

---

the skin, and its thickness is roughly proportional to total body fat. However, not everyone's body fat is distributed in the same way, and as mentioned earlier, excess fat around the abdomen represents a greater risk to health than excess fat elsewhere on the body.[5]

In 1985, the experts met at a conference called specifically to figure out a way to diagnose obesity. They came up with the **body mass index (BMI),** which can be obtained from a mathematical equation involving height and weight. The inside back cover pages Y and Z present a graph developed from the body mass index equation. The graph offers a quick way to find an acceptable range of weights for someone of your height and gender, and it can help you to evaluate your present weight. This chapter's Life Choice Inventory shows you how to use both the traditional tables and the body mass index graph, and it guides you to a tentative answer to the question, "What is an appropriate weight for you?"

Appropriateness depends partly on who you are. A man of normal weight may have, on the average, 15 percent and a woman, 20 percent of the body weight as fat. However, some people have special needs. An endurance athlete needs some minimum of body fat to provide fuel, to insulate the body, and to permit normal fat-soluble hormone activity, but wants no more than that. This athlete desires to be as lean as possible to have the competitive edge in endurance sports. An Alaskan fisherman, on the other hand, needs a blanket of insulating fat to prevent excessive loss of body heat. For a woman starting pregnancy, the ideal percentage of body fat may be different again; the outcome of pregnancy is compromised if the woman starts out with too little body fat. Beyond your needs for functional body fat, you should probably strive to keep body fat as low as possible to minimize your health risks.

The person seeking a single, authoritative answer to the question "How much should I weigh?" is bound to be disappointed. No one can tell you *exactly* how much you should weigh; but with health as a value, you can at

body mass index (BMI) an equation defining appropriate body weight: the weight in kilograms divided by the height (squared) in meters. A BMI of greater than 27.2 in men or 26.9 in women defines obesity.

LIFE CHOICE INVENTORY

What is an appropriate weight for you? Based on physical health alone, a wide range of weights is safe. Within the safe range, the definition of appropriate weight is up to you, depending on factors such as your family history, occupation, physical and recreational activities, and personal preferences.

1. Determine the safe range for a person of your height and gender:

   □ Record your height: _____ feet, _____ inches. Note that height and weight tables (see inside back cover, page X) assume you measured your height in shoes with one-inch heels. If you measured your barefoot height, add an inch; if you wore shoes with heels higher or lower than an inch, adjust accordingly.

   □ Determine your frame size. Record whether you have a small, medium, or large frame: _____ frame.

   □ Look up the appropriate weight for a person of your height, gender, and frame size in the table on the inside back cover, page X. Record the entire range:

   _____ to _____ pounds.
   EXAMPLE: For a man 5 feet 7 inches tall (in shoes) with a small frame, the range of weights is 138 to 145 pounds.

   □ Determine the bottom end of the safe range. A person who is more than 10 percent below the lowest indicated weight for height is considered underweight to a degree that might compromise health. Take ten percent off the bottom end of your range:

   _____ pounds.
   EXAMPLE: Ten percent of 138 pounds is 13.8 pounds (rounded off to 14 pounds). Bottom end of range is 138 minus 14, or 124 pounds.

   □ Determine the top end of the safe range. A person who is more than 20 percent above the highest indicated weight for height is considered obese. Add 20 percent to the top end of your range:

   _____ pounds.
   EXAMPLE: Twenty percent of 145 pounds is 29 pounds. Top end of range is 145 plus 29, or 174 pounds.

   □ Record your safe range here: _____ to _____ pounds.
   EXAMPLE: 124 to 174 pounds.
   If your weight is below the bottom end of this safe range, you need to gain weight; if above the top end, you need to lose weight for your health's sake.

2. If your weight is above the top end of the range, look up your body mass index range (pages Y and Z of inside back cover) to obtain confirmation that you need to lose weight. Use your weight without clothing and your height without shoes.

3. Check your health history for further confirmation. A family or personal medical history of diabetes (non-insulin-dependent type), hypertension, or high blood cholesterol indicates the need for weight loss.

4. Choose a goal weight within the safe range. Answering the following questions should help you to determine where, within the safe range, your personal appropriate weight may be:

   □ Does your occupation demand that you have a certain body shape? Record the weight, within the safe range, that would most nearly approximate this body shape: _____ pounds.

   □ Do you engage in a sport or other physical activity that requires a particular body weight for optimal performance? Consult your instructor or other expert in that sport or activity, and record the weight recommended on that basis: _____ pounds.

   □ Do you hope to start a pregnancy soon? If so, consult your health care provider as to the ideal weight with which to begin a pregnancy:
   _____ pounds.

   □ Undress and stand before a mirror. Do you think you need to gain or lose weight? Add or subtract pounds from your current weight to arrive at a personal goal weight (but be sure to stay within the safe range): _____ pounds.

Now choose a goal weight, giving consideration to each of the weights you just listed above. No formula exists for this estimate: you decide, but don't choose a weight outside the safe range.

YOUR GOAL WEIGHT: _____ POUNDS

■══════■══════════■

Rule-of-Thumb Method of Estimating "Ideal" Weight

To estimate a woman's ideal weight by a quick method, give the height of 5 feet (barefooted) an ideal weight of 100 pounds. For every inch above 5 feet, add 5 pounds. Thus a woman who is 5 feet 4 inches tall would add 20 pounds (4 inches times 5 pounds per inch)

to 100 pounds, making her ideal weight 120 pounds.

For a man, start with 110 pounds at 5 feet, and add 5 pounds per inch above 5 feet. Thus a 6-foot man would have an ideal weight of 170 pounds: $110 + (12 \times 5)$.

---

least use the guideline that your weight should fall within the range that supports your health. Within that range, the weight to pick is up to you. Your own standards are important.

≡▶ *The body weight that is appropriate for a person depends on the person's frame size, body fat distribution, gender, occupation, activities, and health status. Standards based on height or body mass index provide rough approximations of appropriate weight.*

■≡ The Mystery of Obesity

Why do some people get fat? Why do some get thin? And how do some people, amazingly, stay at the same weight year after year?

In general, two schools of thought attempt to explain differences among people's tendencies concerning their weight. One school attributes weight tendencies to inherited metabolic causes and the other school, to behaviors learned from environmental influences. The two views are not mutually exclusive, and both are usually operating, even in the same person. Furthermore, even behavior patterns can have a genetic basis.

Family tendencies are strong in obesity development. For a person who has one parent with a weight problem, the chance of becoming obese is 60 percent; if both parents have weight problems, the probability rises to 90 percent.[6] While this might at first glance seem to support the genetic school of thought, remember that families also not only pass on hereditary traits but also teach behaviors to their children. No doubt, parents who consistently overfeed children on rich snack foods or who permit unlimited television time instead of outdoor play are teaching behaviors that incur obesity.[7]

Genetic theories of obesity are based on the understanding that metabolism, determined by genetic inheritance, varies from person to person. These differences may underlie some people's tendencies to gain fat. One such theory, the **set-point theory,** states that somehow the body chooses a weight that it wants to be and defends that weight by regulating eating behaviors and hormonal actions. The set-point regulators may be appetite control centers in the brain, or possibly controls of fuel-burning activity in

set-point theory the theory that the body tends to maintain a certain weight by means of inherited internal controls and that obesity reflects malfunction of these controls.

body tissues, or both. Researchers suspect that normal weight reflects normal functioning of these set-point regulators and that obesity reflects poor functioning of these regulators.

In contrast, one environmental theory holds that obesity is controlled by environmental stimuli: that people overeat as a response to their surroundings—foremost among them, the availability of a multitude of delectable foods.[8] People who eat at mealtimes even though they aren't hungry, who clean their plates even though they are satisfied sooner, and who partake of food "because it is there" are responding to environmental influences. This is the **external cue theory**—the theory that, at least in some people, outside-the-body factors override internal regulatory systems.

One way researchers have attempted to study what makes people overeat is to investigate **hunger** and **appetite.** Hunger is a drive programmed into us by our heredity. Appetite, which is learned, can teach us to ignore hunger or to overrespond to it. Hunger is physiological, while appetite is psychological, and the two do not always coincide. Some overeaters claim they never feel full. Perhaps because eating can relieve emotional distress, some people overeat not when they are hungry but when they are lonely, bored, or depressed. For an emotionally insecure person, eating when lonely may be less threatening than calling a friend and risking rejection.

One other cause of obesity stands out—lack of physical activity. The control of appetite appears to work well in most healthy, active people; few athletes are obese. But appetite control often fails when activity falls below a certain minimum level. Some obese people eat less than lean people, but they are so extraordinarily inactive that they still manage to have an energy surplus.

Whatever the causes of obesity, it seems clear that prevention is the best solution: not to get fat in the first place. That means adopting lifestyle habits that will promote fitness and appropriate weight from very early in life. And that in turn means that parents and teachers have to be aware of the threat of obesity and willing to put effort into warding it off in children. Most elementary school teachers believe that schools should emphasize healthy eating styles and physical activity more than they do now.[9]

Once obesity has set in, treatment must approach the problem from many angles and address many facets. Foremost among those facets are food choices themselves, physical activity, and responses to environmental stimuli that prompt people to eat. The later section, Weight-Loss Strategies, does just that.

≡▶ *Causes of obesity appear to be both genetic and environmental, and include learned behaviors. Lack of physical activity is a major contributor to obesity.*

■≡ Energy Balance

Whatever theories account for it, some people in the real world are too fat and some are too thin, and the ultimate cause of both is always an unbalanced energy budget.

A day's energy balance can be stated like this:

Change in energy (fat and glycogen) stores equals food energy taken in minus energy spent on metabolic and voluntary muscle activities.

---

external cue theory   the theory that some people eat in response to such external factors as the presence of food or the time of day rather than in response to such internal factors as hunger.

hunger   defined in Chapter 5, the physiological need to eat, experienced as a drive for obtaining food; an unpleasant sensation.

appetite   also defined in Chapter 5, the psychological desire to eat; a learned motivation and a positive sensation.

More simply:

Change in energy stores = energy in − energy out.

People who are too fat have eaten more energy, and people who are too thin, less energy, than they have spent.

Energy Intake

Food energy consumed in a day is the only contributor to the energy intake side of the energy balance equation. Before you can decide how much food energy you need in a day, you must first become familiar with the amounts of energy in foods.

The energy in foods is listed in calories in tables like the ones in this book's Appendix F. Scientists have determined these food energy values by burning foods under controlled conditions and measuring the heat they give off. (When burned, a food releases all of its energy as heat.) The number of calories in a food depends on the amount of each of the energy nutrients the food contains (see margin note). As examples of the numbers of calories associated with foods, an apple provides you with 125 calories; an average candy bar, with 425 calories.

≡▶ *Energy intake must balance with energy output if body weight is to remain constant. Food is the only contributor to energy intake.*

Energy Output

Whether you are sleeping and spending energy only on your ongoing activities of breathing and heartbeats, or whether you are engaging in additional physical activity, the energy you are spending is the energy you have gained from food. As examples of amounts of calories spent, for a 150-pound person, 20 minutes spent walking briskly uses up about 100 calories; 20 minutes spent jogging uses about 200 calories.

Food energy you consume and do *not* spend in activity, you store in body glycogen and fat—mostly fat. You may already know that for each 3,500 calories you eat in excess of expenditures, you store approximately 1 pound of body fat.*

As long as your energy intake from food equals the energy you put out in activities, your weight will stay the same. You eat, then, to meet your energy need.

It is not easy to determine the energy needs of individuals. The RDA (Appendix B) lists recommended energy intakes for various age-gender groups, but the ranges listed are so broad that you can't guess your personal needs from them. To narrow the range, consider some factors about yourself: your lifestyle, personal attributes, and activity levels all affect how much energy you need.

To estimate your total energy expenditure, you must first estimate its two major components and then add them together. The first component is the energy spent on **basal metabolism.** To calculate the energy spent on basal metabolism, use the factor 1.0 calorie per kilogram of body weight per hour

Average energy values of the energy-yielding nutrients and alcohol:

  1 g carbohydrate = 4 cal.

  1 g fat = 9 cal.

  1 g protein = 4 cal.

  1 g alcohol = 7 cal.

1 lb body fat = 3,500 cal.

basal metabolism the sum total of all the involuntary activities that are necessary to sustain life, including respiration, circulation, and new tissue synthesis and excluding digestion and voluntary activities. Basal metabolism accounts for the largest component of the average person's daily energy expenditure. It is measured while lying down, while awake, and at least 12 hours after eating.

*Pure fat is worth 9 cal per gram. A pound of it (450 g), then, would store 4,050 calories. A pound of body fat is not pure fat, though; it contains water, protein, and other materials, hence the lower energy value.

for men or 0.9 for women (men usually have more muscles than do women, and muscles use more energy than other tissues). Example (for a 150-pound man):

1. Change pounds to kilograms:
   150 pounds divided by 2.2 pounds per kilogram = 68 kilograms.
2. Multiply weight in kilograms by the basal metabolism factor:
   68 kilograms times 1 calorie per kilogram per hour = 68 calories per hour.
3. Multiply the calories used in one hour by the hours in a day:
   68 calories per hour times 24 hours per day = 1,632 calories per day.

The man in our example spends 1,632 calories on his basal metabolic activity each day.

The second major component of your energy expenditure is the energy you spend on **voluntary activities.** The following figures are crude approximations of the amounts of energy people spend on voluntary activities. They are based on the amounts of muscular work different people typically perform in a day:

■ Sedentary: men, 25 to 40% of basal metabolic energy; women, 25 to 35%.
■ Light activity: men, 50 to 70% of basal metabolic energy; women, 40 to 60%.
■ Moderate activity: men, 65 to 80% of basal metabolic energy; women, 50 to 70%.
■ Heavy activity: men, 90 to 120% of basal metabolic energy; women, 80 to 100%.
■ Exceptional activity: men, 130 to 145% of basal metabolic energy; women, 110 to 130%.*

To select the activity level appropriate for you, remember to think in terms of the amount of *muscular* work performed; don't confuse being *busy* with being *active.* If you sit down most of the day and drive or ride whenever possible, use the value for a sedentary person. If you move around some of the time, as a teacher or salesperson might during working hours, use the light activity values. If you do some amount of exercise, such as an hour of jogging four or five times a week, or if your occupation calls for some physical work, consider yourself moderately active. A person whose job requires much physical labor, such as a roofer or a carpenter, would be in the heavy activity range. The exceptional activity category is reserved for those few who spend many hours a day in intense physical training, such as professional or college athletes during their sport seasons.

Each energy amount is given as a range—for example, a lightly active man spends, on voluntary activities, about 50 to 70 percent of the amount of energy he spends on basal metabolism. Perform calculations for both extremes to obtain the range of energy intakes appropriate for you. If the 150-pound man we used for an example were lightly active, we could estimate the range of energy he needed for voluntary activities as follows:

1,632 cal/day (basal metabolic energy) × 50% = 816 cal/day.

1,632 cal/day × 70% = 1,142 cal/day.

The man needs from 816 to 1,142 calories per day for his voluntary activities.

voluntary activities   activities (such as walking, sitting, running) conducted by voluntary muscles.

Light activity, for both women and men, means sleeping or lying down for eight hours a day, sitting for seven hours, standing for five, walking for two, and spending two hours a day in light physical activity.

*Percentages derived from the RDA (1989) formula for energy expenditure, accurate within about 20% of total calories.

Now total the two components. The man in our example spends 1,632 calories on basal metabolism, and 816 to 1,142 calories on voluntary activity in a day:

1,632 cal/day + 816 cal/day = 2,448 cal/day.

1,632 cal/day + 1,142 cal/day = 2,774 cal/day.

Express the man's needs as a range (rounded): 2,450 to 2,770 calories per day. On average, he needs about 2,600 calories per day.

This calculation takes care of average daily energy expenditures.* Some college students find, though, that it doesn't account for energy they spend occasionally on vigorous exertions such as 2 hours of handball or a 4-hour basketball practice. To estimate calories for special exercise beyond the averages usually spent, refer to Table 6–1. (If your sport isn't listed in the table, pick one similar to it in the intensity and duration of exertion required.)

As an example, suppose our 150-pound man engaged in 3 hours of bicycling (average, 15 miles per hour) once every weekend. He would calculate this extra energy expenditure as follows:

150 lb × .049 cal/lb/min = 7.35 cal/min.

7.35 cal/min × 180 min = 1,323 cal.

In addition to the energy this man spends on basal metabolism and daily physical activities, he spends 1,323 calories a week bicycling. This, averaged over 7 days, adds 189 calories to his daily energy need. His total energy needs per day, then, must average about 2,600 plus 189, or 2,789—say, 2,800—calories a day.

≡▶ *Energy output can be calculated by adding three amounts together: energy spent on basal metabolism, energy spent on physical activity, and energy spent for unusual exercise beyond the average usually spent.*

■≡ Weight Gain and Loss

The balance between the food energy you take in and the energy you spend on activity determines whether you will gain, lose, or maintain body fat. (For fun, Table 6–2 translates some activity values into food energy terms.) However, when you step on the scale and note that you weigh a pound or two more or less than you did the last time you weighed, this may not indicate that you have gained or lost body fat. A change in body weight may reflect shifts in body fluid content, in bone minerals, or in lean tissues such as muscles. It may also reflect the amount of undigested food in your system; that's why people generally weigh the least before breakfast. It is important for people concerned with weight control to realize that quick, large changes in weight are usually not changes in fat alone, or even at all.

A person who stands about 5 feet 10 inches tall and who weighs 150 pounds carries about 90 of those pounds as water and 30 as fat. The other

■ *FACT OR FICTION:* The dieter who sees a large weight loss on the scale can take this as a sign of success. *False.* A weight loss may reflect loss of water, bone minerals, or lean tissue rather than loss of fat.

---

*The amount of energy spent digesting food is not included either in basal metabolic energy or in voluntary activity energy, but amounts to about 10% added to the sum of the two. For purposes of rough estimation of energy needs such as that demonstrated here, the energy spent digesting food can be ignored.

TABLE 6–1 ■ **Energy Demands of Activities**

Activity	Energy Required	Body Weight (lb)				
		110	125	150	175	200
	(cal/lb/min)[a]	(cal/min)				
Aerobic dance (vigorous)	0.062	6.8	7.8	9.3	10.9	12.4
Basketball (vigorous, full court)	0.097	10.7	12.1	14.6	17.0	19.4
Bicycling						
13 mph	0.045	5.0	5.6	6.8	7.9	9.0
15 mph	0.049	5.4	6.1	7.4	8.6	9.8
17 mph	0.057	6.3	7.1	8.6	10.0	11.4
19 mph	0.076	8.4	9.5	11.4	13.3	15.2
21 mph	0.090	9.9	11.3	13.5	15.8	18.0
23 mph	0.109	12.0	13.6	16.4	19.0	21.8
25 mph	0.139	15.3	17.4	20.9	24.3	27.8
Canoeing (flat water, moderate pace)	0.045	5.0	5.6	6.8	7.9	9.0
Cross-country skiing (8 mph)	0.104	11.4	13.0	15.6	18.2	20.8
Golf (carrying clubs)	0.045	5.0	5.6	6.8	7.9	9.0
Handball	0.078	8.6	9.8	11.7	13.7	15.6
Horseback riding (trot)	0.052	5.7	6.5	7.8	9.1	10.4
Rowing (vigorous)	0.097	10.7	12.1	14.6	17.0	19.4
Running						
5 mph	0.061	6.7	7.6	9.2	10.7	12.2
6 mph	0.074	8.1	9.2	11.1	13.0	14.8
7.5 mph	0.094	10.3	11.8	14.1	16.4	18.8
9 mph	0.103	11.3	12.9	15.5	18.0	20.6
10 mph	0.114	12.5	14.3	17.1	20.0	22.9
11 mph	0.131	14.4	16.4	19.7	22.9	26.2
Soccer (vigorous)	0.097	10.7	12.1	14.6	17.0	19.4
Studying	0.011	1.2	1.4	1.7	1.9	2.2
Swimming						
20 yd/min	0.032	3.5	4.0	4.8	5.6	6.4
45 yd/min	0.058	6.4	7.3	8.7	10.2	11.6
50 yd/min	0.070	7.7	8.8	10.5	12.3	14.0
Table tennis (skilled)	0.045	5.0	5.6	6.8	7.9	9.0
Tennis (beginner)	0.032	3.5	4.0	4.8	5.6	6.4
Walking (brisk pace)						
3.5 mph	0.035	3.9	4.4	5.2	6.1	7.0
4.5 mph	0.048	5.3	6.0	7.2	8.4	9.6

[a]To calculate calories spent per minute of activity for your own body weight, multiply calories/pound/minute by your exact weight, and then multiply that number by the number of minutes spent in the activity. For example, if you weigh 142 lb, and you want to know how many calories you spent doing 30 min of vigorous aerobic dance: 0.062 × 142 = 8.8 cal/min. 8.8 × 30 (min) = 264 total calories spent.

SOURCE: Adapted in part with permission from The Consumers Union of the United States, *Physical Fitness for Practically Everybody: The Consumers Union Report on Exercise* (Mt. Vernon, N.Y.: Consumers Union, 1983), and from G. P. Town and K. B. Wheeler, Nutritional concerns for the endurance athlete, *Dietetic Currents* 13 (1986): 7–12.

30 pounds are the so-called lean tissues—muscles; organs such as the heart, brain, and liver; and the bones of the skeleton.* Stripped of water and fat, then, the person weighs only 30 pounds! This lean tissue is vital to health. The person who seeks to lose weight wants, of course, to lose fat, not this precious lean tissue. And for someone who wants to gain weight, it is desirable to gain lean and fat in proportion, not just fat.

*For a healthy person, 5 feet tall, who weighs 100 pounds, the comparable figures would be 60 pounds of water, 20 pounds of fat, and 20 pounds of lean.

TABLE 6–2 ■ **Activity Equivalents of Food Energy Values**

| Food | Calories | Activity Equivalent for a 150-lb Person to Work Off the Calories (minutes) | | |
		Walk[a]	Run[b]	Wait[c]
Apple, large	125	24	8	75
Regular beer, 1 glass (8 oz)	100	19	6	61
Cookie, chocolate chip	50	10	3	30
Ice cream, 1/2 c	175	34	11	106
Steak, T-bone (6 oz)	475	91	31	288

[a]Energy cost of walking at 3.5 mph: 5.2 cal/min.
[b]Energy cost of running at 9 miles per hour: 15.5 cal/min.
[c]Energy cost of sitting: 1.65 cal/min.

The type of tissue gained or lost depends on how the person goes about gaining or losing it. Some ways of losing weight are dangerous. To lose fluid, for example, one can take a "water pill" (diuretic), causing the kidneys to siphon extra water from the blood into the urine. Or one can engage in heavy exercise while wearing thick clothing in the heat, and lose abundant fluid in sweat—another dangerous practice. To gain water weight, a person can overconsume salt and water; for a few hours the body will then retain water, until it manages to excrete the salt. (This, too, is not recommended.) Most quick-weight-loss diets promote large fluid losses that register temporary, dramatic changes on the scale but that accomplish little loss of body fat. Worse, they also promote breakdown of lean tissue. A later section on strategy stresses physical activity as a recommended means of maintaining lean tissue during weight loss.

Weight Gain and Gradual Weight Loss

Weight gain comes from eating more food energy than you spend. As mentioned, the body stores the excess partly in glycogen, mostly in fat. The energy-yielding nutrients contribute to body stores as follows:

■ Carbohydrate (other than fiber) is broken down to sugars for absorption. In the body tissues, these may be built up to *glycogen* or converted to *fat* and stored.
■ Fat is broken down to glycerol and fatty acids for absorption. Inside the body, these are especially easy for the body to store as *fat* in fat tissue.
■ Protein is broken down to amino acids for absorption. Inside the body, these may be used to replace lost body *protein* and, in a person who is exercising, to build new muscle and other lean tissue. But excess protein cannot be stored as protein. To keep it in the form of protein, the eater needed to put it to use. Any excess amino acids have their nitrogens removed and are converted to *fat*.

Note that although three kinds of energy-yielding nutrients enter the body, they become energy stores only as glycogen and fat. Alcohol also becomes fat if it isn't burned off. Glycogen stores amount to about three-fourths of a pound; fat stores can, of course, amount to many pounds. Note, too, that when excess protein is converted to fat, it cannot be recovered later as protein, because the nitrogen is stripped from it and excreted in the urine.

No matter whether you are receiving your protein by eating steak, brownies, cereal, or baked beans, then, if you eat enough calories of them, any excess protein will be turned to fat within hours.

Some new research suggests that the fat content of food may be more important to body fatness than total calories of food.[10] This makes sense when you consider that fat from food is stored in the body virtually unchanged, with its maximum energy content intact. Carbohydrate, on the other hand, must be dismantled and reassembled into fat before storage, and the chemical labor required to perform these conversions costs energy. Thus after eating 100 calories of fat the body can store a net value of 100 calories, but after eating 100 calories of carbohydrate, the body may net only 75. The total stored energy from excess fat, its "fattening power," is probably greater than researchers once believed; and carbohydrate's "fattening power" is probably far less.

Whether energy values assigned to foods will change to reflect these new understandings is for the future to tell, but you can apply what is known today. If weight gain is your goal, try to choose generous quantities of nutritious foods that provide both fat (mostly unsaturated fat) and carbohydrate as well as protein. If, on the other hand, you wish to lose weight, concentrate on choosing foods with the smallest possible amount of fat, and seek to obtain the calories you need mostly from protein-containing and carbohydrate-rich foods. This may be harder than you think; as the last chapter showed, fat is abundant in the U.S. food supply, and it takes diligence to strip it out of your diet.

It is worth emphasizing these points by repeating them:

■ Any food can make you fat if you eat enough of it. A net excess of energy is stored in the body as fat in fat tissue.
■ Fat from food is especially easy for the body to store as fat tissue.
■ Protein is not stored in the body except in response to exercise; it is present only as working tissue.* Some working protein tissue is lost each day and can be replaced only by protein eaten that day. Excess protein is converted and stored as fat.

When you moderately restrict your calories and consume an otherwise balanced diet, your body will be forced to use some of its stored fat for energy. Gradual weight loss will occur. This is preferred to rapid weight loss, because it spares lean body mass and promotes loss of fat. (You can lose *weight* faster on a total fast, but you can lose *fat* faster on a low-calorie diet.)

▤▶ *To gain weight, add to your diet nutritious foods that contain both fat and carbohydrate. To lose weight, avoid fat-containing foods, moderately restrict energy intake, and eat a balanced diet.*

Rapid Weight Loss

Rapid weight loss, by means of fasting or severely restricting food intake, is not advised. If a person doesn't eat for, say, three whole days or a week, then the body makes one adjustment after another. After about a day, the

---

*Amino acids are present in all body fluids, performing such functions as maintaining the acid-base balance there. The liver is considered by some to be an amino acid storage site.

liver's glycogen is essentially exhausted. Where, then, can the body obtain glucose to keep its nervous system going? Not from the muscles' glycogen, because that is reserved for the muscles' own use. The underfed body must begin to feed on the protein in its own lean tissues.

An alternative source of energy might be the abundant fat stores most people carry, but at this stage these are of no use to the nervous system. The muscles and other organs use fat as fuel, but the nervous system cannot. Most importantly, the body's major fuel, fat, cannot be converted to glucose—the body possesses no enzymes to carry out this conversion.* The body does, however, possess enzymes that can convert protein to glucose. Figure 6–1 reviews how energy is used during both feasting and fasting.

If the body were to continue to consume its lean tissue unchecked, death would ensue within about ten days. After all, not only skeletal muscle but also the liver, the heart muscle, the lung tissue, and the blood cells—all vital tissues—are being burned as fuel. (In fact, fasting or starving people remain alive only until their stores of fat are gone or until half their lean tissue is gone, whichever comes first.) To prevent this, the body plays its last ace: it begins converting fat into ketone compounds that the nervous system can adapt to use and so forestall the end. This is **ketosis.**

In ketosis, ketone compounds circulate in the bloodstream and help to feed the brain, since about half of the brain's cells can make the enzymes needed to use them for energy. Within a few weeks the brain can meet most of its energy needs using this new fuel. Thus indirectly the nervous system begins to feed on the body's fat stores, and this reduces the demand for glucose and the depletion of lean tissue. Thanks to ketosis, a healthy person starting with average body fat content can live totally deprived of food for as long as six to eight weeks.

Fasting has been practiced as a periodic discipline by respected, wise people in many cultures. However, no evidence exists to support the idea that fasting "cleanses" the body, as some believe. Ketosis may harm the body by upsetting the acid-base balance of the blood and by promoting mineral losses in the urine. In addition, people with eating disorders (see

*Glycerol, 5% of fat, can yield glucose but is a negligible source.

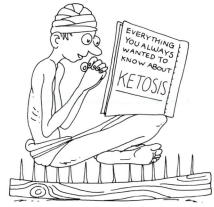

Fasting is an example of how *not* to design a weight-loss diet.

ketosis (kee-TOE-sis)   an adaptation of the body to prolonged fasting or carbohydrate restriction: body fat is converted to ketone bodies, which can be used as fuel for some brain cells.

In early food deprivation:

■ The nervous system cannot use fat as fuel; it can use only glucose.
■ Body fat cannot be converted to glucose.
■ Body protein can be converted to glucose.

FIGURE 6–1 ■ **Feasting and fasting.**

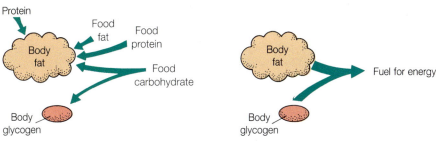

Feasting. Excess energy nutrients from food are mainly stored as fat; a little carbohydrate is stored as glycogen.

Fasting. In times of little food, the body draws on its stored fat and glycogen for the fuel it needs. Note that body stores cannot supply needed protein, even though food protein earlier might have contributed to body fat.

Spotlight) often report that a fast or a bout of severely restricted dieting heralded the beginning of their loss of control over eating. For the person who merely wants to lose weight, fasting is usually not the best way.

≡▶   *When a person fasts or restricts food too severely, the body devours its own lean body tissue to supply the brain with glucose. In time, the body also begins making ketone bodies from fat to feed the brain, but still uses lean tissue as well. Efforts to lose weight rapidly are ill-advised.*

■≡ Weight-Loss Strategies

Although a few people wish to gain weight, and some are satisfied where they are, most desire to lose. How can a person lose weight safely and permanently? The secret is a sensible approach (we didn't say *easy*) that combines diet, physical activity, and behavior modification. It takes tremendous dedication, especially at first, for a person whose habits have all promoted obesity to substitute the hundred or so new behaviors that promote thinness. When people succeed, they do so because they have employed many of the techniques described in this chapter.[11]

To emphasize the personal nature of weight-loss plans, the following sections are written as advice to "you." This is intended to give you the illusion of listening in on a conversation in which an overweight person is being competently counseled by someone familiar with the techniques known to be effective.

Diet

Central to any weight-control plan is diet, and the key to planning a diet *is* control: yours. You are the one who will have to live with the meals, so you had better plan them. If you want to follow a commercial program, choose one that will help you take responsibility, not one that takes it from you. Go to Weight Watchers or a similar program; do not get involved in a scam. The Critical Thinking section that follows and Table 6–3 spell out clues to scams.

No particular diet is magical, and no particular food must be either included or avoided. Don't think of yourself as going "on" a diet, because then you may be tempted to go "off." Think of yourself as adopting an eating plan for life. The plan must consist of foods that you like or can learn to like, that are available to you, and that are within your means.

To be successful, people must first lose weight and then maintain the weight loss. If you adopt an "eating plan" rather than a "diet," you can be practicing maintenance behaviors all the time you are losing weight. You will be ready to succeed for the rest of your life, once you arrive at your goal weight.

Choose a calorie level you can live with. A deficit of 500 calories a day for seven days is a 3,500-calorie deficit—enough to lose a pound of body fat. It is best to do this by both increasing activity and reducing food intake. A rule of thumb for setting the lower limit to your calorie intake is that you need to eat at least 10 calories for each pound of your current weight each day. There is no point in hurrying, because you will never go off the plan—and adequate nutrient intakes can't be achieved on too few calories.

Make your meals adequate. This is a way of putting yourself first. "I like me, and I'm going to take good care of me" is the attitude to adopt. This

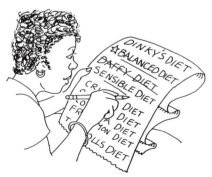

The cautious consumer distinguishes between loss of fat and loss of weight.

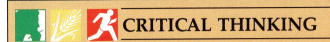

CRITICAL THINKING

Weight-Loss Scams

One survey of 29,000 weight-loss strategies found fewer than 6 percent of them effective—and 13 percent dangerous.[12] People often ask, "Can't the government do something about that?" The government is active in pursuing and cracking down on health swindles, but most agencies have insufficient staff and resources to handle the massive number of reported cases. They can, at best, eliminate only the most dangerous schemes. This results in a free market for other promoters who can rake in billions of dollars on products that are only slightly less dangerous than the worst ones. It is easy for a swindler to get a product on the market and hard for the government or other groups to get it off. That puts the burden of distinguishing frauds from reality on you, the consumer. To keep from getting taken in, remember: If a weight-loss claim sounds too good to be true, it probably is.

If a weight-loss claim sounds too good to be true, it probably is.

means including low-calorie foods that are rich in valuable nutrients: tasty vegetables and fruits; whole-grain breads and cereals; modest portions of lean protein-rich foods like poultry, fish, and eggs; nutritious meat alternates like dried beans and peas; and low-fat milk products such as nonfat milk and yogurt. A recommended pattern to follow is the Daily Food Choices pattern in Chapter 5. A plan that uses the minimum servings suggested by that pattern, without frills, and allows a teaspoon of added fat at each meal provides about 1,200 calories. A 120-pound person could lose weight at a satisfactory rate following such a plan without failing to meet all nutrient needs satisfactorily. Within each food category, learn what foods you like, and use them often. If you plan resolutely to include a certain number of servings of food from each group each day, you may be so busy making sure you get what you need that you will have little time or appetite left for high-calorie or empty-calorie foods.

Slow down when you eat. The signal that you are full is sent after a 20-minute lag, so unless you slow down, you can eat a great deal more than you need before the signal reaches your brain. Foods such as vegetables and whole grains (carbohydrate- and fiber-rich foods) require more chewing than high-sugar or high-fat foods, so they can help you to eat more slowly. Besides, crunchy, wholesome foods offer bulk and satisfy the appetite for far fewer calories than smooth, refined foods. People who eat crunchy, fibrous foods in abundance have been observed to spontaneously eat for longer times and to eat a fourth to a third fewer calories than when eating foods of high calorie density.[13] This switch alone, consistently made, can enable you to reduce your energy intake by 500 or so calories a day. You can eat until you are full and never miss the foods you've omitted.

Measure your dietary fat with extra caution. A slip of the butter knife adds many more calories than a slip of the sugar spoon. Remember that fat may contribute more to body fatness than once believed. Of two diets that offer the same number of calories, the one with less fat will put less fat on the body.[14]

TABLE 6–3 ■ **Clues to Weight-Loss Scams**

---

1. Promises dramatic, rapid weight loss (i.e., substantially more than 1% of total body weight per week).
2. Promotes diets that are extremely low in calories (i.e., below 800 cal/day; diets of 1,200 cal/day preferred) unless under the supervision of competent medical experts.
3. Attempts to make clients dependent upon special products rather than teaching how to make good choices from the conventional food supply (this does not condemn the marketing of low-calorie convenience foods that may be chosen by consumers).
4. Fails to encourage permanent, realistic lifestyle changes, including regular exercise and the behavioral aspects of eating wherein food may be used as a coping device (i.e., programs should focus upon changing the causes of over-weight rather than simply changing the effect, which is the overweight itself).
5. Misrepresents of salespeople as "counselors" supposedly qualified to give guidance in nutrition and/or general health. Even if adequately trained, such "counselors" would still be biased, because they profit directly from products they recommend and sell.
6. Collects large sums of money at the start or requirement that clients sign contracts for expensive, long-term programs. Such practices too often have been abused, as salespeople focus attention upon signing up new people rather than upon delivering continuing, satisfactory service to consumers. Programs should be on a pay-as-you-go basis.
7. Fails to inform clients about the risks associated with weight loss in general or with the specific program being promoted.
8. Promotes unproved or spurious weight-loss aids such as low-carbohydrate diets, water pills, diet pills,[a] expanding pills, body wraps, spa belts and rollers, spa saunas and whirlpools, massages, muscle stimulators, hormones, glucomannan, laxatives, bee pollen, spirulina, lipectomy and suctioning, bypass surgery, stomach stapling, or gastric balloon.
9. Claims that "cellulite" exists in the body.
10. Claims that use of an appetite suppressant or methylcellulose (a "bulking agent") enables a person to lose body fat without restricting accustomed caloric intake.
11. Claims that a weight-control product contains a unique ingredient or component unless it is unavailable in other weight-control products.

---

[a]Including over-the-counter preparations such as phenylpropanolamine and prescriptions such as amphetamines.

SOURCE: Reprinted with permission from *National Council Against Health Fraud Newsletter,* March/April 1987, National Council Against Health Fraud, Inc.

Learn to satisfy your thirst with water. Overeaters often use food to satisfy thirst (food provides water, as you may recall). Instead, drink plenty of water. A generous water intake will do several things for you. It will meet the water need that you formerly met by eating extra food. It will help to fill your stomach between meals, keep your mouth happy, and keep you busy. It will also help you to excrete the waste products of fat breakdown. These waste products are moving out of your fat cells, where the fat has been stored, into your bloodstream, which must deliver them, along with some water, to your kidneys for excretion. Drinking water is a calorie-free plea-sure; cultivate it enthusiastically.

At first it may seem as if you have to spend all your waking hours think-ing about and planning your meals. Such a massive effort is always required when a new skill is being learned. (You spent hours practicing writing the alphabet when you were in the first grade.) Although it is hard at first, after about three weeks, planning your meals will be much easier. Use positive imaging: see yourself as a person who "eats thin." Your new eating pattern will become a habit.

Do not weigh yourself more than every week or two. Gains or losses of a pound or more in a matter of days reverse themselves quickly; a smoothed-out average is what is real. Don't expect to lose continuously as fast as you did at first. A sizable water loss is common in the first week, but it will not happen again. If you have been working out lately, occasional weighings may show no loss, or even a gain. This may reflect a welcome development: the gain of lean body mass—just what you want, if you want to be healthy.

If you slip, don't punish yourself. Positive reinforcement is effective in changing behavior, but punishment seldom works. If you ate an extra 1,000 calories yesterday, don't try to eat 1,000 fewer calories today; it will only propel you into overeating again and set up an endless cycle. Just go back to your plan. On the other hand, you can plan ahead and budget for special occasions. If you want to celebrate your birthday with cake and ice cream, cut a few calories from your bread and milk allowances for several days *beforehand*. Enjoy your treats, then get right back on your plan, and your weight loss will be as smooth as if you had stayed with the daily plan.

If you stop losing weight or start gaining unexpectedly, you may have to get tough with yourself. Ask yourself honestly (no one is listening in), "What am I doing wrong?" Seldom does an unpredicted weight plateau of any duration have no explanation in the dieter's own choices.

Finally, if you stop losing weight or begin to gain, be aware that you may be choosing that course. Your behavior is under your control. Rather than feeling guilty or like a failure, hold your head high and take the attitude, "This is me, and this is the way I am choosing to be right now."

From start to finish, the making of a diet plan must meet the dieter's own needs as well as possible. The pointers given here are summed up in Table 6–4.

TABLE 6–4 ■ **Diet Planning Guidelines**

1. Be involved in planning your own program.
2. Keep in mind that you will want to maintain your lost weight. Practice the needed behaviors as you go.
3. Adopt a realistic plan.
4. Make your meals adequate by emphasizing high-nutrient-density foods that you like.
5. Eat slowly.
6. Make tasty vegetables and fruits central in your meals.
7. Select foods rich in complex carbohydrates and high in bulk.
8. Select low-fat foods regularly.
9. Drink plenty of water.
10. Visualize a changed future self.
11. Take well-spaced weighings to avoid discouragement.
12. Use positive reinforcement. Never blame, never punish.
13. Be honest with yourself.
14. Stress personal responsibility.
15. Maintain self-esteem.

≡▶ *A successful weight-loss program centers on a well-planned diet. In making one, meet personal needs, both for good nutrition and for enjoyment, as creatively as possible.*

Physical Activity

Accompanying diet in successful weight control is physical activity. Activity directly increases energy output. Remember Table 6–1, which shows the calorie costs of each of several activities.

Activity also contributes to energy output in an indirect way—by increasing basal metabolism. It does this in two ways—one today, and the other over the long term. Today, if you exercise vigorously (for an hour, for example), your metabolism may stay speeded up for several hours afterwards, even overnight. That will make a small contribution toward the loss of the pound you are currently working to lose. Over the long term, if you keep repeating such vigorous activity daily for many weeks, your body composition will gradually change to favor more lean tissue. Your metabolic rate will rise accordingly, because lean tissue is more active metabolically than fat tissue—and that, over still more time, will make a contribution toward continued weight loss or maintenance of a healthy weight. The more lean tissue you develop, the more calories you spend, and the more you can afford to eat. Eating more brings you both pleasure and nutrients. Exercise continues to maintain your raised metabolic rate for as long as you keep your body conditioned.

Another thing activity helps with is appetite control. People think that exercising will make them hungry, but this is not entirely true. Yes, active people do have healthy appetites, but immediately after a good workout, most people do not feel like eating. They want to shower; they may be thirsty; but they are not hungry. The reason is that the body has responded to the stress of exercise by mobilizing fuels from storage—glucose and fatty acids are abundant in the blood. (A physiologist would say the body is in a "fed state.") At the same time, the body has suppressed its digestive functions. Hard physical work and eating are not compatible. You must calm down, put your fuels back in storage, and relax before you can eat. Thus exercise helps curb appetite—especially the inappropriate appetite that accompanies boredom, anxiety, or depression, which might prompt you to eat when you really do not need to. (Weight-control programs encourage you to go out and exercise when you're tempted to eat, but not really hungry. It will fill your time, improve your mood, and curb your misguided appetite. Later, when true hunger comes, it will be appropriate to eat.)

Activity also helps reduce stress, as earlier chapters have shown. Since stress, too, is a cue to inappropriate eating behavior for many people, activity can help here, too.

Activity offers still more psychological benefits. The fit person looks and feels healthy, and high self-esteem accompanies these benefits. High self-esteem tends to support a person's resolve to persist in a weight-control effort, rounding out a beneficial cycle.

Weight loss *without* exercise can have a negative effect on body composition. A person who diets without exercising loses both lean and fat tissue, as described earlier. Now suppose the person then regains weight without exercising; the gain will be mostly fat. Finally, suppose the person eats the same amount as before. Because fat tissue burns fewer calories to maintain

■ *FACT OR FICTION:* If an inactive person takes up a daily hour of exercise, the person will end up spending more calories all day, even during sleep. *True.*

Benefits of physical activity in a weight-control program:

Increased expenditure of energy today (including metabolic energy).

Long-term increase (slight) in resting metabolic rate.

Control of inappropriate eating urges.

Stress reduction.

Physical, and therefore psychological, well-being.

High self-esteem.

itself, the person's weight will zoom higher than before, the **ratchet effect,** or **yo-yo effect,** of dieting without exercise (Figure 6–2).

Clearly, then, physical activity is a beneficial part of a weight-control program. What kind of physical activity is best? For the person seeking to *lose* weight, the activities that burn the most *fat*, not necessarily the ones that burn the most *calories*, are the ones to choose. The object is not to get thin at the expense of muscle tissue, but to become fit, with loss of fat and toning of muscles. The next chapter continues emphasizing these distinctions.

This all adds up to a recommendation—the best way to use physical activity to enhance weight control is to cultivate balanced fitness—flexibility, strength, and endurance (and these are the topics of the next chapter). Team up proper nutrition with right physical activity, and the desired body composition will follow.

≡▶ *Physical activity is the second component of a successful weight-control program. Engaged in regularly, it helps promote fat loss, maintain lean body mass, reduce stress, and curb appetite.*

Behavior Modification

The person who weighs too much has engaged in a hundred small behaviors of overeating and underexercising every day, many of which have contributed to, and maintain, the weight problem. The person needs to learn to change all of these behaviors—and behavior modification can help. Figure 1–3 in Chapter 1 showed six strategies you could use to modify your behavior; in relation to eating and physical activity, they might be phrased as follows:

1. Eliminate inappropriate eating cues.
2. Suppress the cues you cannot eliminate.
3. Strengthen cues to appropriate eating and activity.
4. Engage in the desired eating and exercise behaviors.
5. Arrange or emphasize negative consequences of inappropriate eating.
6. Arrange or emphasize positive consequences of appropriate eating and exercise behaviors.

The accompanying Strategies: Modifying Behaviors for Weight Loss show how a person might apply these principles in a weight-control program. Before you begin, establish a baseline, which is a record of your present eating behaviors against which to measure future progress. Keep a diary to learn what your particular eating stimuli, or cues, are.

You may find it helpful to join a weight-loss program, to gain support and reinforcement from fellow dieters. Many colleges offer such programs, often in connection with health or nutrition courses. Many worksites also offer programs,[15] as do self-help groups such as TOPS (Take Off Pounds Sensibly) or Overeaters Anonymous, and private organizations such as Weight Watchers. A modest expenditure for your own wellness is worthwhile (but avoid ripoffs, of course). Many dieters find it helpful to form their own self-help groups. If you are especially sensitive to social situations where you feel you have to eat, it will also help to have some assertiveness training. Learning to say "No, thank you" might be one of your first objectives. Learning not to "clean your plate" might be another.

From all the behavior changes available to you, you can choose the ones to begin with. Don't try to master them all at once. No one who attempts too

ratchet effect or **yo-yo effect**   the effect of repeated rounds of dieting without exercise; the person rebounds to a higher weight and higher body fat content at the end of each round.

Thinness is not the same as fitness.

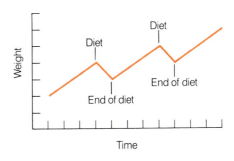

FIGURE 6–2 ■ **The ratchet effect of dieting without exercise.**

Each round of dieting without exercise is followed by a rebound of weight to a higher level than before.

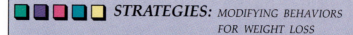

STRATEGIES: *MODIFYING BEHAVIORS FOR WEIGHT LOSS*

1. To eliminate inappropriate eating cues:

   Don't buy problem foods (shop when you are not hungry).

   Don't serve rich sauces and toppings.

   Let your spouse and children buy, store, and serve their own sweets.

   Watch less television; food commercials suggest excessive eating.

   When watching television, change channels or look away during food commercials.

   Shop only from a list, and stay away from convenience stores.

   Carry appropriate snacks from home, and avoid vending machines.

2. To suppress the cues you cannot eliminate:

   Eat only in one place, and in one room.

   Clear plates directly into the garbage or compost.

   Create obstacles to the eating of problem foods (for example, make it necessary to unwrap, cook, and serve each one separately).

   Minimize contact with excessive food (serve individual plates, don't put serving dishes on the table, and leave the table when you are finished).

   Make small portions of food look large (spread food out and serve it on small plates).

   Control states of deprivation (eat regular meals, don't skip meals, avoid getting tired, and avoid boredom by keeping cues to fun activities in sight).

3. To strengthen the cues to appropriate eating and exercise:

   Encourage others to eat appropriate foods with you.

   Keep your favorite appropriate foods in the front of the refrigerator.

   Learn appropriate portion sizes.

   Save permitted foods from meals for snacks (and make these your only snacks).

   Prepare permitted foods attractively.

   Keep your running shoes (hiking boots, tennis racket) by the door.

4. To engage in desired eating or exercise behaviors:

   Slow down when eating (pause for two to three minutes between bites, put down utensils, chew slowly, swallow before reloading the fork, and always use utensils).

   Leave some food on the plate.

   Move more (shake a leg, pace, fidget, or flex your muscles).

   Join in and exercise with a group of active people.

5. To arrange or emphasize negative consequences of inappropriate eating:

   Eat your meals with other people.

   Ask that others respond neutrally to your deviations (make no comment). This is a negative consequence, because it withholds attention.

6. To arrange or emphasize positive consequences of appropriate behaviors:

   Update records of food intake, exercise, and weight change regularly.

   Arrange for rewards for each unit of behavior change or weight loss.

   Ask for social reinforcement (ask to be encouraged).

many changes at one time is successful. Set your own priorities. Pick one trouble area that you think you can handle, start with that, and practice your strategy until it is automatic. Then select another trouble area to work on, and so on.

Enjoy your new, emerging self. Inside every fat person is a fit person struggling to be freed. Get in touch with your fit self, and make that self feel welcome in the light of day.

Finally, be aware that it can be harder to maintain weight loss than to lose the weight. On arriving at the goal weight after months of self-discipline and new habit formation, the victorious weight loser must avoid "celebrating" by resuming old eating habits. They are gone forever—remember? Membership in an ongoing weight-control organization and regular, continued physical activity with others can give indispensable support for the formerly overweight person who wants to remain trim. And see the section on "Weight Maintenance," coming up.

≡▶ *Behavior modification is the third component of a successful weight-control program. Numerous small-step modifications can be useful. Prioritize them and be assertive in carrying them out.*

■≡ Weight-Gain Strategies

It is as hard for a person who tends to be underweight to gain a pound as it is for a person who tends to be overweight to lose one. Like the weight-loser, the person who wants to gain must learn new habits and learn to like new foods.

Here is a special problem. An underweight person must decide, first whether, and then how, to try to gain. To approach the first question: does the underweight represent a healthy or unhealthy state? It is well known that to be slightly under the standard weight, for most people, represents a desirable state. And for most people in their teens and early twenties, especially males, underweight is a temporary state; they simply haven't "filled out" yet, because they are still growing. But if the underweight is due to anorexia nervosa (see "Spotlight: An Obsession with Thinness") or a wasting disease such as tuberculosis or cancer, it may be a dangerous state, and weight gain, if possible, may be indicated. The answer, then, is: If you are healthy at your present weight, stay there; if you are at risk of illness, try to gain. A health care provider's advice can help you to make the distinction.

Some people may wish to gain weight for appearance's sake—provided that the gain is muscle and fat, not just fat. Athletes may wish, or be advised by their coaches, to gain weight to improve their performance. Such people need to be fully aware that a weight gain can be achieved only by physical conditioning combined with a high-calorie diet. A high-calorie diet alone will make a person gain fat only, and even if it makes the appearance more acceptable in the person's own eyes, it is likely to be more detrimental than beneficial to health. Furthermore, some people are unalterably thin by reason of heredity or early environmental influences. Such people find it so difficult to gain weight that it seems not worth the trouble. In increasing food energy intake, such a person might gain some fat and become uncomfortable but would not achieve the desired change in body composition. In an athlete, a weight gain like this might impair performance.

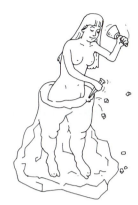

Make your fit self feel welcome in the light of day.

■ *FACT OR FICTION:* It is harder to lose a pound than to gain one. *False.* It is as hard for a person who tends to be thin to gain a pound as it is for a person who tends to be fat to lose one.

Weight gain, like weight loss, is a highly individual matter. In deciding whether to undertake it, be as aware as possible of what your body will permit and tolerate, and be willing to accept what you cannot change.

For the person who wants to gain weight, just as for the one who wants to lose, a combination of diet and exercise is best; but different considerations apply. For your choice of exercise, use strength training primarily, as discussed in Chapter 7. As you add exercise, eat additional calories to support it—otherwise, you will lose weight (body fat). If you eat just enough to support the exercise, you will build muscle, but at the expense of body fat; that is, fat will be burned to support the muscle building. If you eat more, you will gain both muscle and fat.

It takes an excess of about 2,000 to 2,500 calories, in theory, to support the gain of a pound of pure lean tissue.[16] The rate at which a person can build muscle tissue also depends on the person. Both men and women have a mixture of both male and female hormones; those with more male hormones build muscle more easily than others, but the limits are not known. (Chapter 7 provides cautions on the use of steroid hormones.) Conventional advice on diet to the bodybuilder is to eat about 700 to 1,000 calories a day above normal energy needs; this is enough to support both the added exercise and the building of muscle.

If you want to gain weight, you may need to learn to eat different foods. No matter how many sticks of celery you eat, you won't gain weight very fast, because celery simply doesn't offer enough calories. The person who cannot eat much volume is encouraged to use calorie-dense foods in meals (the very ones the dieter is trying to stay away from). Use some of the items colored yellow and red in the Daily Food Choices pattern in Chapter 5. Yes, these foods are high in fat, but if they are contributing energy that will be spent sparing protein, they will not contribute to heart disease. They will help you to build a stronger body. Choose nutritious foods, but choose milk shakes instead of milk, peanut butter instead of lean meat, avocado instead of cucumber, whole-wheat muffins instead of whole-wheat bread. When you do eat celery, put cream cheese on it; add cream and sugar to coffee; use cheese dressings on salads, ice cream on fruit, and sour cream on potatoes. (Because fat contains twice as many calories per teaspoon as sugar, it adds calories without adding much bulk.)

Eat more frequently. Make three sandwiches in the morning, and eat them between classes, in addition to the day's three regular meals. Spend more time eating each meal. If you fill up fast, eat the highest-calorie items first. Don't start with soup or salad; start with the main course. Drink between meals, not with them, to save space for higher-calorie foods. Ask your health care provider for a liquid supplement to drink between meals—or make your own milk shakes. Always finish with dessert. Many an underweight person has simply been too busy (for months) to eat enough to gain or maintain weight. These strategies will help you to change this behavior pattern.

Expect to feel full. Most underweight individuals are accustomed to small quantities of food. When they begin eating significantly more food, they complain of uncomfortable fullness. This is normal and it passes with time.

≡ ▶ *Before taking steps to gain weight, be sure it will promote health. Combine diet (added calories), exercise (strength training), and behavior modification (eating more frequently) to succeed in gaining weight.*

■≡ Weight Maintenance

"I have lost 200 pounds, but I was never more than 20 pounds overweight." This statement expresses the frustration that thousands of dieters experience and that you may have experienced as well—the struggle to *lose* weight and the even greater struggle to *maintain* the desirable weight. Equally frustrating is the realization that hard work invested in *gaining* weight is visibly slipping away. For many, alternating weight loss and weight gain becomes a lifelong pattern. What makes successful, long-term weight maintenance possible? The answers available have to do with formerly-fat people, but many also apply to the formerly-thin.

Characteristics of Those Who Succeed

Researchers have discovered some predictors of success for weight maintenance.[17] The factors center around eating habits, as you might expect, but also believed to be important are changes in thought patterns, body image, family interactions, and activities with friends; details appear in Table 6–5. In addition to these, key traits are an attitude of ownership and responsibility, self-confidence, and self-acceptance.

Regarding ownership, people must come to a full understanding and acceptance that they alone are ultimately responsible for their weight control.[18] No person can control the weight of another, yet many dieters place responsibility for their weight control outside of themselves, on weight-loss programs, on health care professionals, or on pills and potions. This attitude weakens self-confidence and invites failure.

Ownership is learnable. Many previously habitual dieters say that they finally came to a turning point—the point at which they accepted responsibility for their own body weight. Only then were they able to develop workable solutions to maintain desirable weights.

TABLE 6–5 ■ Actions to Promote Weight Maintenance

Social support
  Attend support groups regularly.
  Develop supportive relationships with others.
Physical activity
  Exercise regularly.
Behavioral self-control
  Plan meals, write diet plans, keep records.
  Eat three meals a day at planned times.
  Limit eating after a certain hour in the evening.
  Use high-fiber foods as staple foods.
  Drink eight glasses or more of water a day.
  Eat slowly, and savor each bite.
Attitudes and beliefs
  Use positive self-talk: "You can do it," "You're a success."
  Resist negativity from family members or friends.
  Be realistic about your future body size and shape.
  Stay aware that changes take time.

SOURCE: Adapted from L. Pauley and W. J. Wyatt, Big losers: A compilation of success characteristics, *The Bariatrician*, Fall 1987, pp. 23–27.

Related to ownership is self-confidence—a person's belief that he or she has the ability to respond effectively to a situation by using available skills. Combined with another trait—expectation of success—self-confidence is a powerful tool in maintaining body weight.

Important, too, is self-acceptance. Self-hate predicts failure. A person who feels disgust when looking in a mirror or stepping on a scale can easily fall into a spiral of negative, self-defeating behaviors, including inappropriate eating behaviors. The paradox of behavior change is that self-acceptance (loving the overweight self) is the basis for self-change (liberating the normal-weight self). Letting go of negative feelings frees the person from the self-hate spiral, allowing an unshakable self-worth to take hold and confirm that human worth does not depend on body weight. Self-discipline is most easily sustained when self-acceptance supports it. In fact, clinics find that providing self-worth help for weight-loss clients can greatly improve their chances of success in maintaining desirable weight. Such training makes clients less likely to experience setbacks.

≡▶ *People who succeed at weight maintenance after losing weight are most likely to be those who feel fully responsible for their own weight control, and who have self-confidence and self-esteem.*

Lapse Management and Relapse Prevention

"I did it again," a chronic dieter confided. "I binged again after five years of dieting." Some dieters are forever frustrated by their backsliding behavior: "I feel angry, depressed, and ashamed. All of those meetings! All that therapy! All that work! Why did I go back to my old behaviors?" Disappointment, frustration, and self-condemnation are common in dieters who find themselves stuck in old behaviors.[19]

The term **relapse** describes the end result of a loss of control that results in defeat for dieters, and it doesn't have to happen. Many a relapse begins with just a **lapse,** and dieters need to understand the differences in kind and degree. Lapses happen to people who have been dieting for ten months or ten years. They are a normal part of the behavior-change process and do not indicate lack of willpower. A dieter in a lapse can take corrective action and can thus regain control. However, a lapse can lead to relapse: weight gain due to total abandonment of the weight-control program. If the dieter *perceives* a total loss of control during a lapse, then relapse is likely.[20]

The way people view the habit-change process can influence whether they will ultimately succeed at behavior change or slide into chronic problem behavior.[21] A perfectionistic, "all-or-nothing" attitude is destructive and can lead people to think that a mistake means that control is totally and forever lost. Examples of this erroneous thinking and of right thinking to counteract it appear in Table 6–6. If any of the myths in the table sound familiar, it could be that erroneous thinking is blocking your progress in weight maintenance. Arm yourself with the truth to combat such false, defeating thoughts.

When faced with a lapse into old behaviors, cope with it. Review the behavior modification strategies in the weight-loss section of this chapter. Identify those that apply to the circumstances surrounding your lapse, and redouble your attention to them. For example, if at a party you find that you unexpectedly overate, you might benefit from first adopting an attitude of

relapse the outcome of an uncontrolled series of lapses, such as regaining of weight after successful loss and returning to old patterns of eating.

lapse a falling back into a former condition. In weight maintenance, a temporary, expected backslide into old habits.

TABLE 6–6 ■ **Myths and Truths Regarding Lapses**

Myths contribute to negative thinking that can turn lapses into full-blown relapses. Dieters must be aware of these myths so that they can change them in their own thinking.

Myth: I've been working on this for so long that I shouldn't be making mistakes.

Truth: Even experts make mistakes.

Myth: If I were really doing well, I wouldn't be having these slips.

Truth: Having slips is a normal part of the behavior-change process. I am doing well even though I have slips.

Myth: People wouldn't respect me if they knew I was backsliding like this.

Truth: The important people respect me for my effort to change and know that slips are not reflective of my character.

Myth: Once changed, a behavior is gone forever.

Truth: Old behaviors try to creep back in, even those that were long gone.

Myth: I couldn't possibly be doing this again; I know better.

Truth: Yes, I know better, but even superior knowledge cannot prevent lapses.

Myth: Oh, no! I'm back to square one.

Truth: I may have slipped, but not all the way back to square one. I have made progress, and now I can vault ahead of where I stopped.

---

compassion and forgiving yourself. Then get tough with yourself, and commit to specific actions to control your intake at the next party. Vow to say "no" to food when you're not hungry (to fortify against social pressure), to eat a balanced meal beforehand (to defend against hunger), and to position yourself well away from party buffets (to defuse temptation).

It helps to monitor your behavior with regard to your plan for weight maintenance. For example, set specific tolerance ranges for lapses, and take action should you exceed them. Look for any of the following:

■ A weight gain of from 3 to 5 pounds.
■ A lack of physical activity for more than three days in a row.
■ A second repetition of any destructive behavior.
■ Withdrawal from a support system for a period lasting more than a week.
■ Failure to participate in enjoyable leisure activities for more than a week.

Take action. Review the appropriate steps to behavior modification, and apply them.

Improving behavior is rarely a matter of straight-line progress; it more often follows a path of two steps forward, one step back. For people to succeed in weight control, they must develop healthy attitudes toward lapses. One way to do this is to view lapses as helpful: they help people acquire information about their behaviors. When the normal lapses occur, the healthy person can cope by saying, "Oops! I'm doing it again, but it's okay; I do it less often now, and I'm making progress."

≡▶ *In maintaining a hard-won, healthy body weight, remember that a lapse into old behaviors need not be a full-blown relapse. Maintain high self-esteem, catch lapses early, keep a sense of proportion about them, and keep on trying.*

In weight control, as in life, self-acceptance and compassion create a positive, energizing cycle. Self-care, the fruit of self-acceptance, leads to better feelings and to more self-care; emotional, physical, and nutritional health are built on this positive cycle. The next chapter introduces another element of self-care: developing and maintaining physical fitness.

■≡ For Review

1. Identify the major health risks associated with being overweight or underweight.
2. Identify the social and psychological problems incurred by obesity.
3. Describe how to determine a person's appropriate weight.
4. Describe some physical (hereditary) and psychological (family) factors thought to influence the development of obesity.
5. Explain the concept of energy balance and, in particular, the ways the body spends energy.
6. Explain, in terms of body composition, the various possible ways in which weight may be gained or lost.
7. Describe how the body maintains itself when a person eats:

Too much food.
Just enough food.
Not enough food.
No food.

8. Identify various kinds of weight-loss diets and their effects on the body.
9. Evaluate several diets in terms of their safety and effectiveness.
10. Outline the principles of sound diet planning as they relate to weight loss, weight gain, and weight maintenance.
11. Show how diet, exercise, and behavior modification each can contribute to weight control.
12. List some factors that predict successful weight maintenance.

■≡ Notes

1. G. Kolata, Obesity declared a disease (Research News), *Science* 227 (1985): 1019–1020.
2. J. E. Manson and coauthors, A prospective study of obesity and risk of coronary heart disease in women, *New England Journal of Medicine* 322 (1990): 882–889.
3. C. L. Roch and A. Coulster, Effects of weight cycling, *Nutrition and the MD,* March 1989, p. 7.
4. T. B. Van Itallie, When the frame is part of the picture (Editorial), *American Journal of Public Health* 75 (1985): 1054–1055.
5. Consensus panel addresses obesity question, *Journal of the American Medical Association* 254 (1985): 1878.
6. A. Forse, P. N. Benotti, and G. L. Blackburn, Morbid obesity: Weighing the treatment options—Surgical intervention, *Nutrition Today,* September/October 1989, pp. 10–16.
7. S. R. Rolfes and L. K. DeBruyne, *Life Span Nutrition: Conception through Life,* ed. E. N. Whitney (St. Paul, Minn.: West, 1990), pp. 300–318.
8. This discussion of causes of obesity is adapted from E. N. Whitney, E. M. N. Hamilton, and S. R. Rolfes, *Understanding Nutrition,* 5th ed. (St. Paul, Minn.: West, 1990), Chap. 8.
9. J. H. Price, S. M. Desmond, and E. S. Ruppert, Elementary physical education teachers' perceptions of childhood obesity, *Health Education,* November/December 1990, pp. 26–32.
10. S. R. Rolfes, *A Matter of Fat: Emerging Insights into Obesity Development* (a 1990 monograph in the *Nutrition Clinics* series available from J. B. Lippincott Company, East Washington Square, Philadelphia, PA 19105).
11. The section entitled "Behavior Modification" is adapted from Whitney, Hamilton, and Rolfes, 1990, Chap. 12.
12. M. Simonton, An overview: Advances in research and treatment of obesity, *Food and Nutrition News,* March/April 1982.
13. R. L. Hammer and coauthors, Calorie-restricted low-fat diet and exercise in obese women, *American Journal of Clinical Nutrition* 49 (1989): 77–85; K. H. Duncan, J. A. Bacon, and R. L. Weinsier, The effects of high and low energy density diets on

satiety, energy intake, and eating time of obese and nonobese subjects, *American Journal of Clinical Nutrition* 37 (1983): 763–767.

14. D. M. Dreon and coauthors, Dietary fat:carbohydrate ratio and obesity in middle-aged men, *American Journal of Clinical Nutrition* 47 (1988): 995–1000.

15. D. Dennison, K. F. Dennison, and S. McCann, Integration of nutrient and activity analysis software into a worksite weight management program, *Health Education,* November/December 1990, pp. 4–7.

16. W. D. McArdle, F. I. Katch, and V. L. Katch, *Exercise Physiology: Energy, Nutrition, and Human Performance,* 2d ed. (Philadelphia: Lea & Febiger, 1986), pp. 527–528.

17. L. Pauley and W. J. Wyatt, Big losers: A compilation of success characteristics, *The Bariatrician,* Fall 1987, pp. 23–27.

18. You can lose weight and keep it off, *Tufts University Diet and Nutrition Letter,* March 1989, pp. 1–2.

19. L. W. Turner, Weight maintenance and relapse prevention, *Nutrition Clinics,* January/February 1990.

20. C. L. Rock and A. Coulston, Preventing relapse in dieters, *Nutrition and the MD,* January 1989, p. 7.

21. B. Sternberg, Relapse in weight control: Definitions, processes, and prevention strategies, in *Relapse Prevention: Maintenance Strategies in the Treatment of Addictive Behaviors,* eds. G. A. Marlatt and J. R. Gordon (New York: Guilford Press, 1985), pp. 521–545.

SPOTLIGHT

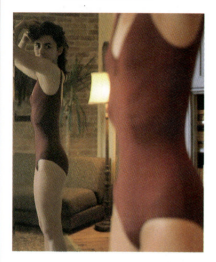

An Obsession With Thinness

An estimated 2 million people in the United States, primarily girls and young women, have been diagnosed with some form of an eating disorder: **anorexia nervosa** or **bulimia** (see the Miniglossary of Eating Disorder Terms for definitions). Still others may not receive a diagnosis but diet to the point of incurring nutritional and other injury.

Society favors thinness in women. Magazines, newspapers, and television display camera-ready women, flaws concealed, unreasonably thin. The message is clear—you are worthy only so long as you are lovely to look at. You should become like the cover girl who doesn't sweat; doesn't grow hair on her slender legs; has firm, small breasts, a flat stomach, a perfect face, small feet; and is always perfectly happy. If *you*, young woman, are not perfectly happy, it is because your body is not beautiful enough. Acceptance of such unreasonable expectations has driven nearly everyone in our society to be engaged in the "pursuit of thinness."

I thought being thin was healthy. Isn't it OK to pursue thinness?

Yes, but within limits. Most evidence supports the idea that thin people enjoy better health and live longer than do fat people.[1]* However, as the chapter pointed out, thinness itself can carry risks of increased infections, of delayed recovery from disease, and of poor tolerance to medical treatments. Eating disorders can expand the risks further, with psychological complications that can be severe.

What happens to someone who has anorexia nervosa?

The story of Julie illustrates this. Julie is 18 years old. She is attractive, she is a superachiever in school, and she prides herself on her fine figure. She watches her diet with great care, and she exercises daily, maintaining a heroic schedule of self-discipline. She is thin, but she is not satisfied with her weight and is determined to lose more. She is 5 feet 6 inches tall and weighs 85 pounds, but she's still trying to get thinner.

How could she possibly think she's too fat, measuring 5 feet 6 inches tall and weighing 85 pounds?

Her self-image is distorted. Her constant complaints of being fat and her obsessive behavior are strong indicators of abnormal mental processes. Against her will, Julie's family insisted that she see a psychiatrist, who tested her. She was given a

*Reference notes are at the end of the Spotlight.

visual self-image test and drew a picture of herself that was grossly distorted. When asked to draw her best friend, Julie rendered an accurate image.

Can't she see that she's hurting her body by being too thin?

Julie is unaware that she is undernourished, and she sees no need to obtain treatment. She stopped menstruating several months ago and has become very moody. Although her eyes lie in deep hollows in her face, and she is obviously close to physical exhaustion, she denies that she is ever tired.

How can someone get so thin and continue to diet?

Julie controls her food intake with tremendous discipline. If she feels that she has slipped and eaten more than intended, she runs or jumps rope until she is sure she has exercised it off, or she takes laxatives to hasten the exit of the food from her system. (She is unaware that laxatives cause dehydration, not loss of body fat.) It is her fierce determination to achieve self-control, not lack of hunger, that prevents her from eating.

What could have caused her to behave this way?

A characteristic cluster of family and social circumstances often, though not always, surrounds the person with anorexia. A family like those described in Chapter 3—that is, a family with dysfunctional interactions between its members—is likely to surround the anorexia victim. Often, the family is dominated by the mother, with the father absent or distant, and it values achievement and outward appearances more than an inner sense of self-worth and self-actualization. The victim of anorexia suffers low self-esteem and thus is susceptible to societal and parental pressure to be thin.

Young women look to their male parents or parent substitutes for important feedback on their self-worth, and when they don't receive it, they tend to be oversensitive to negative cultural messages. Among these negative messages are the worship of thinness and the view of emaciation as beautiful.[2] Julie's father has alcoholism, and her mother left him a year ago.

As a child, when Julie cried with hunger, her parents didn't respond by feeding her. Rather, they fed her on a rigid schedule. They forced food on her at times when she didn't want it, and they withheld it when she was hungry. Julie lost the ability to detect her own hunger signals. Now, she feels she has to control her eating from outside, as her parents did.

What is happening to her physically, and how serious is this condition?

Julie is suffering the physical effects of starvation, in which hormone secretions become abnormal and blood pressure drops. The heart muscle becomes weak and thin and pumps less efficiently; its chambers diminish in size, and its rhythms may change, with a characteristic abnormality appearing on the heart monitor. Sudden stopping of the heart, due to lean tissue loss or mineral deficiencies, accounts for many cases of sudden death among people who are severely emaciated.

Can a person with anorexia be cured?

Treatment outcomes are better than they used to be. Residential treatment centers specializing in eating disorders are often especially successful. Three-quarters of those in treatment may regain weight up to within 25 percent of the desired weight. Half to three-quarters may resume normal menstrual cycles. About two-thirds fail to eat normally on follow-up, but they may eat better than they did before. About 6 percent die, 1 percent by suicide.*

I have a friend who seems to have anorexia nervosa. She's very thin and seems never to eat. How can I tell if she has anorexia, and how can I help her?

On learning of the condition, many people assume that some of their thin friends must have the condition; most times this is not the case. A professional diagnosis is required to identify cases, and even then the diagnosis is difficult. However, sincere concern for your friend is legitimate. Before addressing your fears to the person, be sure to organize your thoughts clearly on why you suspect an eating disorder. Be specific: "Heather has been skipping lunch and exercising two hours each day," rather than "Heather looks thin." Verify your perceptions by discussing them with other concerned friends. Finally, in a gentle, caring way, present your suspicions to your friend, and give the friend the National Anorexic Aid Society (NAAS) hotline number at the bottom of this page.* Then relax,

*This is from a classic review of 19 studies of about 1,000 clients over a five-year period. Other deaths are from infection, heart disease, lung disease, and treatment-related causes including aspiration, electrolyte imbalance from intravenous therapy, and vitamin D poisoning. M. A. Balaa and D. A. Drossman, *Anorexia Nervosa and Bulimia: The Eating Disorders, Disease-a-Month* (Chicago: Year Book Medical, June 1985), p. 34.
*The NAAS hotline number is 1-614-436-1112.

knowing you've done what you could do.

You previously mentioned bulimia. What happens to someone who has this disease?

The case of Sophie illustrates the plight of the person with bulimia. Like the "typical" person with bulimia, Sophie is single, Caucasian, in her early 20s, well educated, and close to her ideal body weight. Sophie is a charming, intelligent woman who thinks constantly about food. She alternatively starves herself and binges, and when she has eaten too much, she vomits.

Her periodic binges take place in secret, usually at night, and they last an hour or more. She seldom lets bingeing interfere with her work or social activities, although a third of all bingers do. She is like most people with bulimia in that she starts the binge after having gone through a period of rigid dieting, so that her eating is accelerated by her hunger. Each time, she consumes thousands of calories (up to 10,000 calories) of easy-to-eat, high-calorie food. (These binges can become quite expensive.) Typically, she chooses cookies, cake, ice cream, or bread, although sometimes she binges on atypical foods—such as vegetables—when she

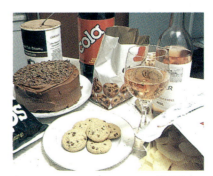

A person may consume up to 10,000 calories during an eating binge.

is dieting. The photo shows foods consumed in a typical binge. The binge is not like normal eating. Often, the hands are used instead of eating utensils. It is a compulsion and usually occurs in several stages:"anticipation and planning, anxiety, urgency to begin, rapid and uncontrollable consumption of food, relief and relaxation, disappointment, and finally shame or disgust."[3]

What are the physical effects of bulimia?

Immediately following a binge, Sophie pays the price of having swollen hands and feet, bloating, fatigue, headache, nausea, and pain. Repeated binges cause more serious consequences. Fluid and electrolyte imbalance caused by vomiting can lead to abnormal heart rhythms and injury to the kidneys. Vomiting causes irritation and infection of the pharynx, esophagus, and salivary glands; erosion of the teeth; and dental caries. The esophagus may rupture or tear, as may the stomach. Sometimes the eyes become red from pressure on vomiting. The hands may be bruised and lacerated from scraping on the teeth while inducing vomiting.

Some people use **cathartics**—laxatives that can injure the lower intestinal tract. Others use **emetics** to induce vomiting; it was overuse of emetics that caused the death of popular singer Karen Carpenter in 1983.

What makes a person become bulimic?

We don't know, but the family dynamics suggest some clues. Much like Julie, who has anorexia nervosa, Sophie has been a high achiever, with a strong feeling of dependence on her parents. Her mother is a bright, well-educated woman who chose to stay home with the children; her father is a powerful and respected, but distant, figure.

Her family often combined hearty eating with much socializing around the dinner table. Food was always involved in celebrations and used to console the family during periods of mourning. Sophie felt it would be disrespectful not to celebrate or mourn by not eating, but equally strong was the demand to be thin, so she tried to do both.

Sophie started bingeing and purging after a diet. She usually conducted these activities in solitude, although at times she involved close high-school friends who admired and emulated her. In college, she started abusing alcohol and often purged after episodes of drinking—again, sometimes with friends who did the same.[4] Other than those friends, she is close to no one; she experiences considerable social anxiety and has difficulty in establishing personal relationships. She is sometimes depressed and often behaves impulsively.

Sophie feels inadequate, because she is unable to control her eating, and so she tends to be passive and to look to men for confirmation of her sense of worth. When she is rejected, either in reality or in her imagination, her bulimia becomes worse. In fact, many women point to male rejection as the event that led to the first binge.[5]

Some people with bulimia engage in antisocial behavior, including compulsive stealing, sexual promiscuity, and drug abuse.[6] These behaviors are more common in bulimia than in anorexia nervosa, and it is thought that bulimia is more of an addictive behavior than anorexia.[7]

How common are anorexia nervosa and bulimia?

Both anorexia nervosa and bulimia occur only in developed nations and become more prevalent as wealth increases. The reported incidence of anorexia in our country and in other industrially advanced countries is steadily increasing. It now is reported to occur in almost 1 of every 100 women.[8] More people than ever before are claiming to have bulimia. In a survey of 300 women shoppers in suburban Boston, over 10 percent reported a history of bulimia, and almost 5 percent were currently practicing it.[9] Among college women, the incidence may range anywhere from 5 to 20 percent.

■ **MINIGLOSSARY**
of Eating Disorder Terms

anorexia nervosa a disorder seen (usually) in teenage girls, characterized by self-starvation to the extreme.
  an = without
  orex = mouth
  nervos = of nervous origin

bulimia (alternative spelling, **bulemia**) (byoo-LEEM-ee-uh) recurring binge eating. Some people call this **bulimarexia** (byoo-lee-ma-REX-ee-uh); others reserve the latter term for bulimia with emaciation probably caused by purging after binging.
  buli = ox
  orex = mouth

cathartic a strong laxative.

emetic (em-ETT-ic) an agent that causes vomiting.

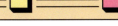

What can be done about this situation?

The causes of both bulimia and anorexia nervosa are unknown, but one school of thought labels them social problems. Perhaps they began when privileged young women internalized a message of their own low worth and adopted the ideal of some unachievable, "perfect" image.

Slowly, society is changing. Recognition of the success and desirability of a growing number of outstanding women in such traditionally male-dominated fields as athletics, science, law, and politics has raised women's collective self-esteem. Perhaps anorexia nervosa and bulimia will disappear as feminine roles and ideals change.

Prevention may be most effective if begun early in children's lives. Warnings to children that the Madison Avenue female figure is simply an advertising gimmick designed to sell products, and not an ideal with which to compare one's own living body, may help. The simple concept—to respect and value your own uniqueness—may be life-saving for a future generation.

■≡ Spotlight Notes

1. E. M. N. Hamilton, E. N. Whitney, and F. S. Sizer, *Nutrition Concepts and Controversies* (St. Paul, Minn.: West, 1991), pp. 469–479.

2. K. McCleary, Eating disorders: Daddy dearest, *American Health,* January/February 1986, p. 86.

3. M. A. Balaa and D. A. Drossman, *Anorexia Nervosa and Bulimia: The Eating Disorders, Disease-a-Month* (Chicago: Year Book Medical, June 1985), p. 38.

4. P. W. Meilman, F. A. von Hippel, and M. S. Gaylor, Self-induced vomiting in college women: Its relation to eating, alcohol use, and Greek life, *Journal of American College Health,* July 1991, pp. 39–41.

5. M. Baskind-Lodahl and J. Sirlin, The gorging-purging syndrome: Bulimarexia, *Psychology Today,* March 1977, pp. 50–52, 82, 85.

6. J. D. Killen, B. Taylor, M. J. Telch, and coauthors, Depressive symptoms and substance abuse among adolescent binge eaters and purgers: A defined population study, *American Journal of Public Health* 77 (1987): 1539–1541; M. S. Gold, Eating disorders linked to chemical dependency, *Alcoholism and Addiction,* May–June 1988, p. 13; J. M. Jonas, M. S. Gold, D. Sweeney, and A. L. C. Pottash, Eating disorders and cocaine abuse: A survey of 259 cocaine abusers, *Journal of Clinical Psychiatry,* February 1987, pp. 47–50.

7. P. de Silva and S. Eysenck, Personality and addictiveness in anorexic and bulimic patients, *Personality and Individual Differences* 8 (1987): 749–751.

8. Balaa and Drossman, 1985, pp. 1–52.

9. H. G. Pope, Jr., J. I. Hudson, and D. Yurgelun-Todd, Anorexia nervosa and bulimia among 300 suburban women shoppers, *American Journal of Psychiatry* 141 (1984): 2, as cited in Balaa and Drossman, 1985.

CHAPTER 7

Fitness

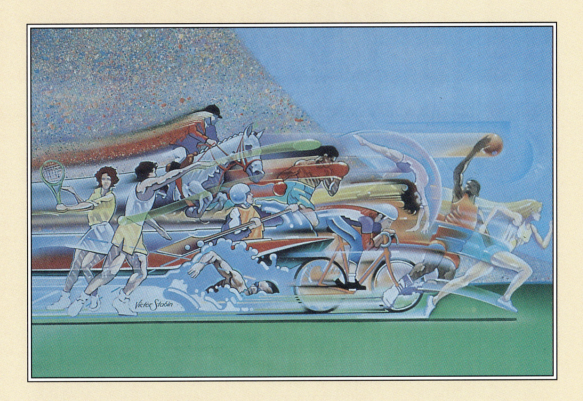

FACT OR FICTION

Just for fun, respond true or false to the following statements. If false, say what is true.

■ You should not overload your body, because overload can cause damage. (Page 172)
■ People born with mostly slow-twitch muscle fibers cannot become competitive athletes. (Page 173)
■ When performing stretching exercises, you should feel tightness but no pain. (Page 177)
■ The person who wishes to gain strength must work with free weights or machines to provide resistance for the muscles. (Page 180)
■ If you feel pain in your feet or legs while running, it is best to keep going and try to work through it. (Page 191)
■ It is best not to interrupt a workout to drink a beverage. (Page 193)
■ Water is the beverage of choice to replace body fluids lost during exercise. (Page 193)

Perhaps you are a physically fit person. If so, the following description applies to you. Your muscles are firm and easily control your body's movements. You are strong and meet physical challenges without strain. Your weight is appropriate for your height, and your body's contours are streamlined. You have endurance; your energy lasts for hours. You can meet normal physical challenges with ease and have plenty of energy in reserve to handle emergencies. What is more, you are likely to be well able to meet mental and emotional challenges, too—for physical fitness undergirds not only physical endurance but also mental and emotional resilience.

If these statements do not describe you as you are today, then you can gain fitness through practice. Activities that promote fitness are themselves enjoyable, and they quickly lead to rewards in terms of physical improvements. Feeling fit can boost your confidence in other areas of life, too: social, academic, professional—you name it.

Narrowly defined, the term **fitness** describes *the characteristics of the body that enable it to perform physical activity*. These characteristics include flexibility of the joints; strength and endurance of the muscles, including the heart muscle; and a healthy body weight. A broader definition of fitness is *the ability to meet routine physical demands, with enough reserve energy to rise to sudden challenges*. This definition shows how fitness relates to everyday life. Ordinary tasks such as carrying heavy suitcases, opening a stuck window, or climbing four flights of stairs, which might strain an unfit person, can be well within the capacity of the fit person. Still another definition is *the body's ability to withstand stressors*, including psychological stressors. There is no contradiction among these three definitions; they are three different expressions of the same wonderful condition of the body. All are attained through regular physical activity.

The body that practices a physical activity *adapts* by becoming better able to perform it after each session—more flexible, stronger, more enduring. Moreover, the body that gains physical fitness also gains in its abilities to take exams in school and take on major responsibilities in society or on the

fitness the characteristics of the body that enable it to perform physical activity; more broadly, the ability to meet routine physical demands, with enough reserve energy to rise to sudden challenges; or the body's ability to withstand stressors of all kinds.

job. Activity promotes fitness; fitness promotes stress resistance in general; and stress resistance benefits health and life in many, many ways.[1]*

Fitness is the reward of a person who leads a physically active life. The opposite of such a life is a **sedentary** life, which means, literally, "sitting down a lot." Today's world permits many people to lead sedentary lives, and even rewards them for it. It provides cars, elevators, escalators, golf-carts, and subways so that people can exert a minimum of physical effort. Unfortunately, the more people use labor-saving devices, the more weak and unfit they become, and the less able to meet life's challenges. The body responds to inactivity by losing muscle and skill, just as it responds to activity by gaining them.

> **≡▶** *Fitness enables the body to meet routine physical demands, to meet sudden challenges, and to withstand stress. Fitness is the product of a physically active life.*

sedentary physically inactive (literally, "sitting down a lot").

■≡ Benefits of Fitness

A fit person benefits in all areas of life (see Figure 7–1). The first and most obvious of the benefits are those in the realm of physical health. Someone who faithfully keeps to a workout schedule, who sleeps soundly, who eats adequately, and who controls weight through diet and activity is one who has every chance for superb health. Physical activity is also one of the most effective strategies against stress-related disease. Equally important to a person's well-being are emotional and mental health, social health, and spiritual health; and fitness also enhances these. Internally, those who are fit have all the advantages—they feel good. Table 7–1 shows how physical activity helps defend against some physical disorders, and also how it helps promote psychological well-being. As for spiritual health, most people experience the "team spirit" of team sports, and find they can do much more than they dream they could do on their own. A person who has climbed a physical mountain gains confidence to scale other kinds of mountains as well, such as finishing difficult intellectual tasks or keeping promises when times are hard. If only half of the rewards listed in the table were yours for the asking, wouldn't you step up to claim them?

Imagine for a moment that the benefits listed in Table 7–1 are associated not with regular exercise but with a newly discovered "miracle pill." A stampede of people would try to buy it. In fact, miracle products claim to offer many of these benefits, and people do spend money in hopes of obtaining them. Why is money so much easier to spend than effort?

Despite evidence of the benefits, only about a third of the U.S. population exercises regularly. Even fewer exercise enough to ensure a healthy heart.[2] Sadly, regular exercise requires more effort than pill taking, and more time. The choice is personal, but this chapter will, of course, try to influence your decision.

More about the relationships of fitness to blood cholesterol, heart attacks, and strokes in Chapter 18.

> **≡▶** *Physical activity promotes fitness, and fitness promotes all aspects of health.*

*Reference notes are at the end of the chapter.

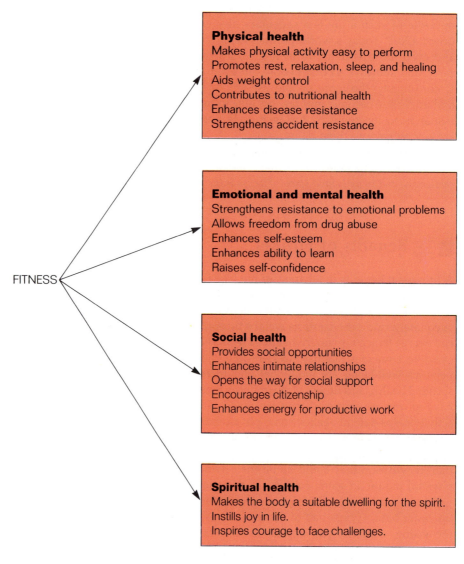

Physical health
Makes physical activity easy to perform
Promotes rest, relaxation, sleep, and healing
Aids weight control
Contributes to nutritional health
Enhances disease resistance
Strengthens accident resistance

Emotional and mental health
Strengthens resistance to emotional problems
Allows freedom from drug abuse
Enhances self-esteem
Enhances ability to learn
Raises self-confidence

FITNESS

Social health
Provides social opportunities
Enhances intimate relationships
Opens the way for social support
Encourages citizenship
Enhances energy for productive work

Spiritual health
Makes the body a suitable dwelling for the spirit.
Instills joy in life.
Inspires courage to face challenges.

FIGURE 7–1 ■ **Fitness contributes to health.**

■≡ The Path to Fitness: Conditioning

To become fit, you don't have to turn yourself into an athlete or a body-builder; you just have to improve your ability to perform physical activity to the point where it supports your health optimally. That means achieving a reasonable weight and enough flexibility, muscular strength, and endurance

TABLE 7–1 ■ **Physical and Psychological Benefits of Physical Activity**

Regular physical activity helps protect against these physical conditions:

- Acne.
- Backaches.
- Cancer (colon cancer, breast cancer, and others).[a]
- Diabetes.[b]
- Digestive disorders (ulcers, constipation, diarrhea, and others).
- Elevated stress hormone secretion.
- Headaches.
- Heart and blood vessel disease (heart attacks and strokes).[c]
- High blood cholesterol and triglycerides, high blood pressure.
- Infections (colds, flu, and many others).
- Infertility (some forms).
- Insomnia[d] (sleep disorders).
- Kidney disease.
- Menstrual irregularities, menstrual cramps, and mood swings associated with the menstrual cycle.
- Obesity.
- Osteoporosis (adult bone loss).[e]

Regular physical activity also benefits people psychologically (sample research findings):

- Physically active people experience less anxiety and depression than sedentary people.[f]
- Fit people deal better with emotionally stressful events than sedentary people.[g]
- Fit people display a positive self-image.
- Depressed people who adopt a routine of regular running become as well and stay as well as others who obtain psychotherapy.[h]

SOURCE:

[a]R. E. Frisch and coauthors, Lower lifetime occurrence of breast cancer and cancers of the reproductive system among former college athletes, *American Journal of Clinical Nutrition* 45 (1987): 328–335.

[b]M. J. Franz, Exercise and the management of diabetes mellitus, *Journal of the American Dietetic Association* 87 (1987): 872–880.

[c]L. G. Ekelund and coauthors, Physical fitness as a predictor of cardiovascular mortality in asymptomatic North American men, *New England Journal of Medicine* 319 (1988): 1379–1384.

[d]K. C. Light and coauthors, Psychological stress induces sodium and fluid retention in men at high risk for hypertension, *Science* 220 (1982): 429–431.

[e]B. Krolner and coauthors, Physical exercise as a prophylaxis against involutional vertebral bone loss: A controlled trial, *Clinical Science* 64 (1983): 541–546, as cited in M. E. Nelson and coauthors, Diet and bone status in amenorrheic runners, *American Journal of Clinical Nutrition* 43 (1986): 910–916.

[f]D. L. Roth and D. S. Holmes, Influence of physical fitness in determining the impact of stressful life events on physical and psychologic health, *Psychosomatic Medicine* 47 (1985): 164–173.

[g]R. M. Hayden, Relationship between aerobic exercise, anxiety, and depression: Convergent validation by knowledgeable informants, *Journal of Sports Medicine* 24 (1984): 69–74.

[h]J. H. Griest, Running as treatment for depression, *Journal of Comprehensive Psychiatry,* January/February 1979, pp. 41–54.

to meet the everyday demands life places on you, plus some to spare. Beyond those goals, you can pursue long-term ideals ("I plan to become able to run for an hour a day" or "I plan to become able to bench-press 100 pounds ten times"), but don't expect too much of yourself too soon. To keep motivation high on the way to your goals, celebrate small day-to-day achievements ("I did better today than yesterday").

Characteristics of Fitness

flexibility   a component of fitness, the ability to bend without injury; it depends on the elasticity of muscles, tendons, and ligaments and on the condition of the joints.

muscle strength   a component of fitness, the ability of muscles to work against resistance.

muscle endurance   a component of fitness, the ability of muscles to sustain an effort for a long time.

cardiovascular endurance   a component of fitness, the ability of the cardiovascular system to sustain effort over a long time.

Different body systems express fitness through different characteristics. With respect to the joints, **flexibility** is important. With respect to the muscles, **strength** and **endurance** are important. With respect to the heart and lungs, endurance is also important: this type of endurance is **cardiovascular endurance**. Athletes go on to describe additional components of fitness related to skill, which they call *performance characteristics*. They describe their goals in terms of agility, balance, coordination, power, speed, and reaction time. The importance of these characteristics varies widely with individual sports, and athletes practice endless hours to develop them. The focus of this chapter is on the health-related aspects of fitness: flexibility, muscle strength and endurance, and cardiovascular endurance.

Fitness follows physical activity, and even routine activities can help to improve it. You can get an estimate of how active you are by answering the questions in this chapter's Life Choice Inventory. Tests that require physical activity would reveal more, and if you were to have measurements taken by a professional, you would obtain an accurate estimate of your fitness.

The path to fitness is physical conditioning, which you acquire through practice or training. Conditioning is the microscopic nuts and bolts of fitness, entailing a multitude of adaptations that cells make to facilitate the work that training demands of them. The sections that follow give general principles governing training and show how training leads to a conditioned body.

First, though, make sure it is safe to begin physical conditioning. Ordinary exercises are not hazardous to any healthy person, but if you answer yes to any of the questions that follow, you should proceed with caution. A fitness professional can test you to make sure you start your program at an intensity level high enough to bring about the desired changes but not so high as to endanger your health. The key questions seem to be:

- Are you over 35?
- Have you been sedentary for a long time?
- Are you more than 20 pounds heavier than you should be?
- Do you now smoke more than a pack and a half of cigarettes per day?
- Do you have any chronic illness?
- Has a health care provider ever said you had heart trouble?
- Did you ever have, or do you now have, a heart murmur?
- Have you ever had a diagnosed or suspected heart attack?
- Do you have chest pains at any time?

If, during exercise, you notice *any* change in your comfort or functioning, or any pain, stop exercising and consult a health care provider before continuing. The rest of this chapter assumes your exercise program will go well.

≡▶ *The components of fitness are flexibility, muscle strength and endurance, and cardiovascular endurance.*

The Overload Principle

Every day the human body works. The stronger and more fit it is, the less it must strain to do that work. If the body is weak, a person can't trade it in as if it were a car too run-down to do its job; but fortunately, there is no need

LIFE CHOICE INVENTORY

How physically active are you? For each question answered yes, give yourself the number of points indicated. Then total your points to determine your score.

Occupation and Daily Activities

1. I usually walk to and from school and work (at least ½ mile each way). 1 point
2. I usually take the stairs rather than use elevators or escalators. 1 point
3. My typical daily physical activity is best described by the following statement (select one):
   a. Most of my day is spent walking to class, sitting in class or at home, or in light activity. 0 points
   b. Most of my day is spent in moderate physical activity—brisk walking or the like. 4 points
   c. My typical day includes several hours of heavy physical activity (football, basketball, gym workout, or the like). 9 points

Leisure Activities

4. I do a few hours of lightly active leisure activity each week (such as slow canoeing or slow cycling). 1 point
5. I hike or bike (at a moderate pace) once a week or more, on the average. 1 point
6. At least once a week, I participate for an hour or more in vigorous dancing, such as aerobic or folk dancing. 1 point
7. I play racquetball or tennis at least once a week. 2 points
8. I often walk for exercise or recreation. 1 point
9. When I feel bothered by pressures at school, work, or home, I use exercise as a way to relax. 1 point

10. Two or more times a week, I perform calisthenic exercises (sit-ups, push-ups, etc.) for at least 10 minutes per session. 3 points
11. I regularly participate in yoga or perform stretching exercises. 2 points
12. Two or more times a week, I engage in weight training for at least 30 minutes. 4 points
13. I participate in active recreational sports such as volleyball, baseball, or softball:
    a. About once a week. 2 points
    b. About twice a week. 4 points
    c. Three times a week or more. 7 points
14. At least once a week, I participate in vigorous fitness activities like jogging or swimming (at least 20 continuous minutes per session):
    a. About once a week. 3 points
    b. About twice a week. 5 points
    c. Three times a week or more. 10 points

Total points earned _____

Scoring:

0 to 5 points—inactive. This amount of exercise leads to a steady deterioration in fitness. Improvement needed.

6 to 11 points—moderately active. This amount slows fitness loss but will not maintain fitness in most persons.

12 to 20 points—active. This amount will maintain an acceptable level of physical fitness.

21 points or over—very active. This amount of activity will maintain a high state of physical fitness.

SOURCE: Adapted with permission of Russell Pate (University of South Carolina, Human Performance Laboratory).

to. Unlike a run-down car, which will break down when overloaded, the body responds to **overload** in a positive way—it gets itself into better shape to meet the demand next time.

Don't do too much too soon. You've heard the expression "No pain, no gain," but pain won't help; effort will. A worthwhile long-term goal is to develop a lifelong fitness program. It doesn't make sense to start with activities so demanding that pain stops the program within two days. Learn to enjoy the small steps along the way, because fitness builds slowly.

overload an extra physical demand placed on the body; an increase in the frequency, duration, or intensity of exercise.

progressive overload principle   the training principle that a body system, in order to improve, must be worked at frequencies, durations, or intensities that increase by increments over time.

frequency   the number of occurrences per unit of time (for example, the number of exercise sessions per week).

intensity   degree (for example, the degree of effort exerted while exercising).

duration   length of time (for example, the length of time spent in each exercise session).

You have to overwork just a little. Pushing the body a little beyond the normal level of demand elicits the release of hormones that stimulate growth of muscle tissue. In 24 to 48 hours, nature repairs any slight injuries the muscles may have incurred during exercise. It also remodels and builds extra tissue in the muscles and bones so that next time the body will meet the more vigorous challenge more easily.

To apply overload, a person can use the **progressive overload principle** in several ways. One way is to do the activity more often—that is, increase its **frequency**; another is to do the activity more strenuously—that is, increase its **intensity**; still another is to do it for longer periods of time—that is, increase its **duration**. All three strategies work well, and exercisers can pick one or a combination, depending on personal preferences. For example, if you love your workout, do it more often. If you lack time, increase intensity. If you hate hard work, take it easy and go longer. Any way you apply it, the progressive overload principle governs improvement of fitness.

Here are some other pointers about applying overload:

■ Exercise regularly.
■ Train hard only once or twice a week, not every time you work out. Between times, do light workouts.
■ Listen to your body and cooperate. If you feel energetic, work hard; if you are tired or in pain, go lightly or stop, even if that was not part of the original plan.

Also, keep in mind that the physical changes that result from overload are specific to the component of fitness being challenged. In other words, stretching develops flexibility, but doesn't build cardiovascular endurance. Therefore, strive for balance in your fitness program.

≡▶   *Overload is extra physical demand that improves fitness. The progressive overload principle states that to improve, one must, over time, increase the frequency, intensity, or duration of exercise.*

The Use-Disuse Principle

Fitness develops in response to demand and wanes when demand ceases— the **use-disuse principle**. When a muscle enlarges after being called upon repeatedly to do a certain type of work, this muscle growth is called **hypertrophy**. When the activity is stopped for a few days, and the muscle group shrinks and loses strength, this is called **atrophy**. A point about atrophy: unused muscles do not "turn to fat," as many people believe. However, with food intake remaining constant, the less a body works, the more fat it collects, and the more muscle it loses. Thus the person who trades activity for an armchair trades fitness for flab.

≡▶   *Fitness develops in response to demand and wanes when demand ceases.*

use-disuse principle   the principle that fitness develops in response to demand and diminishes in response to the lack of demand.

hypertrophy (high-PER-tro-fee)   an increase in muscle size in response to use.
atrophy (AT-ro-fee)   a decrease in muscle size due to lack of use.

Muscle Fibers, Aerobic Work, and Anaerobic Work

The characteristics of muscle tissue depend partly on the kinds of work presented to it. Muscles are made up, largely, of two different types of contracting cells called **muscle fibers**. The two types are **slow-twitch muscle**

muscle fibers   muscle cells.

fibers and **fast-twitch muscle fibers**. Each of these fiber types is best suited to a specific kind of work. Slow-twitch fibers are best suited to **aerobic** work, which is low to moderate in intensity. During this type of exercise, the body can supply enough oxygen to the muscle fibers to sustain their efforts. Fast-twitch fibers are best suited to **anaerobic** work, which is intense enough so that the body cannot deliver sufficient amounts of oxygen fast enough. Without enough oxygen, muscles must rely on their fast-twitch fibers and their special ability to use alternative fuels until oxygen is delivered later. The more of each kind of work (low-intensity or high-intensity) a person performs, the more the muscle fibers adapt to that work in terms of size and capacity. Thus, a jogger develops larger and more efficient slow-twitch fibers, while a weight-lifter develops the fast-twitch type.

The characteristics of muscle tissues also depend partly on heredity. A person's fitness potential or athletic talent is inborn, partly because every person is born with a set number of each type of fiber. In a sense, an individual is born to be either a sprinter or a long-distance runner. A person born with tremendous capacity who chooses to develop it to the fullest can become a great athlete. But even people not born with the ''right stuff'' to be elite athletes can choose to develop fitness to the greatest extent possible by choosing the right exercises.

Slow-twitch muscle fibers (suited for activity of lower intensity and longer duration) depend most on fat, the body's main source of fuel, to provide energy aerobically.* They use some glucose, too, but they draw most heavily on fat. Fast-twitch muscle fibers (suited for high-intensity, short-duration activity) depend mostly on glucose, the body's sugar, for their anaerobic energy fuel. These fibers use a little fat, but lean most heavily on glucose.

Imagine a distance runner on an endless stretch of beach. The runner's steady stride paces off miles of sand with only slight changes in speed, maximizing the distance covered. Now envision a track meet. A sprinter bursts across the starting line in an explosion of energy. The burst lasts only a few seconds, followed by exhaustion at the finish line.

*Fat and glucose provide about 90% of the body's fuel; the other 10% is protein.

slow-twitch muscle fibers muscle fibers best suited to producing energy by aerobic processes for prolonged endurance exercise.

fast-twitch muscle fibers muscle fibers best suited to producing energy by anaerobic processes, to perform high-intensity, short-duration work.

aerobic (air-ROE-bic) refers to energy-producing processes involving the immediate use of oxygen.

■ *aero* = air

anaerobic (AN-air-ROE-bic) refers to energy-producing processes that do not involve the immediate use of oxygen

■ *an* = without

■ *FACT OR FICTION:* People born with mostly slow-twitch muscle fibers cannot become competitive athletes. *False.* People born with mostly slow-twitch muscle fibers are superbly suited to aerobic work and can develop this potential to competitive levels.

These go together:

Muscle fibers—slow-twitch.*

Major fuel—fat.

Energy production—aerobic.

Exercise—low intensity, long duration.

These go together:

Muscle fibers—fast-twitch.

Major fuel—glycogen made available as glucose.

Energy production—anaerobic.

Exercise—high intensity, short duration.

*Slow- and fast-twitch are the two best-known muscle fiber types. There are others.

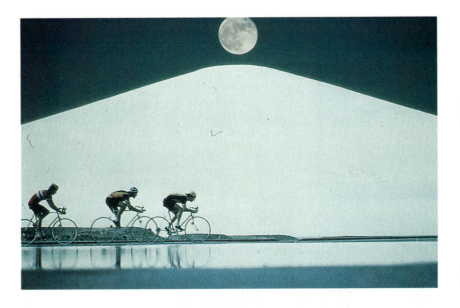

Sustained muscular efforts involve aerobic work.

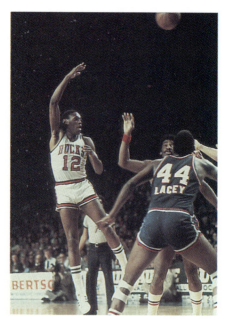

Split-second surges of power involve anaerobic work.

oxygen debt   a deficit of oxygen built up by a body performing exercise so demanding that the circulation cannot bring oxygen to the muscles fast enough for them to completely oxidize their fuel. The debt must be repaid after the activity slows down or stops; rapid breathing delivers the oxygen needed to complete the oxidation process.

The distance runner is engaging largely in aerobic work, which is associated with endurance. The ability to continue swimming until you reach the far bank, to continue hiking until you are at camp, or to continue pedaling until you are home reflects aerobic capacity. This capacity is also crucial to the health of the heart and circulatory system.

The sprinter is engaging in mostly anaerobic activity, which is associated with strength, agility, and split-second surges of power. The jump of the basketball player, the slam of the tennis serve, the weight lifter's heave at the barbells, and the fullback's blast through the opposing line are all anaerobic work. The Spotlight of this chapter revisits the relationships outlined in the margin, for they bear heavily on how well the foods you eat support your chosen activities.

Muscles of all types experience fatigue when they have been worked to capacity. One type of fatigue involves pain in the muscles upon performance of anaerobic work. The accompanying box describes this pain in relation to the phenomenon of **oxygen debt**.

≡▶ *Muscle fibers are of mostly two types—slow- and fast-twitch. Each type is suited to different work, uses a different fuel mix, and produces energy in different ways.*

Oxygen Debt, Lactic Acid, and Muscle Pain

Normally, during aerobic activity, glucose fuel and fat fuel are repeatedly split apart, and the parts are combined with oxygen. The fuels yield smaller and smaller fragments, releasing some energy at each split. In the end, nothing remains except some water and carbon dioxide—tiny waste products that are easily disposed of by way of sweat, urine, and exhaled breath.

Anaerobic activity can use only glucose as fuel. It proceeds by splitting the glucose apart without combining the parts with oxygen. But the splitting of glucose without oxygen can go only so far. Partly broken-down portions of glucose molecules build up, and sooner or later, more oxygen will be needed to break them down completely. The nervous and hormonal systems respond to this buildup of molecules by speeding up the heart and lungs to deliver more oxygen—that's why you pant when you exert yourself.

Your deep, rapid breathing reflects your body's attempt to deliver the needed oxygen to the tissues. But a point comes at which the heart and lungs can't go any faster, and oxygen supply lags behind demand. Faced with the continued accumulation of glucose fragments, and unable to complete their oxidation, the body sets them aside temporarily as lactic acid.

The buildup of lactic acid causes burning pain in the muscles. A strategy for dealing with it is to relax the muscles at every opportunity, so that the circulating blood can wash the lactic acid out of the muscles and bring fresh oxygen in. The oxygen completes the breakdown of the remaining lactic acid to water and carbon dioxide, and it pays off the oxygen debt. This is what mountaineers are doing when they relax their leg muscles at each step (the "mountain rest step").

Principles of Warm-up and Cool-down

The body needs to prepare for exercise. It needs to warm its muscles and connective tissues, so that they will stretch without tearing during the activity. A warm-up activity increases blood flow to muscles and begins the hormonal changes that will liberate the needed fuels from storage. Warmed muscles also stretch easily.

To warm up, take a brisk walk, light jog, or other light exercise followed by a stretching routine. Or do a light version of what you plan to do intensively later. A runner may start out walking; break into a jog; and finally, when it feels right, pick up the pace to an outright run. A person who body builds may start with light weight repetitions; a tennis player, with a few lobs. This strategy is thought to best prepare the main muscle groups required for the task ahead.

The body needs to cool down to ease the transition to relaxation again. A few minutes of light activity facilitates the relaxation of tight muscles and enhances the circulation of blood through them. The circulation in turn brings accumulated heat from the body's core to the surface, where it can radiate away. At the end of the workout, gradually ease up on the intensity of the activity. This is also a good time to stretch, to loosen tight muscles and restore and enhance flexibility.

Cool-down activities can also help to prevent symptoms—dizziness for example—that some people experience if they abruptly stop exercising.[3] A cool-down also can help prevent muscle cramps that might otherwise occur.

Up to now, this chapter has introduced the elements of fitness and described the principles that govern practice. The next few sections provide pointers on how, exactly, one goes about getting fit.

≡▶ *Warm-up activities ready the body tissues for exertion. Cool-down activities help tissues in the transition from exertion to relaxation.*

■≡ Gaining Flexibility

Flexibility depends on the **elasticity** of **muscles**, **tendons**, and **ligaments** and on the condition of the joints (**cartilage** and bone). If the body is flexible, it can move as it was designed to move and will bend instead of tearing or breaking in response to sudden stresses. Flexibility thus becomes especially critical in the later years of life, when falls and the injuries they cause can be life-threatening. In addition, the flexible body can move gracefully. Figure 7–2 shows that body joints are bound by connective tissues loosely enough to permit movement, yet tightly enough to withstand the stresses of vigorous physical activity.

Each body joint has its own movement potential, its **range of motion**, determined by the structure of the joint and the flexibility of its connective tissues. Knees and elbows, for example, bend in one direction only, and if flexible, they move unimpeded through their entire ranges of motion. Figure 7–3 compares an elbow joint, which allows limited one-way motion resembling that of a door hinge, with a shoulder joint, which allows full circular motion more like a ball-and-socket structure. Whatever a joint's potential range of motion, how well the joint moves within its range is determined by the flexibility of the surrounding tissues.

elasticity   the characteristic of being easily stretched or bent and able to return to original size and shape.

range of motion   the mobility of a joint; the direction and the extent to which it bends.

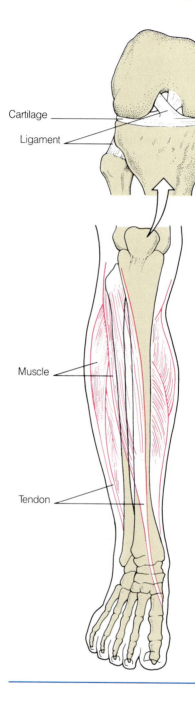

Cartilage

Ligament

cartilage connective tissue that resembles bone but has no embedded minerals; in joints, cartilage reduces friction and cushions the ends of bones.

ligaments flexible straps of connective tissue that connect bones to each other and support joints.

Muscle

muscles tissues made of many fibers (long, thin cells) that have the ability to contract. The muscles of interest here are the **skeletal muscles,** which move the bones. (Other muscles are the heart muscle and the muscles of internal organs.)

Tendon

tendons elastic, flexible straps of connective tissue that anchor the ends of muscles to bones.

FIGURE 7–2 ■ **Muscles, tendons, ligaments, and cartilage.**

As a muscle contracts, it pulls the two bones to which it is attached closer together, creating movement. Joints can bend, and muscles, tendons, and ligaments can stretch, but each has its limits.

Flexibility improves in response to stretching. When you stretch, remember that the goal is to get limber, not to be a contortionist. (Observe a cat stretching, and notice the technique—the stretch is long and luxurious, a few moments of pure pleasure.) Choose easy stretches, and stretch only to the point of resistance—that is, you should feel tightness, but not pain.[4] As you hold the stretch, even the feeling of tightness should gradually ease. If the tightness does not ease, or the stretch becomes painful, you are overstretching.

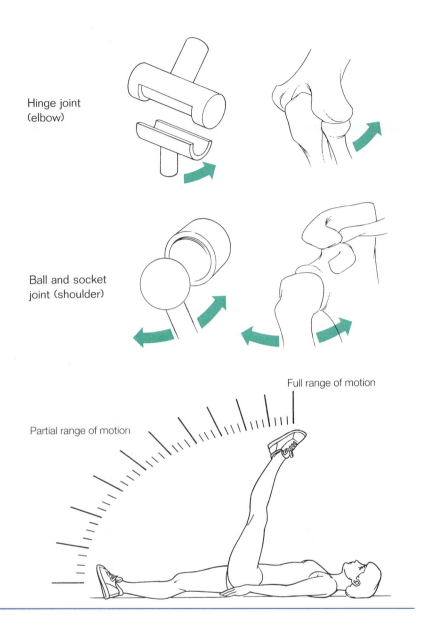

Hinge joint
(elbow)

Ball and socket
joint (shoulder)

Full range of motion

Partial range of motion

FIGURE 7–3 ■ **Examples of joints and their ranges of motion.**

A joint is flexible when it has its full range of motion.

Stretch in smooth motions—do not bounce. Bouncing can easily overstretch or tear a ligament until it can no longer support its joint, making the joint prone to injury. Nerves can overstretch painfully, too, if you are only slightly too enthusiastic. Table 7–2 lists some stretches and exercises to avoid; Figure 7–4 shows the ones that are recommended.

Warm up body tissues with five minutes of light activity or with a hot shower or bath before stretching. Then, to get a full stretch, relax the muscles, allow the body part to move slowly through its full range of motion, and hold each stretch position for 10 seconds. Breathe normally. Repeat the stretch once or twice. To improve, add 2 seconds to the time you hold each stretch until you can hold it for 30 seconds. Choose stretches that work all the major body regions: the neck, the shoulders, all back regions, pelvic regions, thighs (inner, front, and back), calf muscles, and ankles.

■ *FACT OR FICTION:* When performing stretching exercises, you should feel tightness but no pain. *True.*

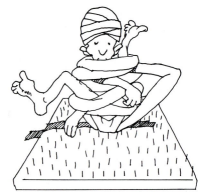

A stretch is long and luxurious, a few moments of pure pleasure.

TABLE 7–2 ■ Stretches and Exercises to Avoid	
Which	**Why**
Unsupervised yoga	May cause many types of injury
Hurdler's stretch (sit on floor with one leg in front, one bent under at the knee, and reach for the toe of the outstretched leg)	May cause knee injury
Toe touching with straight knees	May overstretch tendons and damage major nerves and vertebrae
Deep knee bend and duckwalk (performed so that the buttocks touch the heels)	May cause knee injury
Double straight-leg lift (lie on back and lift both straightened legs)	Aggravates lower back problems
Hyperextension of the back (arch the back and then let it sag, performed to extremes)	May injure lower back
Toe standing	May damage foot arch
Straight-leg sit-up	Aggravates lower back problems
Ballet stretch (designed for dancers)	May cause injuries to many body parts

≡▶ *Flexibility depends on the elasticity of muscles, tendons, and ligaments and on the condition of the joints. Stretching exercises improve flexibility. Flexibility helps prevent injuries, and so is especially important in the later years.*

■≡ Gaining Muscle Strength and Endurance

Strength is familiar to everyone. It is the ability of the muscles to work against **resistance**: to pull weeds from the ground, to push a stalled car, or to open a jar of jam. Many of today's mechanical helpers invented to spare effort rob us of the opportunity to develop strength—for example, a thermostat makes it easy to turn up the heat without chopping firewood. Muscle endurance, closely related to strength, is the ability of a muscle to sustain a contraction for a long time or to perform the contraction repeatedly.

Strength Conditioning

Two ways people gain muscle strength and endurance are through **weight training** and **calisthenics**. Weight training is the most efficient way. Weight training provides resistance in the form of free weights or resistance machines. It strengthens muscles, tendons, ligaments, and bones so that they better protect the body's internal organs from injury. Calisthenics provides resistance by using the body's parts as weights pulled or pushed against gravity.

Typically, weight training has been portrayed as a man's workout technique, but in reality it provides ideal strength training for both men and women. It need not produce big, bulky muscles. Bodybuilders can follow programs specifically designed to do just that, but you can tailor your

resistance a force that opposes another; in fitness, the weight or other opposing force against which muscles must work.

weight training exercise routines for muscular development that employ weights or mechanical devices to provide resistance against which the muscles can work.

calisthenics exercise routines for muscular development that use the parts of the body as weights.

■ *FACT OR FICTION:* The person who wishes to gain strength must work with free weights or machines to provide resistance for the muscles. *False.* The person can work with free weights or machines, but can also do calisthenics, which use the body's own parts as weights.

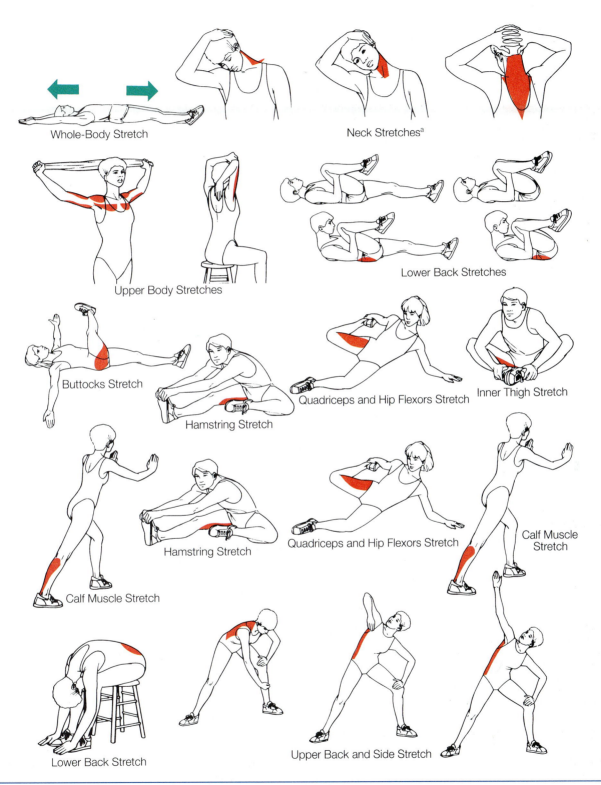

Whole-Body Stretch

Neck Stretches[a]

Upper Body Stretches

Lower Back Stretches

Buttocks Stretch

Hamstring Stretch

Quadriceps and Hip Flexors Stretch

Inner Thigh Stretch

Calf Muscle Stretch

Hamstring Stretch

Quadriceps and Hip Flexors Stretch

Calf Muscle Stretch

Lower Back Stretch

Upper Back and Side Stretch

FIGURE 7–4 ■ **Recommended stretches and exercises.**

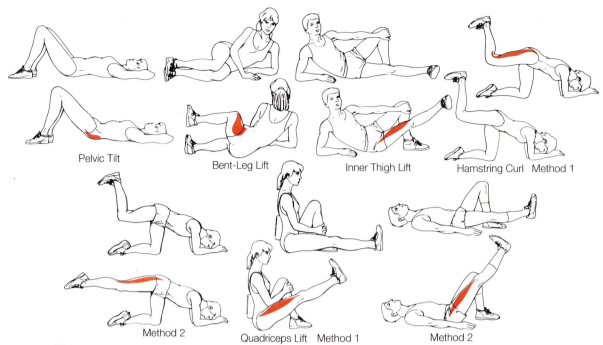

Pelvic Tilt   Bent-Leg Lift   Inner Thigh Lift   Hamstring Curl   Method 1

Method 2   Quadriceps Lift   Method 1   Method 2

FIGURE 7–4 ■ (continued)

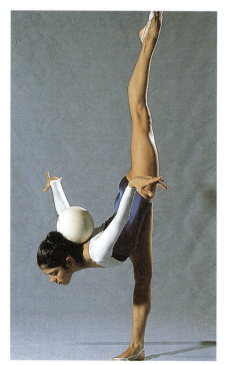

Stretching improves flexibility.

set a group of repetitions in a weight-training routine.

weight routine to meet other goals (use light weights and more repetitions to gain strength without bulk). And weight training need not produce muscle-bound inflexibility; that results from omission of flexibility training.

Figure 7–5 shows exercises that build strength, some using small weights (dumbbells) and others using parts of the body working against gravity to provide resistance (calisthenics). One repetition of any of these exercises is easy to do, so to improve, the exerciser must apply overload. To gain strength, increase the number of repetitions in a set or the number of sets in an exercise session.

Do not hold your breath when you lift heavy weights; it puts pressure on the heart and lungs and can damage them. Exhale as you raise or push the weight away (a way to remember this is to "blow the weight away from you"). Inhale as you lower the weight. Also, raise and lower the weight smoothly. Jerking it up or letting gravity pull it down fails to improve strength and threatens to injure your joints. To develop maximum strength from the smallest number of repetitions, lower the weight especially slowly.[5]* A complete group of ten repetitions of a particular exercise should take about a minute. Such a group of repetitions is called a **set**. Performing many sets with lighter weights mostly increases firmness and endurance, while doing fewer with heavier weights favors bulk and strength.

Small muscles fatigue quickly and can hinder your continuing the workout, so strengthen the larger muscle groups first, then the smaller ones. Make sure to distribute the weight work equally over the arms and legs, both sides—all the muscles. Overdeveloped muscles in one part of the body can stress other, weaker parts and cause damage—especially important with respect to back and stomach muscles. Heavy weights can also be dangerous.

*The raising of the weight is called a *lift;* the lowering is called a *negative.*

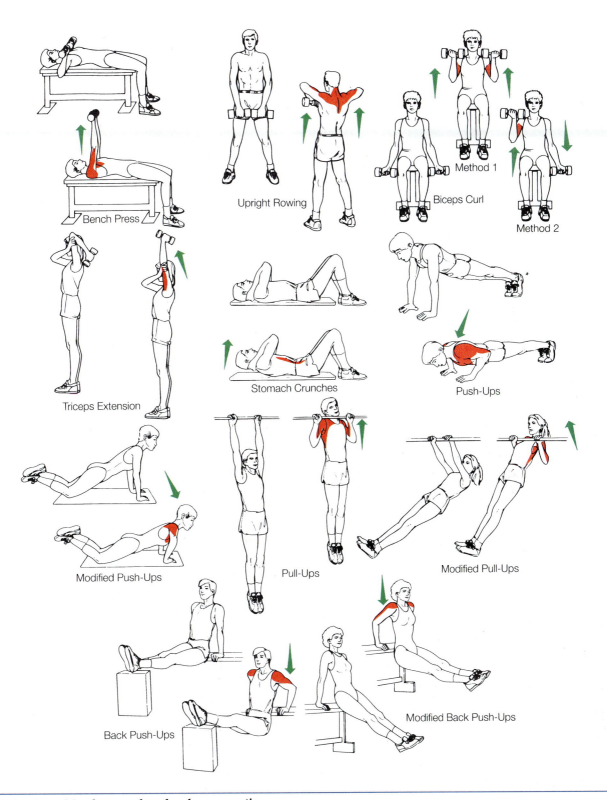

Bench Press

Triceps Extension

Modified Push-Ups

Upright Rowing

Stomach Crunches

Pull-Ups

Biceps Curl
Method 1
Method 2

Push-Ups

Modified Pull-Ups

Back Push-Ups

Modified Back Push-Ups

FIGURE 7–5 ■ **Muscle strength and endurance routines.**
[a]Many of the exercises show people using dumbells. Should you wish to use other equipment to achieve the same effects, consult a reputable trainer.

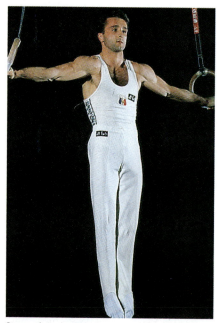

Strength is an important component of fitness.

steroids compounds of a certain chemical type; steroid hormones occur naturally in the body. Anabolic steroids produced by the body promote muscle growth.

Anyone who wishes to begin a program of weight training should seek guidance from a professional trainer who has a reputation for getting the desired results safely. New employees of spas and gyms may be long on enthusiasm but short on knowledge and experience.

Whether the goal is strength, endurance, or a firm body, weight training every other day or so seems to produce the best results. Rest is as important as work; muscles use the time between workouts to repair any small injuries, to replenish their fuel supplies, and to build themselves up. If you like to work out every day, just be sure to work different muscle groups today from those you worked yesterday—give each muscle group a day off. One solution is to alternate between strength workouts and cardiovascular workouts.

Strength develops when muscles work against resistance.

Strength Sought from Steroids and Other Artificial Means

It should go without saying that to use hormones or other drugs to improve strength is a bad idea. Hormones are particularly dangerous, but more athletes are using them today than ever before.[6] Hormone use is tempting, for the reasons presented here.

Men generally develop bulkier muscles than do women in response to exercise. This occurs because men produce larger amounts of the hormones known as **steroids** in their bodies. (These hormones are called *anabolic*, signifying that they promote muscle growth.) These hormones are also available as drugs, used medically to remedy deficiencies in people born without the ability to produce them; and like all drugs, they can be abused. Some athletes, both men and women, self-administer anabolic steroid drugs in the attempt to develop bulkier muscles. Many studies of these practices show that anabolic steroid drugs can increase body weight (especially lean body weight) and, if used in combination with high-intensity weight training, can increase muscular strength in some highly conditioned athletes.[7] No extra aerobic capacity is gained by steroid drug use.[8]

To athletes struggling to excel, the promise of bigger, stronger muscles beyond those that training alone can produce is tempting. Athletes who are not genetic superstar material, and who normally would not be able to break into the elite ranks, can, using steroids, suddenly defeat their former peers and compete with true champions. Such unfair competition compels still other athletes to abuse the drugs. Especially in professional circles, where monetary rewards for excellence are enormous, steroid abuse is common, despite its illegality.

The medical community is concerned about the risks of steroid drug abuse. For one thing, all steroid users experience a sharp change in their blood lipid profiles reflecting an increased risk of heart disease.[9] In addition, steroids are known to cause cancerous liver tumors, liver rupture, and hemorrhage; promote permanent changes in the reproductive system; and alter facial appearance.

Some of the side effects of hormone abuse occur in all people who abuse steroids. In men, the testicles shrink; in women, the breasts shrink, mustache and body hair grows, and the genitals change. People of both genders may experience mood swings, aggressive behavior, and changes in sexual appetite. Steroids bring early sexual maturity in children, they stunt growth in teens who have not yet reached full height, and they may cause acne. Some steroid abusers suffer the most deadly effects promptly; other abusers begin to show symptoms only after 20 years of abuse.

A recent report tells of an ex-football player, Lyle Alzado, who took steroids in an attempt to regain earlier prowess. He now has inoperable cancer at the age of 41. Believing that the steroids depressed his immune system and permitted the cancer to develop, Alzado has gone public with his past steroid abuse. He hopes that his plight might convince other football players to steer clear of steroids.[10]

Because steroids are detectable by urine testing, some athletes have resorted to abusing other hormones that are not detectable, with equally negative effects. Athletes who take **human growth hormone**, for example, develop symptoms of the disease **acromegaly**—huge body size, widened jawline, widened nose, protruding brow and teeth, and an increased likelihood of death before age 50.[11]

The American Academy of Pediatrics and the American College of Sports Medicine condemn the use of hormones by athletes. The federal government agrees. The Food and Drug Administration now classifies steroids with other often-abused prescription drugs and is attempting to limit their availability by requiring that health care providers who wish to dispense them be registered with the Drug Enforcement Administration.[12]

Remember that the start of this chapter talked about miracle pills for fitness? If there were such a thing, people would no doubt gobble them like candy. The use of steroids is just one manifestation of the belief in magic that hooks people into seeking easy ways to hard achievements. Other ways are inspected in the Critical Thinking section that follows.

≡▶ *Hormones promote muscle growth, but self-administering hormones is dangerous to health.*

> **human growth hormone** a nonsteroid hormone produced in the body that promotes growth; also taken as a drug by athletes to enlarge muscles.

> **acromegaly** (ack-ro-MEG-a-lee) a disease caused by above-normal levels of human growth hormone, characterized in adults by thickening of the bones, hands, feet, cheeks, and jaw; thickening of the soft tissue of the eyelids, lips, tongue, and nose; and thickening and rumpling of the skin on the forehead and soles of the feet. Internally, the heart, liver, and other organs become distorted. A child with the condition is said to have *gigantism*, because the bones grow abnormally long.

■≡ Gaining Cardiovascular Endurance

You're exercising. Your heart beats fast, your blood races through your arteries, your breathing delivers great lungfuls of air. How long can your heart and lungs keep going? How developed is your cardiovascular endurance?

At the start of this chapter, Table 7–1 listed some of the benefits of exercise. All of the benefits listed there derive directly from cardiovascular endurance training. Some of the benefits, such as sound sleep, increased lean body mass, and improved self-image, can be promoted by way of flexibility or strength training, but cardiovascular endurance training promotes each and every one. Cardiovascular endurance is, therefore, the component of fitness most important to health and life.

Principles of Cardiovascular Conditioning

Cardiovascular conditioning, that is, improvement in the condition of the heart and blood vessels, comes from workouts that call for cardiovascular

> **cardiovascular conditioning** improvements in the heart and lung function and increased blood volume, brought about by aerobic training.

[a]If you have questions about a fitness product, book, or program, write to the American College of Sports Medicine at its address given in Appendix A.

ergogenic a term that implies "energy giving"; in fact, no products impart such a quality.

CRITICAL THINKING

Pills, Powders, and Potions for Fitness

Athletes and other active people can be easy targets for promoters who sell a tide of products—herbal steroid-drug substitutes, protein supplements, vitamin or mineral supplements, "complete" drinks, "muscle-building" powders, electrolyte pills, and many other so-called **ergogenic** aids. The term *ergogenic* implies that such products have special work-enhancing powers. Actually no food or supplement is ergogenic.

Advertisements for commercial products may read as these do: "SWINDLE amino acids deposit slabs of muscle bulk"; "Hoodwink enzymes ram the body into turbo charge"; "Ultrapotent TECHNO-HYPE vitamins and minerals blast carbs through your system." Fortunately, ads like these are easy to see through—they are transparent in their purpose of trying to pick readers' pockets.

However, some ads, though just as false, create the illusion of credibility to gain readers' trust and thus boost sales. Such ads might have graphs, tables, and a professional-looking "review of the literature" citing such credible sources as the *American Journal of Clinical Nutrition* and the *Journal of the American Medical Association*.

This sounds scientific, and it may be, but don't forget that advertisements are written not to teach, but to sell. A careful reading might reveal that the company has taken the facts out of context. In one such case, ad writers cited an article to support an invalid conclusion: that healthy athletes should take supplements. However, researchers reporting in the cited article had found only that supplements were useful in treating a disease—a true fact. The ad writers had twisted the fact to support sales of their product.[a]

Protein powders can supply amino acids to the body, and many athletes take these powders with the false hope of stimulating muscle growth. Physical overload is the stimulant for muscle growth, and muscles do not respond to excess protein by building up. Any protein taken in excess of the body's need is burned off as energy or is stored as body fat. Besides, extra amino acids place an extra burden on the kidneys to excrete the nitrogen generated from their breakdown.

Amino acid supplements can be especially dangerous and are never needed by healthy athletes. Advertisers like to point out that **branched-chain amino acids** are used as fuel by exercising muscles. What their ads leave out is that compared with glucose and fatty acids, branched-chain amino acids provide minuscule amounts of fuel, and that supplements

branched-chain amino acids amino acids that, unlike the others, can directly provide energy to muscle tissue.

endurance—aerobic training. As a result of this training, the total blood volume increases, so the blood can carry more oxygen. The heart muscle gains size and strength, each beat of the heart pumps more blood, fewer beats are necessary, and the pulse rate slows. The muscles that work the lungs gain strength and endurance, and breathing becomes more efficient. Blood moves easily through the body's arteries and veins, and the blood are unneeded because the liver liberates the right amounts of branched-chain amino acids with precision timing.

Most people assume that pills available over the counter are safe and effective, but the story of what happened to people who bought and used some over-the-counter amino acid supplements shows otherwise. Many people who took pills of the amino acid tryptophan sickened, and at least one person died, from a serious blood condition. The pills were banned from sale, but replacements for tryptophan soon appeared on shelves of health-food stores. These, too, have proved dangerous and have been banned. The point of this story is that pill-taking may seem like a "scientific" approach to nutrition, but even science is limited in its knowledge of how concentrated nutrients interact with the body. Stick with food to provide protein and other nutrients; wholesome food in a balanced diet is virtually guaranteed safe and effective.

Herbs, too, are often peddled to fitness seekers—for example, as legal substitutes for steroid drugs. Sellers falsely claim that these herbs contain hormones, enhance the body's natural hormones, or both. In some cases, an herb may contain some amount of a plant steriod, but not of the type that is active in human beings. The body cannot convert herbal compounds to human steroids, nor does it gain muscle strength from them. The herbs may contain toxins, though, and can have unexpected side effects. Don't make the mistake of equating "natural" with "harmless."

Vitamin and mineral supplements can, if overdone, be even more toxic than herbs, and they are offered to athletes in abundance. As this chapter's Spotlight makes clear, supplements do not enhance the performance of well-nourished people. In spite of this, some athletes may wish to take a supplement anyway. The choices of whether to do so and of which type to take should be made on the basis of the information in the Spotlight of chapter 5, and should not be influenced by glittering words such as "for athletes" or "promotes fitness" written on the label.

In the end, people are left to defend themselves against the lies and half-truths presented to them about fitness products and schemes. Think defensively, then, and keep handy your arsenal of knowledge. Remember to use it when faced with claims that, while they may sound helpful, could rip you off or harm you. The overwhelming majority of potions touted for athletes are frauds.

If pills do seem to work, they probably work by the power of suggestion: don't discount that power, because it is powerful. In fact, use it instead of the pills: imagine yourself as a winner, and visualize yourself as capable in your sport. You don't have to rely on magic for an extra edge, because you already have a real one—your mind.

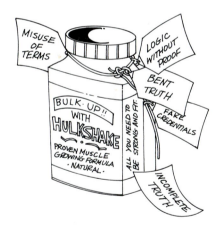

For athletes especially, supplements are silly.

pressure falls. The heart develops extra vessels through which to route its blood supply, **collateral vessels**. Muscles throughout the body become firmer, and like the heart muscle, respond to overload by becoming larger and stronger. Figure 7–6 shows major relationships among the heart, circulatory system, and lungs. A healthy heart and circulatory system reflect a generally healthy person.

collateral vessels alternate blood routes through the heart muscle thought to be important in surviving a heart attack.

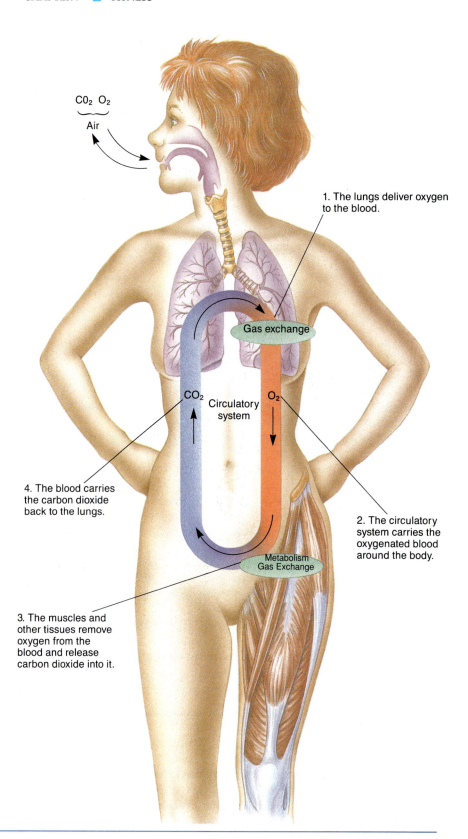

FIGURE 7–6 ■ **Delivery of oxygen by the heart and lungs to the muscles.**

The more fit a muscle is, the more oxygen it draws from the blood. That oxygen is drawn from the lungs, so the person with more fit muscles extracts from the inhaled air more oxygen than a person with less fit muscles. The cardiovascular system responds to the demand for oxygen by building up its capacity to deliver oxygen. Researchers can measure cardiovascular fitness by measuring the amount of oxygen a person consumes per minute while working out, a measure called **VO$_2$ max.**

Labels within figure:

CO_2 O_2
Air

1. The lungs deliver oxygen to the blood.

Gas exchange

CO_2 Circulatory system O_2

2. The circulatory system carries the oxygenated blood around the body.

4. The blood carries the carbon dioxide back to the lungs.

Metabolism Gas Exchange

3. The muscles and other tissues remove oxygen from the blood and release carbon dioxide into it.

VO$_2$ max   the maximum volume of oxygen consumed per minute.

A highly-prized improvement that accompanies cardiovascular conditioning is a lean body composition. Conditioned tissues burn more fat, not just during exercise, but all the time, because they've developed more fat-burning enzymes with which to do the job. The overall effect is reduced body fatness and reduced health risks that accompany overfatness.

A slow resting pulse reflects a healthy cardiovascular system. You may want to perform an informal pulse check right now. As a rule of thumb, the average resting pulse rate for adults is around 70 beats per minute, but the rate can be higher or lower. Active people can have resting pulse rates of 50 or even lower. Instructions for taking your pulse are given in Figure 7–7.

Pulse is an indicator of cardiovascular health, and professional athletes surround themselves with technical trappings to measure it—stopwatches, graphs, and charts. You need not get tangled up in all this, though: just get up and run, dance, or anything you'd like (see the upcoming list in the margin). A guideline for the fitness-minded who do not aspire to the Olympics is to walk, jog, or run for 20 minutes at a rate at which you can talk but not sing. If you can't talk, slow down; if you can sing, speed up. A few of the guidelines that follow are addressed specifically to athletes, but you can translate them all into informal terms.

≡▶ *In response to cardiovascular conditioning, total blood volume increases, the heart muscle gains size and strength, the heart makes extra blood vessels, the pulse rate falls, breathing becomes more efficient, the blood pressure falls, the body becomes leaner as it burns its fat for fuel, and muscles throughout the body become firmer.*

Training for Cardiovascular Endurance

To improve cardiovascular fitness, you must work up to a point where you can exercise aerobically for 20 minutes or more. This requires working with an elevated heart rate (pulse) for that long. The rate to shoot for is considerably faster than the resting rate to "push" the heart, but not so fast as to strain it. Athletes call this the **target heart rate**, and one way you can calculate yours is to start with your age. To calculate your target heart rate, first subtract your age from 220. This provides an estimate of the absolute *maximum heart rate* for a person your age. You should never exercise at this rate, of course. Now multiply your maximum heart rate by 0.75 to get your target heart rate (see the example in the margin). When you first work out, a slow pace may push your heart to the target rate. As your cardiovascular fitness improves, you will have to work at a faster pace to push your heart to beat that fast.

A person who can work out at the target heart rate for 20 to 30 minutes has arrived at this fitness goal. In the building-up stage, **interval training** can ease progress. To use it, a jogger might run at the target heart rate for 2 minutes before tiring, then rest by walking until ready to jog again, run another 2 minutes, then rest by walking, and so on for 20 minutes. At each session the jogger can make the running periods longer and the resting periods shorter. Eventually, in about two months or so, the rest periods will no longer be needed at all. Once up to that level, the exerciser can maintain fitness by repeating the workout about every other day.

You can develop cardiovascular fitness only if you choose aerobic activity. This activity must:

target heart rate   the heartbeat rate that will achieve cardiovascular conditioning for a person—fast enough to push the heart, but not so fast as to strain it.

Target heart rate for a 21-year-old person:

Maximum heart rate = 220 − 21 = 199.

Target heart rate = 199 × 0.75 = 149 beats per minute.

interval training   a pattern for aerobic conditioning that involves exercising at the target heart rate for longer and longer periods of time with breaks between.

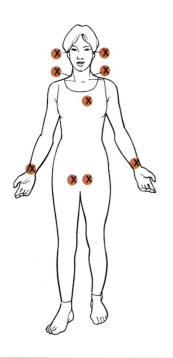

FIGURE 7–7 ■ **How to take your pulse.**
Get a watch or clock with a second hand. Rest a few minutes for a resting pulse. Place your hand over your heart or your finger firmly over an artery in any pulse location shown here that gives a clear rhythm. Start counting your pulse at a convenient second, and continue counting for ten seconds. If a heartbeat occurs exactly on the tenth second, count it as one-half beat. Multiply by 6 to obtain the beats per minute. To ensure a true count:

- Use only fingers, not your thumb, on the pulse point (the thumb has a pulse of its own).
- Press just firmly enough to feel the pulse. Too much pressure can interfere with the pulse rhythm.

low-impact aerobic dance   aerobic dance in which one foot remains on the floor to prevent impact shock to the feet and legs.

- Be relatively low in intensity.
- Use large muscle groups, such as legs, buttocks, and abdomen.
- Be uninterrupted and last for at least 20 minutes.

Walking, aerobic dancing, running, swimming, and cycling all meet these criteria. While many people know a good deal about these activities already, a few facts about them might help.

Walking can be beneficial, but the walker must put some oomph in the pace to achieve an aerobic workout. Strolling along at a pace of 1 or 2 miles per hour might help you to warm up, but striding along at 3.5 to 5 miles per hour is the way to get a workout for your heart. To overload, swing your arms; to progress further, swing 2- to 3-pound weights.[13] People who walk for fitness enjoy practically injury-free workouts (so long as they wear supportive walking shoes and watch for traffic), because walking is easy on the joints and connective tissues. Walkers savor the sights, smells, and sounds they encounter as they move through the world at the original human pace, and they pity the multitudes who miss it all as they whiz through life in their automobiles.

Aerobic dancing is fun and challenging, requires little more equipment than walking, and can provide a balanced, full-body workout as well as a cardiovascular workout. In **low-impact aerobic dance**, one foot always remains in contact with the floor, thus minimizing the chances of injury (see next section). Some dance routines incorporate exercises such as stair climbing, and these can be challenging and fun. Look for classes that are not overcrowded, so that you can move around the room and change direction freely, take long strides, and lift your legs high. These movements, performed with control and vigor, provide a truly effective cardiovascular workout.

What is it about running that makes it a passion for some? The challenge, simplicity, freedom, and mental and physical well-being that come with running keep many people on the road, day after day. However, with the joys come risks, and running injuries are common, as the next section makes clear. Still, running is well-suited to developing cardiovascular fitness, and many programs to reduce risks of heart disease recommend it.

As for swimming and cycling, these too provide the kind of work that strengthens the heart. It's easy to learn to swim and cycle, even for adults, and these activities are almost stress-free for joints and connective tissues. Research shows that swimming ranks high as a means of developing cardiovascular endurance and muscle strength and endurance (especially of the upper body). However, swimming seems not to bring about weight loss in the overweight as efficiently as some other aerobic activities do. Cycling, on the other hand, superbly develops the lower body while it improves cardiovascular endurance, and it promotes weight loss as well. Taken together, the two make a nice conditioning package—swimming for the upper body and heart; cycling for the lower body, heart, and weight control; and both for unique opportunities to enjoy the out-of-doors. Balanced fitness is important, and Table 7–3 can help you to evaluate how well a program of exercise supports it.

The activities just described are but a few of the many that people enjoy while gaining cardiovascular endurance. Don't limit yourself; just use your imagination, and go for it. For a lifestyle that encourages general fitness, this chapter's Strategies offer some novel ways to include exercise in your day.

TABLE 7–3 ■ How Balanced Is Your Fitness Program?

You can evaluate fitness programs objectively by using your knowledge of what fitness is and how it is gained and maintained. The following are some questions that can help in your evaluation. Start with 100 points, and subtract the points indicated for shortcomings.

1. Does the program include sufficient aerobic exercise for cardiovascular fitness (about 20 minutes, three days per week)? If not, **minus 10**.

2. Does the program include exercises that promote muscle strength and endurance, such as sit-ups, push-ups, or weight training? If not, **minus 5**. Are strengthening exercises given for all large muscle groups? If some parts are left out, **minus 5**.

3. Does the program include exercises for flexibility, such as gentle stretches? If not, **minus 10**.

4. Does the program allow for varying initial fitness levels; that is, can you start out slowly and work your way up? If not, **minus 10**.

5. Does the program take a reasonable time at each exercise session—say at least 20 minutes, but less than an hour—at least three days per week? If not, **minus 10**.

6. Does the program include a warm-up and a cool-down period? If no to either, **minus 5**; if no to both, **minus 10**.

7. Can the program be performed with only basic equipment, such as shoes, small weights, or a jump rope? Must you join an expensive club to participate? If specific or unusual products, perhaps sold by the promoters, must be used, or if a large membership fee is required, **minus 10**.

8. Is the program safe? If it suggests bouncy stretches or straight-leg sit-ups, give it a **minus 10**. If it advocates clearly hazardous practices, such as running in heavy or rubber clothing, don't even consider using it: its **total score is 0**.

9. Does the promoter make claims backed up by legitimate research? If unorthodox claims are made, such as "no-work fitness," "redistribute your fat" (or cellulite), or "cures your heart disease" (or other diseases), **minus 10**.

10. Does the program promote a lifetime fitness plan based on a variety of enjoyable activities? If the program is monotonous, it will soon become boring and hard to stay with, so give it a **minus 10**.

≡▶ *Activities that promote cardiovascular endurance are those that raise the heart rate and are sustained for 20 or more minutes. Many activities fit this description.*

■≡ Sports Safety: Preventing Sports Injuries and Accidents

Fitness-minded people talk a lot about shin splints, stress fractures, tennis elbows, sprains, strains and an assortment of other anatomical hobgoblins. The Miniglossary of Sports Injuries lists the injuries that are mentioned most often. These and others can be avoided by following a proper program that builds fitness slowly. Many people could become marathon runners given enough time, but they could do it without joint damage only if they built slowly. Proper equipment and expert advice can help keep you safe. Be sure the "expert" is truly qualified, though. Many employees of spas and health clubs lack knowledge and training, but freely offer advice that might lead to injury.

Some activities that will allow you to reach and sustain your target heart rate are:

Aerobic dancing.
Bicycling.
Cross-country skiing.
Fast walking.
Ice skating.
Jogging.
Rope jumping.
Rowing.
Stair walking.
Swimming.

These sports also help:

Basketball.
Hockey.
Lacrosse.
Racquetball.
Rugby.
Soccer.
Water polo.

■ ■ ■ ■ ■ **STRATEGIES:** *INCLUDING EXERCISE IN A DAY*

To include exercise in a day:

1. Join a corporate fitness program.
2. Join a social fitness club.
3. Make friends with people who help one another stay fit.
4. Play sports in school.
5. Get credit hours for dance, sports, or conditioning courses.
6. Improve your swim strokes.
7. Join a hiking or biking club.
8. Join a YMCA program.
9. Walk to nearby stores.
10. Park a few blocks from your destination, and walk the rest.
11. Take stairs instead of elevators.
12. Stretch often during the day.
13. Lift small weights while watching TV or talking on the phone.
14. Garden.
15. Play with children.
16. Coach a sport.
17. Do your own yard work.
18. Wash your car with extra vigor, or bend and stretch to wash your toes in the bath. Be imaginative.

■ *FACT OR FICTION:* If you feel pain in your feet or legs while running, it is best to keep going and try to work through it. *False.* You may aggravate an injury while running.

Be consistent, too. While too little exercise leads to illness in later years, too much too soon presents a hazard to health and life today. A "weekend athlete," who is sedentary all week and then exercises vigorously on weekends, invites injury, or even a heart attack. Vigorous and sudden demands on out-of-condition muscles, ligaments, and tendons lead to sprains and strains, and sudden demand can damage a weakened heart. Take on a regular program of fitness to develop the strength that safe weekend play demands.

Pain during activity is a signal that something is wrong. For example, if a jogger feels leg pain, a change of posture may be indicated. If the pain persists despite efforts to correct technique, stop the activity until the pain goes away, and then try again slowly, increasing just a little at a time.

To prevent injuries during running, the right shoes are essential. A runner hits the ground with a force of about two to three times the weight of the body, hundreds of times per mile. Running shoes should have an arch support, a flexible sole, and extra cushioning under the heel and the ball of the foot to stabilize the feet and cushion the tremendous impact of each stride. Most injuries in running result from pushing too hard, too fast in an attempt to get fit quickly. To begin a program, start slowly, use interval training, and do not try to rush progress. Run with the traffic, on the left side of the road. If you are a woman running alone, be sure to read and heed Spotlight 12's advice on rape prevention.

In aerobic dance, a good pair of aerobic dance shoes is critical to the safety of the feet and legs. Equally important to safety is the choice of fitness center—check the flooring to make sure that it is made of materials such as

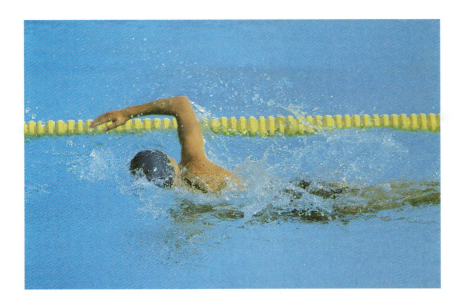

Swimming improves cardiovascular endurance and develops overall muscle strength and endurance as well.

elevated wood floors that absorb shock. Concrete floors are the worst—they are rigid and thus shock the lower body with each step.

As for swimmers and cyclists, following a few common-sense rules can avert the most common forms of injuries. To swim safely, never swim alone, and never when feeling sick, tired, or overfull from eating. Choose carefully a place to swim; be sure it is free of obstructions, such as logs lurking below the surface, before diving in. Stay out of the water if lightning threatens. Cyclists are safest riding with the flow of traffic on a bike equipped with reflectors, and while wearing bright-colored clothing. By far, the most important precaution is to buy a new, high-quality helmet, and to wear it on every ride. (Second-hand helmets may be flawed.) Head injuries account for 85 percent of the nation's 1,000 yearly cycling deaths.[14] Heed the advice of the American Academy of Pediatrics, the National Safety Council, and the Bicycle Federation of America and wear a helmet.

If you have injured yourself, you have two options: to go to a health care provider, or to wait to see whether it clears up by itself. (If you are bleeding or badly hurt, of course, choose the former.) Pain is your guide. If the pain diminishes during the first few hours, chances are the injury is slight. If it increases or stays the same for several hours, you may have a serious condition that requires attention.

If any injury fails to clear up in two or three days, get medical help, but while you are waiting, you can use the RICE principle: Rest, Ice, Compression, and Elevation. To do this, rest the injured part; place an ice pack, wrapped in cloth, on the injury for 15 to 30 minutes at intervals throughout the first day; wrap it comfortably in tape or an elastic bandage; and keep the injured part elevated. The ice reduces fluid accumulation, soothes pain, and promotes healing. Never use heat at first. Tape and bandages provide compression to help reduce swelling. They are not meant to enable you to keep playing despite an injury; to do so is to invite an even worse injury.

RICE:

■ Rest
■ Ice
■ Compression
■ Elevation

Be alert to the dangers of overheating and dehydration. Heat is a by-product of energy fuel breakdown, so muscles heat up during exertion; they are "burning" large amounts of fuel. The body attempts to maintain a normal temperature: blood penetrates the muscles and transports the heat to the skin, where the surrounding air and the evaporation of sweat can carry it away. On humid days, though, sweat does not evaporate well, heat builds up, and the body sweats copiously in an attempt to effect cooling. This excessive sweating can be extremely hazardous, because fluid and electrolyte losses beyond a certain point compromise cellular functioning. It can even be fatal.

The body sends signals of distress, such as cramps, nausea, chest pains, or diarrhea, that warn of overheating: **heat stroke** may be threatening. The most important preventive step is to stop the activity immediately, seek out shade and a cool place, and rest. For the same reasons, it is unwise to exercise in a plastic or rubber suit in hopes of losing pounds. The waterproof material prevents evaporation, causing you to sweat excessively, and brings about a dangerous rise in body temperature. Similarly, too long a stay in a hot whirlpool bath, hot tub, or sauna can cause heat stroke. Pointers to avoid heat stroke:

■ Drink adequate fluid.
■ Recognize dangerous conditions—high humidity, high temperature, or both.
■ Limit intentional exposure to heat.

In potential heat stroke weather:

■ Wear lightweight, loose-fitting clothing.
■ Drink several extra glasses of water in the hours before you exercise heavily.
■ Replace water lost during the activity with a dilute, cold beverage every 15 to 20 minutes. Recommended is about 5 ounces of cold, plain or lightly flavored water or one part fruit juice to four parts water.
■ Recognize your body's distress signals, and heed the message to stop exercising—take a rest in the shade.

Dehydration hampers performance and, if severe, can become life threatening. It can come on faster than most people realize, so remember: if you sweat heavily, you need fluids. Table 7–4 offers a hydration schedule that allows for fluid needs to be met in advance by drinking extra *before* the event. Salt tablets or other forms of salt are almost never heeded and should be given only under medical supervision. Taking salt tablets may make dehydration worse, because they attract water from the tissues into the

heat stroke a dangerous buildup of body heat that can be fatal.

■ *FACT OR FICTION:* It is best not to interrupt a workout to drink a beverage. *False.* It is best to rehydrate as you go.

TABLE 7–4　■　**Fluids before, during, and after Physical Activity**

When To Drink	Amount of Fluids
2 hours before exercise	About 3 c
10 or 15 minutes before exercise	About 2 c
Every 10 to 20 minutes during exercise	About $\frac{1}{2}$ c or more
After exercise	Replace each pound of body weight lost with 2 c fluid

SOURCE: Adapted from J. B. Marcus, ed., *Sports Nutrition* (Chicago: American Dietetic Association, 1986), p. 57.

digestive tract at first. Alcoholic beverages can also cause dehydration. Worse, they rob a person of the judgment needed to stay safe during physical activity. Cold water is the best fluid to drink; most people don't need the salt and sugar in commercial sports drinks. (Endurance athletes, however, may benefit from the sugar they contain.) As for minerals, it is now believed that the best way to replenish those lost in sweat is by consuming ordinary foods and beverages that contain them naturally.

■ *FACT OR FICTION:* Water is the beverage of choice to replace body fluids lost during exercise. *True.*

≡▶ *Most injuries are preventable. The most important preventive measures are to follow proper form, take pain seriously and stop working, and take precautions against heat stroke.*

The progress to fitness is not without setbacks, but setbacks often herald impending success. To deal with them, remember, obstacles only get in your way when you take your eyes off your goals. Don't let them stop you:

- In bad weather, play racquetball or another indoor sport.
- If lonely or depressed, call a friend to go with you.
- If dissatisfied with your progress, look back to see where you started and how far you've come.
- If busy, remember that a workout will boost your energy.
- If sore, enjoy each ache as a badge of courage (and be gentler next time).
- If discouraged, buy yourself a new sweatband or other such symbol to strengthen your identity as "one who does."

"Are you one of those people who can miss a workout because:

- You were expecting a phone call?
- You couldn't find a clean pair of socks?
- They were calling for rain showers?

The problem is you think too much. You know you're going to feel better once you get started with your workout—and *lots* better when you are done. So what's to think about?"

SOURCE: *Executive Edge Newsletter* (see credits).

Physical activity works in harmony with all the other life management skills. It promotes emotional health physically, by improving the chemistry of the brain and circulation to it, and psychologically, by enhancing self-esteem. It aids in stress management: the stress response readies the body for exercise, and exercise discharges the tension. Hand in hand with nutrition, exercise renews and nourishes every body part. Spiritually, play contributes joy.

Your health is worth the time and energy it takes to include physical activity in your day. Jog, play a game, ride a bike. Hike with friends. You work hard every day—you deserve a break every day, too. Go have fun.

■≡ For Review

1. List the benefits that arise from keeping the body physically fit through regular exercise.

2. Describe the components of fitness.

3. Define the terms *overload* and *use-disuse*, and explain how they relate to physical fitness.

4. Name the two predominant types of muscle fibers, and list for each the associated type of work and the associated type of fuel.

5. Describe the relationship of oxygen debt to lactic acid buildup.

6. Describe the benefits derived from both warm-up and cool-down activities.

7. Identify the types of exercises that would best develop each of the following: (1) flexibility, (2) muscle strength, (3) muscle endurance, and (4) cardiovascular endurance.

8. Give some reasons why steroid drug abuse is an unwise practice.

9. Name some factors to consider when evaluating a fitness program.

10. Identify important safety measures for each of several fitness activities.

■ ≡ Notes

1. Much of this discussion is based on L. K. DeBruyne, F. S. Sizer, and E. N. Whitney, *The Fitness Triad: Motivation, Training, and Nutrition* (St. Paul, Minn.: West, 1991).

2. K. E. Powell and coauthors, Status of the 1990 objectives for physical fitness and exercise, *Public Health Reports* 101 (1986): 15–19.

3. C. A. Milesis, M. G. Fougeron, and H. Graham, Effect of active vs. passive recovery on cardiac time components, *Journal of Sports Medicine* 22 (1982): 147–153.

4. B. Anderson, *Stretching* (Bolinas, Calif.: Shelter, 1980), p. 12.

5. K. Hakkinen, M. Alen, and P. V. Komi, Neuromuscular, anaerobic, and aerobic performance characteristics of elite power athletes, *European Journal of Applied Physiology* 53 (1984): 97–105.

6. C. L. Chng and A. Moore, A study of steroid use among athletes: Knowledge, attitude and use, *Health Education* 21 (1990): 12–17.

7. P. G. Dyment and B. Goldberg, Anabolic steroids and the adolescent athlete, *Pediatrics* 83 (1989): 127–128.

8. H. Haupt and G. D. Rovere, Anabolic steroids: A review of the literature, *American Journal of Sports Medicine* 12 (1984): 469–484.

9. M. Alen and P. Rahkila, Reduced high-density lipoprotein-cholesterol in power athletes: Use of male sex hormone derivatives, an atherogenic factor, *International Journal of Sports Medicine* 5 (1984): 341–342; O. L. Webb, P. M. Laskarzewski, and C. J. Glueck, Severe depression of high-density lipoprotein cholesterol levels in weight lifters and body builders by self-administered exogenous testosterone and anabolic-androgenic steroids, *Metabolism* 33 (1984): 971–975.

10. H. Book, Steroids leave Alzado a ruined body and life, *Tallahassee Democrat,* c. March–June 1991.

11. D. R. Lamb, Anabolic steroids in athletics: How well do they work and how dangerous are they? *American Journal of Sports Medicine* 12 (1984): 31–38.

12. Anabolic steroids controlled substances, *FDA Consumer,* May 1991, p. 3.

13. J. M. Rippe and coauthors, Walking for fitness, *Physician and Sportsmedicine,* October 1986, pp. 145–159.

14. Risks to the child as bicycle passenger, *Sports Medicine Digest,* April 1989, p. 5.

SPOTLIGHT

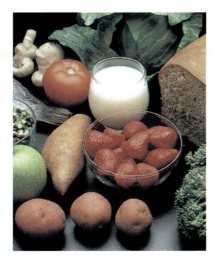

Food For Sport

In the body, fitness and nutrition go hand in hand. The working body demands carbohydrate and fat for energy. It requires protein to build new tissue. It also requires vitamins, minerals, and water to support both these functions. However, while an active body needs *nutrients*, this doesn't mean that it needs *supplements*. Supplements can provide the body with a few of the nutrients it needs, but wise food choices can provide them all.

To obtain the needed nutrients, athletes would do well to heed the proved advice that benefits everyone—eat a balanced diet, control calories, and choose a variety of foods. Beyond these basics, athletes wonder if special foods or nutrients might confer on them special physical prowess. Right away, they should know that no food and no concentrated form of a nutrient has ever been shown to be helpful to the

physical performance of otherwise well-nourished people. However, the diet itself can help or hinder performance.

I work out each day, and I'd like to go out for the track team. Can my diet help me make the team?

The right diet can assist you in your efforts, but it would be an exaggeration to say that diet alone can help you make the team. Rather, the right fuels and other nutrients provide raw materials from which to build muscle and support activity, and enough fluid to allow your body to work hard. Once these things are in place, dedication and hard work can win your spot on the team. Without the right raw materials, you'd be handicapped in striving to make physical gains.

What fuels are best to support my activity? I've heard that carbohydrates are the best.

Yes, carbohydrates are best. At rest, your body uses a mix of about equal parts of fat and carbohydrate. However, when you begin to work physically, the mix of fuels changes. Remember (from the list in the margin on page 173), fat "goes with" aerobic activity—such as casual jogging. Glucose "goes with" anaerobic activity—such as sprinting. So if you are a casual jogger, you'll use mostly fat to provide your energy (but you'll still use some carbohydrate). Long-distance runners, who run hard for more than an hour and a half at a time, use more carbohydrate (although they still use some fat). Sprinters use mostly carbohydrate.

These relationships translate into the body's needs for nutrients. Since the body can store unlimited amounts of fat, and since fat is abundant in the

diet, exercisers need not worry about obtaining enough fat. But carbohydrate is a different story. The body's carbohydrate (glycogen) stores are limited, and must be replenished from food daily.

The availability of glucose to working muscles has a great effect on their performance. Joggers require some carbohydrate to keep going, but they use mostly fat, and their carbohydrate supplies won't normally limit their abilities. Long-distance runners, on the other hand, work at higher intensities (at a faster running pace) and for longer, so they use more carbohydrate than do joggers. Glucose availability can be critical to the completion of a marathon event. A sprinter performs work that can drain away the body's glycogen stores in just a few sprints. In a hot climate, extra glycogen confers an additional advantage on endurance athletes; as glycogen breaks down, it releases water, which helps to meet the athlete's fluid needs.

The athlete who eats more carbohydrate stores more glycogen, and so can perform for a longer time. For many athletes, dietary carbohydrate is the nutrient most critical to performance. Figure S7–1 shows the results of a classic study that still holds true today: a high-carbohydrate diet can triple an athlete's endurance.

What's the best high-carbohydrate food? I assume candy bars would be great.

From the standpoint that candy provides sugar (simple carbohydrate), candy bars might be useful. Candy is available, requires no preparation, and tastes delicious. But before you load up on candy, you should know that most candy contains not just sugar, but a lot of fat. In fact, in most

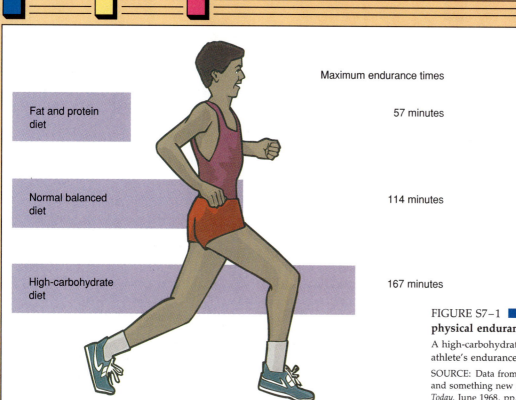

Maximum endurance times

Fat and protein diet

57 minutes

Normal balanced diet

114 minutes

High-carbohydrate diet

167 minutes

FIGURE S7–1 ■ The effect of diet on physical endurance.

A high-carbohydrate diet can triple an athlete's endurance.

SOURCE: Data from P. Astrand, Something old and something new . . . very new, *Nutrition Today,* June 1968, pp. 9–11.

candies, fat calories out number sugar calories. And another thing—candy provides almost no other nutrients. Once in a while, athletes and other active people can afford to indulge in a treat of candy, but when it begins to displace nutritious foods from the diet, the person's overall nutrition suffers. Candy may be quick and easy to eat, but food provides what the body needs and is a better choice.

Are you telling me I should eat more bread, potatoes, and pasta to provide carbohydrate instead of eating candy?

Yes, those are the foods to emphasize along with fruits (almost pure carbohydrate), low-fat milk products, cereals, grains, and vegetables. Olympic training tables are laden with such choices.*

*A balanced diet for athletes consists of nourishing foods that provide between 55 and 65% of calories from carbohydrates.

How can I store a maximum of carbohydrate in my muscles?

Athletes use a technique called carbohydrate loading to trick their muscles into storing extra glycogen before a competition. Don't do this the way they did it in the past, though: don't switch from a low- to a high-carbohydrate diet. Here's the recommended routine. First, increase exercise intensity and eat normally. Next, during the week before competition, cut back on exercise, and on the day before, rest completely while eating a very high carbohydrate diet. You'll store extra glycogen this way, and this can benefit you if you have to keep going 90 minutes or longer at a stretch.

If your work is of shorter duration, just eat a regular high-carbohydrate diet. A high-carbohydrate meal eaten within two hours after physical

activity accelerates the rate of glycogen storage by 300 percent.[1]* Eating the meal after two hours has passed reduces the glycogen synthesis rate by almost half. So after your own workout, you might want to relax with a glass of orange juice and some crackers or other carbohydrate-rich snack, just for your glycogen's sake.

Are there also special foods I should eat?

Don't think in terms of special foods. A better approach is just to eat an athlete's diet every day. Instead of "special foods," think in terms of "special diet," because no one food provides an advantage over any similar food, and none has special powers. What matters is the total

*Reference notes are at the end of the Spotlight.

diet—all three meals, all snacks, eaten each day of every week.

What should I eat before a competitive event to make it go smoothly?

That's a good question, because the foods and liquids taken in during the hours before physical activity affect performance directly. On the day of competition, carefully plan your pregame meal, and eat it three to four hours before the event. It should be light (300 to 1,000 calories) and easily digested. It also should provide fluids to guard against dehydration and heat stroke. As usual, the meal should include many carbohydrate-rich foods such as potatoes, refined pastas and breads, and fruit juices. Not only do these foods supply glucose, but they move out of the digestive tract quickly, so that, during the event, your energy can be directed at competing, not at digesting. (Foods high in fat, protein,

and fiber require long times for digestion.) Tradition may call for a steak dinner before a big game, but the needs of each player are better served by a new tradition—eating a special high-carbohydrate meal before the game, and saving the steaks for later to celebrate the win. Table S7–1 provides some tips for planners of pregame meals.

Speaking of steaks, what about protein? I've always heard that athletes need more than other people do.

Athletes need just slightly more protein than do other people.[2] They use it not only to build muscles, but also for fuel. In particular, the muscles use more branched-chain amino acids for fuel, because these can provide energy in much the same way that glucose does. This makes the body's glycogen stores last longer during physical activity. An ordinary

diet easily provides the amount of protein an athlete needs and offers plenty of branched-chain amino acids, too. Don't take protein powders.

Almost every athlete I know takes vitamin C pills. Do athletes need more vitamin C than food provides?

Your question is part of a large issue: whether athletes need more of *any* vitamin than that amount provided by a regular diet. Athletes need adequate vitamins and minerals to do what they do, but do they need more than the average person? (See Appendix B for amounts of nutrients recommended daily.) The answer is that athletes generally do not need supplements—they get more nutrients because they eat more food. Of course there are exceptions, but health care providers should diagnose these. For example, a certain percentage of athletes are deficient in iron, just as a certain percentage of all people are.

For vitamin C, as for all the other vitamins (including vitamin B_{12} pills and shots, and vitamin E), studies show that more is not better—athletes who take vitamins in addition to an ample diet do not benefit. Besides, anyone eating a reasonable diet would find it almost impossible *not* to receive two or three times the RDA of vitamin C. A person who drinks a small glass of orange juice and eats a baked potato and a serving of broccoli in a day receives about five times the needed vitamin C from these foods alone. When they learn this, people have been known to throw away their pills and learn to cook broccoli.

Some concentrated nutrients may even hurt an athlete's performance. For example, niacin supplements suppress the release of fat, thus forcing the body to use extra glycogen

TABLE S7–1 ■ Pregame Meal Tips

Some Good Ideas for a Pregame Meal	Not Recommended
Angel food cake	Biscuits
Apricot nectar	Butter
Baked white or sweet potatoes	Cheeses
Dry fruit	Creams
Frozen yogurt	Croissants
Gelatin dessert	French fries
Graham crackers	Frosted cakes
Grape juice	Gravy
Honey on toast	Ice cream
Jams	Mayonnaise
Jellies	Meats
Pasta	Muffins
Pineapple juice	Nuts
Popsicles	Onion rings
Sherbet	Pies
Sponge cake	Potato chips
Syrup on pancakes	Salad dressings
	Stuffing

as fuel for activity. This may shorten the time to glycogen depletion and make the work seem more difficult to the exerciser.[3]

I like the drinks and candylike bars that claim to provide "complete" nutrition. Can I relax my diet and rely on them to supply the nutrients I need?

These supplements usually taste good and provide extra food energy, but they are in no way "complete," despite their claim. They lack fiber, many nutrients, and other beneficial components of real food.

   In one instance, though, a liquid meal may be useful. At the pregame meal, a nervous athlete who cannot tolerate solid food might substitute a nutritionally "complete" drink to supply some of the fluid and carbohydrate needed for the event. A milk shake of nonfat milk, ice milk, and a banana blended with flavorings could do the same thing, and less expensively.

Well, in that case, I'd probably drop an egg into mine. Didn't raw egg drinks account for movie boxer Rocky's outstanding performances and help him win matches?

Probably not more than scrambled eggs might have. Raw and cooked eggs are chemically almost identical, both providing high-quality protein and other nutrients. Don't eat raw eggs, though, for several reasons. For one, raw egg whites contain the chemical avidin, which binds a vitamin, biotin. In fact, it is used by scientists in experiments to induce the symptoms of biotin deficiency (skin rashes, leg paralysis, and hair loss).

   Raw eggs present a more imme-

diate threat: a food-borne bacterial infection (*Salmonella*) that produces fever, vomiting, diarrhea, and abdominal pain. Even fresh, grade A, grocery-store raw eggs have been identified as transmitters of such bacteria. To be safe, cook your eggs; in fact, cook all animal and seafood products to avoid the illnesses they would otherwise transmit to you.

So far, you've told me that carbohydrate loading is the only trick that can be helpful to athletes. Are there others?

Yes, there are two. One is to use caffeine in *moderation*. Moderate doses of this mild stimulant (one to three cups of coffee) one hour prior to exercise seem to assist many people's athletic performance. Caffeine stimulates the body's release of fat into the blood early in exercise, thus conserving glycogen. (The Spotlight that follows Chapter 8 provides a list of common caffeine-containing beverages, foods, and medicines.) But remember from the chapter that a warm-up activity stimulates fuel release, too, and offers other benefits as well. And caffeine, taken in excess, causes stomach upset, nervousness, sleeplessness, irritability, headaches, breast disease, and diarrhea. It stimulates urination, causing water loss, which is potentially hazardous for exercisers in a hot environment. Use caffeine-containing beverages, if at all, in moderation, and *in addition* to other fluids, not as substitutes for them. In college, national, and international athletic competitions, the use of caffeine is prohibited in amounts greater than the equivalent of five or six cups of coffee drunk within an hour or two. Urine tests that detect

caffeine in excess of this limit disqualify athletes from competition.

What's the other trick?

The other trick is just to eat right—that is, to eat a balanced diet, as nonathletes do. A healthy diet promotes heart health, helps to guard against some forms of cancer, helps the body fight off infections—and also facilitates athletic performance. It also promotes and maintains a lean body composition. In short, a diet that is low in fat, high in complex carbohydrates, and adequate in protein and other nutrients well serves the needs of human beings, especially those who place physical demands on their bodies. The information of Chapter 5 provided the basics. Figure S7–2 shows how a normal, high-carbohydrate diet can be boosted with

---

■ MINIGLOSSARY
of Sports Injuries

damaged cartilage a joint injury (see Figure 7–2). Cartilage damage is especially troublesome in the knee.

shin splints damage to the muscles and supporting tissues of the shin region from stress. Such damage usually heals with rest.

sprain a joint injury caused when the ligaments of the joint are torn.

strain a muscle injury caused when the muscle is stretched beyond its limit.

stress fractures bone damage resulting from repeated physical force that strains the attachment between ligament and bone.

tennis elbow a painful condition of the arm and joint, usually caused by excessive strain, as from playing tennis.

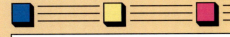

Regular Meal Choices

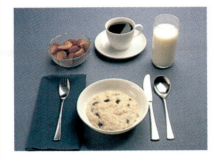

To modify:
The regular breakfast *plus*:
    2 pieces whole-wheat toast
    4 tsp jelly
    ½ c orange juice
    2 tsp brown sugar on the oatmeal
    2% fat milk instead of nonfat

Athlete's Meal Choices

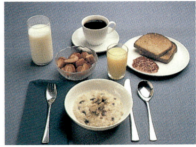

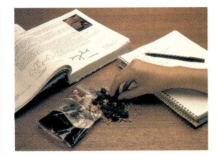

Both enjoy a snack

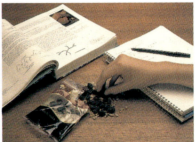

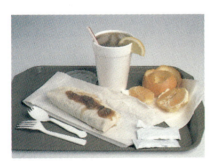

The regular lunch *plus:*
    1 beef and bean burrito
    1 banana

Plus an afternoon snack:
    1 c 2% fat milk
    1 piece angel food cake

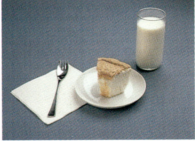

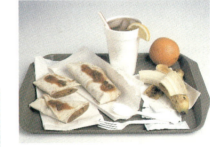

The regular dinner *plus:*
    1 dinner roll
    2 tsp butter
    ¼ c noodles
    ½ c sherbet
    2% fat milk instead of nonfat

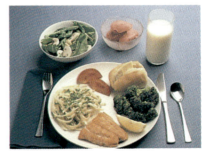

Total cal: 1,759
57% cal from carbohydrate
24% cal from fat
19% cal from protein

Total cal: 3,119
61% cal from carbohydrate
24% cal from fat
15% cal from protein

FIGURE S7–2 ■ **A normal diet and an athlete's diet.**
This figure shows how to modify a regular day's meals, to meet an athlete's needs.

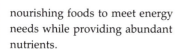

nourishing foods to meet energy needs while providing abundant nutrients.

You can see that the athlete must meet energy needs with the kinds of foods that will support performance—extra helpings of cereals, rice, beans, and bread; more milk and fruit; and even some low-fat sweet snacks such as angel food cake or puddings. Meats provide important nutrients, but people usually choose more than enough of them.

Training and genetics being equal, who would win a competition—the person who habitually consumes too few nutrients or the one who arrives at the event with a long history of full nutrient stores and well-met needs? Be sure you give your active body the food it needs if you expect it to perform its best.

■ Spotlight Notes

1. J. L. Ivy and coauthors, Muscle glycogen synthesis after exercise: Effect of time of carbohydrate ingestion, *Journal of Applied Physiology* 64 (1988): 1480–1485.

2. E. M. N. Hamilton, E. N. Whitney, and F. S. Sizer, *Nutrition: Concepts and Controversies* (St. Paul, Minn.: West, 1991) p. 337.

3. M. H. Williams, The role of vitamins in physical activity, in *Nutrition Aspects of Human Physical and Athletic Performance*, 2d ed. (Springfield, Ill.: Charles C. Thomas, 1985), pp. 147–185.

CHAPTER 8

Drugs as Medicines

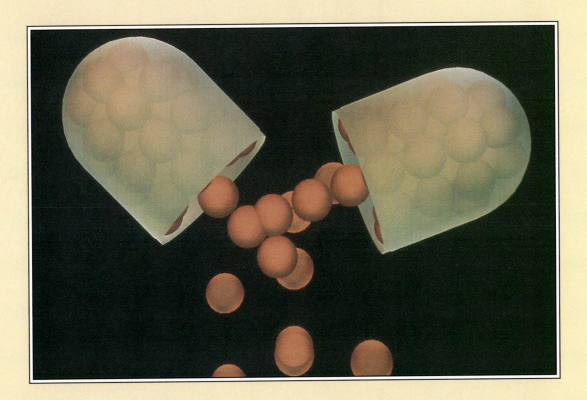

FACT OR FICTION

Just for fun, respond true or false to the following statements. If false, say what is true.

■ People who take aspirin to relieve pain do not receive the same anticlotting effect as people who take it to prevent stroke. (Page 203)

■ A drug taken by mouth acts on the body the same way as the same drug taken by injection. (Page 204)

■ Alcohol drinkers often need higher doses of certain drugs than nondrinkers. (Page 205)

■ Antibiotics are effective in treating colds. (Page 212)

■ All grades of fever are dangerous, and people with fever should always take fever-reducing medicine. (Page 212)

■ Vitamin C can help prevent and cure colds. (Page 213)

■ Generic drugs are exactly the same as their brand name equivalents, only cheaper. (Page 216)

---

drug a substance taken into the body that modifies one or more of its functions.

medicines drugs used to facilitate cure of disease, lessen disease severity, relieve symptoms, prevent disease, facilitate diagnosis, or produce other desired effects.

What are drugs? Most people think of drugs either as illegal, addictive substances or as medicines that help them get better when they are sick. Drugs are both. A **drug** is defined as any substance taken into the body that modifies one or more of its functions.[1]* Illegal addictive substances (such as cocaine and heroin), legal addictive substances (such as alcohol and tobacco), and all **medicines** (such as aspirin and antibiotics) fit that definition; so do many substances that occur naturally in plants, like the caffeine in tea leaves and coffee beans. This chapter presents drugs used as medicines; the Spotlight that follows investigates the effects of caffeine; and the next chapter discusses drugs of abuse.

Drugs used as medicines benefit people in any of several ways:

■ They can facilitate the *cure* of disease.
   Example: Penicillin kills the bacteria that cause pneumonia.

■ They *lessen the severity* of disease.
   Example: Steroid hormones reinforce a bodily defense against arthritis.

■ They *relieve symptoms*.
   Example: Aspirin relieves inflammation, aches, and pains.

■ They help *diagnose* disease.
   Example: A dye is injected into a vein and its rate of travel is measured, to help locate obstructions in the circulatory system.

■ They help *prevent* disease.
   Example: Vaccinations elicit the immune response, which strengthens the body's defenses against disease.

■ They *produce a desired effect* not related to diseases.
   Example: Oral contraceptives prevent conception.

Medical drugs do not "cure" diseases by themselves. Only the body can fully accomplish that, but drugs can help.

---

*Reference notes are at the end of the chapter.

All drugs (whether used medically or abused) affect users physiologically, and their uses involve risks. The next section is about the actions of all drugs.

■☰ The Actions of Drugs

Drugs work by modifying or interfering with the body's own processes. An example of one of the most commonly used drugs illustrates how this works. This drug is familiar to everyone; it is found in tiny, portable boxes or bottles, sometimes right next to the candy counter. It is cheap, ordinary, unglamorous. Consumers reach for a dose over a billion times a year. It is aspirin, unsurpassed for the relief of certain kinds of pain.

Most people think they understand aspirin, because it is so familiar. Their reasoning may go something like this: "Aspirin is cheap and available everywhere. Almost everyone I know takes it for headache or fever. It's not addictive, and it certainly can't be as powerful as the drugs physicians prescribe, therefore it must be safe." If this is how you perceive aspirin, then you will probably be surprised by its far-reaching chemical effects on body systems.

Aspirin works by interfering with powerful, hormonelike chemicals called **prostaglandins.** All body tissues make them. Prostaglandins produce fevers, sensitize pain receptors, cause contractions of the uterus, stimulate digestive tract motion, control nerve impulses, regulate blood pressure, promote blood clotting, and cause inflammation. Aspirin retards the production of certain prostaglandins and so interferes with all these body responses. Thus, among other things, aspirin reduces fever and inflammation, relieves pain, and opposes blood clotting.

You cannot use aspirin for any one purpose without receiving all its effects. A person who is prone to strokes and heart attacks might take aspirin to prevent blood clotting, but this same effect occurs also in people who take aspirin to treat pain. For people who do not expect it, the anticlotting effect may be dangerous, since it can cause abnormal bleeding.*[2] A single two-tablet dose doubles the bleeding time of wounds, an effect that lasts from four to seven days. For this reason, it is important to refrain from taking aspirin before any kind of surgery and in the weeks before childbirth.

These examples illustrate a general characteristic of all drugs: they have **side effects,** some neutral, some harmful. All drugs have many effects, and all of them occur when you take the drugs, whether you want them to or not.

When you take a drug, many factors determine how it will affect you, as the next sections describe. One factor is, of course, the drug itself—the substance. Another is its route of administration. Still another is you—your physiology and your psychology. Another is your past and present drug use; another is your diet. And another is the setting in which you take the drug.

THE DRUG. Each drug has a character of its own. For example, drugs that are liquid may be absorbed faster than those that contain large crystals.

prostaglandins (PROST-uh-GLAND-ins)   a group of hormonelike biological substances that affect the functions of a wide variety of body systems.

■ *FACT OR FICTION:* People who take aspirin to relieve pain do not receive the same anticlotting effect as people who take it to prevent stroke. *False.* Everyone who takes aspirin receives all of its effects, whether or not they seek them.

side effects   any effects of a drug other than the effect that is sought.

---

*Both aspirin and acetaminophen can cause prolonged bleeding.

active ingredients   the ingredients of a drug that bring about the desired effect.

inert ingredients   inactive ingredients in a drug, such as carriers, coloring agents, preservatives, or capsules.

bioavailability   a term used to describe how well a drug is absorbed and how fast it travels to the sites of action.

■ *FACT OR FICTION:* A drug taken by mouth acts on the body the same way as the same drug taken by injection. *False.* A drug may act somewhat differently if administered in a different way.

placebos   inert, or dummy, substances labeled "medicine," used for their psychological effects.

tolerance   a state that develops in users of certain drugs that requires them to take larger and larger amounts of the drug to produce the same effect.

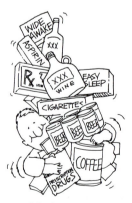

This person might have an unexpected reaction to medicine.

Also, the **active ingredients** may be embedded in a carrier composed of **inert ingredients** that alter their absorption rates. Such factors affect a drug's **bioavailability**—how well it is absorbed and how fast it travels to the sites of action.

THE ROUTE OF ADMINISTRATION. The route of administration affects the drug's action, too. Drugs that are taken by mouth have to pass through the intestinal walls to get into the bloodstream. If injected into muscle or fat, they move slowly into the blood, bypassing stomach or intestinal absorption. Injected into veins, they arrive at their destinations without delay. Drugs held on the skin surface in transdermal patches trickle in slowly and steadily. Drugs that are inhaled enter the bloodstream as quickly as those injected into veins, but they reach the brain even faster, because blood leaving the lungs goes directly to the brain.

YOUR PHYSIOLOGY. Your physiology (which depends on your age, body size, and heredity) also affects the drug's action. For example, older people may metabolize drugs more slowly and so feel their impacts longer. A large person's body dilutes a drug dose more than a small person's body does. And different people's enzymes process drugs differently.

YOUR PSYCHOLOGY. As for psychology, your expectations of a drug can affect its action. Some people, when given fake medicine, or **placebos,** experience great healing and pain relief—this shows the power of suggestion and the power of the mind in healing.

PREVIOUS DRUG USE. A drug may act one way when used in the short term and act entirely differently when used over the long term. When increasing doses of a drug are needed to achieve a desired effect, it is because the body has developed **tolerance** to the drug. Tolerance is an adaptation: the more the body is exposed to the drug, the more enzymes it builds to break it down, and the faster it disposes of it. Many organs may contribute: the liver dismantles the drug faster; the kidney excretes it more quickly; other tissues raise their resistance to its presence. The ability to develop tolerance varies among individuals; some become tolerant to certain drugs easily; others can hardly adjust at all. Tolerance underlies physical dependence.

USE OF OTHER DRUGS. When a person takes two or more drugs at the same time, the drugs may interact with one another in the digestive tract, affecting absorption; in the bloodstream, affecting delivery; in the tissues, affecting metabolism; or in the kidneys, affecting excretion.[3] As an example, consider the metabolism of drugs by the liver. The liver recognizes drugs by their chemical characteristics. Some chemical characteristics are shared by many groups of drugs; thus, for example, the liver's enzymes that break down alcohol may also break down a certain type of sleeping pill. This sometimes can cause trouble, because enzymes can work only so fast. If someone takes two drugs that require the same enzymes, the enzymes' work load is doubled, and each substance is broken down more slowly. In some cases, the enzymes preferentially work on one drug, forcing the other drug to continue circulating in the body, waiting for the enzyme to become available to act on it. Suppose that a person took a sleeping compound and also a dose of alcohol. The liver would deal with the alcohol first, while the sleeping compound would accumulate in the blood and threaten the person's life. This is an example of **synergistic** drug interactions: the effect of two drugs, taken together, is different or greater than the sum of their effects when taken separately. Many drugs react synergistically with alcohol, and such interactions account for many accidental deaths.

The body can also exhibit **cross-tolerance** to drugs. If, for example, a person takes drug A repeatedly, the liver and kidneys must metabolize and excrete it, so these organs build up their supply of enzymes for doing so (the person becomes tolerant to the drug). The person now needs larger doses of drug A to achieve the same tissue level. Then, the person starts taking drug B, and it happens that the enzymes, built to destroy drug A, work just as well on drug B. The person's tolerance to drug A applies to drug B as well, so the person needs larger doses of it, too. Due to cross-tolerance, people who smoke or drink alcohol often may need higher doses of medical drugs.

One drug can also act on another as an **antagonist** by inhibiting or negating the action of the other drug. Such drugs are often useful in the treatment of accidental overdoses or poisoning. Drugs that block the actions of snake venoms are examples of antagonists.

YOUR DIET. Foods or nutrients and drugs interact in many ways:

- ■ Foods can slow down the absorption of drugs from the digestive tract.
- ■ Drugs can make nutrients unavailable for absorption.
- ■ Drugs can alter food intake by modifying taste or the appetite.
- ■ Nutrients can interfere with the action or excretion of drugs.
- ■ Drugs can interfere with the action or excretion of nutrients.

Foods, drugs, and the body are made of chemicals, and so they all interact.

THE SETTING. A final factor influencing a drug's actions is the setting. The chemical environment, such as polluted air that a person might be breathing, can put demands on the body that hamper its ability to deal with drugs. Also, the social environment may affect the expectations with which a person takes a drug. A person who drinks alcohol at a party may feel its effects more intensely than a person who drinks alcohol at home. Clearly, no blanket statement can be made out of context about a drug's effects: they depend on all these factors.

≡▶ *Drugs work by modifying or interfering with the body's own processes. Several factors influence a drug's effects: the drug, the route of administration, the person's physiology and psychology, the person's past and present drug use, the person's diet, and the setting in which the drug is taken.*

■≡ Drug Risks and Safety

Ingredients in drugs are tested both for **safety** and **effectiveness**.[4] The term *safe* means that an ingredient will not hurt you; *effective*, that it will do what the maker claims it will do. Drug manufacturers conduct the initial testing. The Food and Drug Administration (FDA), a watchdog agency of the federal

synergistic (sin-er-JIST-ick) a term that describes the combined action of two agents, when they produce an effect that is different from, or greater than, the effects of the two agents working alone.

cross-tolerance tolerance, developed by the body to one drug, that affects the body's reactions to one or more other drugs as well.

■ *FACT OR FICTION:* Alcohol drinkers often need higher doses of certain drugs than nondrinkers. *True.*

antagonist (an-TAG-uh-nist) a drug that opposes the action of another drug.

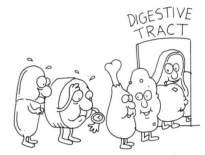

Foods can slow down the absorption of drugs from the digestive tract.

safety the practical certainty that harm will not result from the use of a substance, part of the legal requirement for a drug.

effectiveness having the medically intended effect, part of the legal requirement for a drug.

government, evaluates these tests and grants approval if the studies and results meet specified standards. The FDA continues to maintain records of reported complaints and periodically inspects the company's production plant for as long as the drug is on the market. The FDA cannot possibly sample all drug batches from all of the multitudes of manufacturers it oversees. It is a *monitoring* agency, and as such, it cannot (nor can it be expected to) guarantee 100 percent safety in the drug supply. What it can do is set conditions so that injuries are unlikely, and act promptly when problems or suspicions arise.

No drug is totally safe in any amount. The safety of a substance is related to its dose. People who evaluate the safety of drugs consider the drugs' risks to health in relation to the doses needed for effectiveness.

Drugs that carry low risks to health are most desirable in the treatment of diseases. In fact, scientists use a risk/benefit ratio to assign safety ratings to drugs being considered for use as medicines. The ratio compares the **therapeutic dose** (or *effective dose*) with the **lethal dose,** asking the question, How much drug does it take to help a person compared with the amount that will kill that person? The greater the difference, the greater the margin of safety. A drug's safety margin is called its **therapeutic index,** and Figure 8–1 illustrates how it is derived.

To understand these concepts, consider antibiotic drugs. Some antibiotic drugs work against bacterial infections by stopping cell division. Bacteria divide rapidly, so antibiotic drugs promptly halt their growth. Body cells divide, too, but less rapidly, and antibiotic drugs halt their growth, too, but less promptly. Fortunately, then, bacteria can be inactivated faster than the

therapeutic dose   the amount of a drug required to bring about the desired therapeutic effect—the *effective dose*. Any dose above this is an *overdose*; a dose high enough to threaten health or life is a *toxic dose*.

lethal dose   the amount of a drug necessary to produce death.

therapeutic index   the margin of safety of a drug; the therapeutic dose compared with the lethal dose.

FIGURE 8–1 ■ **The therapeutic index of a drug.**
The dose levels sufficient to kill members of two animal species of different sizes are used to determine the lethal dose for human beings by extrapolation. The therapeutic dose is determined by means of experiments with human beings. The ratio between the therapeutic dose and the lethal dose is the therapeutic index.

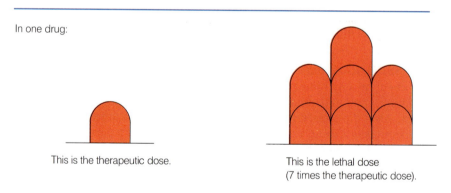

In one drug:

This is the therapeutic dose.

This is the lethal dose (7 times the therapeutic dose).

The therapeutic index is 1/7. This drug has a wide margin of safety.

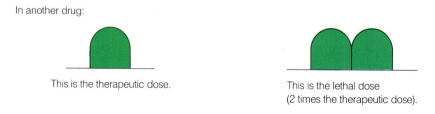

In another drug:

This is the therapeutic dose.

This is the lethal dose (2 times the therapeutic dose).

The therapeutic index is 1/2. The margin of safety is too small; accidents are likely with this drug.

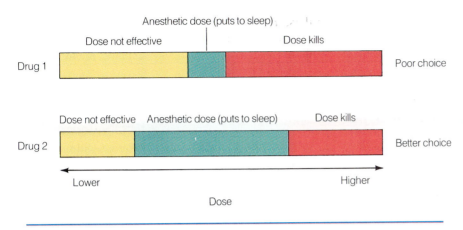

Drug 1

Dose not effective | Anesthetic dose (puts to sleep) | Dose kills — Poor choice

Drug 2

Dose not effective | Anesthetic dose (puts to sleep) | Dose kills — Better choice

Lower ← Dose → Higher

FIGURE 8–2 ■ **Anesthetics.**

An anesthetic has no effect at a low dose. As the dose increases, it puts the person to sleep. A still higher dose stops respiration and heartbeat, and so kills.

With a poor anesthetic (drug 1), the zone of doses within which the person is put to sleep is narrow. A slightly higher dose kills. Alcohol works this way and therefore has been abandoned (except in emergencies) as an anesthetic.

With a better anesthetic (drug 2), the zone within which sleep is induced without killing is wide, thus allowing for some variation in the dose without danger.

body's own cells, and once the drug is out of the system, the body's own cells soon recover. Thus antibiotics have reasonable margins of safety.

Some drugs have narrower margins of safety. An example is the drug alcohol, which was used as an anesthetic during wartime, in surgery, and in childbirth before the development of safer anesthetics. A little alcohol dulls pain, more alcohol produces unconsciousness, and only a little more stops the heartbeat and breathing. The amount of alcohol needed for an anesthetic effect is dangerously close to a lethal dose—making the margin of safety too narrow to tolerate. Today, better painkillers with wider safety margins are used instead (see Figure 8–2).

≡▶ *Ingredients in medicines must be proved safe and effective before they are allowed on the market. People who evaluate the safety of drugs consider the drugs' risks to health in relation to the doses needed for effectiveness. Drugs that carry low risks to health are most desirable in the treatment of disease.*

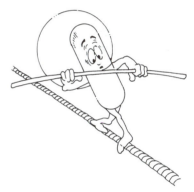

Some drugs have narrow margins of safety.

■≡ Medicine Terms

The FDA divides medicines into two classes: **over-the-counter (OTC) drugs,** sold freely, and **prescription drugs,** obtainable only with a physician's prescription. Both OTC drugs and prescription drugs are referred to by two terms. First, the **generic name** is the chemical name of a drug, and it carries this name no matter what company makes it. (Generic names never begin with capital letters.) Second, the **brand name** is the name given to a drug by the company that produces it (and it is always capitalized). A brand name also has a circled R by it, indicating "registered trademark." One generic drug may have several brand names. Table 8–1 lists the generic names of several common painkillers, and the Miniglossary of Medicine Terms defines classes of drugs used as medicines.

≡▶ *Medicines are divided into two classes: over-the-counter (OTC) drugs and prescription drugs. Both classes of drugs are referred to by two terms: generic names (the chemical names of drugs) and brand names (the names given to the drugs by the companies that produce them).*

over-the-counter (OTC) drugs drugs legally available without a prescription.

prescription drugs drugs available only with a physician's order.

generic (jeh-NEHR-ick) **name** the chemical name for a drug, as opposed to the brand name.

brand name the name a company gives to a drug; the name by which it is sold.

Brand names of the three most common painkillers:

Advil, Motrin, Nuprin, Rufen (all of these have the generic name *ibuprofen*).

Anacin-3, Datril, Panadol, Tylenol (these have the generic name *acetaminophen*).

Bufferin, Bayer's Aspirin (these have the generic name *aspirin*).

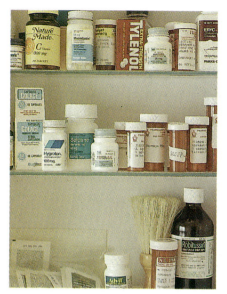

Medicines can be overused.

OTC drugs have these characteristics:

■ They are relatively safe with regard to accidental misuse.

■ The dose is fairly universal.

■ They can be used without guidance; instructions are not complex.

■ They have a low abuse potential; they do not induce addiction.

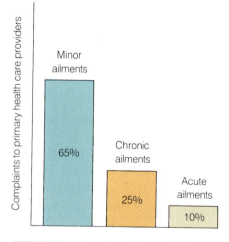

Complaints to primary health care providers

Minor ailments
65%

Chronic ailments
25%

Acute ailments
10%

FIGURE 8–3 ■ **Ailments benefiting from self-care.**

Of people visiting general health care providers, perhaps about 65 percent have minor ailments; another 25 percent have chronic ailments; and only 10 percent have acute conditions that demand dramatic medical treatment. Thus 90 percent of these people could appropriately select their own medicines and administer their own self-care.

TABLE 8–1 ■ Generic Names of Selected Common Painkillers	
Generic Name	**Common Brand Names**
Acetaminaphen	Anacin-3
	Datril
	Panadol
	Tylenol
Aspirin	Bayer's Aspirin
	Bufferin
Ibuprofen	Advil
	Motrin
	Nuprin
	Rufen

■≡ Nonprescription (Over-the-Counter) Medications

People buy OTC medicines in the belief that these drugs will help fix what ails them. Fortunately, some OTC drugs are effective and inexpensive, as well as freely available, making them useful for people who choose to treat their own minor ailments. Figure 8–3 shows that, if people took advantage of these medicines, they could avoid 9 out of every 10 trips to health care providers.

Other OTC medicines are unnecessary and may be quite costly. Net sales for OTC medicines are in the multibillion dollar range every year.

Unfortunately, people don't use OTC medicines appropriately, and they greatly overuse them.[5] Drug manufacturers encourage these errors. Advertisers train people to identify minor complaints and then to seek cures through pills. For example, many a person with a headache simply takes an aspirin instead of trying to identify the cause of the headache. Maybe the person's headache is from hunger or tension. Pain or other discomfort is a signal that something in the body is out of balance. Often, simply getting more sleep, eating better, exercising regularly, or using some stress-reduction technique can help relieve ailments and help people avoid the risks and expenses of OTC medication. Before heading for the medicine cabinet for every minor ailment, stop and listen to your body, and try to relieve the pain by seeking the cause. Instead of taking a tablet for indigestion, try eating more slowly, and see if that relieves your discomfort.

Sometimes people not only overuse OTC medicines but use them with misguided expectations for the wrong purposes. Again, advertisers encourage these errors. They are not allowed to use drug labels to seduce people this way, but they find other cunning ways to do it (see Critical Thinking: Legal Lies).

≡▶ *OTC drugs are usually effective and inexpensive. OTC drugs are relatively safe, the doses are fairly universal, the instructions for use are not complex, and they have a low abuse potential. Being freely available, OTC drugs are greatly overused and sometimes used with inflated expectations.*

■ MINIGLOSSARY
of Medicine Terms

Abusable drugs among the medicines are marked with an asterisk (*) and are discussed in Chapter 9.

acetaminophen (ah-SEET-ah-MIN-o-fen) an analgesic drug.

***amphetamine** (am-FET-uh-meen) a type of stimulant drug. Examples are Benzedrine, Dexedrine, and Ritalin.

analgesic (AN-ul-JEE-zick) a drug that relieves pain and fever, such as aspirin, ibuprofen, or acetaminophen.

anesthetic a drug that produces loss of sensation, with or without loss of consciousness.

antacid a drug that neutralizes stomach acid.

antibiotic a drug used to fight bacterial infection.

anticoagulant (an-tee-coh-AG-you-lant) a drug used to prevent blood clotting.

antidiarrheal (an-tee-dye-uh-REE-ul) a drug used to relieve diarrhea.

antiemetic (an-tee-uh-MET-ick) a drug used to treat nausea and vomiting.

antifungal a drug used to treat fungus infections.

antihistamine a drug that counteracts the effects of histamine, one of the chemicals involved in allergic reactions.

antipyretic (an-tee-pie-RET-ick) a drug that reduces fever.

aspirin an analgesic drug.

***barbiturate** (bar-BIH-chur-et) a type of depressant drug.

bronchodilator (BRONK-oh-DYE-lay-tor) a drug that opens the bronchial tubes within the lungs.

caffeine a stimulant drug.

***codeine** a narcotic drug.

cough suppressant a drug that acts on the nervous system to suppress the cough reflex.

decongestant a drug used to relieve nasal and sinus congestion.

***depressant** a drug that depresses the central nervous system. Types include sedatives, tranquilizers, barbiturates (such as Seconal), and alcohol.

diuretic (DIE-you-RET-ick) a drug that increases the urine produced by the kidneys, used to rid the body of excess fluid.

expectorant a drug that stimulates the flow of mucus and promotes coughing, used to eliminate phlegm from the respiratory tract.

ibuprofen (EYE-byoo-PRO-fen) an analgesic drug.

laxative a drug that increases the frequency and ease of bowel movements.

muscle relaxant a drug that relieves muscle spasms, used for disorders such as backache.

***narcotic** medically, a drug that slows down functioning of the central nervous system; narcotics include heroin, opium, morphine, methadone, codeine, paregoric, Demerol, and Darvon. Legally, the term includes any drug with potential for abuse.

***sedative** a type of depressant drug.

***stimulant** any of a wide variety of drugs that speed up the central nervous system, including amphetamines, caffeine, and others.

thrombolytic (THROM-boh-LIT-ic) a drug that helps dissolve and disperse blood clots.

***tranquilizer** a drug that has a calming effect; *major tranquilizers* are used to control people with severe psychosis; *minor tranquilizers* (such as Valium and Librium) are mild versions.

■≡ Strategies: Nonprescription Medications

Nonprescription, or over-the counter, medicines are those you buy, yourself, when you want to treat a condition. To select such medicines wisely, you need to know how to read their labels.

Drug companies are required to include only approved active ingredients in their products. The FDA lists only a few hundred approved active ingredients, yet 50,000 OTC drugs are on the market. How can there be so many, each claiming to be unique? The answer is that in addition to the active ingredients, each manufacturer adds other, inert ingredients. Some are useful and necessary substances that carry the active ingredient, or add bulk to the medicine. Others may be there simply because they have fancy chemical names that will lead buyers to believe the products are superior.

The drug label lists:

■ Name and statement of identity of the product.
■ What the product will do.

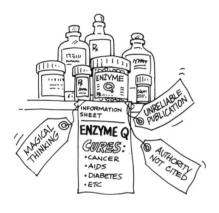

Lies on labels are illegal, but "information" sheets can say anything and claim freedom of the press.

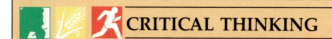 **CRITICAL THINKING**

Legal Lies

Sometimes, misleading information may remain on a label for a while after it has been noticed or reported, because the FDA hasn't had time to act. For example, a medication was marketed for many years that claimed to benefit the liver, when, in fact, no such benefit was ever proved. The FDA took the company to court, and 14 years after proceedings began, the word *liver* was finally removed from the label. You can't depend on a label to conform to the law; the law may not have been enforced yet.

Even if the label conforms to the law, unscrupulous manufacturers may place "information" sheets near the display shelf where the product is being sold. Often, false information appears on these sheets and entices people to buy the products. This trick is especially common in places that sell "health" or "natural" products, but such sheets can appear in regular drugstores and grocery stores, too. Be suspicious of claims of cures or benefits on any printed matter near products.

A similar trick is used in some magazines. You might open a magazine and start reading an article that contains a list of authentic-looking references and is written by Dr. Rip Off, M.D., who says, with absolute certainty, that zinc improves sexual performance. Already you have become uneasy—*the claim seems too good to be true.* As you scan the next page, an advertisement jumps out at you: "Full-Life zinc tablets—only $6.95 per bottle." The advertisement says only that the company sells zinc tablets, a legal claim. But if you were to search for the origins of the article on the previous page, chances are you would find that the Full-Life Company sent it, as well as the advertisement, to be published. The article is a hoax, but its publication is legal. The law bars companies from printing lies in advertisements, but no law forbids lies in other writing. Your first clue to the hoax is the claims in the article; your second is the advertisement for the product in close proximity.

■ Quantity of contents.
■ Active ingredients and, usually, inactive ingredients.
■ Name and address of the manufacturer, distributor, or packer.

It also lists directions:

■ The correct amount of each dose.
■ How frequently to take it.
■ How to take it (by mouth, with water, and so on).
■ How to store it.
■ When to throw it away (the expiration date).

Finally, it lists warnings:

■ A limit on how long to use it.
■ Side effects, if any (drowsiness, constipation, and the like); see Table 8–2.

TABLE 8–2 ■ **Some Side Effects of OTC Drugs**

Drug	Possible Hazard
Acetaminophen	Bloody urine, painful urination, skin rash, bleeding and bruising, yellowing of the eyes or skin (even for normal doses)
	Difficulty in diagnosing overdose, because reaction may be delayed up to a week after ingestion of medication
	Severe liver damage and death (for dose of about 50 tablets)
	Liver damage from chronic low-level excesses
Antacids	Reduced mineral absorption from food
	Possible concealment of ulcer
	Reduction of effectiveness of anticlotting medications
	Prevention of certain antibiotics' functioning (for antacids that contain aluminum)
	Worsening of high blood pressure (for antacids that contain sodium)
	Aggravation of kidney problems
Aspirin	Stomach upset and vomiting, stomach bleeding, worsening of ulcers
	Enhancement of the action of anticlotting medications
	Potentiation of hearing damage from loud noise
	Severe allergic reaction in some people
	Association with Reye's syndrome in children and teenagers[a]
	Possible prolonged bleeding time when combined with alcohol
Cold medications	Loss of consciousness (if taken with prescription tranquilizers)
Diet pills, decongestants, and caffeine[b]	Organ damage or death from cerebral hemorrhage
Ibuprofen	Allergic reaction in some people with aspirin allergy
	Fluid retention or edema
	Liver damage similar to that from acetaminophen
	Enhancement of action of anticlotting medications
	Digestive disturbances (half as often as with aspirin)
Laxatives	Reduced absorption of minerals from food
	Creation of dependency
Toothache medications	Destruction of the still-healthy part of a damaged tooth (for medications that contain clove oil)

[a]Reye's (pronounced RISE) syndrome is a rare and potentially life-threatening condition linked to aspirin use associated with chicken pox or flu. Children and teenagers should never take aspirin—their illnesses might turn out to be chicken pox or flu. They should be treated with acetaminophen.

[b]These three OTC drugs are often combined in street varieties of abused drugs because they produce a high. They are sold in capsules called "look-alikes" that resemble prescription mind-altering drugs. See Chapter 9.

■ Circumstances that may require a health care provider's advice before use.

■ A warning to the pregnant woman discouraging her use of the product without the advice of her health care provider.

Once you know how to read drug labels, you have half of the information you need to treat your ailment. The other half is a good understanding of the ailment itself. Say you have a cold. First, you might consult a home-reference medical guide. A cold is a self-limiting respiratory infection caused by any of many different viruses, which lasts from one to two weeks. The symptoms usually occur in progression, starting with a sore throat, sneezing, and a runny nose. In a few days the nose may be stuffed up and the eyes watery. Aches and pains may accompany these symptoms, along with tiredness and sometimes a fever. A cough usually develops during the later stages. Health care experts suggest that the best treatment for a cold is bed rest, abundant fluids, plain aspirin* (or acetaminophen or ibuprofen) if body aches are present, and a box of soft facial tissues (tissues help prevent transmission of colds). Since colds are caused by viruses, antibiotics are useless against them.

If you have a fever, you should know a few things about it before you reach for fever-relief medicine. People fear fever because it is associated with dangerous diseases, but the fever itself may actually assist the immune system.[6] Clearly, fever stresses the body—it raises the heart rate and increases the tissues' demands for oxygen. A weak heart could be damaged by such a strain. High temperatures (over 104 degrees Fahrenheit or, in some cases, lower) can cause convulsions and should be treated by a health care provider, not only to control the fever but to determine and treat the underlying condition. Generally, though, a mild fever should be allowed to do its job of assisting the immune system.[7] If the temperature goes above about 100, you can lower it with aspirin, acetaminophen, or ibuprofen.

Suppose, now, that you decide to treat your cold yourself. You head for the drugstore, but knowing that no cold medicine (or vitamin supplement) will prevent, cure, or even shorten a cold, you seek OTC medicine only for relief of symptoms. You feel achy, so you study first the array of painkillers.

Being a shrewd consumer, you comparison-shop, ignoring the brand names and reading the labels to discover the active ingredients in each. You overlook the claims of "extra strength," because you know you can adjust your dose yourself. (If you want an extra-strength dose, you can take two and a half pills of a regular-strength medicine; if you want a combination of pain relievers, you can take one and a quarter pills of each.) You also ignore the claims that "buffered" products protect your stomach, knowing that you can drink a full glass of water with any common pain reliever to achieve the same protection. (If aspirin irritates your stomach, though, switch pain relievers, or use coated pills.) The prices of aspirins, acetaminophens, and ibuprofens vary threefold; you choose the cheapest, store-brand, regular-strength medicine.

You pause by the vitamin counter, but remember promptly that vitamin C won't cure your cold, even if the cold came on partly because your diet was

■ **FACT OR FICTION:** Antibiotics are effective in treating colds. *False.* Colds are caused by viruses, so antibiotics are not effective in treating them.

■ **FACT OR FICTION:** All grades of fever are dangerous, and people with fever should always take fever-reducing medicine. *False.* The guidelines are:

■ Up to 100 degrees Fahrenheit, fevers need no treatment.

■ Between 100 and 104 degrees, treat if you wish.

■ At or above 104 degrees, they require medical attention.

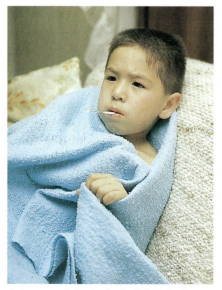

A fever can help the body fight infection.

*Children and teens should never take aspirin, due to the risk of Reye's syndrome, explained in Table 8–2.

low in vitamin C. An adequate intake of *all* nutrients is essential to your recovery and your health thereafter. Your best bet is not to take vitamin pills but to eat balanced meals and drink juice to meet your extra fluid needs. That way, all your nutrient needs will be well covered, and you'll resist future colds better.

Your nose is runny, so you buy a box of soft tissues that will not irritate it. You refrain from buying a nasal decongestant spray, because your nose is not stopped up. Overuse of sprays can make nasal passages swell, necessitating medical treatment. You do not buy a spray for later, either, because medicines expire. You also refrain from buying "nighttime cold medicines." The labels list ingredients you do not need—antihistamines for relief of allergy (not cold) symptoms, cough suppressants (you are not coughing)—and these medicines are loaded with alcohol, which can dehydrate you and disturb your sleep.

You have a sore throat, so you buy some anesthetizing spray. You plan to suck lozenges or gargle with warm saltwater just for comfort, but you need no costly mouthwashes. Most sore throats are caused by viruses, and mouthwashes do not kill viruses. You ask whether your painkiller and spray interact; the pharmacist assures you that they do not. Lastly, you buy some juices and soups to boost your liquid intake. As you leave the store, you pat yourself on the back for a shopping job well done.

Because drugs can mask symptoms, sick people who take them can be tempted to carry on with their regular routines, risking prolonged illness or relapse. You plan to rest in bed until you are well. You have made wise decisions based on hard facts. You have not spent money on wishful thinking, but only on the best relief for your particular cold.

The strategies described here apply to your selection of all OTC medications. To see how well you apply them, try this chapter's Life Choice Inventory. A Strategies section at the end of the chapter goes on to instruct you on use and storage of all medicines, both OTC and prescription.

≡▶ *To treat a minor illness with nonprescription medication, you need to learn to read drug labels, and to understand the ailment you have contracted. Next, you need to purchase medication based on knowledge of ingredients, not on advertisements. Following directions carefully is also important in self-care.*

■≡ Prescription Medications

Prescription drugs can only be obtained on physicians' orders. They are true miracles of our time—when they are used correctly. As an example, for a person whose cells do not absorb glucose from the blood, insulin is literally a life-saving treatment.

Before prescribing a drug, the wise physician asks questions about nutrition, exercise, sleep, social life, and work, because drugs and lifestyle factors can work either in harmony or in conflict with one another. For instance, in the treatment of a person with a lung condition brought on by smoking, drugs may help a little, but for a full cure, the person must stop smoking. Another example: some people with diabetes can reduce their need for insulin by exercising regularly.[8]

■ **FACT OR FICTION:** Vitamin C can help prevent and cure colds. *False.* No vitamin can prevent or cure colds, although deficiencies can weaken resistance to them.

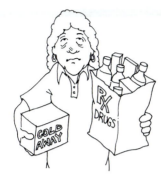

What *do* you need to buy for a cold?

Several home medical guides are suggested at the end of Spotlight 1, page 29.

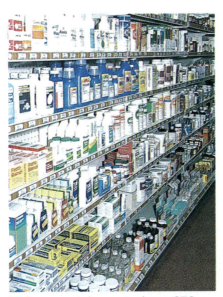

It takes a smart shopper to choose OTC drugs wisely.

LIFE CHOICE INVENTORY

How wisely do you choose over-the-counter medications? Answer these questions to find out.

1. When I have an ailment, I do not go straight to the drugstore. First, I ask myself honestly if there's a life-style change I need to make, such as getting more sleep, eating better, or exercising more. If so, I make the change.   4 points.
2. If I have an ailment that I think would respond to self-care, I first consult a medical book to check my suspicions.   3 points.
3. In buying OTC drugs to treat an ailment, I buy just the ones specific to my symptoms (for example, a cough suppressant, not an inflammation reliever, for a cough).   3 points.
4. I read drug labels and buy by chemical names, not by brand names.   3 points.
5. In taking medicines, I reread their labels and follow directions as to dose, timing, and duration.   3 points.
6. I do not overbuy, and I throw away drugs after their expiration dates have passed.   2 points.

7. Before taking two or more drugs, I check with my health care provider or pharmacist to be sure there is no cross-reaction.   3 points.
8. If my symptoms persist, I see a health care profes-sional.   2 points.

Scoring: For each "yes" or "true" answer, give yourself the number of points indicated.

23:	Perfect score! You are a wise user of OTC medicines.
18–22:	Very good. Identify the questions you missed, and raise your score to 23.
13–17:	Not so good. You could be undermining your health or wasting money by making unwise or unnecessary drug purchases.
12 or under:	Improvement needed. Think, revise your behaviors, and then take this quiz again.

Prescription drugs have these character-istics:

■ They may be dangerous if misused.
■ The dose must be adjusted to body weight, age, or other drug use.
■ Their correct use requires following complex directions.
■ They have potential for abuse.

Prescription medicines can be abused. Drug companies advertise them aggressively to physicians, who are led to overprescribe them. The tranquil-izer Valium is an example, and its overuse leads to addictions. The risks of using prescription medicines may be as great as the benefits. In fact, as noted earlier, that is why they are available only by prescription: to select them properly and adjust their doses to individuals who need them requires medical training. That does not mean a client can leave the responsibility entirely to the physician, though. The client has a part to play, too, and the next section describes it.

≡▶   *Prescription medications are different from over-the-counter drugs in that they may be dangerous if misused, the dose must be adjusted, they require complex directions, and they have potential for abuse.*

■≡ Strategies: Prescription Medications

Suppose you have cold symptoms that do not go away after two weeks of rest and OTC medication. You begin to wonder if your illness is more seri-ous than a cold, and you wisely decide to see a health care professional. After an examination, your physician writes a prescription for you and begins to leave the room. "Not so fast," you say; being a wise consumer, you

---

■ ■ ■ ■ □ *STRATEGIES: TAKING AND STORING MEDICATIONS*

To take medication safely, you must:

1. Ask your physician or pharmacist before substituting generic for brand name medicine.
2. Read and follow instructions on labels or on package inserts.
3. Do not share prescription medications with other people. The underlying causes of their symptoms can be different, and a drug or dose that is safe for you may be dangerous for someone else.
4. Do not use two or more drugs (including OTC and other drugs) without checking first with your physician or pharmacist.
5. Drink no alcohol when using medication.
6. Do not drive if you are taking medicine that causes drowsiness.
7. Take no medicine beyond its expiration date. Drugs break down into unknown, untested chemicals as they age.
8. If the drug isn't doing what you expect it to, call your physician.
9. If you experience side effects, call your physician.
10. When taking medicine at night, turn on the light to see the label and your dose.
11. Take the medication for the specified number of days, even if you feel better right away. After the symptoms are gone, the underlying cause may still remain, so the total prescription must be taken to completely treat the condition.

To store medication properly:

12. Store drugs in a cool, dark place. Be especially careful in the summertime—medicines left in a hot car can turn into who-knows-what. Some drugs must be refrigerated and others protected from light.
13. Keep the drug in its original container.
14. Keep all medicines where young children can't get them.

---

have some questions for your physician. Before leaving, be sure that you know:

■ The diagnosis of your condition.
■ That your physician is aware of all other drugs you are taking, including birth control pills and alcohol.[9]*
■ The name of the medicine the physician has prescribed.
■ How often, how long, and in what doses you should take it.
■ When to take it in relation to meals.
■ Whether side effects are likely to occur, and what they are.
■ What you should do if you forget to take a dose on time—double the next one, take it late, or omit it entirely.

A wise consumer also reads the prescription. Table 8–3 explains some common prescription symbols.

---

*Antibiotics reduce the effectiveness of birth control pills; alcohol reduces the effectiveness of antibiotics.

TABLE 8–3 ■ **Some Common Prescription Symbols**

Latin	Abbreviation	Meaning
ad libitum	ad lib.	freely, as needed
ante cibum	a.c.	before meals
bis in die	b.i.d.	twice a day
capsula	caps.	capsule
gutta	gtt.	drop
hora somni	h.s.	at bedtime
per os	p.o.	orally
quaque 4 hora	q.4 h.	every four hours
quater in die	q.i.d.	four times a day
ter in die	t.i.d.	three times a day
ut dictum	ut dict., ud	as directed

■ *FACT OR FICTION:* Generic drugs are exactly the same as their brand name equivalents, only cheaper. *False.* Generic drugs contain the same active ingredients as name brands but may contain different inactive ingredients that can affect their action in the body.

You can often save money by using a generic drug rather than the same drug sold with a brand name. Ask your physician or pharmacist first, though. A generic drug contains the same active ingredients as the brand name drug, but it may have different inactive ingredients—this may affect its absorption. If the exact timing of absorption is important, the physician may choose a particular brand name drug. Other strategies for taking medications, both OTC and prescription, and for storing them, are summed up in the accompanying "Strategies: Taking and Storing Medications."

≡▶ *Taking prescription medication is not a simple task. It is wise to understand the diagnosis, the medication being prescribed, and the instructions for taking the medication. The wise consumer takes the medication exactly as prescribed and follows other guidelines carefully.*

Drugs used as medicines can do wonders for those who need them—if they are selected and used appropriately. They also possess the potential to do harm if incorrectly used. The risk of harm is even greater (without any medicinal benefits) in the case of drugs of abuse, the subject of the next chapter.

◼☰ For Review

1. Define *drug.*
2. List the roles drugs play as medicines.
3. List the factors that affect a drug's actions in the body.
4. Explain why all drugs present both risks and benefits.
5. Describe the proper uses of OTC medications.
6. List some considerations in selecting OTC medications.
7. Tell how generic and brand name drugs are similar and how they differ.
8. List strategies for taking and storing prescription medication.

◼☰ Notes

1. C. L. Thomas, ed., *Taber's Cyclopedic Medical Dictionary,* 14th ed. (Philadelphia: Davis, 1981), p. 431.
2. W. R. Bartle and J. A. Blakely, Potentiation of warfarin anticoagulation by acetaminophen, *Journal of the American Medical Association* 265 (1991): 1260.
3. Alcohol, caffeine, and tobacco are drugs, too, *Consumer Reports Health Letter,* February 1991, pp. 12–14.
4. D. Farley, Benefit versus risk: How FDA approves new drugs, *FDA Consumer,* December 1987/January 1988, pp. 7–10.
5. Over-the-counter drugs: "Nonprescription" doesn't mean harmless, *The University of Texas Lifetime Health Letter,* December 1990, pp. 1–3.
6. M. S. Kramer, L. Naimark, and D. G. Leduc, Parental fever phobia and its correlates, *Pediatrics* 75 (1985): 1110–1113.
7. H. D. Jampel and coauthors, Fever and immunoregulation, 3: Hyperthermia augments the primary in vitro humoral immune response, *Journal of Experimental Medicine* 157 (1983): 1229–1238.
8. M. J. Franz, Exercise and the management of diabetes mellitus, *Journal of the American Dietetic Association* 87 (1987): 28–34.
9. Multiple medication danger, *Health Gazette,* March 1990, p. 2; Warning: Alcohol and nitroglycerin don't mix, *Tufts Diet and Nutrition Letter,* October 1990, pp. 7–8.

SPOTLIGHT

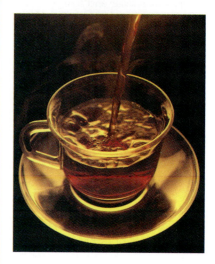

Caffeine

Most people have been using caffeine, in one form or another, since their first cola drink, cup of tea, or chocolate bar. People are exposed to caffeine in coffee, and in wake-up pills and other medications. Lately, though, some people have been cutting back on caffeine because they fear it may cause harm.

What exactly does caffeine do?

Caffeine is a stimulant drug believed to work largely by interacting with the central nervous system. The familiar "pick-me-up" effects are reduced drowsiness and fatigue and a sharper focus on tasks at hand. To what extent you experience these effects depends on how much you ingest and how much you're used to, as well as on your individual makeup. Most people experience the accelerated heart rate and skeletal muscle tension associated with nervous system stimulation if they take the equivalent of two to five cups of brewed coffee within half a day.

Does caffeine have side effects?

Yes. The nervous system stimulation itself is a stress effect, and in excess it can tire the body. There's also a diuretic effect (frequent urination). Caffeine stimulates stomach acid secretion and so will irritate the stomach of a person prone to ulcer. (Decaffeinated coffee does the same thing, because it contains caffeine relatives, so people with ulcers are advised to drink no coffee, whether decaffeinated or regular.) The most severe effect of caffeine is outright poisoning, but that occurs only with massive doses. For example, if a child accidentally ate thirty or so wake-up pills, medical treatment would be necessary to prevent death.

How can I tell if I'm getting too much caffeine?

If you take more caffeine than the amount in about five cups of coffee, you may experience irregular heartbeats, insomnia, headaches, trembling, nervousness, and other symptoms of anxiety. These symptoms could, of course, arise from anxiety itself, but if you've been taking a caffeine-containing substance, chances are that it's the culprit.

All of caffeine's symptoms seem to affect children the most. If a child is cranky or unable to sleep, try to determine how many caffeine-containing foods and beverages that child consumed during the day. As people age, they again become sensitive to caffeine, and older people are therefore advised to reduce their caffeine consumption.

I've heard people say, as a joke, "I'm addicted to cola!" Is caffeine addictive?

Yes, although not dangerously so, in comparison with other addictive drugs. People who take large amounts of caffeine daily build up a tolerance to it. If they suddenly stop, they are likely to experience uncomfortable withdrawal symptoms: anxiety, muscle tension, and a headache that no painkiller can relieve. (It's interesting that the symptoms of caffeine withdrawal are the same as some of those produced by a sudden large dose of caffeine.) A dose or two of caffeine makes them feel better, and they soon learn that they can avoid withdrawal by taking the drug.

Is that why they put caffeine in headache medicines, then?

Yes. Someone with a caffeine-withdrawal headache may try plain pain relievers, but of course they fail to cure the headache. When the person tries an "extra-strength" kind that includes caffeine, the headache disappears. The person may easily be led to believe (wrongly) that those pills are indeed stronger against pain in general, and so may buy them regularly.

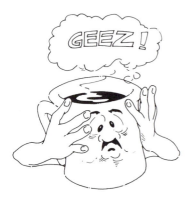

The caffeine withdrawal headache is a symptom of addiction.

Does caffeine harm the body?

Caffeine is unlikely to be abused to extremes, because it does not produce pleasant sensations. Researchers have been exploring possible links between caffeine and such disorders as birth defects, heart disease, adult bone loss, cancer, and a painful breast condition called fibrocystic breast disease. Most of these are still under investigation, but at present the researchers think that caffeine does not *cause* any of them. In excess, it may, however, *aggravate* heart disease by raising the blood pressure and triggering the release of stress hormones, which in turn raise the concentration of the risk-posing blood lipids.[1]* Caffeine may hasten adult bone loss by causing increased calcium excretion,[2] and it may intensify fibrocystic breast disease.[3] Research does not support a connection with birth defects or cancer.

Do you think we should all do without caffeine?

Most likely not. The equivalent of one or two cups of coffee a day is probably safe for any adult. In fact, more may well be safe, but pregnant women might be wise not to exceed

*Reference notes are at the end of the Spotlight.

Table S8-1 ■ Caffeine Contents of Beverages, Foods, and OTC Drugs

Item	Caffeine (mg)	
	Average	*Range*
Drinks and Foods		
Coffee (5-oz cup)		
Brewed, drip method	130	110–150
Brewed, percolator	94	64–124
Instant	74	40–108
Decaffeinated, brewed or instant	3	1–5
Tea (5-oz cup)		
Brewed, major U.S. brands	40	20–90
Brewed, imported brands	60	25–110
Instant	30	25–50
Iced (12-oz glass)	70	67–76
Soft drinks (12-oz can)		
Dr. Pepper		40
Colas and cherry colas: Regular		30–46
Diet		2–58
Caffeine-free		0–trace
Jolt		72
Mountain Dew, Mello Yello		52
Big Red		38
Fresca, Hires Root Beer, 7-Up, Sprite, Squirt, Sunkist Orange		0
Cocoa beverage (5-oz cup)	4	2–20
Chocolate milk beverage (8 oz)	5	2–7
Milk chocolate (1 oz)	6	1–15
Dark chocolate, semisweet (1 oz)	20	5–35
Chocolate-flavored syrup (1 oz)	4	4
Drugs[a]		
Cold remedies (standard dose)		
Dristan		0
Coryban-D, Triaminicin		30
Diuretics (standard dose)		
Aqua-ban, Permathene H_2Off		200
Pre-Mens Forte		100
Pain relievers (standard dose)		
Excedrin		130
Midol, Anacin		65
Aspirin, plain (any brand)		0
Stimulants		
Caffedrin, NoDoz, Vivarin		200
Weight-control aids (daily dose)		
Prolamine		280
Dexatrim, Dietac		200

[a]Because products change in formulation, contact the manufacturer for an update.

SOURCE: C. Lecos, The latest caffeine scoreboard, *FDA Consumer,* March 1984, p. 14; Measuring your life with coffee spoons, *Tufts University Diet and Nutrition Letter,* April 1984, pp. 3–6; Expert Panel on Food Safety and Nutrition, Institute of Food Technologists, *Evaluation of Caffeine Safety,* 1986 (a publication available from the Institute of Food Technologists, 221 N. LaSalle St., Chicago, IL 60601).

this limit. Parents may want to limit their children's intakes—just because the research is unclear. People at risk for adult bone loss and heart disease should also be moderate in their use of caffeine. If you want to monitor your intake, consult Table S8–1 for the amounts of caffeine in beverages, foods, and drugs.

Can you suggest some alternatives to beverages that contain caffeine?

No doubt you are aware that some cola products contain no caffeine, and of course, decaffeinated coffee is an old standby. (By the way, there is no truth in the popular belief that processing chemicals remain in decaffeinated coffee in dangerous amounts. They evaporate from the beans long before they can be ground into the coffee.) Other beverages include decaffeinated tea or teas made from mint or other herbs. When selecting

herbal teas, though, be aware that many herbs contain *other* chemicals that act as drugs, whose effects may be harmful. Therefore, choose only herbal teas produced by major companies, whose reputations rest on the safety and purity of their products, and use even those in moderation. Don't forget that refreshment can be found in a glass of ice cold water, juice, or milk—the "natural" drinks with a health bonus.

■≡ Spotlight Notes

1. G. A. Pincomb, W. R. Lovallo, and R. B. Passey, Effects of caffeine on vascular resistance, cardiac output and myocardial contractility in young men, *American Journal of Cardiology* 56 (1985): 119–122.

2. E. N. Hamilton, E. N. Whitney, and F. S. Sizer, *Nutrition Concepts and Controversies,* 5th ed., (St Paul, Minn.: West, 1991), pp. 272–282.

3. Hamilton, Whitney, and Sizer, 1991, pp. 429–436.

CHAPTER 9

Drugs of Abuse

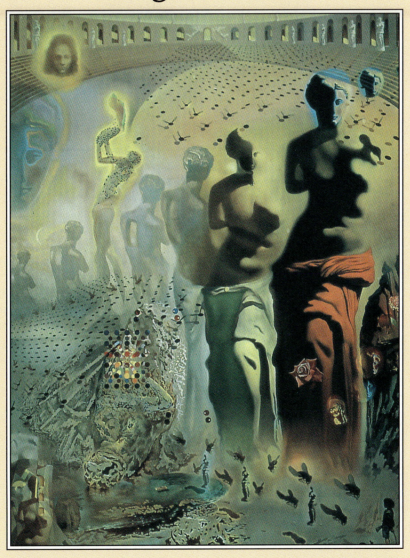

A concerned mother tells her husband that she is upset about her son's use of marijuana—his drug abuse. The situation has her so uptight that she takes prescribed Valium to calm her nerves.

A young man comes home from a stressful day at his high-pressure job and drinks a six-pack of beer to relax. On the 11 o'clock news, he hears a report of a local cocaine drug bust. He thinks to himself, "Those people who abuse drugs should be locked up."

What is drug abuse? People trying to define drug abuse often end up in emotional and controversial discussions. Would it surprise you to know that in the two scenarios just described, the people complaining about drug abuse were also engaging in it?

■ ☰ Drug Abuse Defined

Definitions of drug abuse vary. The medical community and the FDA have created one set of formal definitions; society has created another set; and individual people have created others that reflect their own drug histories and attitudes.

The FDA makes these distinctions: **drug use** is the taking of a drug as medicine, correctly—that is, for a medically intended purpose, and in the appropriate amount, frequency, strength, and manner. In contrast, **drug abuse** is the deliberate taking of a drug for a nonmedical purpose and in a manner that can result in damage to a person's health or ability to function. Both legal and illegal drugs can be abused. The FDA also defines **drug misuse** (with respect to legal drugs only) as the taking of a drug for its medically intended purpose, but not in the appropriate amount, frequency, strength, or manner. Recreational use of drugs is not defined by the FDA.[1]* Medical terminology describes drug abuse simply as any nonmedical use or overuse of any drug.[2] These definitions classify any use of drugs for nonmedical reasons as drug abuse; there is no such thing as mere "use"—for example, to produce pleasure or hallucinations. Medically speaking, then, a person who drinks alcohol excessively to get high or who uses tobacco is

drug use the taking of a drug for its medically intended purpose, and in the appropriate amount, frequency, strength, and manner.

drug abuse the deliberate taking of a drug for other than a medical purpose and in a manner that can result in damage to a person's health or ability to function.

drug misuse the taking of a drug for its medically intended purpose, but not in the appropriate amount, frequency, strength, or manner.

*Reference notes are at the end of the chapter.

abusing a drug. Someone who takes too large a dose of a prescription or over-the-counter drug is misusing the drug. Such drug misuse can lead to drug abuse.

Society's view of drug use is reflected in its laws. Society disapproves of mind-altering drugs except for alcohol. Other mind-altering (**psychoactive**) drugs—that is, those that produce **euphoria**—are available; most are available only by prescription or are outright illegal. By making its laws, society has defined the use of mind-altering drugs, except alcohol, as abuse.

Some individuals see drug use differently. Many people call themselves drug users, not abusers, when they take mind-altering drugs. They label their use of drugs **recreational drug use;** they claim it produces no harmful health effects, and they think it causes no deterioration of function in terms of job, family, or society. (People who call themselves *social drinkers* make the same distinction.) This term does not hold much meaning, because people who are not informed about the risks of drug abuse are not qualified to make such statements.

A student who considers using an illegal drug faces harsh punishment for its possession or sale. No one embarks on drug abuse intending to become an addict or a criminal, but every step in the abuse of illegal drugs is a step in that direction. This chapter is about some of the most commonly abused illegal drugs, but keep in mind that the most abused drug in the United States is still alcohol. Chapter 10 is devoted entirely to it.

≡▶ *Drug abuse is the deliberate taking of a drug for a nonmedical purpose and in a manner that can result in damage to a person's health or ability to function. Both legal and illegal drugs can be abused. Psychoactive drugs have a high potential for abuse because they produce euphoria.*

■≡ Why Do People Abuse Drugs?

Different factors may lead different people to abuse drugs. Among them are the nature of the person, the legal consequences, and the nature of the drug.

The nature of a person influences the person's relationships with drugs in several ways. One is genetic, or physical. Some researchers are looking to people's genetic makeups in hopes of finding inborn tendencies toward drug abuse. Others are exploring the personalities of youngsters to identify traits that predict such tendencies.[3] These traits may be hereditary, may result from the way parents raise their children, or both.

Curiosity can be a strong motivator promoting drug abuse. Some people try drugs to see what they are like. Of these who experiment, some continue to use drugs and become drug dependent.

The desire to fit in socially motivates many people to abuse drugs. Drugs are often part of social events. Everyone needs to have a sense of belonging to some group, and drug-taking can provide a reason for being together.

A person's self-perception may be a fourth influence on drug abuse. People with narcissistic personality traits (self-obsession) are likely to abuse cocaine.[4] People may gravitate toward drugs because they pride themselves on their deviance from the rest of society. Drugs thus fit their image.

Self-esteem is another factor. A person with high self-esteem finds it easy to refuse drugs when offered. Many education programs designed to curtail

psychoactive mind altering; a term used to describe drugs that produce pleasure or hallucinations.

euphoria (you-FORE-ee-uh) an inflated sense of well-being and pleasure brought on by some drugs, popularly called a *high*.

recreational drug use a term not defined by authorities, but used by people who claim their drug taking produces no harmful social or health effects.

■ *FACT OR FICTION:* Alcohol is the most commonly abused drug in the United States. *True.*

drug abuse teach refusal skills.[5] A person with low self-esteem is more easily influenced by others and may use drugs to improve self-image.

Not only does a person's nature affect the choice to abuse a drug or not, but also the person's perception of how severely society punishes people for drug abuse affects the choice. Tolerant drug policies may spread drug addiction.* Research has shown that education about drug hazards is not effective against drug abuse—physicians, despite their superior knowledge, have narcotic addiction rates at least 30 times higher than members of the general population.[6] The reason is unknown, but perhaps easy access to drugs combined with a false sense of security (they think they can handle it) overwhelm even a superior education.

The nature of the drug, too, is a factor influencing drug abuse. Those that give pleasure, or produce euphoria, are most likely to be abused. When animals are fitted with an apparatus to receive cocaine, they visit the device often. In fact, when they are offered either food or the drug, they consistently choose the drug until eventually they starve.[7] The feeling of pleasure the drug produces makes them forget to eat or sleep. Cocaine can have that effect on people, too.

A few drugs produce addictions without euphoria. Nicotine, the subject of Chapter 11, is one; caffeine (in the Spotlight that follows Chapter 8) is another.

≡▶ *People abuse drugs for many reasons: the nature of the person, the person's perception of the legal consequences, and the nature of the drug. Drugs that give pleasure are the most likely to be abused.*

■≡ Addiction

Seeking pleasure is an inborn instinct, universal to all creatures on earth. In nature, this instinct normally drives creatures to act in ways that benefit them without harming them. Eating is a pleasure that, in nature, leads to nourishment of the body. Sexual activity is pleasurable and leads to propagation of the species. Exercising and then relaxing after exertion are pleasurable, and lead to improved fitness and high energy.

All of these activities can themselves be abused, and can lead to harm—overeating causes obesity, indiscriminate sexual activity can lead to unwanted pregnancy and sexually transmitted disease, and overexercising can lead to injury. All these concerns are addressed elsewhere in the book; the point here is that reasonable pleasure seeking by healthy means is beneficial, but that obsessive pleasure seeking through risky behaviors can be harmful.

The acts of eating, engaging in sexual activity, exercising, and relaxing produce pleasure by stimulating the brain to produce **endorphins,** pleasure-producing chemicals. These chemicals are similar to mind-altering drugs, but there is a key difference—they are continuously produced in response to *healthful activities.* The taking of a mind-altering drug produces pleasure

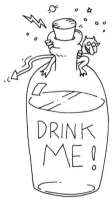

Many people who use drugs to chase away unpleasant feelings are unaware that the unpleasant feelings are the aftereffects of the drugs themselves.

endorphins   pleasure-producing, pain-relieving chemicals produced in the brain in response to a variety of activities.

*England and Sweden tried to combat addiction by making heroin legally available to addicts, with resulting epidemics of drug addiction. In both countries the policies were ultimately reversed. N. Bejerot, *Addiction, an Artificially Induced Drive* (Springfield, Ill.: Charles C. Thomas, 1972), pp. 46–59.

directly in the brain, but intermittently, and causes the brain to produce fewer endorphins on its own. When the effects of the drug wear off, there is a lack of endorphin production. The drug-taker feels the low endorphin concentration as an unpleasant sensation, known as **dysphoria.** The person may then use drugs to chase away the dysphoria, unaware that the unpleasant feelings are the aftereffects of the drugs themselves.

The repeated attempt to ease dysphoria often leads to a drug **addiction.** This state can be either physiological or psychological. (see the Miniglossary of Addiction terms). In **physiological addiction,** the body changes chemically so that it demands the presence of the drug not for pleasure but in order to function normally in many ways. As the body begins to clear the drug from the system, the altered body chemistry disrupts normal functioning, and the symptoms of **withdrawal,** including dysphoria, ensue.[8] Depending on the drug, these symptoms may include disrupted vision, muscle activity, digestion, perception, and temperature regulation (see Table 9–1, later in this chapter). This creates an urgent need for another dose of the drug. By this time in the addiction process, the drug may be producing little or no euphoria; the person now requires it to relieve pain.

A drug is physiologically addictive if, when it is withheld, brainwave patterns change, mood alters, and drug-seeking behavior follows (just as food-seeking behavior follows food deprivation).[9] Physiological addiction also involves tolerance, necessitating *increasing doses.*[10] (Tolerance was discussed in Chapter 8.) The downward spiral of physiological addiction is described in Figure 9–1.

Physiological addiction always has a psychological component—a strong craving for the drug. But **psychological addiction** can occur without

dysphoria (dis-FORE-ee-uh) unpleasant feelings that commonly follow drug-induced euphoria.

withdrawal the process of ceasing to use a particular drug, with accompanying physiological effects.

■ *FACT OR FICTION:* When people become addicted to drugs, the primary reason they continue to use them is to experience pleasure. *False.* People continue abusing drugs to avoid the pain of withdrawal symptoms.

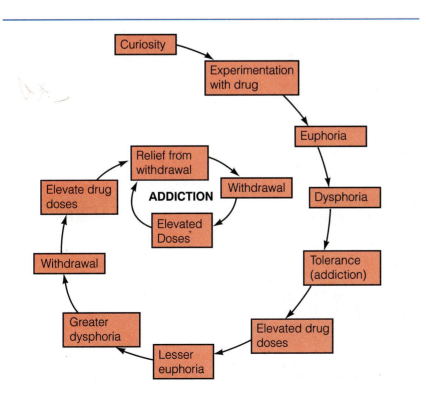

FIGURE 9–1 ■ **The downward spiral of physiological addiction.**

■ MINIGLOSSARY
of Addiction Terms

addiction   an artificially induced strong desire for something; can be either physiological or psychological. Also called *dependence.*

physiological addiction   a change in the body's biochemistry so that it demands the presence of a substance (drug) in order to function normally.

psychological addiction   compulsive use of a substance or behavior to avoid facing emotional pain.

---

denial   refusal to admit, or failure to see, that a problem exists.

physiological addiction, and the craving can be for some other habit or behavior, such as excessive sexual activity, overwork, or overexercise. Almost any behavior can be employed in a psychological addiction, and such an addiction can be as powerful as a physiological addiction.

People with psychological addictions have not learned healthy ways to cope with emotional pain. They crave relief from emotional hurt and use a substance or behavior to distract themselves. The underlying motive is the same, regardless of the behavior used to relieve pain. People who use behaviors or drugs this way achieve temporary numbness and receive short-term relief, but if the behavior is destructive, they have negative consequences to face after indulging in it. If the person repeatedly turns to the behavior or substance, the person is caught up in the cycle depicted in Figure 9–2.

Drug addiction is a staggering problem in the United States.[11] Addiction not only impairs physical health, but also disrupts the personal, social, and financial lives of those addicted and their families. Drug addiction is alarmingly widespread. According to the National Institute of Drug Abuse, three million people are addicted to narcotics or cocaine, and 33 percent of Americans over age 12 have experimented with some sort of illegal drug.[12] Recovery rates from drug addiction are depressingly low.

You might think that a person, once caught up in the cycle of addiction, would admit to the problem, try to break out of it, and seek help, if necessary, in doing so. In reality, though, most people deny their addictions; in fact, **denial** is a hallmark of the addiction syndrome. If you state that a drug problem has extensively damaged a person's family, work, social life, and health, the person may well respond, "Who, me? No, I don't have a drug

FIGURE 9–2 ■ **The cycle of psychological addiction.**

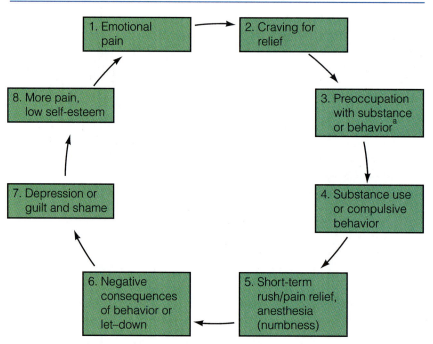

a Examples: Abuse of nicotine, alcohol, or other drugs; over-exercise; obsessiveness in relationships or sex; overeating; compulsive working; gambling.

problem. I'm just having a little bad luck, that's all. I can control my use of the drug."

Denial often continues to prevent people's seeking treatment or accepting help long after their problems have become unmanageable. That is why recovery depends first and foremost on addicts' admitting their problems, as the conclusion of this chapter, "Kicking the Habit," demonstrates.

Drug addiction is unexpected. Probably no one who starts out using a substance intends to get hooked, but it happens nevertheless. A person tries a drug for one reason but continues taking it because addiction has set in. For example, someone may begin to smoke cigarettes to look grown-up—but 30 years later, the person is still smoking. The original reason is long gone; the addiction has taken over.

People who experiment with drugs often want to believe that the craving won't get to them, only to others who are somehow inferior. The truth is that no one is exempt, not people, not animals—no one. The only way to escape drug addiction is to refrain from experimenting with drugs that produce it.

≡▶ *For any drug that produces withdrawal symptoms, the repeated attempt to ease dysphoria often leads to addiction. Addiction can be physiological and/or psychological. No one is exempt from developing an addiction.*

■≡ Commonly Abused Drugs

This section discusses commonly abused drugs and compares the actual effects with the popular beliefs about them. Table 9–1 presents details regarding medical uses, addictiveness, effects, and withdrawal symptoms.

Marijuana and Other Cannabis Drugs

Marijuana plants are harvested and dried, and then the flowers, as well as some of the leaves and small stems, are rolled into cigarettes (joints) or smoked in pipes. The constituents are rapidly and completely (90 percent) absorbed from the lungs and then travel in the blood to the various body tissues that process them. The ingredient in marijuana that produces euphoria is delta-9-tetrahydrocannabinol, or THC for short. This constituent lingers for several weeks in body fat before being excreted. THC can remain in the body for up to a month after marijuana use. Today's drug tests can detect trace amounts of THC for as long as six months after use.

THC circulates to all the tissues, affecting hearing, touch, taste, and smell, as well as perceptions of time, of space, and of the body; it also produces changes in mental sensations and sleep patterns. Among the taste changes apparently induced is a great enjoyment of eating, especially of sweets ("the munchies"), but it is not known how this effect occurs.[13]

THC is sometimes used as a medicine to treat nausea in people with cancer or to reduce eye swelling from the disease glaucoma. However, a variety of other drugs, many of which are considered more effective, are also used for these purposes.

The percentage of THC in marijuana today is considerably higher than in the 1960s, when its use became popular. Today's marijuana averages 3 to 4

TABLE 9–1 ■ Abused Drugs

Class	Drug (with selected brand or other names)	Medical Use	Physiological Addiction
Depressants	Barbiturates (phenobarbital, Alurate, Butisol, Nembutal, Secobarbital, Seconal, Tuinal), chloral hydrate (Noctec)	Anesthetic, anticonvulsant, sedative, hypnotic	Yes
	Glutethimide (Doriden), methaqualone (Quaalude, Sopor)	Sedative, hypnotic	Yes
	Benzodiazepines (Ativan, Clonopin, Dalmane, Diazepam, Librium, Serax, Tranxene, Valium), others (Equanil, Miltown, Noludar Placidyl, Valmid)	Anxiety reliever, anticonvulsant, sedative, hypnotic	Yes
Designer Drugs	Ecstasy, Ex, MDMA	None	Varies
Hallucinogens	Lysergic acid diethylamide (LSD, acid, microdot), mescaline and peyote (mesc, buttons, cactus)	None	No
	Amphetamine variants (2,5-DMA, PMA, STP, MDA, MMDA, TMA, DOM, DOB)	None	Unknown
	Psilocybin and related mushroom species (mushrooms, shrooms)	None	Unknown
	Phencyclidine hydrochloride (PCP, angel dust, hog)	Veterinary anesthetic	Unknown
	Others (PCE, PCPy, TCP, DMT, DET, morning glory seeds)	None	No
Inhalants	Hydrocarbon vapors from many sources, such as plastic cement, gasoline, spray cans (glue, gas, poppers, locker room, rush, odor of man, Aspirols, Vaporal, amyl nitrite, butyl nitrite, nitrous oxide, laughing gas, whip-its)	Amyl nitrite relieves angina pectoris nitrous oxide relieves anxiety	Yes
Marijuana and Other Cannabis Drugs	Marijuana (pot, Acapulco gold, grass, weed, dope, reefer, sinsemilla, Thai sticks), tetrahydrocannabinol (THC), hashish (hash), hashish oil (hash oil)	Relieves glaucoma and cancer therapy side effects	Unknown
Narcotics	Opium (Dover's Powder, paregoric, Parepectolin), morphine (Pectoral Syrup), codeine (Empirin with Codeine, Robitussin A-C), others (Levo-Dromoran, Percodan, Tussionex, Fentanyl, Sublimaze, Darvon, Talwin, Lomotil)	Analgesic, antidiarrheal, antitussive	Yes
	Heroin (diacetylmorphine, H, black tar, horse, smack)	Pain reliever	Yes
	Hydromorphone (Dilaudid), meperidine (pethidine) hydrochloride (Demerol)	Analgesic	Yes
	Methadone hydrochloride (Dolophine, methadone, Methadose)	Analgesic, heroin substitute	Yes
Stimulants	Cocaine (base, coke, crack, flake, rock, snow)	Local anesthetic	Possible
	Amphetamines (biphetamine, speed, uppers, black beauties, white crosses, Desoxyn, Dexedrine, Mediatric), phenmetrazine hydrochloride (Preludin), methylphenidate hydrochloride (Ritalin), others (Adipex, Bacarate, Cylert, Didrex, lonamin, Plegine, Sanorex, Tenuate, Tepanil)	Used to treat hyperkinesis, narcolepsy, weight control	Possible
	Amphetamine look-alikes (crystal, crank)	None	Possible
Others	Clove cigarettes rolled from high-nicotine and high-tar tobacco, clove oil, cocoa, licorice, and other ingredients (Djarum, Kreteks)	None	Possible

SOURCE: Adapted from R. D. Thompkins, *Before It's Too Late: The Prevention Manual on Drug Abuse for People Who Care* (Englewood, N.J.: Family Information Services, 1981), pp. 16–17.

TABLE 9–1 ■ continued

Psychological Addiction	Tolerance	Usual Method of Administration	Possible Effect	Effect of Overdose	Withdrawal Syndrome
Yes	Yes	Oral, injected	Slurred speech, disorientation, drunken behavior without odor of alcohol	Shallow respiration, cold and clammy skin, dilated pupils, weak and rapid pulse, coma, possible death	Anxiety, insomnia, tremors, delirium, convulsions, possible death
Yes	Yes	Oral, injected			
Yes	Yes	Oral, injected			
Varies	Varies	Varies	Varies	Varies	Varies
Unknown	Yes	Oral, injected	Illusions and hallucinations, poor perception of time and distance, nausea, vomiting	Longer, more intense "trip" episodes; psychosis; possible death	None reported
Unknown	Yes	Oral, injected			
Yes, rarely	Yes	Oral			
Yes	Yes	Smoked, oral, injected			
Unknown	Yes	Smoked, oral, injected, sniffed			
Yes	Yes	Sniffed, vapors concentrated and inhaled	Altered time sense; brief euphoria; nausea; vomiting; dizziness; headache; liver, brain, and kidney cancer	Loss of consciousness, death by suffocation, cerebral hemorrhage	None reported
Yes	Yes	Smoked, oral	Euphoria, relaxed inhibitions, increased appetite, disoriented behavior	Fatigue, paranoia, possible psychosis	Insomnia, hyperactivity, decreased appetite
Yes	Yes	Oral, smoked, injected			
Yes	Yes	Injected, sniffed, smoked	Euphoria, drowsiness, respiratory depression, constricted pupils, nausea	Slow and shallow breathing, clammy skin, convulsions, coma, possible death	Watery eyes, runny nose, yawning, loss of appetite, irritability, tremors, panic, chills and sweating, cramps, nausea
Yes	Yes	Oral, injected			
Yes	Yes	Oral, injected			
Yes	Possible	Sniffed, injected, smoked			
Yes	Yes	Oral, injected	Increased alertness, excitation, euphoria, increased pulse rate and blood pressure, insomnia, loss of appetite, skin lesions	Agitation, increase in body temperature, hallucinations, convulsions, possible death	Apathy, long periods of sleep, irritability, depression, disorientation
Yes	Yes	Oral			
Unknown	Unknown	Unknown	Nausea, vomiting, respiratory dysfunctions and bleeding, allergic reaction	Possible death from severe lung infection	None reported

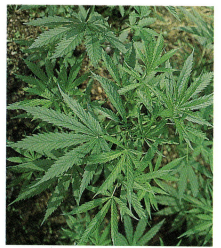

The marijuana plant.

amotivational syndrome loss of ambition and drive; a characteristic of long-term users of marijuana.

▪ *FACT OR FICTION:* Smoking marijuana is more damaging to the lungs than smoking tobacco cigarettes. *True.*

percent THC (with some samples exceeding 10 percent), compared with the marijuana of the 1960s, which contained less than 0.05 percent.[14]

In addition to THC, scientists have identified at least 400 different chemicals in marijuana, and their ratios differ by genetic strain and even within the same strain from season to season. These differences in chemical composition affect users' experiences.

Besides the potency and chemical composition of marijuana, personal factors also influence the high. People's expectations of how they will feel, their surroundings, and frequency of marijuana use can all combine to vary users' reactions. Reactions range from a mild euphoria and giddiness to hallucinations. Users may feel less inhibited or, on the other hand, may feel paranoid and more inhibited. They may feel graceful (but act clumsy), they may feel like excellent drivers (but actually become impaired), they may feel brilliant or witty (but make no sense). Marijuana may dull sexual pleasure and is more likely to make people feel sleepy than sexy. The morning after an evening of smoking is, for many, a morning of tiredness and irritability, and for many, time to roll another joint to get rid of unpleasant feelings (dysphoria), thus setting out on the road to being a habitual user.

Some people who use marijuana falsely believe that it provides a harmless high. Research indicates, however, that harmful health effects are associated with its use.

Marijuana causes alteration in heart action, including rapid and sometimes irregular heartbeat. Marijuana may also reduce the body's immune response and, in young men, may reduce the sex hormone level and sperm count. It also causes short-term memory loss, overestimation of the passage of time, and loss of ability to maintain focused attention on a task. Like other drugs, marijuana presents the greatest potential hazard to those who use it most heavily and frequently.

Some people respond to long-term use by losing ambition and drive, the so-called **amotivational syndrome.**[15] Some people find that giving up the drug is extremely difficult and require formal therapy to succeed.

Another risk associated with marijuana use is that of escalation to the use of more powerful drugs. Users looking for a "better high" sometimes shift to hashish, a concentrated marijuana resin collected from the flowering top of the plant. With hashish, the risks probably increase dramatically, because the user receives a stronger dose.

Marijuana smoking, to a greater degree than cigarette smoking, sets the stage for lung damage, including lung cancer. Smoking three to four marijuana cigarettes produces damage equivalent to that from more than 20 tobacco cigarettes.[16] Other hazards are significant: marijuana may be contaminated with pesticides, poisonous molds, or herbicides. It may contain dangerous drugs such as the animal tranquilizer phencyclidine hydrochloride (PCP or "angel dust"), which is added to low-grade marijuana by sellers to deceive buyers into believing that its potency is high.

A dangerous side effect of using marijuana is its interference with driving ability. Even in doses that people use socially, the drug impairs driving performance, and the effect persists long after the high is gone.

≡▶ *Marijuana affects hearing, touch, taste, and smell, as well as perceptions of time, of space, and of the body. Marijuana is not a harmless high. Its use causes physical complications and interferes with driving ability.*

Depressants: Sedatives and Barbiturates

Sedatives and barbiturates are examples of drugs that exert a depressant effect on many body systems, in a number of different ways. Some sedatives slow the heart; some, the brain and nervous system; some, both. They may be used to calm agitation, dull sensation, or induce sleep, so they are useful tools in the hands of medical professionals but potentially dangerous when self-administered. Some are more dangerous than others, but none are safe.

Barbiturates are a group of chemically related compounds that all have similar effects. They depress the nervous system, the heart rate, the respiration rate, the blood pressure, and the body temperature. They, too, have their medical uses, but they are easily abused. Long-term use can cause depression, forgetfulness, reduced sex drive, and many other adverse effects, including addiction; overdoses kill.

≡▶ *Sedatives and barbiturates act as depressants, slowing the body's systems. They have their medical uses but are easily abused and potentially dangerous when self-administered. Long-term use causes many adverse effects, including addiction.*

Stimulants: Amphetamines and Cocaine

In this high-speed society, drugs that reportedly provide some extra get-up-and-go might tempt even the most cautious.

AMPHETAMINES Amphetamines are stimulants—drugs that stimulate the central nervous system, increasing activity, suppressing fatigue and hunger, and producing euphoria. They are available by prescription to treat diseases such as intractable obesity, uncontrollable sleeping, or, in children, hyperactivity.*

People may start using amphetamines to lose weight; to combat fatigue so they can work at night or study for exams; to party all night; or to offset the sleepiness brought on by alcohol, marijuana, or sedatives. Sometimes a daily cycle develops in which people use depressants such as barbiturates to relieve amphetamine overstimulation and then more amphetamines to pick themselves up again. Physical tolerance to amphetamines builds up in just a few weeks, and soon the user may be taking several hundred times the normally prescribed dose to achieve the desired effect. At this point, drug addiction is extreme.

Most amphetamine abusers take the drugs by mouth; although some inject the substances into their veins. The risks of using any drug increase dramatically when the drug is injected. Overdoses are likely. Needles may not be sterile, or the skin may not be clean. The needle puncture may introduce life-threatening microbes or a fatal air bubble into the bloodstream. People who share needles share infections such as AIDS or hepatitis (a dangerous, often incurable liver condition).

More about AIDS in Chapter 17.

A person injecting amphetamines experiences an intense, short-lived euphoria. The drug-taker may feel unusually strong; this, coupled with drug-induced hyperactivity and paranoid delusions, can lead to dangerous behavior against self and others. The user may repeat the injection ten times

*In the case of hyperactivity, the amphetamine acts not to stimulate the child but to stimulate a brain center that filters out distractions, so that the child can concentrate.

daily for several days consecutively, with no sleep and very little food. This behavior sets the stage for the impairments of nutrition status that typically appear with most drug addictions.[17]

The euphoria wears off much more quickly than the drug's other effects. Accidents are likely, because the user is unaware of fatigue until suddenly overwhelmed by it, perhaps while driving or crossing the street. When fatigue or confusion becomes so great that injection is no longer possible, the drug binge is over and the person sleeps for days, awakening with voracious hunger. Severe dysphoria and psychological depression follow, and the person may turn again to the drug for relief. When injected, moderate doses of amphetamines can cause acute anxiety, psychosis, and malnutrition. High doses can cause convulsions, lack of oxygen, loss of consciousness, dangerously elevated temperature, brain hemorrhage, high blood pressure, and death.

People taking amphetamines may think they have desirable traits that they really do not have. The undrugged self pales by comparison. They continue to take the drug to maintain their illusions, and in doing so, abandon real life, where they could become genuinely more sensitive, more fun, more intelligent, better lovers, or whatever else might improve the quality of their lives.

COCAINE The leaves of the coca bush are processed to yield the isolated drug cocaine. In coca-growing cultures, people chew the leaves to receive small doses of the stimulant to help them work longer. In other cultures, the isolated chemical is usually mixed with other white powders—some inert, some not—before it is sold. If an unwary consumer happens upon pure cocaine and uses it in the same quantity as the diluted product, the reactions are severe or fatal.

People may use any of a number of methods to self-administer cocaine. One route is snorting—that is, sniffing the powder into the nose. Others may inject or smoke the drug. Many a person who starts by snorting a little escalates by increasing the doses, going on binges, and moving to the more direct administration routes—injection or smoking. Such people have been known to rip through thousands of dollars worth of cocaine *each week.* (See the box The Cocaine Craze for the history of cocaine abuse.)

One smokable form of cocaine is "base"; cheaper forms are "crack" or "rock." Crack opened whole new drug markets because of its low price, and deaths from the drug followed.

Cocaine's effects, when subjected to scientific examination, are found to be similar to those of two groups of medical drugs: the local anesthetics and the stimulants. The short-lived burst of exhilaration produced by cocaine is followed by intense irritability—dysphoria. The intensity of the high and the low depends partly on the drug dose, partly on the route of administration, and partly on the user's expectations. Repeated use of the drug shuts off all drives, including the sex drive, and replaces them with the drug-seeking drive.

Cocaine stimulates the sympathetic nervous system, the system responsible for the stress response, and causes constriction of blood vessels (and thus elevation of the blood pressure), dilation of the pupils of the eyes, and increased body temperature. It also banishes fatigue and hunger. Cocaine levels in brain tissues remain high long after euphoria has faded, and the stored drug is released slowly as blood levels start to fall.

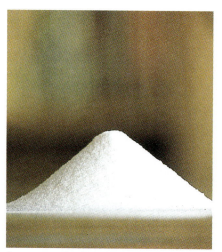

Cocaine, in the form of white powder.

■ *FACT OR FICTION:* Repeated use of cocaine stimulates the sex drive. *False.* Repeated use of cocaine shuts off the sex drive.

The Cocaine Craze

Contrary to popular belief, cocaine is not a new drug. The United States experienced its first cocaine epidemic in the late 1880s. Sigmund Freud tested and praised the drug in 1884. Other medical authorities claimed cocaine was valuable in curing opiate addictions and it became widely used in the form of coca leaves. With no laws restricting the sale, consumption, or advertising of cocaine (or any other drugs), manufacturers made cocaine available as a popular liquid potion.

Besides being available in the form of coca leaves and elixirs, the drug was also available in several other forms. Coca Cola contained minute amounts of cocaine (.0025 percent in 1900), enough to act as a significant stimulant (it has since been replaced by caffeine). Coca Cola was marketed as a healthful soft drink and a "brain tonic" to relieve headaches, and cure all nervous afflictions. Cocaine was also widely available as an antidote for toothache pain. It was offered to treat asthma and became the official remedy of the American Hay Fever Association. Then the widespread use of cocaine brought on alarming problems of addiction among many of its users of all social classes. In 1903, cocaine addiction became a problem in the poor community and caused rampant crime. In 1910, President Taft presented a State Department report to Congress declaring cocaine a public enemy: "The illicit sale of [cocaine] and the habitual use of it temporarily raises the power of a criminal to a point where in resisting arrest there is no hesitation to murder. It is more appalling in its effects than any other habit-forming drug used in the United States." Shortly after that came the passing of the Harrison Act in 1914, a law that tightly regulates the distribution and sale of drugs.

America's first great cocaine epidemic went through three distinct phases. During the first phase it was introduced and readily accepted, during the second phase its use spread and its ill effects came to light and during the final stage it became the most feared of all illicit drugs.

Does this story of cocaine's first epidemic have a familiar ring to it? Enough time passed so that the nation forgot cocaine's early tainted reputation. By the late 1900s, America was ready for another fling with this most seductive and dangerous drug, which was to parallel the events of the early part of the century. Thus, around 1980, the United States entered its second cocaine craze. Many prominent Americans touted the use of this "harmless" agent, and the young and the rich made cocaine their favorite leisure pharmaceutical. Then cocaine overdoses killed several celebrities—including actor John Belushi and college basketball star Len Bias—and cocaine's popularity began to dwindle. By 1988, the drug had turned out to be a factor in countless crimes and had claimed several other lives. People who once viewed cocaine as glamorous and safe began to regard it as a devastating menace. As a result, cocaine abuse has dramatically declined among the middle and upper classes. Perhaps it will again fade away, as it did 80 years ago.

SOURCE: Adapted from D. E. Musto, America's first cocaine epidemic, *The Wilson Quarterly*, Summer 1989, pp. 59–64.

By constricting the blood vessels, cocaine erodes nasal tissues in habitual snorters. At first, this causes such symptoms as sinus infection, runny nose, and nosebleeds. With increasing use, nasal tissues die, leaving a hole between the nostrils. Just over half of chronic users report nasal problems.

More commonly, people report chronic fatigue (yet they claim coke peps them up), poor sexual performance (but they claim coke is good for sex), and severe headaches. In one study, over a third of chronic cocaine users reported having considered suicide, and about a tenth had made suicide attempts.[18] The use of cocaine during pregnancy is linked to birth defects and infant deaths. Expectant mothers who take cocaine can be prosecuted for damaging their unborn babies.

For many, cocaine abuse is a destructive habit embedded within other harmful behaviors such as consuming alcohol and other drugs to excess and eating poorly.[19] When cocaine abusers suffer physical damage, then, they do so not only from the harmful effects of the drug itself, but from all their poor health habits combined. When cocaine causes death, it is often by heart attack, stroke, or seizure in an already damaged body system.[20]

Cocaine abuse is a problem for over 1 million Americans.[21] Between 60 and 80 percent of users questioned believe themselves to be addicted, unable to turn the drug down if offered and unable to limit cocaine use.[22] A person who is addicted to cocaine can lose the ability to work, to keep a job, to play, or to stop using the drug.

≡▶ *Amphetamines are stimulants. Withdrawal from amphetamines causes severe dysphoria and psychological depression. Cocaine is a stimulant and anesthetic. It produces short-term, intense pleasure that is followed by extreme irritability and dysphoria. Adverse effects are numerous, and the most severe is death.*

Inhalants

Three categories of chemicals are sometimes inhaled to produce a high: solvents, propellants, and drugs. The solvents people use are organic liquids that vaporize at room temperature. Examples are fumes from gasoline, glue, lighter fluid, cleaning fluid, and paint thinner.

Propellants are compounds added by manufacturers to products so that they can be sprayed. Examples of products people use are spray paints, spray deodorants, hairsprays, whipped-cream sprays, and spray oils. All these products bear labels that warn against inhaling their fumes because of the hazards they present. A person who experiments with them, even once, risks permanent disability or death from heart failure or suffocation.

Examples of the drugs people use as inhalants are chloroform, ether, nitrous oxide (laughing gas), and others. Amyl nitrite, a heart pain medicine, is sometimes abused this way, and so is butyl nitrite, sold legally as a "room odorizer." Some claim that sniffing the nitrites is a sexual stimulant; research shows that these chemicals interfere with erection and bring on headache, dizziness, accelerated heart rate, nausea, nasal irritation, or cough.

Inhalants' effects on brain cells are unpredictable and depend on the doses of the chemicals present. In general, even short-term abuse brings on vision disturbances, impaired judgment, and reduced muscle and reflex control that may be impossible to reverse. Many cases of permanent brain and nerve damage have resulted from sniffing; the kidneys, blood, liver, and bone marrow also suffer. Suffocation occurs when the lungs fill with gases that contain no oxygen or when the product coats the lungs' absorptive surfaces and thus blocks oxygen transfer to the blood.

≡▶ *Three categories of chemicals are used as inhalants: solvents, propellants, and drugs such as chloroform and nitrous oxide. People who experiment with inhalants risk permanent disability or death from heart failure or suffocation. Inhalants' effects are unpredictable.*

Narcotics

Narcotics (also called opiates) are used medically to relieve pain and induce sleep. They are abused by people to achieve the effects of euphoric relaxation.

Some common narcotics include opium, morphine, heroin, and methadone. Opium is derived from an oriental poppy plant, morphine is the active ingredient in opium, and heroin is synthesized from morphine. Heroin is the most commonly abused narcotic, and of all drugs, it is commonly injected by drug abusers, hence, more than any other drug, it is associated with the risks of contracting diseases such as AIDS. Methadone, a synthetic narcotic, is a milder drug prescribed to assist heroin addicts in their progress toward rehabilitation.

Narcotics produce both physiological and psychological tolerance and addiction. They cause euphoria, drowsiness, respiratory depression, and sometimes nausea. Convulsions, coma, or even death are possible on overdose.

≡▶ *Narcotics are used medically to relieve pain and induce sleep but are also abused to achieve a euphoric relaxation. Narcotics produce addiction and death by overdose.*

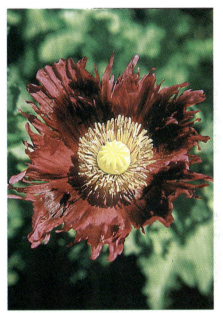

Drug dependence is unexpected. Plants like the opium poppy look innocent.

Hallucinogens

Hallucinogens are drugs that create perceived distortions of reality, or hallucinations. People who take hallucinogens label their experiences of distorted reality "trips," some reported as pleasant, some as negative.

Some common forms of hallucinogens are lysergic acid diethylamide (LSD, produced in the laboratory), mescaline (from a cactus), and psilocybin (from mushroom extracts). Physiological addiction is not reported in connection with hallucinogen abuse because tolerance apparently does not develop. More commonly observed is psychological addiction.

≡▶ *Hallucinogens are drugs that produce distortions of reality and may cause psychological addiction.*

Look-alikes

Another group of easily accessible drugs is the so-called look-alikes. Drug pushers, masquerading as companies, use OTC drugs and other legal substances to produce pills and powders that look like the prescription medications and illegal drugs that abusers seek. For example, magazines publish ads for "legal stimulants" ("mail-order speed") that mimic the prescription drugs' appearance almost exactly, with one important difference: the capsules or tablets contain a combination of OTC stimulants, decongestants, antihistamines, and other drugs instead of amphetamines.

Because look-alikes are weaker than the drugs they mimic, users tend to take a lot of them. As a result, users may experience sleep disturbances, heartbeat irregularities, and sudden rises in blood pressure. The most dangerous situation occurs when a user can't tell the difference between the look-alike and the real thing; when such a person gets some of the more potent drugs and takes the same number of pills, a fatal overdose results.

The look-alikes are legal, so there are no limits on their sale and distribution. Those who sell them make huge profits at the expense of the consumer's health. But so it is with all street drugs—no one is looking out for the consumer. This chapter's Critical Thinking box explores this issue.

≡▶ *Look-alikes are made from legal substances to look like the prescription medications and illegal drugs that abusers seek. As with all illegal drugs, no agency monitors the contents of these drugs, so the user takes risks when using them.*

Designer Drugs

Designer drugs are laboratory-synthesized compounds that closely resemble illegal drugs in chemical structure. In the past, each drug was defined as legal or illegal based on its exact chemical formula. Therefore, designer drugs, having new formulas, were at one time, able to escape this definition. Until recently, designer drugs were sufficiently different from the chemical formulas of illegal drugs that they could escape governmental control. Today, in order to curtail the making and selling of designer drugs, laws have been made less specific as to the exact formulas of drugs. Ecstasy (designer cocaine) is an example of a popular designer drug.

A case with a devastating outcome shows what actually can happen with designer drugs.[23] A fumbling amateur chemist, using a crude basement laboratory in California, tried to produce a batch of designer heroin. His inept attempt at chemistry produced, instead, a substance so toxic to brain cells that when the heroin addicts who purchased it injected the stuff, they were immediately and permanently paralyzed.* The substance left them with Parkinson's disease—destruction of the parts of the brain that control motor activity. The police found and arrested the "designer"; he too had developed parkinsonism from his creation, because he had absorbed the chemical through his skin and lungs. Now, the same chemical is showing up in other chemists' drugs, under the names of designer heroin and designer cocaine.

This story accentuates the problem all users of street drugs face: lack of standardization. People who use them, or even simply handle them, are risking exposure to highly toxic chemicals.

≡▶ *Designer drugs are laboratory-synthesized compounds that closely resemble other illegal drugs in chemical structure. Lack of standardization presents enormous risks to users.*

*The substance is MPTP, a side product that usually arises in small amounts during chemical transformations to produce designer heroin. This particular batch was 90% MPTP. One of the early symptoms of MPTP exposure is an uncharacteristic burning at the site of entry, such as at the injection site or in the nasal passages.

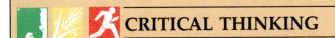

CRITICAL THINKING

Street Drug Surprises

No watchdog agency such as the FDA screens illegal drugs for safety, purity, or concentration, and this has implications for those who abuse drugs. The substances provided by an illicit source are of unpredictable composition, and they vary from batch to batch. Illegal drugs provide a profit at each level of sale, so sellers tend to mix them liberally with extenders at every turn. For example, "consumer-quality" cocaine is expected to contain some quantity of white powder other than pure cocaine, usually talcum powder or the powdered sugar lactose. However, some sellers of cocaine maximize profits by adding enormous quantities of sugar and then masking the weakened effect of the cocaine with cheaper drugs, such as amphetamines, caffeine, or anesthetics that mimic some of cocaine's effects. As great a danger as the drugs themselves may pose to the users, greater still may be the dangers from unknown substances they contain.

Medical drugs are standardized; street drugs can contain nasty surprises.

■≡ Drugs and Driving

Mind-altering drugs, including alcohol, marijuana, tranquilizers, and barbiturates, impair people's judgment of speed and slow down their reactions. In simulator tests, people on drugs crash more frequently than others.[24] In the case of alcohol and marijuana, the impairment of driving lasts for hours *after* the high from the drug has worn off—even to the next day.[25]

Amphetamines are drugs that speed up the nervous system. You might think they would improve people's driving, but accident studies show otherwise. Heavy amphetamine use allows fatigued people to override their feelings of exhaustion; driving ability declines even though they think they are doing well.

≡▶ *Use of mind-altering drugs impairs people's judgment of speed, slows their reactions, and hinders driving ability.*

■≡ Strategies: Freedom from Drugs

How can you tell whether someone close to you is abusing drugs? Here are some behavioral signs:

■ Pallor and perspiration.
■ Dilated pupils.
■ Runny nose and nosebleeds.
■ Jitters and hyperactivity.
■ Ability to go without food or sleep for long periods of time.
■ Lack of interest in sex and inability to perform.
■ Paranoia, anxiety, suspiciousness.
■ Loss of memory.

■ Increase in energy and talkativeness, followed by lethargy and depression.

■ Sudden carelessness about personal appearance.

■ Broken appointments, broken promises, lying.

■ Inability to explain what happened to the paycheck or other money.[26]

Extreme caution should be used in attributing any of these signs to drug abuse; they may be caused by hundreds of other things as well. Probably the best way to find out if a person is abusing drugs is to express concern and ask questions. If you care, this is a way to show it.

If a drug is causing you chronic difficulty, face the problem. A way to recognize a drug problem is to give up the drug for a month. (Of course, if the drug is a medicine, the physician should decide whether it is safe to do without it.) Coffee, colas, cigarettes, OTC drugs, prescriptions, and alcohol, as well as illegal drugs, all qualify for this test. Try doing without one, and write down your responses to this chapter's Life Choice Inventory.

Kicking the Habit

When people realize they have a drug problem, they have taken one important step: admitting it. They have broken through their denial of a problem. Now comes a hard choice: continue to suffer, or quit. To quit involves suffering, too, but the suffering ends. Recovery entails much more than is presented here, and the dynamics are more fully covered, with respect to recovery from alcohol addiction, in the Spotlight that follows Chapter 10.

For those who face the problem and choose to quit, the next step is to get help. Rarely do people recover from drugs on their own. Help comes in many forms—hospitalization, drug-quitting groups, psychological therapy, and drug therapy.*

An example of a drug therapy is the use of methadone as treatment for heroin addiction. Methadone is an addictive drug, as heroin is, but it is cheaper, and its effects are milder and longer-lasting. Taking a ''maintenance'' drug such as methadone or one of its relatives allows people addicted to heroin to recover socially—that is, they no longer must struggle to purchase expensive, illegal drugs to hold off withdrawal. Yet, they still have to cope with the psychological component of the addiction, so they will have a greater chance of success if their recovery program addresses both parts of the dependency.

Another useful drug treatment employs drugs called narcotic antagonists, which the person takes daily so as to renew the commitment to abstinence. The antagonists block the effects of the addicting agent, and each administration protects the taker for the next day or so. The same drugs are used to treat overdoses.

Few people who attempt recovery make it all the way. Instead of the normal life that awaits those few who make it, most people get caught in something like a revolving door: undergoing treatment, giving up the drug, getting out of treatment, taking the drug again, going back into treatment—and so on indefinitely. Many factors contribute to this pattern, a major one being the addicted person's failure to make necessary lifestyle changes.

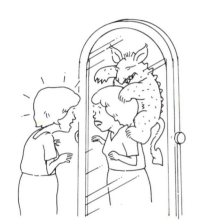

A person who faces up to a drug problem has taken the first important step.

*For help, call the National Drug Information Clearinghouse at 1-800-336-4797; the National Cocaine Hotline at 1-800-COCAINE, or the National Institute on Drug Abuse Hotline at 1-800-662-HELP.

LIFE CHOICE INVENTORY

Do you have a drug problem? For whatever drug comes to mind, this exercise is an informal way to find out. Give up the drug for a month, and answer these questions:

1. Do you miss the drug?
2. Are you experiencing withdrawal effects?
3. Does life seem less full or less fun without the drug?
4. Are you suddenly aware of problems in your life that you had been ignoring?
5. Are you feeling more tense or anxious than usual?
6. Are you feeling depressed?
7. Do you feel better without the drug?
8. Do you have more problems concentrating or meeting goals and deadlines than usual?
9. Do you find that you spend a lot of time thinking about the drug?
10. Did you ensure quick access to some of the drug just in case you missed it too much?

If you were unable to give up the drug for a month, you have a drug problem. If you answered yes to many of these questions, you may have a drug problem. If you gave up the drug for a month, you may want to kick the habit permanently. You need not figure it out alone; you may want to get someone to help you to do so.

SOURCE: Adapted from S. J. Levy, *Managing the "Drugs" in Your Life* (New York: McGraw-Hill, 1983), p. 41.

When the person first becomes free of the drug, problems are not only more numerous than ever, but now must be handled without the escape that drugs once provided. The person who develops a support system to facilitate confronting the problems has the best chance of staying free of drug abuse.

Another factor is the loss of the reinforcement the person was accustomed to receiving while on the drug. This took three forms. There was the association with fellow drug-takers, a sort of support group, which now is a negative influence. And there was the stimulation of the negative attention that people gave the drug habit. Then in the initial stages of recovery, there was strong positive reinforcement from the treatment staff. When ex-drug-takers leave treatment, all forms of attention disappear, and they still crave the drug. Thus they often fall back into drug abuse.

Still, some people make it. The first part is the hardest, for life seems empty without the drug; but later, looking back, the recovered person finds that the rewards of sanity and health outweigh whatever the drug seemed to offer (see Drug-free Highs). A great reinforcer of recovery is to turn and offer a helping hand to others.

▶ *Admitting a drug problem is the first step to overcoming it. Getting help comes in many forms: hospitalization, drug-quitting groups, psychological therapy, and drug therapy. Few people who attempt recovery make it all the way, but those who do find that the rewards far outweigh whatever the drug seemed to offer.*

Helping Someone Kick the Habit

If you care about a person with a drug problem, you will be willing to make the effort to help, even if this means being tough. You may have to risk

---

■ ■ ■ ■ ■ **STRATEGIES:** *FINDING DRUG-FREE HIGHS*

Pleasure is there for the taking, for those who know where to look. To get high:

1. Run, walk, or skip across an open field, through a park, or along a beach.
2. Ask one of your grandparents what life is about.
3. Play with a baby.
4. Give a friend a gift that you made with your own hands.
5. Get involved in worthwhile activities with groups in which you feel you are contributing and are needed.
6. Work hard at something, and see it through to completion.
7. Have a good cry about that thing you have been hiding from for too long.
8. Learn to meditate.
9. Eat nourishing food.
10. Write some poetry for yourself (it doesn't have to rhyme).
11. Climb a mountain.
12. Visit a river.
13. Say "thank you" more often.
14. Beat the feathers out of a pillow next time you are very angry.
15. Stop biting your nails (or shed another bad habit).
16. Read a good book.
17. Give someone a long hug.
18. Call your parent and say, "I love you."

SOURCE: Partially inspired by S. J. Levy, *Managing the "Drugs" in Your Life* (New York: McGraw-Hill, 1983), p. 104.

---

confrontation, standing against your peers, and maybe even loss of a friend in the effort to save the person's health or life. Things you can do include:

■ Making sure the person knows you won't endorse the drug habit.
■ Making available all the information you can gather on the health effects.
■ Making sure the person knows, on choosing to seek help, where to go for it.

Drug addiction does not mean a person is inferior. Blame can only make people feel guilty, it can't help them get better. Drug-addicted people pay heavily enough for past choices. If you want to help, you won't judge or blame. Blame can weaken self-esteem, and it is a form of negative attention.

No amount of effort on your part, however, can supply the crucial ingredient in someone else's choice to give up drugs: the will to quit. In fact, the toughest job for many people whose lives are affected by drug abusers is to learn how to manage their own lives without being dragged down. Often they have to learn simply to accept the other person's choice, painful as that may be. Beyond caring, you have to let go. To watch a person self-destruct with drugs is to witness a tragedy—but once you have done all you can, your best choice is to live your own life as fully as possible while it is yours to live.

≡▶ *You cannot make someone quit a drug habit; the person has to have the will to quit. The toughest part for those close to an addicted person is to learn how to manage their own lives without being dragged down.*

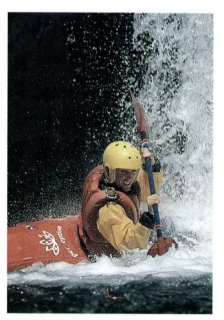

Life without the substance may be better.

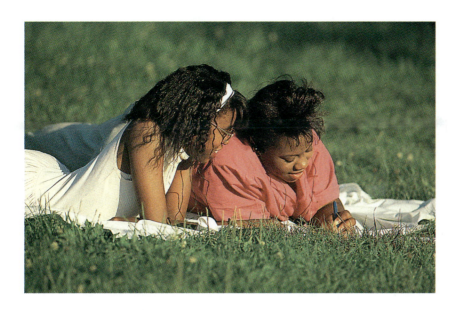

Honest talk helps people face problems.

This chapter defined drug abuse, discussed reasons why people abuse drugs, and presented commonly abused drugs and the associated health risks. It presented ideas for recovery and how to help someone with a drug problem. The next chapter discusses the most commonly abused drug in the United States: alcohol.

■≡ For Review

1. Give the medical definitions of *drug use, drug misuse,* and *drug abuse.*
2. Describe some of the hazards of abusing drugs (for example, marijuana, depressants, stimulants, inhalants, narcotics, hallucinogens, look-alikes, and designer drugs).
3. Describe the effects of drugs on driving.
4. Describe some signs that indicate that a person might have a drug problem.
5. State ways a person can help someone give up drugs.

■≡ Notes

1. R. O'Brien and S. Cohen, *The Encyclopedia of Drug Abuse* (New York: Facts on File, 1984), p. 1.
2. C. L. Thomas, ed., *Taber's Cyclopedic Medical Dictionary,* 14th ed. (Philadelphia: Davis, 1981), p. 431.
3. G. M. Smith, Adolescent personality traits that predict young adult drug use, *Comprehensive Therapy* 12 (1986): 44–50.

4. W. R. Yates, A. I. Fulton, J. M. Gabel, and C. T. Brass, Personality risk factors for cocaine abuse, *American Journal of Public Health,* July 1989, pp. 891–892.
5. A. R. Tarlov and R. W. Rimel, Drug abuse prevention—The sponsoring foundations' perspective, *Journal of School Health* 56 (1986): 358.

6. F. Bruno, *Combatting Drug Abuse and Related Crime: Comparative Research on the Effectiveness of Socio-legal Preventive and Control Measures in Different Countries on the Interaction between Criminal Behavior and Drug Abuse* (Rome: Fratelli Palombi Editori, 1984), p. 160.
7. Among many studies that show cocaine to be an effective reinforcer:

T. G. Aigner and R. L. Balster, Choice behavior in rhesus monkeys: Cocaine vs. food, *Science* 201 (1978): 534–535.

8. C. A. Dachis and M. S. Gold, Pharmacological approaches to cocaine addiction, *Journal of Substance Abuse Treatment* 2 (1985): 139–145.

9. J. Henningfield, Addiction Research Center, National Institute of Drug Abuse, as cited in D. D. Edwards, Nicotine: A drug of choice? *Science News,* 18 January 1986, pp. 44–45.

10. Thomas, 1981, p. 431.

11. M. E. Mohs, R. R. Watson, and T. Leonard-Green, Nutritional effects of marijuana, heroin, cocaine, and nicotine, *Journal of the American Dietetic Association* 90 (1990): 1261–1267.

12. L. J. Kolbe, Preventing drug abuse in the United States: Integrating the efforts of schools, communities, and science, *Journal of School Health* 56 (1986): 357.

13. R. W. Foltin, J. V. Brady, and M. W. Fischman, Behavioral analysis of marijuana effects on food intake in humans, *Pharmacology, Biochemistry and Behavior* 25 (1986): 577–582.

14. D. Sperling, Pot: More punch than in the '60s, *USA Today,* March 1986, p. 1a.

15. E. Hollister, Health effects of cannabis, *Pharmacological Reviews* 38, March 1986, pp. 1–20.

16. T. Wu, D. P. Tashkin, B. Djahed, and J. E. Rose, Pulmonary hazards of smoking marijuana as compared with tobacco, *New England Journal of Medicine* 318 (1988): 347–351.

17. M. E. Mohs, R. R. Watson, and T. Leonard-Green, Nutritional effects of marijuana, heroin, cocaine, and nicotine, *Journal of the American Dietetic Association* 90 (1990): 1261–1267.

18. From a self-administered questionnaire in a study of cocaine users in M. S. Gold, *800-Cocaine* (New York: Bantam, 1984), pp. 10–11. The book title is actually a national cocaine hotline number, 1–800-COCAINE.

19. F. G. Castro, M. D. Newcomb, and K. Cadish, Lifestyle differences between young adult cocaine users and their nonuser peers, *Journal of Drug Education* 17 (1987): 89–111.

20. J. M Isner and S. K. Chokshi, Cocaine and vasospasm, *New England Journal of Medicine,* 7 December 1989, pp. 1604–1606.

21. D. M. Barnes, Drugs: Running the numbers, *Science* 240 (1988): 1729–1731.

22. Gold, 1984.

23. *The Case of the Frozen Addict,* a transcript of a "Nova" program, 18 February 1986, available from WGBH Transcripts, 125 Western Ave., Boston, MA 02134.

24. A. Smiley and coauthors, Effects of drugs on driving: Driving simulator tests of secobarbital, diazepam, marijuana, and alcohol, *Clinical and Behavior Pharmacology Research Report,* DHHS publication no. (ADM) 85–1386, 1985.

25. G. T. Johnson, Marijuana: What are the risks? *Harvard Medical School Health Letter,* June 1980, pp. 1–3; D. Pine, Hungover driving, *Health,* May 1984, p. 12.

26. The list of symptoms of drug abuse comes from a letter to Ann Landers, *Tallahassee Democrat,* 14 January 1986.

SPOTLIGHT

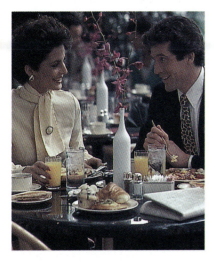

Social Health

Every definition of health mentions several dimensions of a person: physical, mental, emotional, interpersonal, social, and spiritual. And in talking about optimal health, or high-level wellness, such definitions describe a life of high quality—a life that has a purposeful direction, in which each dimension is healthy, and in which all of the dimensions work together in a balanced way.[1]* Emotional health was described in Chapter 2. Physical fitness was described in Chapter 7. This Spotlight presents social health, an important dimension of wellness. The lack of social health is related to the causation of illness.[2]

What is social health?

Social health is a state of well-being that results from a person's skill in

*Reference notes are at the end of the Spotlight.

interacting with other people and with society as a whole.[3] A person has the best chance of being socially healthy if the person knows how best to get along with other people and to function effectively in social groups. It also helps if the person has a social conscience—if the person believes, for example, that "peace on earth begins with me," or if, on perceiving that a social problem exists, the person tries "to be part of the solution, rather than part of the problem." Progress toward a person's highest potential as a contributing member of a society or culture is progress toward high-level social health.

Is social health the same as mental and emotional health?

Social health and mental and emotional health are related. People with mental health have the ability to learn and to reason. People with high-level emotional health are energetic, enthusiastic, and optimistic about life. They are relaxed, confident, and comfortable with their natural tendencies to be extroverted or introverted. They welcome new experiences and are curious about people. They refrain from stereotyping new people they meet. They accept their negative as well as positive traits.

A high level of social health is built on a foundation of sound mental and emotional health. One must accept and like oneself and value one's own emotional integrity if one is to accept, like, and get along with others. The process of maturing socially includes developing unselfishness, generosity, and a feeling of belonging in society.

When one's emotional health is impaired, one's social health is impaired. Impaired social health leads to social problems such as divorce,

abuse of alcohol and other drugs, crime, delinquency, even accidents.[4] People suffering from emotional problems lack high-level social health and may miss out on many things that make life worth living: love, happiness, creativity, accomplishments, and contributions.

Is social health mostly concerned with relationships?

Yes, one part of social health is the ability to have healthy relationships with family, friends, peers, and others such as teachers. This ability prepares people to develop much-needed support systems as they move away from their families and childhood friends and into new cities and communities.

Another part of social health is concerned with the ability to find one's place in society as a whole. Contributing to the well-being of society is a way to gain a sense of ownership of society's characteristics. If the society is attempting to become more democratic, for example, the member who shares that value tries to contribute toward the effort. If the society is persecuting some of its own members, the person who values equality for all takes responsibility for assisting society to change in the desired direction. A person who has a sense of ownership also tends to have a sense of responsibility—a feeling of *having* to contribute.

How do people gain a sense of ownership of society?

Some ways to develop a sense of ownership include:

1. Volunteering time in organizations that could not stay in business if they had to pay staff people for the services.

2. Giving volunteer time to further aesthetic, cultural, or political causes that are valuable to the larger community or to future generations, such as efforts to minimize the waste of natural resources or to reduce environmental pollution.

3. Supporting with time and money the institutions and organizations that are meaningful to you and that you hope will be preserved for posterity.

These opportunities also allow people to meet others who share in their values, to develop friendships that will really last, and to develop support systems that will hold up in times of need. Participating in these kinds of activities provides evidence not only of citizenship (being responsible—a social strength) but also of altruism (selfless giving—a spiritual strength). It has been said that the service we render is the rent we pay for the space we occupy on the earth.

How do you describe people with high-level social health?

People with high-level social wellness give more to their society or community than they take from it.[5] They have an internal locus of control and take precautions against becoming a burden on society. They are able to adapt to changes in support systems as their life courses change.[6]

A person with strong social health responds and reacts appropriately in social situations. Can you identify these characteristics in yourself? Do you:

■ Meet people easily?
■ Accept differences in other people?

■ Make friends easily with people of both genders?
■ Participate in social and recreational groups?
■ Communicate your own ideas and wishes successfully to other members of groups?
■ Listen well and hear clearly their ideas and wishes?
■ Accept other people's suggestions when working in a group?
■ Continue to take part in group activities even when your own suggestions are not accepted by the group?
■ Have the ability to deal with different people?

According to scientists who study social relationships (sociologists), effective communication may be the single most important element of effective social functioning.

How do sociologists describe effective social functioning?

Sociologists have found that its basic features are communication, cooperation, and compromise.

Communication is a two-way street. Individuals who communicate well have the ability to listen—really listen—as well as the ability to take their turns speaking.

Cooperation is working together for the good of all. This is known as teamwork. Working as a team builds strong relationships. To be a good team player, you need to have an open mind and a willingness to carry a part of the load.

Compromise is the result of each person's giving up something in order to reach a solution that can be accepted by all. This is known as "give and take." This does not mean letting people take advantage of you,

or giving up strong moral beliefs, or giving in to others when the results are harmful. It means expressing your view and hearing another view, and then reaching a final decision that is somewhere in between.

Chapter 2 has already discussed interpersonal communication skills such as the ability to be assertive, rather than aggressive or submissive, in expressing feelings. Interpersonal skills are key to functioning well, whether in a social club, on a volunteer committee, or in a task force at the workplace. People who understand group dynamics and the various roles played by members of a group are best prepared to work in a group toward any goal, whether in planning a charity ball or completing a group class assignment. Communication, cooperation, and compromise are present in all effective group dynamics.

What are group dynamics?

Group dynamics are the interactions that take place during group deliberations. The communication, cooperation, and compromise taking place during group processes define the dynamics of the group. Leaders, managers, administrators, and every member of a group need to understand the group's dynamics in order to make the group work effectively together. Power, prestige, and skills in influencing others are also factors that affect group dynamics. Some people do not distinguish between their social group skills and their roles in teams or professional group settings. Workplace management and public relations are important areas of study. Getting along in work settings is as important as, if not more important than, the technical skills needed to do a job. Getting along in settings other than the workplace demands a sense of good manners and etiquette.

Who decides what manners and etiquette are appropriate in a given setting?

This is decided by the culture, the values, and the standards of the social groups in that setting. Most people begin learning manners and etiquette within the social life of their own families, at family and community gatherings. In new social settings, however, a person may be unsure of what social behaviors are expected.

In some social situations, people want very much to do what is considered correct. When you are dating somebody who is important to you, for example, you may want to know what the person's family considers to be good manners, so that you don't accidentally offend them. When you are seeking entry into a new group, you may need to adopt its customs so as not to appear rude.

Some behaviors are almost universally expected and appreciated, no matter what the social group. Most societies expect their members to consistently say "Please," "Thank you," and "Excuse me," or the equivalent; to hold doors open for others; to refrain from blocking people's views of events or passage along aisles; to be on time for appointments; to refrain from disrupting conversations, movies, or religious services; to write letters saying thank you after receiving gifts or visiting people's homes; and in general to behave in ways that help others feel comfortable.

Some aspects of another group's etiquette may seem unnecessary or even silly at times, but etiquette provides a framework within which everyone knows how to operate and what to expect from each other. Long conversations about the weather may seem trivial, for example, and yet a keen observer may discover that beneath the apparent superficiality, an important process is going on. Two people who seem to be discussing whether it will rain today are actually, subtly, expressing a willingness to listen to each other, to find common interests, and to express understanding of each other's concerns and hopes. A newcomer to the society who appreciates the function of such conversations will not scoff at them but will learn the rules and sensitively join in.

How can a person find out what a society considers to be good manners or etiquette?

Guidelines provided by the writings of Miss Manners or Letitia Baldridge can help people learn etiquette, build confidence, and avoid embarrassing social blunders. These sources provide rules that people may not learn in their own families, rules that may be unimportant in one setting but indispensable to acceptance in another.

What if your family behaves one way and another group you belong to behaves another way? My date expects me to exhibit manners that differ from my family's manners.

It is possible to function well in different social groups, by the rule "When in Rome, do as the Romans do." To adopt a group's customs while in that group does not make you a hypocrite; it reflects your desire to get along well within the group. Just as speaking the language of a country you are visiting is a sign of respect for the culture, so is adopting the manners of the group while you are part of it. This is not hypocritical; you are not abandoning a value but expressing a value—honoring people's customs that are different from your own.

A custom that differs among different groups is that of responding to invitations. Sometimes an RSVP is requested. RSVP is French for "Répondez s'il vous plaît," meaning "The favor of a reply is requested." In some social circles, a written reply is considered the most correct response to a written invitation. Much of today's society, however, may consider a telephone response acceptable. In any case, to ignore an RSVP may lead to being branded rude, and to being excluded from future gatherings. Table manners, too, can be important in the same way.

Learning social skills can permit entry into areas where a person can fulfill cherished aspirations and make valued contributions. Failing to learn the manners and etiquette of a given society often leads to exclusion from that society and loss of the opportunity to realize these hopes. It might seem, on first consideration, as if social skills were useful only to please others, but on further thought it becomes obvious that they are indispensable to a person's own high-level wellness.

■≡ Spotlight Notes

1. H. L. Dunn, *High-level wellness* (Arlington, VA: Beatty 1961), pp. 4–5.

2. J. S. House, K. R. Landis, and D. Umberson, Social relationships and health, *Science* 241 (1988): 540–544.

3. M. Minkler, The social component of health, *American Journal of Health Promotion* 1, No. 2 (Fall, 1986): 33–38.

4. M. B. Merki, *Teen Health* (Mission Hills, Calif.: Glencoe, 1990), pp. 96–99.

5. W. M. Kane, Sr. Consultant, and co-consultants, *Understanding Health* (New York: Random House, 1987), pp. 5–6.

6. S. Cohen and S. Syme, *Social Support and Health* (New York: Academic Press, 1985), p. 15.

CHAPTER 10

Alcohol: Use and Abuse

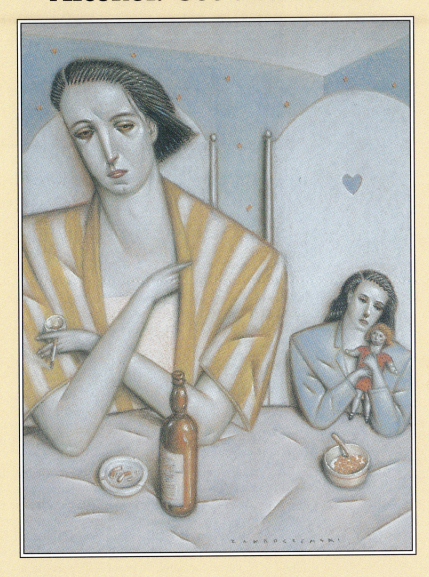

Just for fun, respond true or false to the following statements. If false, say what is true.

■ Alcohol kills brain cells. (Page 248)
■ Drinking alcohol can help a shy, inhibited person learn to be outgoing, carefree, and bold. (Page 252)
■ People who drink only beer or wine cannot become problem drinkers. (Page 254)

■ People who drink only on social occasions are not problem drinkers. (Page 254)
■ Alcohol is a stimulant. (Page 255)
■ Alcohol enhances sexual relations. (Page 257)
■ A person can die from drinking too much alcohol at one sitting. (Page 258)

What are you doing this Friday night? Going drinking? The typical college student is said to reserve weekends for drinking alcohol— usually to excess. Some claim that excessive drinking on weekends is part of the college social experience.

Is drinking harmful to health? What are the risks of alcohol consumption? What is responsible drinking? This chapter explores these questions and others by presenting the facts about alcohol. Whether or not you drink, or drink to excess, it makes sense to learn about alcohol, for everyone has many choices to make in relation to it. And alcohol profoundly affects many people you know, whether you realize that or not.

■≡ Alcohol

The **alcohols** are a class of chemical compounds. The term *alcohol*, as commonly used, refers to the active ingredient of alcoholic beverages—**ethanol**, or **ethyl alcohol**.

Ethanol arises naturally from carbohydrates when certain microorganisms break them down in the absence of oxygen—a process called **fermentation**. Since all plants contain carbohydrates, all can serve as the starting material for fermentation. Different societies use many different plants to produce alcoholic beverages; the most familiar are grapes and grains.

The percentage of alcohol in distilled liquor is stated as *proof:* 100-proof liquor is 50 percent alcohol; 90 proof is 45 percent, and so forth. A **drink** is a dose of any alcoholic beverage that delivers 1/2 ounce of pure ethanol:

3 to 4 oz wine.

10 oz standard wine cooler.

12 oz standard beer.

1 oz hard liquor (whiskey, gin, rum, vodka).

Alcohols affect living things profoundly, partly because they act as fat solvents. They can dissolve the fats out of cell membranes, thereby killing the cells. Most alcohols are toxic, or poisonous; ethanol is one of these. Taken in large enough doses, it kills brain cells. On the average, adults who

alcohols a class of chemical compounds. Ethanol, or ethyl alcohol (commonly called *alcohol*) is one member of the class of chemical compounds known as alcohols, the alcohol of alcoholic beverages.

fermentation the breakdown of carbohydrate in the absence of oxygen, a process that yields ethanol.

drink a dose of any alcoholic beverage that delivers ½ oz pure ethanol.

■ *FACT OR FICTION:* Alcohol kills brain cells. *True.*

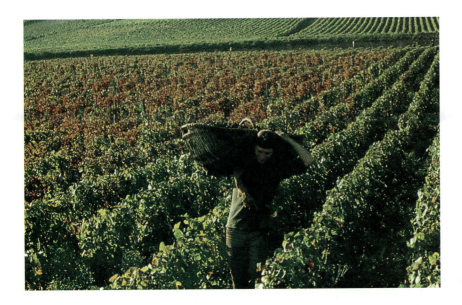

Grapes provide most of the world's wine.

drink alcohol lose about 100,000 brain cells before reaching age 35.[1]* However, sufficiently diluted and taken in small enough doses, alcohol produces **euphoria** not without risk, but with a risk some people consider acceptable, possibly because they are not well informed.

Alcohol is a drug—that is, a substance that can modify one or more of the body's functions. Ethanol happens to be the only nonprescription euphoria-producing drug that is legal in our society. It also happens to be a classically abusable drug. Like the other euphoria-producers, alcohol can be addicting. The cycle of addiction, both physiological and psychological, entraps about one out of every ten users of alcohol and not only ruins their lives but also disrupts the lives of all who surround them in the family and on the job.

According to the U.S. surgeon general, alcohol use is increasing among teenagers. More than half of the students in the nation's junior and senior high schools are alcohol drinkers. Of those who drink, 8 million consume alcohol weekly, 5.4 million have binged on occasion, and nearly half a million go on weekly binges, guzzling five or more drinks in a row. This is a staggering problem, killing many teens in car accidents and starting addiction in many more.[2]

> ≡▶ *Alcohol, the product of fermentation of plant carbohydrate, is toxic in excess, but small doses present a risk that some people consider acceptable. It is the only legal nonprescription euphoria-producing drug and like other such drugs, it can cause addictions.*

■≡ Why People Drink

Drinkers give many reasons for drinking alcohol: to celebrate, to unwind, to get high, or because they like the taste of alcoholic beverages. Many people drink because peer pressure demands it, and young people may drink

euphoria a sense of well-being and pleasure, a high (also defined in Chapter 9).

A drug is a substance that produces physical, mental, emotional, or behavioral changes in the user.

*Reference notes are at the end of the chapter.

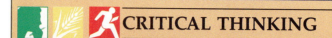 **CRITICAL THINKING**

Deceptive Appeals

Billboards, magazine ads, and other advertisements; TV dramas and movies project an image of the alcohol drinker in a variety of appealing ways to encourage excessive alcohol consumption and increase alcohol sales. All of these appeals have two things in common. First, they suggest that consuming alcohol can help people achieve the qualities they most desire. (In reality, consuming alcohol hinders obtaining these desired traits.) Second, they conceal facts that would steer people away from their products. (In reality, alcohol consumption can be dangerous and sometimes deadly.)

SOPHISTICATION APPEAL. Some forms of alcohol promotion show drinkers as members of select cliques—this appeals to people who yearn for high-society class and respect. Social sophistication seems to radiate from the expensive attire of actors or models who are shown drinking cocktails in plush surroundings. Captivating slogans reinforce the glamorous images shown. Special brands of wine, beer, and liquor are advertised as expensive, so using them shows affluence. Ads for liquor are not allowed on television, but the liquor industry still pressures the makers of television dramas to show drinkers, and to display them as smiling, healthy, beautiful, strong, and young.

SOCIAL AND SEX APPEAL. Similarly, to draw the high-school and college-aged groups' dollars, the industry promotes the image of the alcohol drinker as a "happy-go-lucky party animal." The alcohol drinker is shown as carefree, outgoing, with no worries or concerns. This drinker is popular with members of the other sex, and sexual activity is freely available to this imaginary person. One advertisement strategy is to supply posters to gas stations and college drinking places, to be given away to students. These posters show sexy young women in bathing suits, definitely a feast for the eyes. Students are likely to take free posters home and use them to decorate their dorm room walls. They are happy to have pictures of sexy women and usually totally unaware of the unconscious message being embedded in their brains daily: drinking alcohol will enhance your social life and provide a means of obtaining sex. The alcohol industry pays top dollar to its sharpest marketing executives to deliver this subtle but strong message in just the right form to rack in sales.

Many alcohol advertisements directly tie sexual availability to alcohol use. An example: the message "This will get you what you want" is

because they think drinking shows their maturity. Still younger people use it as a way of rebelling against authority. In many societies, people yield to social pressure that heavily favors drinking; in the United States, private industry encourages people to drink. Some people use drinking as a way of escaping life's pressures.

displayed on a billboard that shows a sexually available, seductive woman and a beer can.

A person dazzled by the sexual excitement of these cunning advertisements never guesses that they are blatantly deceptive. The reality of excessive alcohol consumption involves a dark side indeed: it leads some people to addiction, and that in turn leads to tragic life-destroying consequences. Also, the casual sexual activity that often occurs under the influence of alcohol directly leads to people's contracting incurable, life-threatening, and life-changing sexually transmitted diseases.

The peddlers of all drugs push them this way. They tell lies.

SPORTS APPEAL. Drinking alcohol is also promoted as a way to become manly, rugged, even athletic. This appeals to men who long for these qualities. For instance, beer consumption is associated with certain sports, partly through famous athletes' appearance in beer advertisements. These ads show off attractive images of the athletes, who want their fans to see them in a glowing light, and the ads seduce the fans into identifying their sports idols with alcohol use. The tragic result: the advertisements entice both athletes and fans into alcohol abuse. Alcoholism sometimes destroys athletes early in their careers. "Some guys don't learn how to handle it," says Clete Boyer, the former coach of baseball's Oakland A's. Numerous famous baseball players have developed alcoholism. Says one, who now runs an alcoholism clinic, "We just didn't understand and winked at each other as we drank each other to death."[3]

These and other appeals, which make alcohol drinking attractive or acceptable, have found their way into almost every area of life. Greeting cards and comedy routines portray drinking and even getting drunk as funny, and the "in" thing to do. A comedy movie shows a drunken, laughing man driving around town, arriving at his destination with ease. The movie does not show what happens in reality when people drive drunk: they can kill themselves and others as well.

Looked at with a rational eye, alcohol use hinders attainment of all the qualities used to promote it. A person striving for sophistication and for rewarding social and sexual interactions needs not to lose control, but to gain it by practicing social skills. A person seeking sports success will not find it by drinking beer on the couch, but by faithfully practicing the sport. The ads, though, deceive people by lying: they suggest that people can obtain the desired qualities in an easy way—by drinking alcohol.

All such advertisements strengthen the emotional impulse to consume alcohol. With alcohol, as with any other product, learning to recognize these appeals for what they are can help consumers distinguish fake from fact and decide whether they really want what is offered.

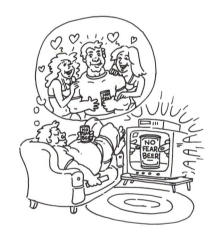

Advertisers tie alcohol to people's cherished fantasies, but the alcohol itself produces unwanted realities.

A common reason college students give for drinking alcohol is to overcome shyness. Many people long to have the courage to meet new friends, particularly members of the other sex, but have not developed the social skills or confidence to do so with ease. They claim drinking alcohol makes them feel more confident, and they are able to be outgoing, carefree, and

■ *FACT OR FICTION:* Drinking alcohol can help a shy, inhibited person learn to be outgoing, carefree, and bold. *False*. Drinking alcohol is more likely to make a person giggly, foolish, and careless and often delays the learning of social skills.

congeners (CON-jen-ers)   ingredients in alcoholic beverages, other than the alcohol itself, that confer flavor and other properties and that may have irritating effects on the nervous system either alone or in combination.

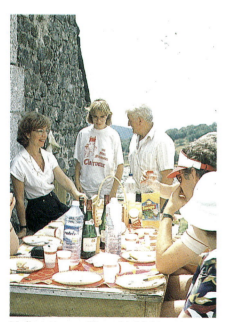

Moderate, responsible social drinking can enhance life's enjoyments.

bold under its influence. They do add, however, that some problems often result: they usually consume too much, so instead of making a positive first impression, they become intoxicated, embarrass themselves, and suffer bruised egos the next day. People who use "liquid courage" to help with socialization when young discover later that they still have not learned the skills necessary for successful social interaction. If drinkers discover later that they regret having gotten involved with alcohol, they are not alone. Our whole society seems geared to promoting alcohol use and abuse (see Critical Thinking: Deceptive Appeals).

Some people drink because alcohol is an anesthetic and thus eases pain. It does this by affecting the system that produces endorphins, and as described in the last chapter, it causes the body to make less of its own natural painkillers. Physiologically, it works better to involve yourself in activities that cause your body to soothe pain naturally.

Like all drugs, alcohol offers both benefits and hazards. In moderation, it can affect the appetite. Sometimes alcohol reduces appetite, making people unaware that they are hungry, but in people who are tense and unable to eat, a glass of wine taken 20 minutes before meals improves the appetite. Certain acid compounds in the wine, known as **congeners**, are credited with this effect. Thus wine may benefit undernourished people and people with severely depressed appetites, by facilitating eating. Because the congeners are at least partially responsible, even dealcoholized wine may enhance appetite.

Some evidence indicates that both men and women who use alcohol moderately over a lifetime have a lower risk of heart attack and a longer life than either nondrinkers or people who drink to excess.[4] This is probably not because of any direct physical effect of alcohol, but because of the life full of friendships and social stimulation that such people often enjoy. A person who relaxes with friends at intervals may suffer less tension at work and less social isolation, and thereby sustain fewer of the life-shortening effects of stress. Of course, one can learn to live such a life without alcohol, but in a drinking society, the two may often be found together.

It has been thought, incorrectly, that part of the reason moderate drinkers have a lower risk of heart attack than nondrinkers involved blood lipids. Moderate alcohol use raises the blood concentration of HDL (high-density lipoproteins), the indicator of a low risk of heart attack (see Chapter 18).[5] However, two classes of HDL exist—one class associated with lowered heart disease risk and a different class associated with moderate drinking. Alcohol does raise one type of HDL, but it is not the type that reduces heart disease risk.[6] Some researchers claim that the concept that moderate alcohol consumption is protective against heart disease ignores the abundant evidence showing a relationship between alcohol consumption and poor health, discussed at greater length later in this chapter.[7]

Alcohol, *when taken in moderation and used responsibly,* can be socially, psychologically, and physiologically beneficial.[8] For those who choose to drink, the goal is learning to drink responsibly, in moderation.

≡▶ *People drink for various reasons, many of which have to do with social pressure and deceptive appeals by advertisers. Alcohol offers some benefits when taken in moderation, but causes many problems when taken to excess.*

⬛≡ Moderate, Social, and Problem Drinking

Just what is **moderation** in the use of alcohol? No one exact amount of alcohol per day would be appropriate for everyone, because people differ in their tolerance levels. Authorities have, however, attempted to set a limit that is appropriate for most healthy people. They suggest not more than three drinks a day for the average-sized, healthy man or two drinks a day for the average-sized, healthy woman.[9] (See page 248 for the definition of "a drink.") This amount is supposed to be enough to produce euphoria without incurring any long-term harm to health. Doubtless some people could definitely not handle nearly so much without significant risk; others could perhaps consume slightly more. Wherever the line is drawn, on the other side of it is **alcohol abuse**.

Everyone could quarrel with this definition of moderate drinking. People who oppose the use of any alcohol at all argue that there is nothing moderate whatever in taking three drinks a day for a lifetime, and medical evidence indicates that, indeed, harm to health can result from this level of intake. Habitual heavy drinkers could argue that three beers between, say, noon and midnight is *light* drinking, and that six beers might more appropriately be called moderate. We do not have space to present all the differences of opinion but think it important to convey two things. First, a wide range of drinking styles falls between total abstinence and alcoholism. Second, the danger increases as the amount of alcohol consumed increases. Each person must monitor and evaluate his or her own drinking behavior.

Many factors determine how much alcohol a person can tolerate without harm to health. One is gender: women, who on the average have smaller livers than men, can process alcohol less rapidly, and so are more affected by a given dose of alcohol than men of the same age and weight.[10] Genetics and health are other influential factors. Terms that describe people who drink are used in this book as follows; their complete definitions are in the margin.

A **moderate drinker** is someone who does not drink too much. Behaviors typical of moderate drinkers include: They drink slowly (no fast gulping). They know when to stop drinking; they don't drink to get drunk. They eat before or while drinking. They do not drive after drinking. They know and obey laws related to drinking. They respect nondrinkers. They do not consider alcohol consumption proof of adulthood or virility. Their activities do not focus on alcohol consumption. They do not view intoxication as stylish, comic, tolerable, or socially acceptable.[11]

A **social drinker** is someone who may or may not drink too much. Some are moderate drinkers, some are problem drinkers.

A **problem drinker** or **alcohol abuser** is someone who drinks too much and who, as a direct result, has problems functioning. Behaviors typical of problem drinkers are: They drink to get drunk. They try to solve problems by drinking. They drink to seek relief from stress. They experience personality changes; they may become loud, angry, and violent or silent, remote, and reclusive. They drink when it is unsafe or unwise to do so (before driving or going to class or work). They cause other problems, such as physically or emotionally harming themselves, family, friends, and strangers.[12] They pressure others to drink. They gulp or "chug" their drinks, or

moderation with respect to alcohol use, consumption of an amount of alcohol sufficient to produce euphoria without causing harm to health. A possible guideline: not more than three drinks a day for the average-sized, healthy man and not more than two drinks for the average-sized, healthy woman.

alcohol abuse drinking to excess, or to an extent that produces long-term harm to health.

alcoholism the extreme of alcohol abuse, a disease. See page 254 for complete definition.

moderate drinker a person who does not drink excessively; that is, one who behaves appropriately on drinking occasions, and whose health is not adversely affected by alcohol over the long term.

social drinker a person who drinks only on social occasions. Depending on the amounts of alcohol such a person consumes, the person may be a moderate or problem drinker.

problem drinker a person whose drinking is beginning to cause social, emotional, family, job-related, or other problems; a person on the way to alcoholism. Other terms for this kind of drinker: **alcohol abuser**, **pre-alcoholic drinker**.

alcohol addict a person with alcoholism.

alcoholism the disease of addiction to alcohol. It is chronic, progressive, and potentially fatal, characterized by tolerance, physical addiction, and organ damage caused directly or indirectly by alcohol consumption.

■ *FACT OR FICTION:* People who drink only beer or wine cannot become problem drinkers. *False.* People who only drink beer or wine may be problem drinkers, depending on how much they drink, their reasons for drinking, their behavior while drinking, and the consequences of the drinking behavior.

■ *FACT OR FICTION:* People who drink only on social occasions are not problem drinkers. *False.* Social drinkers may be problem drinkers, depending on the amount they drink, their reasons for drinking, their behavior while drinking, and the consequences of the drinking behavior.

drink two or more drinks per hour. They use alcohol while taking prescription or OTC medication.

An **alcohol addict** is a person with the full-blown disease of **alcoholism.** This person's problems, caused by alcohol abuse, are out of control. The old term for this kind of drinker is an *alcoholic.*

The old term *alcoholic* is a poor choice of words, because it implies that the person *is* the problem, a destructive, judgmental, and unhelpful attitude. *Person addicted to alcohol* or *person dependent on alcohol* are preferable terms, because they imply that the person *has* the problem and can recover from it.

How *much* people drink is not the only factor that defines problem drinking. Other factors include their *reasons* for drinking, their *behavior* while drinking, and the *consequences* of their drinking. Also, the type of alcoholic beverage consumed is irrelevant: people who drink only beer or wine can be problem drinkers. And contrary to popular opinion, a person who only drinks socially can be a problem drinker.

Problem drinking among college students leads to consequences such as inability to keep up with schoolwork, followed by falling grades, class absences and failures, and dropping out of school. In families, it disrupts relationships, contributing to the many emotional problems described in Chapter 3.

One way of looking at a drinking problem is to try to classify it in one of three ways: social, psychological, or physical. This chapter's Life Choice Inventory helps to make the distinction.

▶ *Moderate drinking produces no long-term harm to health. Beyond it lies problem drinking, and beyond that, alcohol-addicted drinking (alcoholism).*

■≡ Effects of Alcohol on Body and Behavior

The drug alcohol has both short- and long-term effects, and they differ depending on whether the dose is moderate or excessive. To use alcohol without harm, the drinker needs to know just how it acts on the body.

Moderate Drinking: Immediate Effects

The little ethanol molecule acts in many ways in the body. It is extremely small, as molecules go. It can move fast, and it can mix with both fatty and watery substances. This means that it meets with no barriers in the body; it can go anywhere.

From the moment a person swallows it, alcohol is active in a multitude of ways. From the stomach and intestines it moves rapidly into the bloodstream, and from the blood it enters every cell. Within minutes after the first sip of a drink, alcohol is acting in the brain, muscles, nerves, glands, and the small blood vessels of the skin. It also passes through a vast bed of capillaries in the liver, the only organ equipped with enzymes to convert alcohol to harmless waste substances the body can excrete. The liver goes to work on it right away but can handle only about one drink (one ounce of 100–

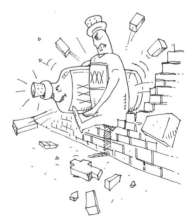

Alcohol meets with no barriers in the body; it can go anywhere.

LIFE CHOICE INVENTORY

What is your drinking style? Some people drink primarily for social reasons. They may or may not drink to excess. Some drink for psychological reasons—for the mood change alcohol induces; they may be, or may become, psychologically dependent on alcohol. Some drink because they are physically addicted.

Answer each of the questions below. For each statement, circle the number that describes how often you drink that way: 4—always; 3—frequently; 2—occasionally; 1—seldom; 0—never.

1. I drink to be socially accepted.   4 3 2 1 0
2. I drink to be more myself.   4 3 2 1 0
3. I feel more comfortable at a party
   when drinking.   4 3 2 1 0
4. I down (gulp) my alcohol
   beverage.   4 3 2 1 0
5. I have had memory losses (blackouts)
   during or after drinking.   4 3 2 1 0
6. I drink when depressed, frustrated,
   or angry.   4 3 2 1 0
7. I accept a drink when pressured
   by friends.   4 3 2 1 0
8. I have gotten into fights or
   arguments when drinking.   4 3 2 1 0
9. I feel superior when
   drinking.   4 3 2 1 0
10. I drink when I am bored.   4 3 2 1 0
11. I feel more popular when
    relaxed with alcohol.   4 3 2 1 0
12. I like to drink alone.   4 3 2 1 0

Scoring: Be sure you have answered all 12 questions. Add up your scores for questions 1, 3, 7, and 11. These questions refer to the *Social Dependence Index;* the higher your score, the more likely you are to depend on alcohol for social reasons.

Now add up your scores for questions 2, 6, 9, and 10. These questions refer to the *Psychological Dependence Index*. The higher your score, the more likely you are to depend on alcohol for psychological reasons.

Questions 4, 5, 8, and 12 refer to the *Physical Dependence Index*. Higher scores for these questions indicate a physical dependence on alcohol.

SOURCE: Adapted from an inventory contributed by Professor Martin Turnaver, Radford University, Radford, Virginia. Original source unknown.

proof liquor) an hour. If a person drinks faster than this, the excess keeps recirculating, affecting all the cells, until the liver can oxidize it.

The effects of which the drinker is most conscious, naturally, are those that result from alcohol's action on the nervous system. Alcohol acts first on some of the brain's fine-tuning inhibitory nerves—those that normally set limits on behavior. It puts those nerves to sleep, thus releasing other nerves from the anesthetized nerves' controlling influence. Thus a person slightly under the influence of alcohol will talk or laugh more loudly and gesture more vigorously after these controls are released. The loud buzz of animated conversation that you start to hear half an hour into a cocktail party reflects this effect.

The inhibition-releasing effect of one drink has given people the impression that alcohol is a stimulant. It is not; it is a depressant. The ethanol molecule never stimulates any process within the body. In fact, it acts like an anesthetic such as ether or chloroform.

Soon after a few sips of alcohol, the drinker can feel it seeming to warm the skin. Nerves normally keep skin capillaries constricted to prevent heat

■ *FACT OR FICTION:* Alcohol is a stimulant. *False.* Alcohol is a depressant drug; it slows people down. Its inhibition-releasing effect is due to its anesthetizing the brain.

loss by radiation, but alcohol relaxes these controls. (For this reason, it is *not* a good idea to drink alcohol when you are dangerously cold. It may make you feel warmer, because the skin's temperature receptors feel warm blood flowing past them and send messages saying "warm" to the brain; but in reality, your body is losing heat from its core to the surroundings.)

Alcohol also disturbs sleep, even after just one drink. It takes two nights with no alcohol in the body to restore the ability to sleep normally. Alcohol also causes abnormal respiratory events in some people during sleep: they stop breathing for dangerously long periods, then gasp for breath.[13]

Another effect, after even one drink, is reduced ability to perform mental tasks. To think clearly requires concentration, and that means you have to focus on one task and screen out distractions. Certain nerves screen out extraneous stimuli, but these nerves are put to sleep by alcohol, leaving you undefended against distraction and unable to concentrate.

Another early effect of alcohol in the brain is sedation of the cerebral cortex (see Figure 10–1), where conscious thinking takes place. The drinker loses certain kinds of consciousness, including consciousness of unpleasant recent events, worries, insecurity, discomfort, and pain. Simultaneously, the brain's speech and vision centers are being narcotized.

People sometimes wonder why they urinate more when drinking alcohol. Alcohol inhibits the brain's pituitary gland, which ordinarily secretes a hormone (the antidiuretic hormone) that prevents excessive water loss via urination. Without the action of this hormone, one loses more water than

FIGURE 10–1 ■ **Alcohol's effects on the brain.**

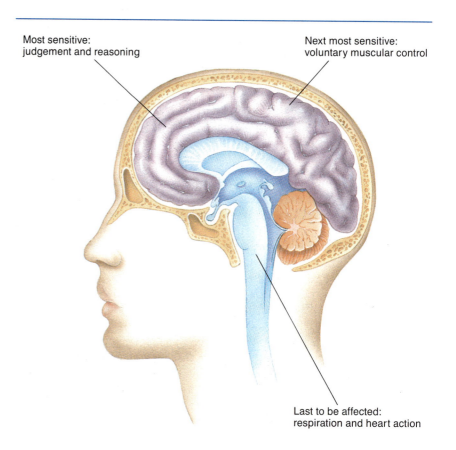

Most sensitive:
judgement and reasoning

Next most sensitive:
voluntary muscular control

Last to be affected:
respiration and heart action

usual. The body excretes only a little alcohol in the urine, but the person becomes dehydrated and thirsty. A thirsty person may respond by drinking another alcoholic beverage, receiving too much alcohol and too little water.

As the blood alcohol content rises, it affects deeper brain centers—among them, the center that controls emotions. The brain stops inhibiting the awareness and expression of emotions. Thus the person expresses love, joy, sorrow, anger, lust, and hatred more easily than before.

Responsible social use of alcohol involves achieving and maintaining a blood level high enough to enjoy the mood-heightening effects but low enough to prevent loss of control. The way to do this is to consume exactly as much alcohol per unit of time as the body can destroy in that time (about one drink an hour), so that a plateau is maintained.

≡▶ *Alcohol affects the whole body. In the brain it releases inhibition by sedating the inhibitory nerves. Moderate doses disturb sleep, impair concentration, and stimulate urination. Slightly higher doses release normally suppressed emotions.*

Excessive Drinking: Immediate Effects

With increasing doses, behavior becomes unpredictable. People may act on their impulses against their own better judgment, because their consciousness of that judgment is now gone. Against all reason, people may get in fights, or attempt dangerous physical exploits—with painful or even tragic consequences. They may even have unprotected sexual intercourse, risking pregnancy or sexually transmitted diseases. Or one may force another into sexual activity: date rape is almost invariably preceded by excessive alcohol consumption by one or both of the people involved. The reason people take such risks when intoxicated is clear from the map of the brain in Figure 10–1: judgment would prevent the behavior, but the judgment center has been put to sleep.

Judgment also would tell a person not to have another drink—but again, judgment is anesthetized. This is why a person may continue drinking to the point of passing out. The person no longer has the ability to perceive the need to stop.

After the loss of judgment, alcohol disables speech, vision, and coordination. The cells of the brain that govern large muscle movement lose control; at this point, people stagger or weave when they try to walk.

Once coordination is affected, you might think judgment would tell the drinker not to drive—but remember, the judgment center is asleep. Beyond a certain point, drinkers cannot tell that they should not drive. Everyone has seen the out-of-control driver, weaving back and forth on the highway, out of touch with the cues that show how fast to go and how to steer. The driver is more entertained than frightened, though; lacking the perception that classifies the risks as life-threatening, this person may find such dangerous mistakes amusing.

Some people believe falsely, that alcohol enhances sexual relations. Actually, excessive drinking causes many people to lose the ability to perform– the effect described in the famous lines from Shakespeare's play *Macbeth*: Alcohol "provokes the desire, but it takes away the performance."

With still more drinking, the conscious brain is completely subdued, and the person passes out. Now, the person can drink no more—luckily, because

More about sexually transmitted diseases in Chapter 17.

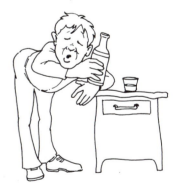

A person who has drunk too much alcohol too fast no longer can perceive the need to stop.

■ *FACT OR FICTION:* Alcohol enhances sexual relations. *False*. Alcohol may provoke sexual desire, but it hinders performance.

an only slightly higher alcohol level would anesthetize the deepest brain centers that stimulate breathing and heartbeat.

You may recall that alcohol was described earlier as an anesthetic. Alcohol is a poor choice among anesthetics, though; it is like heroin in that it does not reliably keep people under, yet it can kill them. The zone between unconsciousness and death is too narrow for safety (see Figure 8–2 in Chapter 8).

Because the brain centers respond to alcohol in the order just described, the drinker's life is often protected. People usually pass out before they can drink a lethal dose. It is possible, though, to drink so fast that the blood level of alcohol continues to rise after one has passed out, and even to rise so high as to stop the heart and lungs. Drinking contests are common among college groups, and it is important to recognize that gulping or "chugging" contests can be lethal. Table 10–1 shows the blood alcohol levels that correspond with progressively greater intoxication, and the box First Aid for Acute Alcohol Intoxication shows how to deal with alcohol overdoses.

While fast drinking is proceeding, the drinker's body is processing alcohol as fast as it can, and trying to protect itself in other ways, too. Alcohol is a toxin, and the body defends itself against ingested toxins in several ways. For one thing, straight alcohol stings as it goes down and triggers the choking reflex that keeps the drinker from swallowing too much at a time (you can gulp water easily, but it is difficult to gulp pure alcohol). A second protective device is the stomach, which rejects a too-large dose. The drinker vomits and expels at least part of the dose before it can be absorbed. What alcohol does get into the blood, other body systems metabolize or excrete it as quickly as they can.

The less food the stomach contains, the more rapidly alcohol enters the bloodstream. This is why a person who drinks alcohol on an empty stomach can feel the effects on the brain within a minute. (Conversely, if you want alcohol to trickle into the body rather than flooding it suddenly, eat first, then drink.)

Alcohol entering the stomach and intestines diffuses rapidly into the bloodstream (unless food is present to slow down its absorption). From there, it proceeds directly to the liver, which filters all the alcohol it can handle out of the blood before releasing the blood to the rest of the body. The liver thus gets the chance to remove toxic substances before they go on to other body organs such as the heart and brain, but the liver itself faces a

■ *FACT OR FICTION:* A person can die from drinking too much alcohol at one sitting. *True.*

TABLE 10–1 ■ **Effects of Various Blood Alcohol Levels**

Blood Alcohol Level (%)	Effect
0.04	Increased heart rate
0.06	Impaired judgment
0.10	Blurred vision, slurred speech, impaired coordination
0.30	Drunkenness, loss of control
0.40	Unconsciousness
0.50	Amnesia, eventual death

NOTE: Data are for an average-sized person under ordinary circumstances. Effects vary greatly from person to person, from day to day, and from one circumstance to another.

First Aid for Acute Alcohol Intoxication

"Chug! Chug! Chug!" The chanting at the dormitory party encourages the participants to "chug" (or gulp) large amounts of beer in a short time. People who engage in this rapid downing of alcohol often do not realize that this behavior can kill them. Drinking large amounts of alcohol quickly causes blood alcohol levels to rise dangerously, resulting in *acute alcohol intoxication,* or alcohol poisoning. Part of responsible drinking involves knowing about the physical signs and symptoms of alcohol poisoning and when to call for help in the case of emergency.

The first danger signs are the signs typical of shock, indicating failure of many vital body functions. The victim is in an unconscious state—unable to be aroused from a deep stupor. The pulse is weak and rapid (over 100 beats per minute); the skin, cool and damp; the breathing, fast (once every three or four seconds) and irregular. The skin color is pale or bluish; in a dark-skinned person this pallor appears in the mouth and corners of the eyes. Whenever these signs are present, seek emergency help immediately: call an ambulance. Meanwhile, administer first aid.

Involuntary vomiting helps rid the body of alcohol, but can threaten the life of a person who has lost consciousness. Vomiting can block the airway, so the person can die from asphyxiation. To provide first aid, position the person lying on his or her side to minimize the chance of airway obstruction. Watch closely anyone who "passes out" from heavy drinking. Instead of carrying drunk people to bed and forgetting about them, monitor their physical condition at regular intervals until the symptoms have disappeared and they are out of danger. You could save a friend's life.

hazard. Given too much of any toxin, the liver is the first organ to be damaged. Figure 10–2 shows where the liver is located along the blood's route and presents a few details about its services to the body.

The liver possesses a set of enzymes that can metabolize alcohol and other drugs. Like all enzymes, they are made of protein, and like all body proteins, they break down when a person fails to eat. Fasting for as little as a day can reduce the rate of alcohol metabolism by half. Drinking on an empty stomach thus not only lets the drinker feel the effects more promptly, but also raises the blood alcohol level higher for longer times and anesthetizes the brain more profoundly. The drinker who does not know the risks of drinking on an empty stomach may be in for a dangerous surprise.

While in the system, alcohol causes some vitamins and minerals to be destroyed, excreted, or both. Thus the person who drinks 300 calories of empty-calorie alcoholic beverages not only loses the nutrients that might have been delivered by 300 calories of food taken instead, but loses more nutrients besides.

Whenever alcohol is being metabolized in the body, some is used as fuel, and some is converted to fatty acids. Fat accumulates in the liver during a

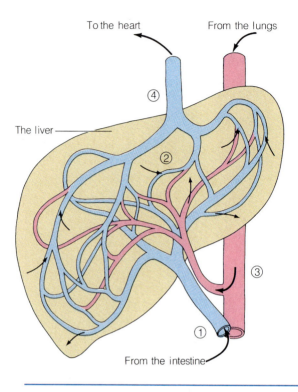

To the heart   From the lungs

④

The liver

②

③

①

From the intestine

1. All blood from the intestines has to pass through the liver before it goes anywhere else. It arrives by way of the portal vein.

2. The liver removes toxins and other materials for processing. It manufactures fats and other compounds for the body's use and releases them into the blood.

3. The liver has its own supply of freshly oxygenated blood that is conducted to it by way of the hepatic artery.

4. Blood leaving the liver has been filtered and its composition adjusted. It travels back to the heart by way of the hepatic vein.

FIGURE 10–2 ■ **The liver.**

single night of drinking. Some research conducted on this process, using beer-drinking fraternity brothers on a college campus, showed that more fat could accumulate in the liver in a single night of heavy drinking than the body could clear away in a single day. People who drink as heavily as these young men were doing, and who do so every night, will therefore experience progressive accumulation of fat in their livers, even if they eat well and are otherwise strong and healthy.

The first stage of liver deterioration, **fatty liver**, interferes with the distribution of nutrients and oxygen to the liver cells. If drinking episodes are so close together that the liver cannot recover between times, then the fat-stuffed liver cells stop functioning, and liver disease develops—as described in the section on long-term effects of excessive drinking later in this chapter.

People sometimes ask if excessive drinking, confined to weekends, permits sufficient recovery between times for a person to retain overall health. Perhaps for a while, in the sense that the liver may regain full function during the week, but a price is paid in brain cell loss, nutrient loss, and loss of time that might have been productive. This price is not repaid.

≡▶ *Excessive drinking produces self-destructive behaviors as increasing doses of alcohol sedate successive brain functions. Unconsciousness follows high doses, and fast drinking of high doses can kill. Long-term excessive drinking produces liver disease.*

The Hangover

The hangover—the awful feeling of headache pain, unpleasant sensations in the mouth, and nausea that one has the morning after drinking too

fatty liver an early stage of liver deterioration characterized by the accumulation of fat in the liver cells.

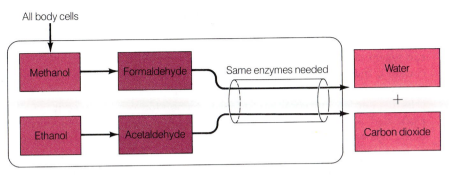

FIGURE 10–3 ■ **The hangover.**

methanol an alcohol produced in the body continually by all cells.

acetaldehyde (ass-et-AL-deh-hide) a substance to which ethanol is metabolized on its way to becoming harmless waste products that can be excreted.

much—is a mild form of drug withdrawal. The worse form is a delirium with severe tremors that warns of a danger of death and demands medical management. Hangovers are caused by several factors. One is the toxic effects of congeners, already mentioned, that accompany the alcohol in alcoholic beverages. The congeners in gin are different from those in vodka, which in turn are different from those in bourbon or rye whiskey. So if one particular kind of liquor produces a hangover in a person, it's possible that another kind may not. However, this is only one of several factors that produce hangovers, and mixing or switching drinks will not prevent them if too much is drunk.

Dehydration of the brain is a second factor: alcohol not only causes the body to lose water, but actually reduces the brain cells' water content. When they rehydrate the morning after, nerve pain accompanies their swelling back to their normal size.[14] Another contributor to the hangover is **formaldehyde**, the same chemical as is used in medical laboratories to preserve dead animals. Figure 10–3 shows where it comes from.

formaldehyde a substance to which methanol is metabolized on the way to being converted to harmless waste products that can be excreted.

Time alone is the cure for a hangover. Simple-minded remedies clearly will not work: for example taking vitamins or tranquilizers, drinking more alcohol, breathing pure oxygen, exercising, eating, drinking something awful, or taking painkillers. (Tylenol, or acetaminophen, can actually accelerate liver damage in alcohol drinkers, and aspirin can make the stomach bleed.) The headache pain, unpleasantness in the mouth, and nausea of a hangover come simply from drinking too much. Drink less next time.

≡▶ *Hangovers are caused by the congeners in alcoholic beverages; by dehydration and rehydration (swelling) of the brain; and by formaldehyde that accumulates when alcohol is metabolized. Time alone cures hangovers.*

Excessive Drinking: Long-Term Effects

Unfortunately, excessive drinking one night often leads to more excessive drinking on subsequent nights, for, as already described, alcohol is addictive. Long-term abuse of alcohol wreaks havoc on the body. It causes the greatest damage in one person's liver, another person's brain, and another person's pancreas, but it always damages all organs and organ systems to various extents.

Probably the most common disease to occur among abusers of alcohol is liver disease. We have already mentioned the effect of excessive drinking for one night: the liver cells start to fill with fat. If time between drinking bouts

fibrosis an intermediate stage of liver deterioration in which fibrous scar tissue invades the liver.

cirrhosis (seer-OH-sis) advanced liver disease, in which liver cells have hardened, turned orange, and died.

is not sufficient to permit this fat to be transported away to storage sites, then the fat-stuffed liver cells die, and inert, fibrous scar tissue invades the area (this is **fibrosis**, the second stage of liver deterioration). Some liver cells can regenerate with nutrition support and abstinence from alcohol; if they couldn't, many more drinkers would die. In the next (last) stage of liver disease—**cirrhosis**—though, regeneration becomes impossible. The liver cells die, harden, turn orange, and lose function forever. Cirrhosis is usually associated with alcoholism, and its victims often die, typically by massive blood loss when veins near the hardened liver burst from high blood pressure.

Since the liver is a crossroads for all of the working compounds that travel in the blood, its injury results in many ill effects elsewhere in the body. Foremost among them is high blood pressure, which sets the stage for heart damage and stroke. Another is brain and nervous system damage, for a healthy liver, by filtering the blood's contents before they reach the rest of the body, is a major protector of these organs.

Malnutrition usually accompanies heavy drinking, for drinkers obtain many of their calories from alcohol, leaving a smaller energy allowance within which to obtain needed nutrients. But eating well, even eating a superbly nutritious diet, although of course it benefits health to some extent, does not protect the drinker from alcohol-induced damage; one has to stop drinking alcohol for complete protection.[15]

Nerve and gland tissues are particularly sensitive to all these effects of long-term drinking.[16] The brain shrinks, even in people who drink only moderately.[17] The damage from alcohol is localized primarily on the brain's left side, and the extent of the shrinkage is proportional to the amount drunk.[18] Abstinence, together with good nutrition, reverses some of the brain damage—in fact, all of it, if heavy drinking has not continued for more than a few years—but prolonged drinking beyond an individual's capacity to recover can severely and irreversibly impair vision, memory, learning ability, and other functions.[19] Deep, healing sleep becomes impossible.

Prolonged drinking in combination with poor nutrition causes major brain diseases. Combined with smoking and malnutrition (as it often is), prolonged heavy drinking destroys vision: the optic nerve degenerates.[20] In addition, a head injury that occurs while alcohol is in the system is likely to incur far more severe brain damage than it would otherwise.[21]

Gland tissue is closely similar to nerve tissue, and the body's glands respond similarly to alcohol abuse. Pancreatic failure is common, and leads to a failure of blood sugar regulation and digestion; some people develop diabetes from alcohol abuse.[22] Damage to the adrenal glands leads to failure of testicular function, prostate gland damage, feminization, and sexual impotence in men; and to failure of the ovaries and early menopause in women.[23]

This description of the physical damage caused by heavy drinking has only covered the liver, brain and nervous system, and the hormonal system, and those only superficially. Table 10–2 sums up other physical effects on the drinker, which would otherwise occupy many pages. And still, these are only the physical effects on drinkers themselves. There are also psychological effects: a major one is depression.[24] Then, there are the effects on others—notably, the unborn children of alcohol abusers; and the families.

TABLE 10–2 ■ **Effects of Alcohol Abuse on Body Systems**

All organs—malnutrition and direct toxic effects of alcohol.
  Protein deficiencies.[a]
  Vitamin and mineral deficiencies.[a]
  Fat deposits in liver, arteries, and heart muscle, which interfere with function.[b]
All organs—increased risk of cancer of the mouth, throat, esophagus, rectum, and
  lungs; and of polyps in the large intestine.[c]
All organs—increased likelihood of adverse drug reactions (alcohol-drug
  interactions are the second most frequent cause of drug-related medical crises in
  the United States).[d]
Bones—osteoporosis.
Brain and nervous system—brain and nerve damage.
Cardiovascular system
  Heart muscle breakdown.[e]
  High blood pressure.
  Fat deposits (atherosclerosis).
  Reduced capacity for exercise; heart pain sooner during exercise.[d]
Digestive system
  Inflammation of the intestines.[d]
  Ulcers of the stomach and intestines.[d]
Hormonal system—damage to hormone-producing glands.
Immune system
  Slowed synthesis of important proteins.[f]
  Lowered defenses against disease and infection.[f]
  Increased susceptibility to lung infections—flu, pneumonia, tuberculosis.[d]
  Sedation of the bone marrow, which normally produces both red and white
  blood cells, with consequent blood abnormalities.[d]
Liver—fatty liver, fibrosis, and cirrhosis.
Muscles—skeletal muscle breakdown.[e]
Skin—Failure to maintain the skin's health: skin rashes and sores.[d]
Urinogenital system
  Bladder damage.[d]
  Kidney damage.[d]

---

[a]E. H. Jung, Y. Itokawa, and K. Nishino, Effect of chronic alcohol administration on transketolase in the brain and liver of rats, *American Journal of Clinical Nutrition* 53 (1991): 100–105.

[b]C. S. Lieber and L. M. DeCarli, Animal models of ethanol dependence and liver injury in rats and baboons, *Federation Proceedings* 35 (1976): 1232–1236.

[c]E. S. Pollack and coauthors, Prospective study of alcohol consumption and cancer, *New England Journal of Medicine* 310 (1984): 617; G. N. Stemmermann, L. K. Heilbrun, and A. M. Y. Nomura, Association of diet and other factors with adenomatous polyps of the large bowel: A prospective autopsy study, *American Journal of Clinical Nutrition* 47 (1988): 312–317.

[d]M. J. Eckardt and coauthors, Health hazards associated with alcohol consumption, *Journal of the American Medical Association* 246 (1981): 648–666.

[e]A. Urbano-Marquez, R. Estruch, F. Navarro-Lopez, J. M. Grau, and coauthors, The effects of alcoholism on skeletal and cardiac muscle, *New England Journal of Medicine* 320 (1989): 409–415.

[f]Alcohol intake and immunity, *Nutrition Today,* July/August 1988, p. 33.

The damage alcohol can do to the fetus carried by a pregnant woman who abuses alcohol may last long after the woman herself has died, for **fetal alcohol syndrome (FAS)**, lasts a lifetime. FAS includes mental and physical retardation and birth defects; Chapter 14 describes the syndrome in detail, and concludes that women should not drink alcohol at all during pregnancy.

fetal alcohol syndrome (FAS) a cluster of birth defects including irreversible mental and physical retardation and a characteristic set of facial abnormalities in children born to mothers who abuse alcohol during pregnancy.

Finally, a constellation of other effects, familial and social, surround the drinker. Dysfunctional family dynamics have already been described (Chapter 3), and are often induced or worsened by alcoholism. The children of people with alcoholism carry scars well into adulthood, and indeed, throughout life unless teachers or health care providers intervene,[25] or unless, as adults, they take the responsibility of making efforts to recover.

The concept that an adult aged 20, 30, 40 or more might still carry a wounded child within may be unfamiliar to some, but it has validity borne out by research. "Adult children" of people with alcoholism have banded together in groups all across the country and are working actively to help themselves and each other recover from the scars of their childhoods. These groups, known as ACOA groups (for "Adult Children of Alcoholics") have documented the damage done to them in their childhoods in statistics that show higher rates of health care costs; of hospital admissions; of substance abuse; and of mental disorders, injuries, poisonings, respiratory ailments, diseases of the digestive system, and complications in pregnancy and childbirth.[26] Recovery from the wounds caused by alcoholism is possible, however, and this chapter's Spotlight suggests ways to get started.

To sum up, alcohol abuse is globally damaging to health and wellness. The hazards are so well recognized that Congress requires the producers of alcoholic beverages to cite health warnings on their products. Even social drinking, if it is not moderate, is associated with an increased risk of death from all causes; social drinkers are thus at risk even though they may never appear drunk.[27] The vast weight of evidence is against alcohol for its health effects; the only points in its favor seem to be those we mentioned at the start of this chapter—the social benefits and the appetite-enhancing effect of wine.

≡▶ *Long-term alcohol abuse causes liver, heart, and brain disease, as well as many other disorders. Most devastating are fetal alcohol syndrome and dysfunctional family dynamics.*

■≡ How to Drink, How to Refuse, How to Give a Great Party

Those who choose to drink need to learn to handle drinking well. Those who choose to abstain need to learn to do so with ease.

Those who succeed in drinking moderately drink at appropriate times and in appropriate settings only. They limit their intake, and they enjoy being in control. They acknowledge that they have a responsibility not to damage themselves or society, and they know that being intoxicated is irresponsible drinking behavior.[28] Among the skills they report they've had to learn are the following:

■ "I get together with my friends and we decide ahead of time who will drive us home. The designated driver agrees not to drink at all at the party."

■ "I decide in advance how much I'm going to drink. If it's BYOB (bring your own bottle), I take only two drinks with me."

■ "If they're serving beer by the pitcher, I still order it by the glass. I read a report that ordering beer by the pitcher tends to double a drinker's intake."[29]

■ "I eat before and during a party, and then I drink slowly."

■ "I allow time to metabolize the alcohol I've drunk before I drive home."

■ "I sip my drinks; I add ice cubes or water; and if I'm thirsty, I drink water."

■ "I use fruit juices for mixers. They meet my calorie need and keep my blood sugar up."

■ "When I want dessert, I eat ice cream. A piña colada has too many calories."

■ "Now and then I skip a round. I don't accept drinks I don't want."

■ "I go slowly with unfamiliar drinks."

■ "If I need sleep, I sleep—I don't drink. If I need to relax, I relax—I don't drink."

■ "I know my capacity, and I don't exceed it."[30]

Those who choose not to drink have every right to make that choice. The choice is personal, it is yours, and it is no one else's business. A perfectly legitimate statement is: "I don't drink because I don't want to drink." Nevertheless, some social groups give people a hard time for refusing to participate in drinking, because it is a shared experience. Pointers for the nondrinker appear in the Strategies that follow on the next page.

Whether or not you drink, you may give a party at which alcohol is served. Comments made by people who give great parties include the following:

■ "What's a good party? One that's remembered with unqualified pleasure. Do we come together just to drink, or to have a good time socially? Alcohol shouldn't have to be used to make a party go."

■ "I keep the cocktail hour short. And I keep the music turned down. Music that makes it impossible to talk makes people drink more."

■ "I provide plenty of snacks with drinks. I don't serve drinks too early or too generously, and I don't offer refills too often."

■ "I'm careful about whom I ask to tend bar. I've noticed that problem drinkers tend to push drinks at people."

■ "I provide nonalcoholic beverages so people can pace themselves. When they've had enough alcohol, they can switch."

■ "I don't make nondrinkers feel like outsiders. They may be pilots, surgeons, recovering alcohol addicts, Moslems—whatever their reason, it's their business."

■ "If I notice someone drinking too fast, I offer that person coffee. He or she usually gets the hint."

■ "I limit alcohol consumption by providing filling calories with it—punch. If this disappoints anyone, I don't take it personally. Their disappointment is a reflection on their drinking problem, not on my hospitality."

If a friend has drunk too much, you can't hasten the return of sobriety by, say, taking your friend for a walk around the block. Walking forces the muscles to work, but since muscles cannot metabolize alcohol, they cannot help clear it from the blood. Time is the only thing that will do the job; each person's blood is cleared of alcohol at a steady but limited rate.

Nor will it help to give your friend a cup of coffee. Caffeine is a stimulant, but it won't help metabolize alcohol. The police say ruefully, "A drunk who drinks a cup of coffee won't get sober but may become a wide-awake drunk."

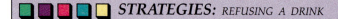

STRATEGIES: REFUSING A DRINK

To refuse an unwanted drink gracefully:

1. *Don't apologize.* It may take guts to say, ''No, thanks.'' Say it calmly, casually, firmly. Keep it brief; don't give excuses, explanations, or arguments. A discussion period is a good time for explanations; a party is not.
2. *Expect others to respect your choice.* When you're confident of your own choice, you will take it for granted that your ''No, thanks'' will receive respect from others. Your firm manner will make your confidence clear to them, and respect is what you'll get. But if you're hesitant, you pave the way for others to tease or argue; they think you really want them to persuade you to accept.
3. *Respect the drinker's choice to drink.* Give the person who drinks the same acceptance you want to receive. If you don't—if you sneer or argue or shake your head sadly—you're backing the person into a corner. People who are cornered have to fight their way out; probably the person will try to embarrass you for your decision not to drink.
4. *Consider another group of friends.* If you continue to receive pressure to drink from those who are drinking, even after trying the above suggestions, consider developing other friendships. Those who push alcohol on nondrinkers are using alcohol irresponsibly, and they often are problem drinkers, uncomfortable if those around them are not drinking. If they base the friendship on your drinking behavior, you may benefit from looking elsewhere for quality friendships.

SOURCE: Adapted from U.S. Department of Health and Human Services, *Thinking about Drinking*, HHS publication no. (ADM) 74-27, 1974; R. C. Engs, Responsibility and alcohol: Teaching responsible decisions about alcohol and its use for those who choose to drink, *Health Education*, January/February 1989, pp. 20–22.

Other suggestions for dealing with someone who is intoxicated:

■ Don't respond to emotions stirred by drink.
■ Do show concern.
■ Refuse or allow another drink based on your judgment, not your friend's.
■ Take your friend's car keys away.
■ If your friend insists on driving, don't get in the car.

Some states have passed laws that hold a host accountable for alcohol-related accidents or damage caused by the host's guest. Learning to serve alcohol responsibly is thus worthwhile for both social and legal reasons. Learning to give enjoyable parties that *don't* include alcohol is also worthwhile.

For someone who has had too much to drink, we repeat, time is the only real cure. One-half pint takes 10 hours to leave the system, and a person needs 24 hours to sober up completely after having passed out. Keep an eye on such people, in case they show the danger signs described earlier, but let them sleep, don't let them drive, and never offer a drink for the road.[31]

≡▶ *People who are successful in remaining moderate drinkers have mastered many social skills to resist social pressure to drink too much. Abstainers can enjoy social events that involve drinking by employing a corresponding set of skills. Hosts and friends of drinkers can help protect them from dangerous consequences of excess drinking.*

■☰ Drinking, Driving, Accidents, and Violence

Drinking slows reactions. Drinking before and while driving kills motorists; it is the leading cause of highway death.[32] Of all fatal automobile accidents occurring on the roads today, 40 percent involve alcohol intoxication.[33] Alcohol addicts have more collisions than non-addicts.[34] In automobile accidents with survivors, when alcohol is involved, more severe injuries occur.[35]

The hazards associated with drinking and driving have led to laws that forbid driving under the influence of alcohol. Under these laws, it is a punishable offense to be **DUI** (driving under the influence of alcohol) or **DWI** (driving while impaired by an abusable substance). The *influence* of alcohol is considered proved if the driver's blood alcohol level is between 0.05 and 0.10 percent (depending on state laws).[36] The blood alcohol level can be determined using a **breathalyzer test**. A driver's *impairment* is measured using tests of coordination and can occur at blood alcohol levels as low as 0.04 percent or even lower. Lobby groups such as MADD (Mothers Against Drunk Drivers) and SADD (Students Against Drunk Drivers) are putting pressure on legislators to make the laws stricter, because they have lost too many cherished sons, daughters, and friends in alcohol-related accidents on the highways.[37] Parents have also successfully prosecuted colleges and other institutions on occasions when their sons or daughters have been injured in episodes involving alcohol abuse, forcing the institutions to take greater responsibility. And students in many colleges and universities, in cooperation with their health centers or student activities centers, have formed many kinds of organizations that promote responsible drinking.

Driving under the influence of alcohol is especially hazardous for young drivers, who are inexperienced at both driving and drinking. Drivers younger than 20 represent fewer than 8 percent of the nation's licensed drivers, but they are involved in more than 25 percent of all collisions,[38] and drinking-driving accidents are the leading cause of death in young people up to 24 years of age. At the urging of the Federal Transportation Safety

DUI driving under the influence (of alcohol or any other abusable substance).

DWI driving while impaired by any abusable substance—a crime by law.

breathalyzer test a test used to determine blood alcohol level. About 10% of the alcohol in the blood is excreted through the breath, so the amount of alcohol in the breath accurately reflects the amount in the blood.

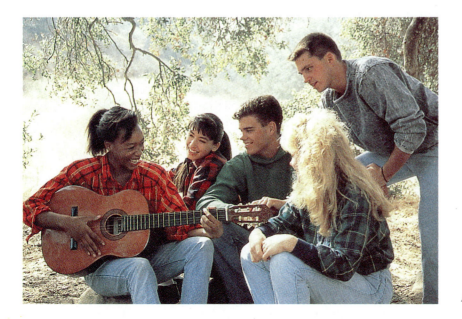

Alcohol isn't needed to have a good time.

Alcohol also is involved in:

55% of arrests.

53% of fire deaths.

45% of drownings.

36% of pedestrian accidents.

22% of home accidents.

Board, as well as of concerned parents, teachers, and young people themselves, all states have now adopted a legal minimum drinking age of 21.

After the blood alcohol level has fallen back to zero, a person still cannot drive safely for several hours. You should abstain, even from moderate alcohol consumption, for at least four to five hours before driving.[39] Some say you should even abstain from driving the morning after an evening of moderate drinking, for your driving ability may still be impaired by as much as 20 percent—a finding based on research on moderate drinkers aged 19 to 38.[40]

Not only auto accidents, but all accidents, are more likely when people overconsume alcohol. Violent crimes are, too. Abuse of alcohol on college campuses leads to acts of violence on the part of people who would never otherwise commit them. Parties intended just for relaxation and fun can, with too much alcohol, become brawls, complete with dangerous fights, injuries, rapes, vandalism, and other crimes.

The party begins.

I can drive when I drink.

2 drinks later.

I can drive when I drink.

After 4 drinks.

I can drive when I drunk.

After 5 drinks.

I can driv when I driv

7 drinks in all.

I can drv edn dmv

The more you drink, the more coordination you lose. That's a fact, plain and simple.

Still, people drink too much and then go out and expect to handle a car.

When you drink too much you can't handle a car. You can't even handle a pen.

The House of Seagram

Alcohol impairs coordination.

Most violent crimes are committed by people who have drunk heavily enough to achieve levels of alcohol in their blood from 0.10 to 0.30 percent. (With levels higher than that, people pass out.) Remember, these people are not necessarily violent to begin with, but under alcohol's influence, they become violent. Violent behavior attributed to alcohol misuse accounts for one-third to two-thirds of all murders, assaults, rapes, suicides, spouse abuse, and child abuse.[41]

≡▶   *Drinking alcohol and driving don't mix. The rates of all accidents and violence are accelerated by alcohol abuse.*

■≡ Alcoholism

Alcoholism, or alcohol addiction, is one of the nation's most serious health problems and is a major social, economic, and public health problem throughout much of the world.[42] Approximately 10 percent of the adult population in the United States is addicted to alcohol.[43] The annual cost to the nation, including work time lost to alcohol abuse and health expenses related to alcoholism, is estimated to be in the hundreds of billions of dollars.[44]

Alcoholism is a disease of addiction to the substance alcohol itself. Many misconceptions are attached to the term *alcoholism*. First of all, alcoholism is not related to the kind of beverage drunk. Second, it is not defined by how much is drunk. Nor is alcoholism tied to a particular age. Nor is it always obvious: it is easy to hide, even well into the advanced stages. People have been amazed to learn that a good friend, whom they have respected and thought of as a fully functioning member of society, has reached a late stage of alcoholism undetected.

To be drunk is not the same thing as to be a victim of alcoholism. Anybody can get drunk, simply by drinking too much alcohol, but that does not necessarily signify alcoholism. (It may, but authorities use other criteria to make the diagnosis.)

As defined by the American Medical Association (AMA), the American Psychiatric Association (APA), and other authorities, alcoholism is a disease. It is chronic, progressive, and potentially fatal, characterized by tolerance and physical addiction or organ damage caused directly or indirectly by alcohol consumption.[45]

The sequence of symptoms in alcoholism are well defined. It typically progresses from the first drink, usually in the teens, through increasing involvement with alcohol, to a point where alcohol comes to dominate the person's life, damaging family and friendships, work life, and physical health. Full-blown alcoholism typically takes from three to ten years to develop after heavy drinking has begun. Less time is required, though, if the abuser is young, and some teenagers are clearly already alcohol addicted.[46]

A key feature of alcoholism is denial: the person with the disease refuses to acknowledge it. As a result, a diagnosis made by someone else usually cannot lead to effective treatment, for the person with the disease won't cooperate. The best diagnosis for alcoholism, therefore, is self-diagnosis; this is why experts encourage the widespread use of self-tests, and why

Alcoholism is globally damaging to people and society.

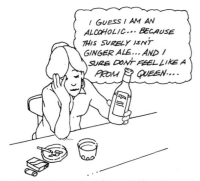

The diagnosis of alcoholism is usually made by the person himself or herself.

blackout episodes of temporary retrospective amnesia, characteristic of the person with alcoholism after periods of drinking.

they emphasize certain symptoms such as blackouts (described later), which only the person experiencing them can recognize.

The causes of alcoholism are varied and not completely understood. It is not even clear whether the disease is inherited. Alcoholism does tend to run in families, but families, of course, give their children both their genes and their environments, so this finding does not help to reveal the disease's cause.

On the genetic side, it is known that people with alcoholism metabolize alcohol differently than others, suggesting that they have inherited a physiological difference that leads to the disease.[47] The sons of men with early-onset alcoholism clearly have such an inherited predisposition to alcoholism.[48] But on the environment's side, dysfunctional family dynamics clearly also foster the development of problem behaviors that increase the risk of becoming addicted to alcohol. Dysfunctional family dynamics seem to both result from and cause alcoholism (see Chapter 3). Outside the family, a major environmental factor is the free availability of alcohol itself, which makes it easy to start and to continue drinking.

Not knowing the cause makes alcoholism hard to prevent, and hard to treat. Researchers interested in prevention have worked on predicting who will develop alcoholism, based on factors in their families and environments. A person who has one parent with alcoholism is four times as likely to develop alcoholism as one without such a parent, whatever the cause, so efforts at prevention focus on such families.

Efforts at prevention and treatment also focus on key steps along the path to full-blown alcoholism. The steps are shown in Figure 10–4, which illustrates how mysterious it is that one person may follow the whole downward spiral while another gets off it early. One key step is the beginning of **blackouts**, which many researchers consider a key sign that someone is becoming alcohol addicted.

Blackouts are episodes of amnesia that occur after, not during, times when a person is drinking. During an event, the drinker may function perfectly normally—not appear drunk, and certainly not pass out (a blackout in no way resembles passing out). No one can tell that anything is wrong, or even if the drinker is drinking at the time. But afterwards (typically the morning after), the drinker will remember nothing about the event. Blackouts are so striking that the discovery that one is having them is often enough to make a person quit drinking for life.

Some authorities say that blackouts are the single most useful diagnostic feature of alcoholism. This statement is open to question, but blackouts are certainly a sign of alcoholism.

The dangerous thing about blackouts is that a person experiencing one may do something terrible and afterwards be unaware of it. A person may experience a blackout while driving, and kill someone. The following morning, the person might awaken completely unaware of what transpired the previous evening. A dent and some blood on the front of the car might be the only clues to the previous night's events. No one else can tell that someone is having a blackout; that is why diagnosis hinges on a person's own admission of the problem.

Just as people with diabetes or cancer come in all sizes, shapes, and varieties, so do people with alcoholism. The disease is no respecter of income, education, social class, or physical attractiveness: it is an equal-

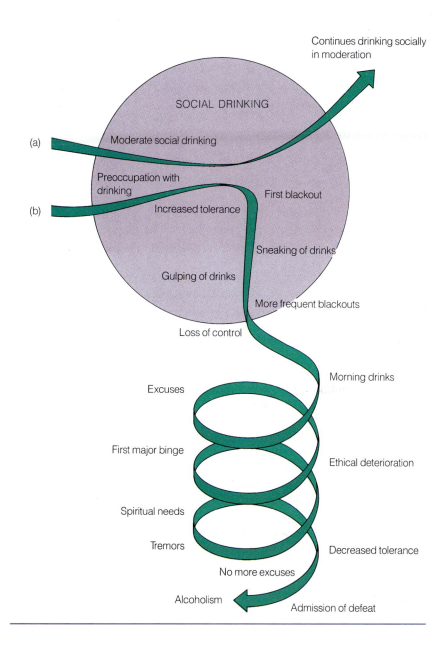

FIGURE 10–4 ■ **The fates of two drinkers.**

opportunity destroyer. The person you most admire from a distance is just as likely to be dependent on alcohol as the person you most despise. One does not have to be morally degenerate to be susceptible to alcoholism; one is just susceptible to alcoholism.

Alcoholism is not the addict's fault, but it is the addict's responsibility. If you want to be helpful remember this distinction. Learn to separate the *person* from the *behavior*: consider the person worthwhile, even if you oppose what the person *does*. Use language that reflects this attitude: speak of "the person with alcoholism," not of "the alcoholic." The person is not "an alcoholic" any more than a person with cancer is "a canceric." After all, if treatment is successful, the person may become a person *without* active

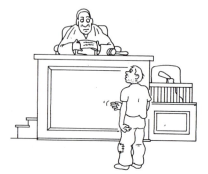

You can't tell just by looking which of these people might have an alcohol problem.

alcoholism. It is probably not correct to think alcoholism can be cured, but certainly the disease is treatable. And it can be arrested, as long as the person steers clear of alcohol.

Although the person with alcoholism is not at fault, the person is responsible for the disease. If a person with alcoholism chooses to continue engaging in the addictive behavior, then it is that person, not others, who should suffer the consequences. Experts say that this is neither an unfeeling, nor a judgmental statement; it is simply true. They call it "tough love": if you love someone with alcoholism, let the person experience the pain it causes, fully enough to become motivated to seek treatment and stop drinking. This may mean abandoning the person to go it alone, the hardest thing in the world to do, but often the only thing that will help. (You can go back when recovery is well under way.) Unfortunately, people seek treatment only when the pain of *not* doing so exceeds the pain of giving up the substance alcohol.

Family members who do otherwise, even with the best of intentions, are making the situation worse, not better. They may think they are helping, but it is not helpful either to deny that a problem exists, or to "help" by enabling the drinker to keep on drinking. Denial and enabling are the two behaviors family members engage in that most powerfully perpetuate the problem of alcoholism.

"But what if the person has children?" people often ask. If a spouse or other relative can take care of the children while the addict is making the choice to get worse or get better, that can facilitate resolution of the problem. Helping agencies can help families make decisions of this kind.* If the children are teenagers, they can request assistance on their own.** And for the spouse or closest family member, assistance is also available in the form of groups that show people how to draw the line between what they can control and what they can't, and how to achieve serenity and even joy in the midst of lives that do not meet their original expectations.†

If the person with alcoholism seeks treatment, recovery is possible. First and foremost, the person has to give up the drug, but many more steps must follow before success can be claimed. Recovery for the person addicted to alcohol and for the family members is the topic of this chapter's Spotlight.

≡▶   *Alcoholism is a progressive and potentially fatal disease. Key features are denial and blackouts. Alcoholism's causes are unknown, although it tends to run in families. Diagnosis and recovery require that the victim take responsibility.*

Although the drug alcohol, used in moderation and with great skill, can possibly enhance life, its use without such skill and in excess produces devastating harm to health, family life, and society. In-depth education on the facts about alcohol helps defend people against that harm. The next chapter describes the effects of another legal, addictive drug—nicotine, found in tobacco.

---

*Look up "Alcohol" or "Mental health" in the telephone book or call the National Clearinghouse for Alcohol Information, (301) 468–2600; or the Alcohol Hotline: (800) ALCOHOL.
**Look up "Alateen" in the telephone book or call the hotlines just listed.
†Look up "Alanon" or "ACOA" in the telephone book or call the hotlines just listed.

■☰ For Review

1. Explain what "proof" means with respect to alcoholic beverages.
2. Describe social and other pressures that promote people's drinking.
3. Describe a positive effect of moderate alcohol use.
4. Describe how one or two alcoholic drinks immediately affect the body and mind.

5. Describe the hazards associated with drinking too much too fast.
6. Identify some of the long-term effects of alcohol abuse on health, including the health of the unborn infant.
7. Describe the behaviors of a responsible drinker or host.

8. List ways to refuse alcohol without offending the host.
9. Describe how drinking alcohol affects driving.
10. Define alcoholism, and describe the problems it involves.
11. Describe the roles that denial and enabling play in alcoholism.

■☰ Notes

1. *Shattering Myths about Drinking,* 1977 (a booklet available from the Florida Department of Health and Rehabilitative Services, Alcoholic Rehabilitation Program, 1309 Winewood Blvd., Tallahassee, FL 32301).

2. Department of Health and Human Services, *Alcohol Practices, Policies, and Potentials of American Colleges and Universities* (Rockville, Md.: Department of Health and Human Servies, 1991), pp. 11–15.

3. Ryne Duren, as quoted by L. Herberg, Alcoholism: The national pastime, *Arizona Republic*, 30 March 1980, p. F1.

4. M. J. Stampfer and coauthors, A prospective study of moderate alcohol consumption and the risk of coronary disease and stroke in women, *New England Journal of Medicine* 319 (1988): 267–273; T. Gordon and W. B. Kannel, Drinking habits and cardiovascular disease: The Framingham Study, *American Heart Journal* 105 (1983): 667–673; A. L. Klatsky, G. D. Griedman, and A. B. Siegelaub, Alcohol consumption before myocardial infarction: Results from the Kaiser-Permanente Epidemiologic Study of myocardial infarction, *Annals of Internal Medicine* 81 (1974): 294–301; K. Cullen, N. S. Stenhouse, and K. L. Wearne, Alcohol and mortality in the Busselton Study,

International Journal of Epidemiology 11 (1982): 67–70.

5. N. A. Frimpong and J. A. Lapp, Effects of moderate alcohol intake in fixed or variable amounts on concentration of serum lipids and liver enzymes in healthy young men, *American Journal of Clinical Nutrition* 50 (1989): 987–991.

6. National Academy of Sciences, National Research Council, Food and Nutrition Board, Committee on Diet and Health, *Diet and Health: Implications for Reducing Chronic Disease Risk* (Washington, D.C.: National Academy Press, 1989), pp. 443–444.

7. A. G. Shaper, G. Wannamethee, and M. Walker, Alcohol and morality: The myth of the U-shaped curve, *Lancet* 2 (1988): 1267–1273.

8. R. C. Engs, Responsibility and alcohol: Teaching responsible decisions about alcohol and its use for those who choose to drink, *Health Education,* January/February 1989, pp. 20–22.

9. National Academy of Sciences, National Research Council, Food and Nutrition Board, *Toward Healthful Diets,* as reprinted in *Nutrition Today,* May/June 1980, pp. 7–11. Another nutritionist defines moderation as 10% of calories from alcohol energy, which translates roughly to about two drinks per day for the average woman

and three drinks per day for the average man. J. McDonald, Moderate amounts of alcoholic beverages and clinical nutrition, *Journal of Nutrition Education* 14 (1982): 58–60.

10. *The Responsible Use of Alcohol: Defining the Parameters of Moderation* (American Council on Science and Health, January 1991).

11. All items except the last three in the discussion of moderate drinking behaviors are from *Adult Children of Alcohol Abusers,* 1988 (a brochure available from the American College Health Association, 15879 Crabbs Branch Way, Rockville, MD 20855); the last three items in the list discussion from Engs, 1989.

12. All items except the last three in the discussion of problem drinking behaviors are from *Adult Children,* 1988.

13. P. Gunby, A drink a night keeps good slumber at bay, *Journal of the American Medical Association* 246 (1981): 589; Of frogs and fizzy blood: Alcohol is good/bad for your health, *Health Picture* 1 (1983): 60–62.

14. G. Mirkin, The dynamics of drinking, *Health,* July/August 1981, pp. 44–45, 58.

15. G. A. Roa and E. C. Larkin, Alcohol-induced injury to the liver, *New England Journal of Medicine* 320 (1989): 1353; C. S. Lieber and L. M.

DeCarli, Animal models of ethanol dependence and liver injury in rats and baboons, *Federation Proceedings* 35 (1976): 1232–1236.

16. M. E. Charness, R. P. Simon, and D. A Greenberg, Ethanol and the nervous system, *New England Journal of Medicine* 321 (1989): 442–454.

17. Getting pickled, *Scientific American*, April 1985, p. 76.

18. D. W. Walker and coauthors, Neuronal loss in hippocampus induced by prolonged ethanol consumption in rats, *Science* 209 (1980): 711–713.

19. Alcohol-induced brain damage and its reversibility, *Nutrition Reviews* 38 (1980): 11–12; L. A. Cala and coauthors, Alcohol-related brain damage: Serial studies after abstinence and recommencement of drinking, *Australian Alcohol/Drug Review*, July 1984, pp. 127–140.

20. M. Victor, Tobacco-alcohol amblyopia, *Archives of Ophthalmology* 70 (1963): 313–318.

21. M. Albin of the University of Texas Health and Science Center, San Antonio, as quoted in A double for the road, *Executive Fitness Newsletter*, 19 March 1983.

22. D. A. Roe, Alcohol-induced malabsorption, *Nutrition and the MD,* August 1984.

23. M. J. Eckardt and coauthors, Health hazards associated with alcohol consumption, *Journal of the American Medical Association* 246 (1981): 648–666.

24. Eckardt and coauthors, 1981.

25. S. S. Mull, Help for the children of alcoholics, *Health Education*, September/October 1990, pp. 42–45.

26. Information on the survey that produced these statistics is available from Children of Alcoholics Foundation, Inc., P.O. Box 4185, Grand

Central Station, New York, NY 10163–4185; telephone (212) 315–2680.

27. E. Rubin, The "social" drinker (Questions and Answers), *Journal of the American Medical Association* 248 (1982): 2179.

28. Engs, 1989.

29. E. S. Geller, in a study of 256 college students, as cited in S. Cunningham, Drunker by the pitcher, *Psychology Today,* March 1985, p. 80.

30. Some of the items in this list were adapted from *How to Be a Good Host: A Guide to Responsible Drinking* (a booklet available from the Bureau of Alcoholic Rehabilitation, P.O. Box 1147, Avon Park, FL 33825).

31. Partly excerpted from *How to Be a Good Host*.

32. J. K. Worden, B. S. Flynn, D. G. Merrill, and coauthors, Preventing alcohol-impaired driving through community self-regulation training, *American Journal of Public Health* 79 (1989): 287–290.

33. Department of Health and Human Services, *Seventh Special Report to the U.S. Congress on Alcohol and Health from the Secretary of Health and Human Services* (Rockville, Md.: Department of Health and Human Services, 1990), pp. 13–41, 163–179, as cited in J. G. Modell and J. M. Mountz, Drinking and flying—The problem of alcohol use by pilots, *New England Journal of Medicine* 323 (1990): 455–461.

34. J. A. Waller, Health status and motor vehicle crashes, *New England Journal of Medicine* 324 (1991): 54–55.

35. G. J. Wintemute, J. F. Kraus, S. P. Teret, and M. A. Wright, Death resulting from motor vehicle immersions: The nature of the injuries, personal and environmental contrib-

uting factors, and potential interventions, *American Journal of Public Health* 80 (1990): 1068–1070.

36. W. Darby and A. Heinz, *The Responsible Use of Alcohol: Defining the Parameters of Moderation,* January 1991 (a booklet available from the American Council on Science and Health, 1995 Broadway, 16th Floor, New York, NY 10023–5860).

37. Tougher alcohol rules urged, *Tallahassee Democrat*, 18 February 1986.

38. Statistics provided by the U.S. Department of Transportation, National Highway Traffic Safety Administration.

39. Darby and Heinz, 1991.

40. D. Pine, Hungover driving, *Health,* May 1984, p. 12.

41. *Facts on Alcoholism* (available from the National Council on Alcoholism, Inc., 2 Park Ave., New York, NY 10016).

42. Charness, Simon, and Greenberg, 1989.

43. M. Rudzinski and J. A. Stankaitis, Recognizing the alcoholic patient, *New England Journal of Medicine* 320 (1989): 125.

44. Charness, Simon, and Greenberg, 1989.

45. A. Silverstein and V. B. Silverstein, *Alcoholism* (Philadelphia: Lippincott, 1975), pp. 61–68.

46. N. Bejerot, *Addiction: An Artificially Induced Drive* (Springfield, Ill.: Charles C. Thomas, 1972), p. 27.

47. B. Tabakoff, P. L. Hoffman, J. M. Lee, and coauthors, Differences in platelet enzyme activity between alcoholics and nonalcoholics, *New England Journal of Medicine* 318 (1988): 134–139.

48. Charness, Simon, and Greenberg, 1989.

SPOTLIGHT

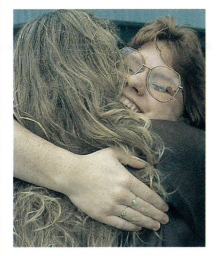

Addiction Recovery and Facilitating Recovery

This Spotlight is about recovery from all addictions, although alcohol addiction serves as a useful example. Alcohol is the best known of all the drugs to which people become addicted. Recovery from alcohol addiction is similar to recovery from any drug addiction. Recovery involves two parts: first, learning to abstain from the substance, and second, overcoming the problems that contributed to the addiction as well as the problems the addiction caused.

I thought a person who had stopped abusing a substance had recovered. Are you saying that to be fully recovered, a person has to do more?

A common misconception is that once substance abuse stops, all problems are solved. Abstinence is necessary for physical healing, but it doesn't fix other problems; it doesn't address what happened to the family as a result of the substance abuse, nor does it address the circumstances that contributed to the addiction in the first place. Stopping drinking (or using another drug) is just the first step; many other adjustments in all realms—emotional, social, job-related, and even spiritual—have to take place before a stable state of true sobriety is attained.

Recovery sounds like an unsurmountable task. Do many addicts succeed?

Recovery is an overwhelming task. Few make it, but those who do usually emerge with an enormous amount of character, depth, humility, and understanding. Estimates of the success rate in alcoholism recovery programs range from 1 in 3 to 1 in 33. Success rates depend, among other things, on the quality of the program and on the length of time the person stays in treatment.

How long does recovery take?

The progression back to normality from addiction may take years, if the damage done by the drug has progressed for years and every aspect of life has been affected. The first stage—learning abstinence—is characterized by its own sequence of events, as shown in Figure S10–1 which illustrates the recovery from alcoholism. The person stops drinking, begins to regain health, becomes able to eat and regains appetite, begins to function better socially, returns to functioning on the job, and regains health. The second part of recovery—addressing the problems that preceded and resulted from the problem drinking—takes even longer, usually between three and five years.

Can certain drugs help recovery?

Yes. Methadone and other drug antagonists help with recovery from some drug addictions. An aid to therapy for alcohol-addicted people is a prescription medicine, *Antabuse*. The person who takes a single pill of Antabuse each day cannot drink alcohol without becoming violently ill. Antabuse completely eliminates drinking on impulse; one has to stop taking it for five days before drinking.

Antabuse is inexpensive and can be started within three days after a person has stopped drinking. It is infallible; it never fails to react with alcohol. It is not addictive, and it has no side effects. Some people recovering from alcoholism take it for years. It is most effective when used in connection with psychological therapy.

How does therapy help in addiction recovery?

Therapy helps in both stages of recovery. Giving up a drug is a grief experience. For reasons the non-addicted person cannot possibly fathom, the addicted person is extremely attached to the drug and cannot imagine life without it. It is a friend, a lover, a comfort, even a god. To give it up necessitates going through the stages of grief (already discussed in Chapter 3). An early stage is denial. Another is bargaining. Then come rounds of anger and guilt, and finally acceptance. The recovering addict needs professional support to pass through these stages of grief.

Psychological therapy also helps in the second stage of recovery, in which the addict examines the problems that led to the addiction and learns new ways to cope with these problems. Emotional healing is crucial in addiction recovery (see the Spotlight following Chapter 3).

The most helpful therapy seems to be group therapy, which puts the person in touch with other people who are recovering and have recovered. No one is so persuasive in assisting a person recovering from substance abuse as one who has been through the experience and succeeded. The worldwide self-help recovery group Alcoholics Anonymous (AA) is based on this principle. In AA, thousands of people have helped one another recover from alcoholism without cost or publicity. The AA program is particularly effective because it takes a positive approach—12 steps to recovery that promote spiritual growth and culminate in the person's actively helping others.* For drug addictions, comparable groups exist, such as Narcotics Anonymous (NA). Table S10–1 describes a typical 12-step program.

What can I do if I have a friend or family member with a substance abuse problem?

The most important thing you can do is *not* enable the person to escape the problems resulting from the substance abuse. If you know someone with an alcohol or other drug addiction (or who is otherwise irresponsible) and you look at the people in that person's life, you will likely find someone who is making it easy for that person to continue to be irresponsible. This person is called an enabler (or codependent).

Enabling behavior was defined and described in Chapter 3. An enabler

*AA and NA are listed in most telephone books under "AA," "NA," "Alcohol," and "Narcotics." The world address of AA is P.O. Box 459, Grand Central Station, New York, NY 10017.

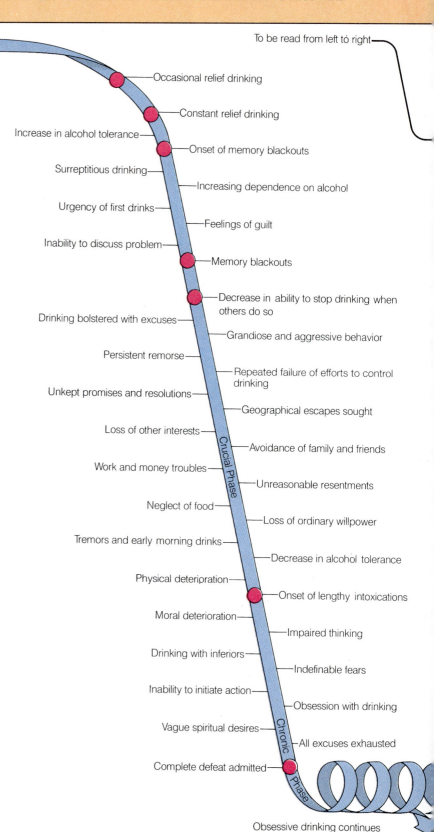

To be read from left to right

- Occasional relief drinking
- Constant relief drinking
- Increase in alcohol tolerance
- Onset of memory blackouts
- Surreptitious drinking
- Increasing dependence on alcohol
- Urgency of first drinks
- Feelings of guilt
- Inability to discuss problem
- Memory blackouts
- Decrease in ability to stop drinking when others do so
- Grandiose and aggressive behavior
- Drinking bolstered with excuses
- Persistent remorse
- Repeated failure of efforts to control drinking
- Unkept promises and resolutions
- Geographical escapes sought
- Loss of other interests
- Avoidance of family and friends
- Work and money troubles
- Unreasonable resentments
- Neglect of food
- Loss of ordinary willpower
- Tremors and early morning drinks
- Decrease in alcohol tolerance
- Physical deterioration
- Onset of lengthy intoxications
- Moral deterioration
- Impaired thinking
- Drinking with inferiors
- Indefinable fears
- Inability to initiate action
- Obsession with drinking
- Vague spiritual desires
- All excuses exhausted
- Complete defeat admitted

Crucial Phase

Chronic Phase

Obsessive drinking continues

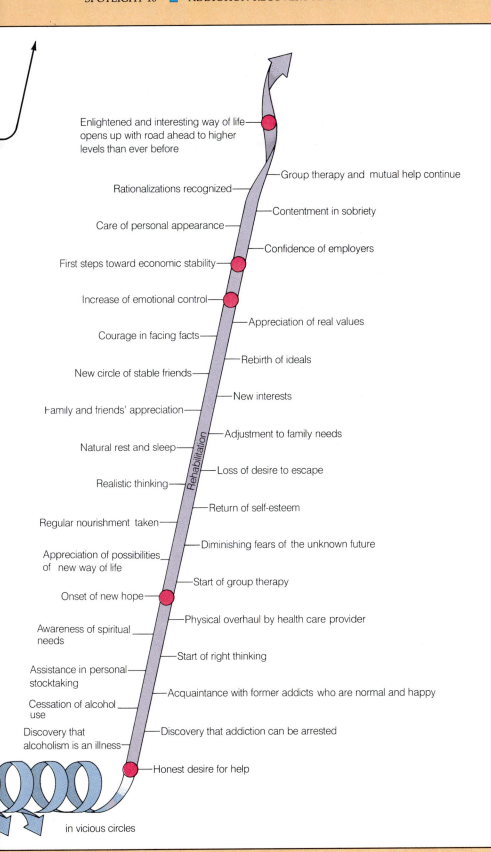

Enlightened and interesting way of life opens up with road ahead to higher levels than ever before

Group therapy and mutual help continue

Rationalizations recognized

Contentment in sobriety

Care of personal appearance

Confidence of employers

First steps toward economic stability

Increase of emotional control

Appreciation of real values

Courage in facing facts

Rebirth of ideals

New circle of stable friends

New interests

Family and friends' appreciation

Adjustment to family needs

Natural rest and sleep

Loss of desire to escape

Realistic thinking

Rehabilitation

Return of self-esteem

Regular nourishment taken

Diminishing fears of the unknown future

Appreciation of possibilities of new way of life

Start of group therapy

Onset of new hope

Physical overhaul by health care provider

Awareness of spiritual needs

Start of right thinking

Assistance in personal stocktaking

Acquaintance with former addicts who are normal and happy

Cessation of alcohol use

Discovery that alcoholism is an illness

Discovery that addiction can be arrested

Honest desire for help

in vicious circles

FIGURE S10–1 ■ **The way back.**

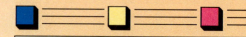

TABLE S10–1 ■ **Typical 12-Step Program**

1. We admitted we were powerless over the obsession or compulsion (such as drinking alcohol, using other drugs, gambling, overworking, overexercising, overeating, or excessively depending on other people)—that our lives had become unmanageable.
2. We came to believe that a power greater than ourselves could restore us to sanity.
3. We made a decision to turn our will and our lives over to the care of God as we understood him.
4. We made a searching and fearless moral inventory of ourselves.
5. We admitted to God, to ourselves, and to another human being the exact nature of our wrongs.
6. We were entirely ready to have God remove all these defects of character.
7. We humbly asked him to remove our shortcomings.
8. We made a list of all the persons we had harmed, and became willing to make amends to them all.
9. We made direct amends to such people wherever possible, except when doing so would hurt them or others.
10. We continued to take personal inventory, and when we were wrong, promptly admitted it.
11. We sought through prayer and meditation to improve our conscious contact with God as we understood him, praying only for knowledge of his will for us and the power to carry that out.
12. Having had a spiritual awakening as the result of these steps, we tried to carry this message to other people who suffer from the same compulsions, and to practice these principles in all our affairs.

(or codependent) is a misguided helper, a rescuer who tries to save the substance abuser from the consequences of his or her behavior. The rescuer is well-intentioned, but actually does harm by supporting a troubled person's continued self-destructive behavior. By paying the price for the substance abuser, the enabler keeps the abuser from taking responsibility for his or her own behavior. Enabling takes many different forms— for example, coming up with money when it's owed, helping make excuses ("I'm sorry to have to tell you this, Boss, but my spouse is sick today"), and doing the other person's work.

How can I tell if I'm enabling?

Sometimes it is difficult to identify enabling behavior. Four guidelines may help you determine if you are enabling or if you are helping in a healthy way. You are probably enabling if:

■ The behavior you are "helping" with is repeated.
■ You view your "helping" as saving someone from severe consequences.
■ You allow the person to behave inappropriately toward you.
■ You feel some degree of resentment after "helping."

If one of these describes your behavior, you may be enabling; if all four describe you, you are definitely enabling.

Aside from not enabling, how can I help a close person with an addiction?

You can refuse to tolerate the inappropriate behavior. Assertive communication is needed. Some guidelines for communicating to an addict about inappropriate behavior include:

■ Maintain a context of personal concern. (Convey the message, "I care about you. I see you as a worthwhile person but I object to your behaviors.")
■ Be prompt. Speak as immediately after each episode as possible. (But be sure to give yourself enough time to cool off when you are angry.)
■ Point out the behavior, but do not attack the person. (Do say, "You

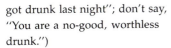

got drunk last night"; don't say, "You are a no-good, worthless drunk.")

■ Be specific; name and describe behaviors; don't judge. (Do say, "You fell and broke the standing lamp"; don't say, "You made a fool of yourself.")

■ Report how the behavior affects you. (Describe how you feel about the behavior.)

■ Clearly, calmly, and firmly state what behavior you will or will not accept. Describe what action you will take if the irresponsible behavior does not stop. (Say, "If you do not stop coming home drunk at three o'clock in the morning, I will move out.")

■ Be prepared to follow through with what you will do if the disrespectful behavior continues. (Don't just make empty threats; the person won't take you seriously.)

What else can I do as a concerned friend or family member?

Other strategies for helpers include:

■ Seek a support group (Al-Anon for adult family members, Alateen for teenaged children, or ACOA for adult children, of people with alcoholism).

■ Build your self-esteem. Know your personal bill of rights (see Table S10–2).

■ If you have a close family member with a drinking problem, watch your own drinking behavior:

TABLE S10–2   ■   Personal Bill of Rights

1. I have a right to joy in this life, right here, right now—not just a momentary rush of euphoria, but something more substantive.
2. I have a right to relax and have fun in a functional and nondestructive way.
3. I have a right to actively pursue people, places, and situations that will help me in achieving a good life.
4. I have the right to say no whenever I feel something is not safe or I am not ready.
5. I have a right to not participate in either the active or passive emotionally unhealthy behavior of parents, siblings, friends, roommates, or any others.
6. I have a right to take calculated risks and to experiment with new strategies.
7. I have a right to "mess up," to make mistakes, to "blow it," to disappoint myself, and to fall short of the mark.
8. I have a right to leave the company of people who deliberately or inadvertently put me down, lay a guilt trip on me, manipulate me, or humiliate me, including my parents, siblings, other family members, roommates, or any others.
9. I have a right to put an end to conversations with people who make me feel put down and humiliated.
10. I have a right to all my feelings.
11. I have a right to trust my feelings, my judgment, my hunches, my intuition.
12. I have a right to develop myself as a whole person emotionally, spiritually, mentally, physically, and psychologically.
13. I have a right to express all my feelings in a nondestructive way and at safe times and places.
14. I have a right to a mentally healthy, sane way of existence, though it may deviate in part, or all, from others' prescribed philosophy of life.
15. I have a right to carve out my place in this world.
16. I have a right to follow any of the above rights, live my life the way I want, and not wait until those around me get well, get happy, seek help, or admit there is a problem.

---

children of alcoholics are four times more likely to develop alcoholism.

Beyond these strategies, codependents should go about living and enjoying their own lives to the best of their ability, minimizing the other person's influence on their happiness. The substance abuse problem is not their problem. They cannot solve it, change it, take it away, or assume responsibility for it; but they do have the responsibility for their own lives.

CHAPTER 11

Smoking and Smokeless Tobacco

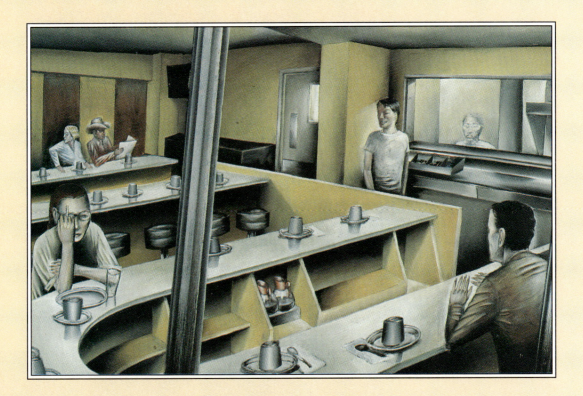

FACT OR FICTION

Just for fun, respond true or false to the following statements. If false, say what is true.

■ After someone has started smoking, enjoyment is the reason he or she continues to smoke. (Page 284)

■ Nicotine is a highly addictive drug. (Page 284)

■ Smoking wrinkles the skin. (Page 291)

■ To live with a smoker is to invite the risk of lung cancer. (Page 293)

■ One effective way to reduce the risk of cancer from smoking is to switch from cigarettes to chewing tobacco or snuff. (Page 295)

■ Most people who successfully quit smoking do it for their family and friends. (Page 297)

Undeniably, tobacco brings rewards to some people. Otherwise they wouldn't use it, because, as nearly everyone knows, many health hazards accompany tobacco use. If you use tobacco, you are probably aware of both the pleasures and the hazards. If you don't use it, you need to understand why some people do. This chapter therefore begins with the tobacco user's viewpoint before going on to look at the health effects of smoking and smokeless tobacco. The last section focuses on how to quit using tobacco and how to help the quitter. This chapter tries to present all the facts, both pro and con, with honesty. The health evidence, though, is one-sided—con.

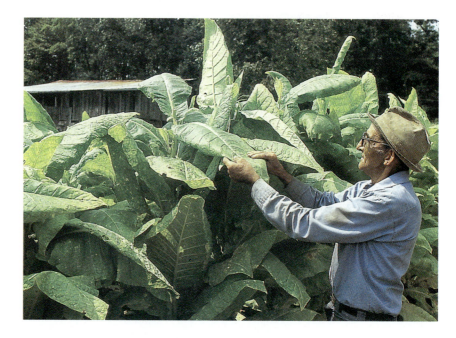

Tobacco farmers make the effort to produce high-quality green tobacco.

■≡ Why People Use Tobacco

The tobacco industry distributes highly persuasive advertisements. Ads associate tobacco use (by suggestion) with stereotypes: handsome, macho cowboys; successful executives; athletic, dynamic-looking women. These stereotypes undermine people's individuality, but people don't always see through them. Even cigarettes' brand names reflect carefully chosen images—Slims, Kool, Satin, More, Eve, Vantage, Bucks. Cigarette company advertisements deliver double messages: although required to acknowledge that smoking harms health, they show healthy people smoking. And they falsely associate smoking with healthy activities, which confuses people, especially children, about the unhealthy effects. Young people, searching for role models, imitate those they admire, and take up the habit of smoking or chewing tobacco. Then they show off their new behavior, enticing their peers into the same habits.

A person whose mind is open to using tobacco begins by trying it once. That one time may be followed by another, and in a short while, because nicotine is a powerfully addictive drug, the person becomes a regular user. Tobacco companies know that once they've got people started, they've got them hooked, and so they aim their ads at the young. They must attract children and young teenagers in order to replace the more than 2 million adult smokers who die each year worldwide from lung cancer and other smoking-related diseases.

Statistics on smoking are impressive. Each day, 5,000 children light up for the first time—some of them only seven or eight years old, in a hurry to grow up. If the current rate of tobacco use by young people continues, the U.S. surgeon general warns that 5 million of today's children will die of smoking-related illnesses in their later years.[1]*

Cigarette smoking among high school seniors peaked in the mid-1970s, declined until 1980, and seems to have leveled off. About one in five high school seniors smokes regularly, and more than 3,000 teenagers become regular smokers each day.[2]

A folder written by young people for young people describes how smokers rationalize their choice to smoke:

■ I'm young now. Why not smoke? I can quit later.
■ I don't inhale. Smoking can't hurt me.
■ Smoking makes me look grown-up and mature.
■ Smoking gives me self-confidence.
■ I smoke filter cigarettes; that will protect me.
■ My parents smoke. Why shouldn't I?
■ If I don't spend the money on cigarettes, I'll spend it on something else.
■ All my friends smoke. Why shouldn't I?
■ It keeps me from biting my nails.
■ It keeps me from putting on weight.
■ It gives me something to do when I'm mad or bored or hurt or unhappy or restless.
■ I know I'm going to die of something. At least I know what it will be.[3]

*Reference notes are at the end of the chapter.

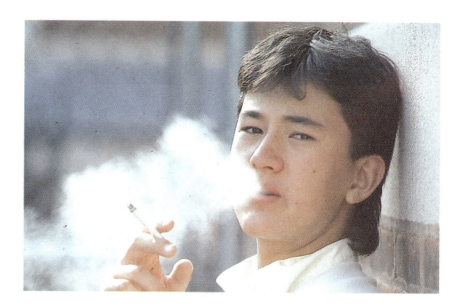

Young smokers imitate role models they admire.

All of these reasons are invalid, but the new smoker believes them. (Remember the phenomenon of denial, first mentioned in Chapter 9? These statements are classic examples of rationalizations.)

About half of all adults smoke or have smoked at one time or another; only one in four succeeds in quitting. Smoking is widespread among all races, all across the world. In this country, as many women as men smoke. And, as a health expert has said: "Women who smoke like men, die like men who smoke."[4]

Why do people keep on using tobacco? The first use of tobacco is, to most people, a noxious experience. Chewing tobacco in the mouth tastes unpleasant, and the body reacts to tobacco smoke inhaled into the lungs as to any smoke—by coughing to expel the foreign, unwelcome substance.

nicotine an addictive drug present in tobacco.

If this were all there were to it, no one would get hooked. Yet users keep coming back for more, mainly for the drug **nicotine,** to which they have developed an addiction. The addiction is so strong that users who give up or can't obtain one form helplessly switch to others—cigarettes to a pipe, pipe to chewing, chewing back to smoking.

■ *FACT OR FICTION:* After someone has started smoking, enjoyment is the reason he or she continues to smoke. *False.* The main reason for continuing to smoke is addiction to nicotine.

Nicotine has multiple effects on the body, especially affecting the major communication networks (the nervous and hormonal systems), the circulatory system, and the digestive system. Nicotine stimulates epinephrine secretion, which speeds up the heart rate and raises the blood pressure. Nicotine changes the brainwave pattern, calms the nerves, reduces anxiety, increases tolerance to pain, facilitates concentration, dulls the taste buds, and reduces hunger. Depending on the pattern of use, it arouses or calms the smoker. Nicotine acts on many different brain centers, so it elicits different responses from different people.[5] As a result, different people use tobacco for somewhat different reasons, and so there is no one way to help everyone stop.

Epinephrine is one of the stress hormones; see Chapter 4.

Because it is taken into the lungs rather than eaten or injected, a dose of nicotine reaches the brain all at once, rather than gradually. The user notices the pleasant effects immediately, but even more noticeable are the unpleasant effects of withdrawal as the dose wears off: a slowed heart rate, reduced

■ *FACT OR FICTION:* Nicotine is a highly addictive drug. *True.*

Addiction Is the Key

How can I tell you how serious smoking is? Look: the 350,000 premature deaths *per year* caused by cigarette smoking exceed all other drug and alcohol abuse deaths combined, seven times more than all automobile fatalities per year . . . and more than the combined American military fatalities in World War I, World War II, and Vietnam.

More than 60 percent of these yearly deaths *represent persons who became addicted to nicotine as adolescents, before the age of legal consent.*

SOURCE: Adapted from W. Pollin, Addiction is the key step in causation of all tobacco-related diseases (Editorial), *World Smoking and Health,* Spring 1985, pp. 2–3.

---

blood pressure, nausea, headache, irritability, restlessness, anxiety, drowsiness, inability to concentrate, and a craving for another dose.[6]

Many users take the next dose in order to avoid the letdown from the last one—a pattern revealing that they are addicted to nicotine. The addiction becomes so strong that they are unable to quit even in the face of the obvious physical evidence of their own impaired health, to be described in the next section.

Physical addiction, although the most significant reason, is not the only reason people continue to use tobacco. Psychological dependence also plays a role, because nicotine both increases pleasure and reduces pain. People enjoy the behavior itself: it provides an excuse, in a busy routine, to take a break and relax. Important, too, it immediately relieves small stresses. A person who is embarrassed and doesn't know what to say can light up a cigarette. A person who is angry and needs to cool off before speaking can pack a pipe. For these and many other reasons, people use tobacco. But they pay a tremendous price.

➡▶ *People begin using tobacco for a variety of reasons: influence of advertisements, peer pressure, or rebellion. All people continue to use tobacco for the same reason: they become addicted to the drug nicotine. Withdrawal from nicotine is extremely unpleasant.*

■≡ Health Effects of Smoking

Anything burned releases a multitude of chemicals not present in the original raw material. The damage people inflict on themselves by smoking is primarily from the *burning* ingredients of cigarettes—more than 4,000 hazardous compounds make their way into the lungs of smokers and into the air that everyone breathes.[7]

The most harmful ingredients are the **tars,** which are similar to the tars used on roads. These are notorious **carcinogens,** known to be responsible for most cases of lung cancer and for cancers of many other organs. Smokers who puff 20 to 60 cigarettes per day collect anywhere from ¼ to 1½ pounds

tars one of a class of chemical compounds present in (among other things) tobacco. Burning tars contain many carcinogens.

carcinogens cancer-causing agents.

of the sticky black tar in their lungs each year.[8] Tars are also primarily responsible for emphysema, another major disease of the lungs.

Many other ingredients in cigarettes also harm smokers. Cigarette manufacturers select from an array of some 1,400 additives to enhance the appeal of their products—flavoring agents, agents to moisten the tobacco, agents to prevent cigarettes from extinguishing themselves, and others. Among the flavoring agents are cocoa, licorice, prune juice, and raisin juice. You might think these would be harmless, but both cocoa and licorice, when burned, form carcinogens. Many of the other ingredients in cigarettes probably do, too, but they are company secrets, so scientists cannot conduct research on their effects. Perhaps a first step toward finding out the risks these ingredients present will be to insist that the industry disclose the ingredients in cigarettes.[9]

The smoke that reaches smokers is a little different from the smoke that reaches those in the room with them. The **mainstream smoke** from a cigarette is the smoke that passes through the cigarette and then enters the smoker's lungs; the **sidestream smoke** is the smoke that enters the air from the burning tip of the cigarette. Figure 11–1 shows the chemical composition of mainstream smoke and a few of its vapors and particles. Clearly, when people smoke, they inhale a multitude of harmful compounds. Naturally, the organ most affected by smoke is the lungs.

mainstream smoke   the smoke that flows through the cigarette and into the lungs when a smoker inhales.

sidestream smoke   the smoke that escapes into the air from the burning tip of a cigarette (and may then be inhaled by the smoker or by someone else).

FIGURE 11–1   ■   **Chemical composition of mainstream smoke.**

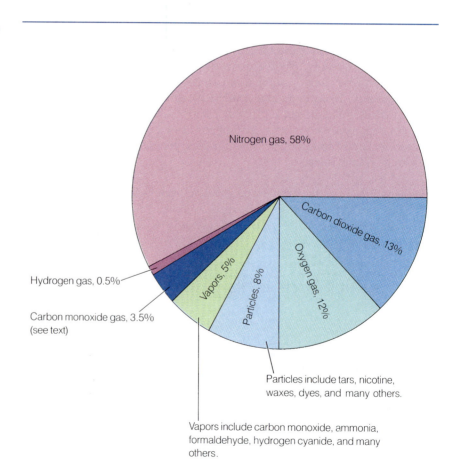

Nitrogen gas, 58%

Carbon dioxide gas, 13%

Oxygen gas, 12%

Particles, 8%

Vapors, 5%

Hydrogen gas, 0.5%

Carbon monoxide gas, 3.5% (see text)

Particles include tars, nicotine, waxes, dyes, and many others.

Vapors include carbon monoxide, ammonia, formaldehyde, hydrogen cyanide, and many others.

The Lungs

A diagram of the lungs appears in Figure 11–2(A). The lungs receive blood pumped from the heart and add oxygen to it; then the oxygenated blood returns to the heart to be distributed to all the body's cells. Every cell has to breathe; the lungs transmit oxygen to the cells so they can stay alive.

The lungs are huge, compared with the heart, they are rich with blood vessels, and they fill the chest. Twelve to fourteen times a minute they draw in air deeply and, like a sponge, soak up oxygen and squeeze out carbon dioxide.

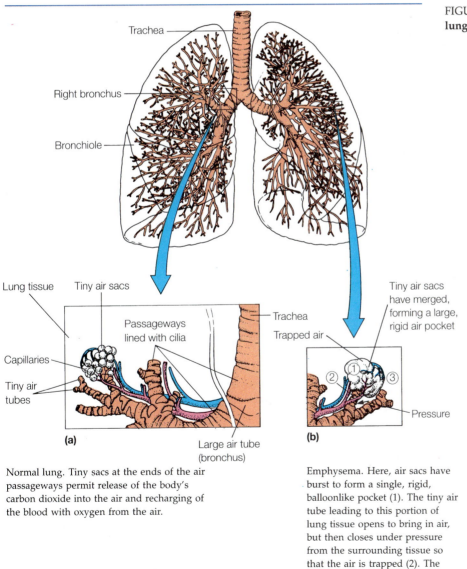

FIGURE 11–2 ■ **Normal lung versus lung with emphysema.**

Trachea

Right bronchus

Bronchiole

Lung tissue   Tiny air sacs

Passageways lined with cilia

Capillaries

Tiny air tubes

Trachea

Tiny air sacs have merged, forming a large, rigid air pocket

Trapped air

Pressure

(a)

Large air tube (bronchus)

(b)

Normal lung. Tiny sacs at the ends of the air passageways permit release of the body's carbon dioxide into the air and recharging of the blood with oxygen from the air.

Emphysema. Here, air sacs have burst to form a single, rigid, balloonlike pocket (1). The tiny air tube leading to this portion of lung tissue opens to bring in air, but then closes under pressure from the surrounding tissue so that the air is trapped (2). The capillaries are breaking down (3).

bronchi (BRONK-eye; singular, **bronchus,** BRONK-us)   the two main airways in the lungs; branches of the trachea.

mucus (MYOO-cuss)   a slippery secretion, produced by cells of the body's linings, that protects the underlying tissues.

cilia (singular, **cilium**)   hairlike structures extending from the surface of cells that line body passageways such as the trachea and upper lungs. The cilia wave, propelling the mucous coat along to sweep away debris.

trachea (TRAY-kee-uh)   the main air passageway from the nose and throat to the lungs, sometimes called the windpipe.

bronchitis (bron-KITE-us)   a respiratory disorder involving irritation and inflammation of the bronchi, with thickened mucus and deep, harsh coughing.

emphysema (em-fih-ZEE-muh)   a disease of the lungs in which many small, flexible air sacs burst and form a few large, rigid air pockets; as a result, the lungs' absorbing surface is reduced, and breathing is both difficult and ineffective.

Healthy **bronchi,** the major breathing tubes leading to each lung, are lined with cells coated with slippery **mucus** and little waving hairs (**cilia**). The mucus catches particles and bacteria that would otherwise lodge in the lungs, and the cilia sweep the mucus in a constant stream, up to the **trachea,** the windpipe. Cilia also line the trachea, and they sweep the mucus all the way up to the throat. When you clear your throat and swallow or spit, you remove a bit of this mucus, with its burden of contaminants, from your air passages and dispose of it.

Smoking damages the lung tissue in many ways. The tars in cigarette smoke make the mucous coat abnormally thick and inhibit the action of the cilia so that they become sluggish in sweeping out the accumulated debris. Irritation builds, making the smoker feel like coughing; but each puff on a cigarette paralyzes the cilia for a while, so the smoker feels *less* irritation. The need to cough feels like a need to smoke; the very thing that harms also soothes.

Some people who smoke ultimately get one or more chronic diseases of the lungs, such as **bronchitis** or **emphysema.** Bronchitis is familiar to most people as inflammation of the bronchi, which become infected and clogged with heavy mucus; the irritation causes deep, harsh coughing and wheezing. Bronchitis, which develops in virtually all cigarette smokers after about ten years, increases the smoker's susceptibility to other respiratory infections.[10]

Emphysema takes longer to develop than chronic bronchitis, but its effects are more devastating. Emphysema does not strike only smokers; people who live in smoggy cities or who are exposed to polluted air for other reasons (for example, coal miners or workers in smoky factories) may get it, too. A few genetically susceptible people will contract emphysema whether they smoke or not, but most get emphysema from smoking. At present, no reliable method exists to determine who is susceptible to emphysema.[11]

In contrast with Figure 11–2(A), which shows normal lung tissue, Figure 11–2(B) shows lung tissue damaged by emphysema. As you can see by comparing the two, the normal tissue is intricately laced with multitudes of tiny, bubblelike air sacs. These provide a huge surface across which oxygen and carbon dioxide can be exchanged. A tiny air tube leads to each little sac. As the lung expands, the sac expands and draws air in through the tube. As the lung deflates, the sac collapses and squeezes air back out.

In emphysema, the air sacs lose their intricate structure and balloon out to become empty pockets of air. (This is much like what happens when 50 tiny soap bubbles merge to form one big bubble.) These rigid, bulging pockets put pressure on the tubes that conduct air to and from them. As the lung expands, the pockets still draw air in, but as the lung deflates, the stiffened tissue around the air tubes shuts them down so that air can't escape. Bubbles of air are trapped in the lungs; they burst and tear lung tissue, making the pockets larger and more rigid, and creating more pressure. Thus lung damage occurs, not because people can't breathe in, but because they can't breathe out. Anyone who has seen exactly how the disease affects the lung tissue will never forget it.

The merging of the sacs also greatly reduces the surface area of the lungs available to absorb oxygen. Thus not only does emphysema make it hard to breathe, but each breath delivers less oxygen to the person panting for it.

You can get some idea of what it is like to try to breathe with emphysema-damaged lungs if you run up a long flight of stairs and then clamp a wet towel over your nose and mouth. You are out of breath, your chest is heaving, but you cannot get enough air. The person with emphysema pants for oxygen 30 times a minute at rest, compared with the normal adult's 20 times, but never gets the satisfaction of taking a deep breath. It's a crippling, depressing, debilitating condition. It ruins the quality of life, and ultimately it kills. Death in emphysema is from slow suffocation—or from heart failure, because the heart muscle itself is deprived of oxygen at the same time it is being given the signal to pump harder because the blood lacks oxygen.

Bronchitis, emphysema, and a few other diseases of the lungs are often termed **chronic obstructive pulmonary disease (COPD),** because less and less air flows in and out of the lungs. Smoking-related obstructive lung diseases such as bronchitis and emphysema kill an estimated 57,000 people a year in the United States. The Surgeon General concludes that ''the contribution of cigarette smoking to COPD death far outweighs all other factors.''[12]

Another disease of the lungs—cancer—is much more common in smokers than in nonsmokers. The carcinogens in cigarette smoke cause cancer not only in the lungs but also in the nose, lips, mouth, tongue, throat, and esophagus. Some of the carcinogens get into the bloodstream and travel elsewhere in the body, so they can cause cancer in any other organ as well; smokers have higher rates of bladder, pancreatic, and kidney cancer than nonsmokers (see Table 11–1). Lung cancer has now surpassed breast cancer as the leading killer among cancers in women, who are the victims of an ''epidemic of smoking.''[13] Evidence is mounting that cigarette smoking places men at risk for precancerous colon polyps and young women at risk for cervical cancer.[14] As a result of all this, cigarette smoking is the

chronic obstructive pulmonary disease (COPD) a collective term for several diseases that interfere with breathing; also known as *chronic obstructive lung disease (COLD).* Asthma, bronchitis, and emphysema are examples of COPD.

TABLE 11–1 ■ **The Risks of Smoking**

Disease	Smokers Increase Their Risk of Dying by
Lung cancer	7 to 15 times
Throat cancer	5 to 13 times
Oral cancer	3 to 15 times
Esophagus cancer	4 to 5 times
Bladder cancer	2 to 3 times
Pancreatic cancer	2 times
Kidney cancer	1½ times
Heart disease	1½ to 3 times
Emphysema and other chronic airway obstructions (excluding asthma)	10 to 20 times
Peptic ulcer diseases	2 times

[a]A person who smokes one pack of cigarettes or less per day assumes the risk at the lower end of the spectrum. Those who smoke more than a pack a day assume risks at the higher end. Most important, *the smoker assumes risks of all these diseases at the same time.*

SOURCE: Adapted from American Council on Science and Health, *Smoking or Health: It's Your Choice,* January 1984 (a report available from the American Council on Science and Health, 97 Maple St., Summit, NJ 06901).

major single cause of cancer mortality in the United States. Smoking inflicts higher rates of lung cancer on blacks than on any other population group in the country.[15]

Smoking combined with certain other factors creates a far greater hazard than smoking by itself. For example, the risk of developing cancer of the esophagus, lips, tongue, mouth, pharynx, or larynx increases dramatically for people who drink alcohol and smoke.[16] For another example, asbestos plus smoking add up to a deadly hazard. Asbestos by itself constitutes a lung cancer hazard; asbestos workers are 5 times more likely to contract lung cancer than are members of the general population. Smokers who do not work with asbestos are 10 times more likely. But people who both smoke and work with asbestos are 50 times more likely to contract lung cancer. Unfortunately, many asbestos workers do smoke.[17]

Smokers know that lung cancer is a risk, but many are sure it won't happen to them. Others believe that if cancer arises, x-ray tests can catch it in time to save their lives. Unfortunately, by the time a cancerous spot in the lung is only a millimeter across—just large enough to be seen on an X ray—it is already too late to stop it. (Chapter 19 offers more on cancer.)

≡▶   *Smoking cigarettes is associated with a multitude of health hazards: bronchitis; emphysema; chronic obstructive lung disease; and cancers of the lungs, nose, lips, mouth, tongue, throat, esophagus, bladder, pancreas, and kidney. Drinking alcohol and smoking intensifies the risk of cancer.*

The Heart and Circulatory System

Smoking is as damaging to the heart and circulatory system as it is to the lungs. It causes about one-fifth of all deaths from heart disease and stroke.[18] Smoking burdens the heart in five concurrent ways:

1. Nicotine stimulates epinephrine secretion, which speeds up the heart rate. This increases the heart's work load, so the smoker's heart requires more oxygen than does the nonsmoker's heart.
2. Epinephrine also raises the blood pressure, and the heart has to push blood around the body against this pressure. This, too, increases the heart's work load and requirement for oxygen.
3. Simultaneously, smoking reduces the amount of oxygen the blood can carry. Every time the smoker inhales, the blood receives a dose of **carbon monoxide** from the smoke. The carbon monoxide displaces oxygen from the protein hemoglobin in the red blood cells, forming **carboxyhemoglobin.** This reduces the red blood cells' ability to transport oxygen, and thus reduces the heart muscle's oxygen supply.
4. Nicotine also damages tiny particles in the blood, called **platelets,** and promotes the formation of clots. When clots lodge in arteries that feed the heart muscle, they kill portions of that muscle—heart attacks. When they lodge in arteries that feed the brain, they kill parts of the brain—strokes.
5. Conclusive research shows that smoking drastically reduces the blood flow in the heart's own major arteries, the coronary arteries. When this effect is severe enough, the result is heart attack.[19]

It is ironic that the two major ingredients of cigarettes, nicotine and tars, damage the body's two major life-support systems. Tars reduce the lungs'

carbon monoxide   a gas formed when oxidation or burning of carbon compounds is not complete enough to form the normal waste product, carbon dioxide.

carboxyhemoglobin (car-BOX-ee-HE-mo-gloh-bin)   a compound formed when carbon monoxide displaces oxygen on hemoglobin.

platelet (PLATE-let)   a tiny particle in the blood, important in blood clotting.

ability to supply oxygen; nicotine increases the heart's need for it. (Chapter 18 offers more on heart disease.)

≡▶ *Smoking burdens the heart and circulatory system in several ways. Smoking reduces the body's ability to supply oxygen while increasing the heart's needs for it. Smoking is directly associated with heart disease.*

Other Effects of Smoking

Smoking damages other organs besides the lungs and the heart. In fact, it harms every organ. Smoking:

- Shuts down circulation in capillaries, causing cold hands and feet and wrinkling of skin, and in some cases, necessitating amputation of limbs.[20]
- Increases risks of ulcers and makes dying from ulcers more likely.[21]
- Increases the body's drug tolerance, requiring larger doses for illness and pain, and rendering vaccinations ineffective.
- Interacts with oral contraceptives so as to greatly increase risks of heart attack and stroke (see Figure 11–3).
- In pregnancy, deprives developing fetuses of oxygen, resulting in smaller babies, premature births, spontaneous abortions (fetal deaths), and increased risks of infants' dying early in life.[22]
- Impairs fertility and estrogen production in women; causes early menopause, increased bone loss, and osteoporosis.[23]
- Reduces oxygen supply to the brain, impairing memory.[24]
- Thickens mucus, increasing the risk of chronic **sinusitis** (painful infection of the sinuses). The infection can spread to the brain and spinal cord—a life-threatening condition.
- Suppresses immunity by altering the numbers and actions of white blood cells and by affecting the chemistry of the antibodies, making colds and flu likely.
- Interferes with normal sleep. (Quitters sleep better within three nights of quitting.)[25]
- Delivers radiation to the chest. (Smoking one and a half packs of cigarettes a day for one year delivers radiation equal to that from 300 chest X rays.[26])
- Increases the likelihood of abnormal sperm production.[27]
- Causes progressive hearing loss, in low sound frequencies.[28]
- Causes increased **plaque** formation on the teeth, with accompanying gum (periodontal) disease.[29]
- Is associated with an increased risk of leukemia.[30]

Beyond all these physiological effects is the matter of personal appearance. Besides wrinkling the skin, smoking causes bad breath and yellows the teeth. The smell of stale smoke clings to the smoker's hair, clothes, dwelling, and car, so people who find the smell unpleasant want to avoid both the person and the surroundings. Many nonsmokers refuse even to date people who smoke. Then there is the cost: at upwards of $2 a pack, smoking can cost the heavy smoker from $1,000 to $2,000 a year. Should you

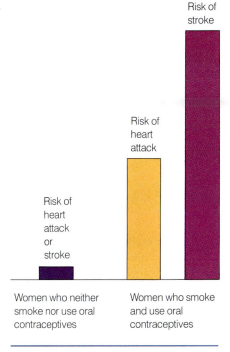

FIGURE 11–3 ■ **Smoking and oral contraceptives.**

sinusitis (sign-us-EYE-tus) infection of the sinuses, spaces in the bones of the skull.

■ *FACT OR FICTION:* Smoking wrinkles the skin. *True.*

plaque (PLAK) a buildup of material on a surface. Dental plaques build up on tooth enamel.

contribute that much to a personal pleasure fund instead, you could visit Hawaii every two years.

Finally, there is the danger of fire. Fires started by dropped or carelessly discarded cigarettes cause some 2,000 deaths and 4,000 injuries a year.[31] Altogether, smoking is the single greatest cause of preventable death in the United States today.

Despite the seemingly obvious hazards smoking presents, some smokers remain totally unaware that it increases risks. One poll showed that 13 to 17 percent of smokers don't know that cigarette smoking is hazardous at all, even though cigarette packages carry warnings. A survey of more than 15,000 high school seniors revealed that nearly one-third did not perceive any great risk associated with smoking.[32] Especially distressing is that nearly half of all teenagers are unaware that nicotine is an addictive drug. Children see adults smoking and think that smoking is OK.

Low-tar, low-nicotine cigarettes are no better than the regular cigarettes just described. Studies of smokers who switch to them show that some compensate for the reduction of tar and nicotine by smoking more cigarettes, smoking to a shorter butt, puffing more frequently, or inhaling more deeply. Studies of women who smoke low-yield cigarettes show that they incur the same risks of heart attack as smokers of regular cigarettes.[33]

Pipe smoking also presents unacceptable risks. Pipe smokers who do not inhale tend to have lower rates of lung cancer, emphysema, and heart disease than do cigarette smokers, but they are susceptible to cancers of the lips and tongue. People who switch from cigarettes to pipes tend to inhale more smoke, and thus have higher blood levels of nicotine than people who have smoked only pipes.[34] Pipe smoke is higher in tar than cigarette smoke, so the risk of lung cancer from pipes may actually be higher than from cigarettes.[35]

Quitting altogether is clearly the best alternative. The sooner, the better, too. The risk of heart attack in both men and women declines rapidly and approaches the nonsmoker's risk within a few years. The risk of dying from lung cancer declines steadily in people who quit smoking; after ten years of abstinence, the risk is about half of that for continuing smokers.[36] In short, people who quit smoking live longer than those who continue to smoke. Still, reducing the number or the strength of the cigarettes smoked is preferable to doing nothing. The less a person smokes, the smaller the risks. Every cigarette counts.

≡▶ *Smoking harms every organ of the body. It is the single greatest cause of preventable death in the United States today. During pregnancy, smoking harms the developing fetus and increases the risk of the infant's dying early in life. Smoking wrinkles skin; yellows teeth; causes bad breath; makes clothes, skin, hair, and surroundings smell bad; and is expensive.*

■≡ Passive Smoking

Does environmental tobacco smoke, or passive smoking, cause lung cancer? In 1981, the *British Medical Journal* published the first major report that said yes: spouses of people who smoked had an increased risk of dying of lung cancer. A hullabaloo arose; the tobacco industry claimed that the study was

---

Warnings required by law on cigarette packages:

SURGEON GENERAL'S WARNING: Smoking causes lung cancer, heart disease, emphysema, and may complicate pregnancy.

SURGEON GENERAL'S WARNING: Quitting smoking now greatly reduces serious risks to your health.

SURGEON GENERAL'S WARNING: Smoking by pregnant women may result in fetal injury, premature birth, and low birth weight.

SURGEON GENERAL'S WARNING: Cigarette smoke contains carbon monoxide.

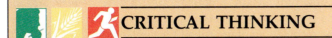

CRITICAL THINKING

Destructive Double Messages

Smoking, the very habit children need most to be warned against, is promoted to them as something that will make them grown up, cool, and "in." Robert Keeshan, TV's Captain Kangaroo, remembers as a 17-year-old U.S. Marine being told by his buddies that if he did not smoke cigarettes, he was not a real Marine. "I wanted to be just like John Wayne," he says, "and so I started smoking cigarettes. It took me 25 years to grow up and break the habit."[37]

To counter the images advertisers promote, Keeshan has introduced into his programs a campaign entitled "Smoking—YUCK!" Many more such efforts are needed. A suggested warning on cigarette packages might be the following: "TEENAGERS: Smoking is addictive. Never starting means never having to try to quit."

In contrast to the glamorous, cool, healthy images advertisers use to promote smoking and tobacco use, hard reality reveals these habits as unglamorous, uncool, and unhealthy. A user's body is neither fit nor beautiful; it is debilitated, weakened, aged, and unappealing. See through double messages. No matter what they say, smoking is unattractive and dangerous.

Shoot down tobacco ads by recognizing their lies and double messages.

invalid, but a follow-up study, reported in 1983, confirmed that the spouses of cigarette smokers have a 60 percent higher risk of lung cancer than the spouses of nonsmokers.[38] In 1986, the U.S. surgeon general and the National Academy of Sciences reviewed the evidence and reached similar conclusions: environmental tobacco smoke, or passive smoking by nonsmokers, causes disease in healthy adults and children.[39] Smokers do indeed expose their living and working companions to a deadly hazard. You may choose not to smoke, but if you live with a smoker, you are a smoker, too—an involuntary, passive smoker.

Passive smoking raises not only cancer risks, but also the risks of heart disease. Nonsmokers who live with smokers are subject to both short-term and long-term insults to their hearts and circulatory systems. For example, passive smoking reduces exercise tolerance in both healthy individuals and those with existing heart disease, probably because it reduces blood flow to the heart. Passive smoking also raises heart attack risk in the long term.[40]

In many ways besides cancer and heart disease risk, living or working with a smoker creates a hazard for the nonsmoker. It worsens allergic symptoms, asthma, and sinus conditions. Smoking irritates the eyes, especially if contact lenses are worn, and causes headaches, dizziness, and nausea. Smoking near children doubles their risks of pneumonia or bronchitis (up to age one), causes permanent lung damage, and brings on asthma attacks. The infant born to a woman who lived with a smoker during her pregnancy faces many of the same risks as the infant born to a woman who smoked, herself, during pregnancy. These risks include stillbirths, death in the first

■ *FACT OR FICTION:* To live with a smoker is to invite the risk of lung cancer. *True.*

six weeks of life, low birthweight, a doubled risk of birth defects, and impaired mental and physical development up to age 11. So there is no question about it: other people's smoking is bad for nonsmokers. In fact, 53,000 deaths a year are attributed to passive smoking, making it the third leading preventable cause of death in the United States, behind active smoking and alcohol.[41]

The harm to passive smokers comes from sidestream smoke, which contains 40 known carcinogens as well as other compounds. One of its gases is carbon monoxide, and in a closed room with smokers, this may raise the amount of carboxyhemoglobin in a nonsmoker's blood fivefold. Figure 11–4 shows the levels of carbon monoxide considered acceptable for human exposure and the amounts that a person may be exposed to in the presence of people who are smoking. (A hazard of sitting in idling traffic, as you probably know, is the high concentration of carbon monoxide emitted from the exhaust pipes of the surrounding cars. And as you also know, a person who inhales these fumes in a closed car dies within minutes. Carbon monoxide has no smell, so it can't be detected, but one sign of exposure is yawning.)

A nonsmoking section in any closed space contains just as much carbon monoxide as the smoking section, because carbon monoxide is a gas and diffuses rapidly and freely. Proper ventilation could disperse the carbon monoxide but is lacking in airplanes and many workplaces. Thus many nonsmokers rightly demand that smoking not be permitted in environments

FIGURE 11–4 ■ **Carbon monoxide sources compared.**

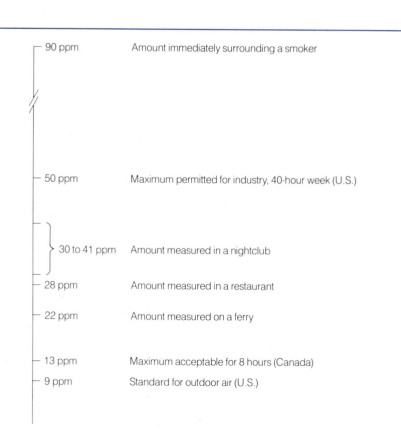

90 ppm — Amount immediately surrounding a smoker

50 ppm — Maximum permitted for industry, 40-hour week (U.S.)

30 to 41 ppm — Amount measured in a nightclub

28 ppm — Amount measured in a restaurant

22 ppm — Amount measured on a ferry

13 ppm — Maximum acceptable for 8 hours (Canada)

9 ppm — Standard for outdoor air (U.S.)

they share with smokers. Thanks to the efforts of nonsmokers' rights associations, many restaurants now forbid all smoking, and a federal law bans smoking on all domestic airline flights.* Almost every state restricts smoking on public transportation and in hospitals, elevators, schools, and libraries, and many workplaces also limit smoking.)

If you object to people's smoking near you, you can practice asserting yourself. Without being aggressive or insulting to the smoker, simply say, "Please don't smoke. It bothers me."

≡▶ *Passive smoking raises the involuntary smoker's risk of cancer, heart disease, and all other associated risks. Passive smoking is the third leading cause of preventable death in the United States.*

■≡ Smokeless Tobacco

Some people use **smokeless tobacco** products—snuff or chewing tobacco. Snuff dipping involves placing and retaining a pinch of moist, shredded tobacco between the gum and cheek, where it gradually releases its nicotine. The user salivates heavily and spits out the contaminated saliva at intervals. Snuff is also available as a dry powder that is inhaled. The moist variety is the most popular form of snuff in the United States. Chewing tobacco comes in two forms: loose leaf and plug. As its name implies, loose leaf chew is loose in the container or pouch it comes in. Plug chewing tobacco is sold in pressed or cake form. Both types are held in the cheek in a wad or **quid.**[42]

The use of smokeless tobacco by high school athletes is on the rise. Although most young users are aware of the health risks, as many as one out of three high school athletes has tried or used smokeless tobacco.[43]

Smokeless tobacco products produce the same dependency as smoked products, because they deliver the addictive drug nicotine just as cigarettes do. Users attain the same blood concentrations of nicotine.[44] Laboratory studies on both human beings and animals have shown that such products alter mood, are self-administered voluntarily, and are sought repeatedly, as are other addictive drugs.

The tobacco industry introduces smokeless tobacco products to new users just as dealers introduce illegal drugs. A typical advertisement for a smokeless tobacco product suggests: Use this sparingly at first, because it will irritate the gums. After a few weeks, the irritation will decrease. Start slowly and increase exposure over time, because, as with alcohol, it takes time to get accustomed to strong products and large doses.[45] (The person who is alert to double messages will recognize that this one says the product is dangerous.)

Smokeless tobacco use is linked to health problems ranging from minor mouth sores to cancer. Snuff dipping is associated with cancerous tumors in the nasal cavity, cheek, gum, and throat. Tobacco chewing incurs a *greater* risk of mouth cancer than does tobacco smoking. Cancer-causing compounds called nitrosamines in snuff and chewing tobacco can occur at concentrations

smokeless tobacco tobacco used for snuff or chewing rather than for smoking.

quid a small portion of any form of smokeless tobacco.

■ *FACT OR FICTION:* One effective way to reduce the risk of cancer from smoking is to switch from cigarettes to chewing tobacco or snuff. *False.* The risks of cancer of the mouth and throat are greater for people using smokeless tobacco products than for smokers.

*The national U.S. organization is Americans for Nonsmokers' Rights, 2054 University Ave., Suite 500-H, Berkeley, CA 94704. The Canadian organization is the Non-Smoker's Rights Association, 455 Spadina Ave., Suite 426A, Toronto, Ontario M55 2G8, Canada.

1,000 times the limits the government allows in foods.[46] Moderate users of smokeless tobacco products have a fourfold increase in the risk of developing oral cancer; heavy users have a sevenfold increase compared with nonusers. One of baseball's legends, Babe Ruth, was a heavy user of snuff and chewing tobacco; he died of throat cancer at the age of 52.

The dentist who examines a person's mouth for signs of oral cancer looks for **leukoplakia**—whitish or greyish patches of cells that form in the mouths of tobacco chewers and tend to become cancerous. They develop where the quid is held.

Smokeless tobacco presents its users with a unique problem: it is not always convenient or socially acceptable to spit out the contaminated saliva. At such times, some users swallow it, exposing their digestive tracts and all body systems to the entire contents. Others refrain from chewing in such situations but yield to their nicotine cravings by bumming cigarettes, thus becoming addicted to smoking and subjecting themselves to the associated risks.

Less lethal drawbacks to tobacco chewing and snuff dipping include bad breath, discolored teeth, and blunted senses of smell and taste. Tobacco chewing also makes the gums recede, wears the tooth surfaces, and destroys the supporting bones, so that in later life loss of teeth becomes likely.

≡▶ *Smokeless tobacco produces an addiction to the drug nicotine. These health problems are associated with smokeless tobacco: mouth sores and cancerous tumors of the mouth, nasal cavity, cheek, gum, and throat. Users of smokeless tobacco often become smokers. Smokeless tobacco causes bad breath and discolored teeth.*

■≡ The Decision to Quit

A smoker who couldn't quit asked a successful quitter how to do it. The quitter replied, "I just got my inner self and my outer self together. When they had completely agreed that we should quit, we did. It was easy."

What makes a person ready to take a major step like this? It seems to be different things for different people. For example, one man could not quit smoking until the night his young daughter said to him, "Daddy, I don't want to kiss you anymore because your breath smells."[47] Over 30 million people in the United States have quit in the last 20 years or so, and many teenagers are deciding not to start. Of people who still smoke, nine out of ten would like to stop but say they "can't." Still, people do arrive at the decision point, and once they are there, they can use some of the following information. The next section is written in terms of "you," to personalize the presentation. It is addressed to smokers, but it might apply to the users of smokeless tobacco as well.

How to Quit Smoking

Kicking the smoking habit is famous for being difficult to do. A newspaper columnist invited his smoking readers to explain why they persisted in using cigarettes. He expected a flood of angry letters scolding him for his strong antismoking stance and praising the pleasures of smoking. Instead, he received many letters like this one:

leukoplakia (loo-koh-PLAKE-ee-uh)   whitish or greyish patches in the mouth that develop in response to exposure to tobacco and indicate a probability that cancer will follow.

Warnings required by law on smokeless tobacco products:

WARNING: This product may cause oral cancer.

WARNING: This product may cause gum disease and tooth loss.

WARNING: This product is not a safe alternative to cigarettes.

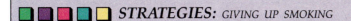

STRATEGIES: *GIVING UP SMOKING*

To give up smoking:

1. Ask yourself whether *you* really want to quit.
2. Believe in your ability to succeed.
3. Review the health benefits of quitting smoking.
4. Expect to be challenged.
5. Plan your strategy.
6. Find new ways to relax.
7. Make a list of alternative activities; prepare to engage in them.
8. Commit yourself.
9. Seek support.
10. Tune in to the immediate rewards.

Don't refer to what we do as "smoking"—refer to it as "nicotine addiction." Don't refer to "quitting"—refer to "nicotine detoxification." Nobody really likes smoking all that much. It's the nicotine surges that we get hooked on. I am trying to quit. Detoxification is truly the most difficult thing I've ever experienced—and I haven't had a particularly uneventful life. If I give in to the addiction, I know I'll die with a cigarette in my hand.[48]

In other words, people don't continue smoking because they want to, but because they are hooked. Whenever they try to quit, they face withdrawal: irritability, restlessness, anxiety, and of course, a craving for nicotine. Nicotine withdrawal symptoms usually peak within one to two days of cessation and gradually subside over the next two to four weeks.[49]

Quitting is hard. Before you start, ask yourself whether *you* really want to do it. Research shows that successful quitters are really ready to quit; they are doing it for themselves, not for anyone else.[50] Then look at the "Strategies: Giving Up Smoking," for a preview of what is ahead.

Successful quitters believe they can succeed. They are confident they can resist the urge to smoke. With each day's success they gain more confidence and resist more easily. Remind yourself again and again of the health benefits—both immediate and long term—that you gain when you stop smoking. Smoking cuts life short by an average of 18 years. The truth is, there just are not many 85-year-old smokers—they died many years before.

Be prepared for obstacles along the way—especially the nicotine withdrawal symptoms. Knowing and expecting that you will be challenged—especially at first—can help you rise to the challenge successfully. Also, analyze your smoking style to find out what kinds of pleasures smoking gives you. This chapter's Life Choice Inventory enables you to identify the ones you especially value—stimulation, handling the cigarette, relaxation, or others. When you quit, pay special attention to meeting those needs in other ways. The Life Choice Inventory also offers suggestions for each type of smoker.

For many people, smoking is one way to relax. Your chances of quitting successfully improve, then, if you find new ways to relax. A long, hot bath or some light stretching may help release tension (see Chapter 4 for more on relaxation, and Chapter 7 for stretching exercises.)

■ *FACT OR FICTION:* Most people who successfully quit smoking do it for their family and friends. *False.* Successful quitters do it for themselves.

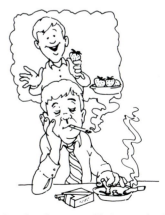

Imagine the pleasures of being smoke-free.

LIFE CHOICE INVENTORY

Why do you smoke? (If you don't smoke, this quiz may help you understand a friend or acquaintance who does.) Here are some statements people make to describe what they get out of smoking cigarettes. How often do you feel this way when smoking? Circle one number for each statement. Important: *Answer every question.*

		Always	Frequently	Occasionally	Seldom	Never
A.	I smoke cigarettes to keep myself from slowing down.	5	4	3	2	1
B.	Handling a cigarette is part of the enjoyment of smoking.	5	4	3	2	1
C.	Smoking cigarettes is pleasant and relaxing.	5	4	3	2	1
D.	I light up a cigarette when I feel angry about something.	5	4	3	2	1
E.	When I have run out of cigarettes, I find it almost unbearable until I can get more.	5	4	3	2	1
F.	I smoke cigarettes without being aware of it.	5	4	3	2	1
G.	I smoke cigarettes to stimulate myself, to perk myself up.	5	4	3	2	1
H.	Part of the enjoyment of smoking a cigarette comes from the steps I take to light up.	5	4	3	2	1
I.	I find cigarettes pleasurable.	5	4	3	2	1
J.	When I feel upset, I light up a cigarette.	5	4	3	2	1
K.	When I'm not smoking, I am very much aware of it.	5	4	3	2	1
L.	I light up a cigarette without realizing I still have one burning in the ashtray.	5	4	3	2	1
M.	I smoke cigarettes to give myself a lift.	5	4	3	2	1
N.	When I smoke a cigarette, part of the enjoyment is watching the smoke as I exhale it.	4	3	2	1	
O.	I want a cigarette most when I am comfortable and relaxed.	5	4	3	2	1
P.	When I feel blue, I smoke cigarettes.	5	4	3	2	1
Q.	I crave a cigarette when I haven't smoked for a while.	5	4	3	2	1
R.	I've sometimes found a cigarette in my mouth and don't remember putting it there.	5	4	3	2	1

When you want to reach for a cigarette, you may find it helpful to reach for a list of substitute activities instead. Sit down ahead of time and make this list.

Now, commit yourself. There are two ways to quit—tapering off or quitting all at once ("cold turkey"). A way to taper off is to start smoking each

continued
How to score:

1. Enter the numbers you have circled for each question on the lines below.

_____ + _____ + _____ = _____ Stimulation.
   A   G   M

_____ + _____ + _____ = _____ Handling.
   B   H   N

_____ + _____ + _____ = _____ Pleasure/relaxation.
   C   I   O

_____ + _____ + _____ = _____ Crutch/tension reduction.
   D   J   P

_____ + _____ + _____ = _____ Craving/psychological dependence.
   E   K   Q

_____ + _____ + _____ = _____ Habit.
   F   L   R

2. Add up your scores. For example, the sum of the numbers on lines A, G, and M gives you your score on Stimulation; lines B, H, and N, your score on Handling; and so on. Scores can vary from 3 to 15. Any score 11 or above is high; any score 7 or below is low. The higher your score, the more important this source of satisfaction is to you. When you give up smoking, you will have to find another way to get this satisfaction:

□ *Stimulation.* Safe substitutes are brisk walking or other moderate exercise.
□ *Handling.* Toy with a pen or pencil. Try doodling. Play with a coin, a piece of jewelry, or plastic straws.
□ *Pleasure/relaxation.* Substitute chewing gum, healthful snacks or beverages, and social or physical activities.
□ *Crutch/tension reduction.* Physical exertion, healthful snacks or beverages, chewing gum, or social activity may help in times of tension.
□ *Craving/psychological dependence.* Isolate yourself completely from cigarettes until the craving is gone—or use nicotine gum as described later in the chapter. Giving up cigarettes may be so hard and cause so much discomfort that once you do quit, you will find it easy to resist the temptation to go back to smoking. If you do start smoking again, you know that someday you will have to go through the same agony again.
□ *Habit.* It may be easy to quit if you can break your habit patterns. Become aware of each cigarette you smoke. Ask yourself, "Do I really want this cigarette?" You may be surprised at how many you do not want.

You must make two important decisions: (1) whether to try to do without the satisfactions you get from smoking or find an appropriate, less hazardous substitute and (2) whether to try to cut out cigarettes all at once or taper off. Your scores should guide you in making both these decisions.

SOURCE: Adapted from Test III of the Smoker's Self-Testing Kit developed by Daniel H. Horn, Ph.D., and originally printed by the U.S. Department of Health, Education, and Welfare, National Clearinghouse for Smoking and Health, HEW publication no. (NIH) 79–1822, 1979. The wording of the test interpretation has been edited.

day an hour later than you did the day before. Another is to take up a fitness activity that will squeeze the smoking out of your days; in fact, such a choice can even lead someone to quit without initially intending to do so. The person takes up jogging, discovers that smoking limits endurance, cuts down on smoking, experiences the reward of improved performance, and ultimately cuts out smoking altogether. Another motivator is to start spending time with someone who doesn't smoke or to take a job in a nonsmoking company. The more time you spend not smoking, the more apparent the rewards will be.

While tapering off works well for some people, most are more successful quitting cold turkey, because the difficult part passes more quickly. Two weeks after quitting, people who quit cold turkey have fewer and less intense cravings for cigarettes than those who cut back gradually. If you plan to quit cold turkey:

■ Promise yourself that you will not smoke at all for a week, even if the sky falls. More than a week is too much to handle; less would make it too tempting to fall back.

■ Inform everyone who is close to you. This puts your reputation at stake; you will lose face if you break your word.

■ Get a friend to quit with you. Make a friendly wager, agree to celebrate each week, call each other, or agree on other ways of giving each other support.

■ Ask for special consideration at first, in case you're irritable (or get your health care provider or a friend to ask in your behalf). You'll need it.

■ Keep busy—very busy—in whatever way you can. After two weeks, you can begin to relax and let down your guard.

■ If you do smoke, don't smoke just one. Smoke a whole pack in rapid succession; make yourself sick with smoking so that you will want to quit again.

Now, start noticing the immediate rewards. At first, you will be keenly conscious of the craving to resume smoking. You will have to fight the temptation to light up again. Tuning in to the pleasures of *not* smoking will raise the odds in favor of success. Quitters list small and big pleasures:

■ I can breathe again—deep breaths of clean air.
■ I don't have to carry cigarettes and matches wherever I go.
■ The guilt is gone. I can look my friends and family members in the eye.
■ Foods taste better, and I can smell flowers again.
■ My breath, clothes, and hair don't smell like smoke anymore.
■ I don't get out of breath so quickly when I walk.
■ I can talk on the phone without panicking if my cigarettes are out of reach.
■ There are no dirty ashtrays around me.
■ I'm not burning holes in my clothes anymore.
■ I have more money to spend on other things.
■ That attractive nonsmoker who sits next to me in class has started showing interest in me.

No matter why you decided to quit, what makes you persevere is that you feel better after only two or three days: better physically, and better about yourself.

Whenever you crave a smoke, breathe deeply. Pantomime the smoking process. Relax. You can have all the pleasures of smoking a cigarette, except the cigarette. You may find that what you really want is a moment of relaxation and a deep breath, not a cigarette after all.

When you feel like reaching for a smoke, reach for the radio instead, or for the telephone, to make a date with a friend. And take up some form of

12 THINGS TO DO INSTEAD OF SMOKING CIGARETTES.

Jump. Swim. Smell. Play. Dance. Ride. Listen. Talk. Sing. Jog. Draw. Nothing.

American Cancer Society

physical activity that will get your heart and lungs in shape again: hiking, skiing, aerobic dance, swimming, or the like. Great pleasure comes from the rapid recovery of breathing that occurs early in a training program for the person who has just quit smoking: "The first day, I could swim across the pool only once, and then I was panting. Now, only three days later, I can swim six lengths and still feel like doing more."

If you can't make it alone, or if you don't choose to, you can get help. Classes are offered by Smokenders, the American Cancer Society, the American Lung Association, and the American Heart Association. A class can

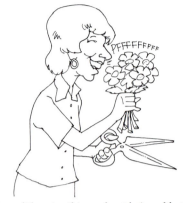

One of the nice things about being able to breathe is that you can smell things.

help you identify your smoking style and tailor your quitting strategy accordingly.

You may be afraid that if you quit, you will gain weight. Some people actually lose weight, but most quitters do gain—usually about 4 to 5 pounds, but sometimes more—for two reasons. One is psychological: smoking is an oral behavior, and to cope with the stress of giving it up, some smokers turn to another oral behavior, eating. The other reason is physiological: the enzymes that store fat are less active in smokers, and they resume normal activity when smokers quit.[51] But you don't have to gain. If you wish to prevent weight gain:

■ Diet at first, until your smoke-free life and weight have both stabilized.
■ Drink lots of liquids, especially water, sparkling water, iced tea, diet beverages, and low-calorie fruit juices, in place of smoking. The liquid will help fill you up; excreting it will help rid your body of toxins from smoking; and the sweetness will please your recovering awareness of sweet tastes.
■ If you crave sweet or crunchy things, eat fruits or low-calorie vegetables instead of candy or chips.
■ Add physical activity to your daily routine. Now that you can breathe again, activity will both bring you pleasure and help to keep your weight down.

If you do gain a few pounds, it's worth it, to give up cigarettes. Once you are secure in being an ex-smoker, you can take the weight off; Chapter 6 offers more on how to do this. Others have done it; you can, too.

Nicotine-containing gum is an aid available to smokers as a stepping-stone to freedom from smoking. This gum, available by prescription, delivers the same amount of nicotine as two or three cigarettes. The user must make a firm commitment to stop smoking and to chew the gum instead, at the rate of about six to eight pieces a day. The instructions say to chew each piece slowly, making it last a half-hour or more, thus delivering nicotine to the body at a steady rate. When chewing the gum, it is best to drink no beverage but water. Coffee, cola, and other beverages interfere with nicotine absorption.[52]

After several weeks of using the gum, the user will have lost all the habits associated with smoking: handling the cigarettes, lighting them, puffing on them, and so forth. Now (the theory goes) it will be relatively easy to taper off the use of the gum, since nicotine addiction is the only problem left. Nicotine-containing gum proves successful in a significant number of cases.

≡▶ *The smoker must make a firm decision to quit smoking. Many programs and strategies are available to help a determined smoker quit. Quitting is not easy, but the rewards of a smoke-free life are worth the work.*

How to Help the Smoker Quit

What if you are a sympathetic bystander who wants to help a smoker quit? First, you must realize that smokers can quit only when they are ready. Your job, then, is to help them get ready. You cannot force them to quit.

The key to effective helping is "tough love"—a term borrowed from alcoholism treatment. The idea is this: if you really care about a person, you will not keep quiet about a dangerous habit. Assert yourself. Confront the person. At the same time, show that you care, and make the distinction

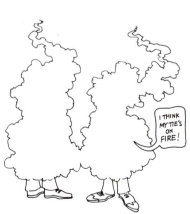

Another reward is that you don't burn holes in your clothes anymore.

clear: it is the behavior you reject, not the person. Express concern about the risks of the behavior. Express your dislike of the habit itself. Offer whatever information comes your way—research news on the effects of smoking and the benefits of quitting. Identify reasons appropriate to the listener: tell the high school student, for example, that smoking impairs sports performance and that it is unattractive.

Do not be surprised, though, if the smoker does not "hear" these messages. The person is committed to smoking, at least at present. The person ignores health warnings, giving only lip service to their existence: "Yes, I know." If the person continues to smoke, then protect your own health. Insist, "Don't smoke around me," and let it go. Don't be discouraged. You may think your efforts have been in vain, but they may have been gradually tipping the scale in favor of health. One day, the last piece will be added, and the person will quit.

Employers can help by prohibiting smoking on the job or refusing to hire smokers at all. This may seem unfair to the smoker, but it is fair to nonsmokers, protects their health, and is legal. Studies show that smokers take more breaks and are absent from work more often than nonsmokers.[53] Magazines, films, and other mass communicators can help by refusing to advertise tobacco—a decision that takes courage, because advertising is so profitable. Even children can help, by asking parents who smoke to stop.

Many organizations have mounted opposition to the marketing and sales of tobacco—cancer societies; medical, lung, and heart associations; and others. The American Council on Science and Health has been especially effective, in part by conducting a campaign against the many magazines that advertise cigarettes. The council points out that, because these magazines accept advertising money, they are under pressure not to publish information on the hazards of smoking, a phenomenon the council calls "the conspiracy of silence."*

Many agencies share in working toward the goal of a smoke-free society by the year 2000. Many communities have passed no-smoking ordinances, and laws on advertising are getting stricter. Although many people still smoke, and many young people are still starting, numbers of both are diminishing. The only group that opposes this trend is, of course, the tobacco industry.

≡▶ *If you want to help smokers quit, remember, smokers can quit only when they are ready. Express your concern for people who smoke and for their health. If they are not willing to quit, protect yourself by insisting that they do not smoke around you.*

In aggressively marketing tobacco, the industry is doing what any industry must do to be successful: maximizing profits and developing markets to foster its own growth. But unfortunately, to expand the market means having to persuade more people to use tobacco. This destroys health, so every effort the tobacco industry makes in this direction is unethical, and those who would promote health must directly oppose the tobacco industry's interests. The accompanying box, "Tobacco and Profits," reveals the global damage that results from the tobacco industry's efforts to promote tobacco sales both at home and abroad, and shows how your tax dollars support those efforts. The Spotlight that follows illustrates, among other things, an especially dramatic example of the tobacco industry's use of double messages to promote its interests at the expense of the nation's and the world's health.

*Write to the council at 47 Maple St., Summit, NJ 07901.

Tobacco and Profits

The tobacco industry is big business and represents immense financial interests, not only in the United States, but all across the world. Here are some of the facts on the worldwide marketing of tobacco:

■ Taxpayers' money supports the tobacco industry. Without tax dollars it could not exist.

■ The U.S. Department of Agriculture gives out millions of dollars in subsidies every year to support the growth of more tobacco than U.S. consumers can use. The excess is sold abroad.

■ In other countries, too, the U.S. government supports tobacco production, again using taxpayers' dollars.

■ The United States threatens to refuse to trade with countries that won't sell U.S. tobacco within their borders. This threat has forced Japan, Taiwan, and South Korea to import U.S. tobacco, and as a result, many more women and young people in those countries have started smoking. The cigarettes sold there are higher in tar and nicotine than those allowed domestically.

■ Tobacco is the most widely grown nonfood crop in 120 countries; they depend on the tobacco industry for their cash. They gain in dollars, but their health-care costs for smoking-related diseases are soaring. Also, tobacco-growing takes up land and labor that could be used to grow food for 10 to 20 million people. Labor for the production of tobacco is needed in spurts, diverting it from farms where it is needed continuously. As a result, food crops are neglected and fail, while laborers are out of work between times of working on tobacco crops.

■ Tobacco-growing costs the environment, too. To cure an acre of tobacco, the growers have to fell and burn an acre of trees; Malawi has already cut a third of its trees for this purpose. Tobacco-growing countries are suffering massive deforestation, which contributes to global warming (see Chapter 21). Fertilizers, herbicides, and pesticides spread on tobacco crops run into streams and rivers and work their way through whole ecosystems. Pests become resistant to pesticides used on tobacco, then attack food crops and cannot be controlled.

■ Globally, smoking causes 2.5 million deaths a year. Of those now alive, 500 million will be killed by tobacco.

What to do about all this? The American Medical Association (AMA) recommends the economic strategy known as divestment (the opposite of investment). Do not invest money in funds that include tobacco companies, and persuade your broker, credit union, college, church, synagogue, bank, city council, and all other businesses you deal with to take their money out of such funds.[a]

[a]Call the AMA's Tobacco Divestment Project at (617) 266–6130.

SOURCES: Information from C. B. Popescu, The Third World: Marlboro Country's final frontier, *ACSH News and Views*, May/June 1984, pp. 6–7; M. Barry, the influence of the U.S. tobacco industry on the health, economy, and environment of developing countries, *New England Journal of Medicine* 324 (1991): 917–920; K. E. Warner and G. N. Connolly, The global metastasis of the Marlboro man, *American Journal of Health Promotion*, May–June 1991, pp. 325–327.

◼≡ For Review

1. Describe how people get started smoking, why they continue, and why they find it hard to quit.

2. Describe the effects of nicotine on the body and the sensations associated with withdrawal.

3. Identify some of the substances in mainstream cigarette smoke, and describe some of their effects.

4. Describe some of the immediate effects of smoking on the lungs, the heart, and other organs.

5. Itemize some of the many long-term health hazards associated with smoking.

6. Describe the major health hazards smoking presents to women who smoke.

7. Cite some evidence that associates passive smoking with harm to health.

8. Compare the risks of cigarette smoking with those of pipe smoking, tobacco chewing, or snuff dipping.

9. Name some of the early rewards that can motivate a person to persist in the effort to quit smoking.

10. Describe strategies smokers can use to succeed in quitting and strategies people who care about them can use to help them quit.

◼≡ Notes

1. Smoking warning given, *Tallahassee Democrat,* June 1, 1990; more smokers listening to surgeon general's warnings, *Executive Fitness*, May 1989, p. 7.

2. Data are from the national surveys of roughly 17,000 high school seniors entitled "Monitoring the Future: A Continuing Study of the Lifestyles and Values of Youth," funded by the National Institute on Drug Abuse, conducted every spring since 1975, as cited by L. D. Johnston, P. M. O'Malley, and J. G. Bachman, Psychotherapeutic, licit, and illicit use of drugs among adolescents, *Journal of Adolescent Health Care* 8 (1987): 36–51.

3. All but the last two bulleted items are adapted from U.S. Department of Health and Human Services, *8 Reasons Young People Smoke,* HHS publication no. 200–75–0516 (Washington, D.C.: Government Printing Office, 1975); the fourth bulleted item also comes from S. Clayton, Gender differences in psychosocial determinants of adolescent smoking, *Journal of School Health* 61 (1991): 115–120.

4. Joseph Califano, former secretary of the U.S. Department of Health, Education, and Welfare, as cited in Smoking and health: A 25-year perspective (Editorial), *American Journal of Public Health* 79 (1989): 141–143.

5. O. F. Pomerleau and C. S. Pomerleau, Neuroregulators and the reinforcement of smoking: Toward a biobehavioral explanation, *Neuroscience and Biobehavioral Reviews* 8 (1984): 503–513.

6. W. Pollin, Tobacco: #1 drug of dependence, *World Smoking and Health* (an American Cancer Society journal), Summer 1983, pp. 45–46.

7. K. H. Ginzel, What's in a cigarette? *Priorities for Long Life and Good Health* (a publication of the American Council on Science and Health), Fall 1990, pp. 10–12.

8. Ginzel, 1990.

9. C. B. Popescu, Cigarettes' secret ingredients, *ACSH News and Views,* January/February 1983, pp. 1–3.

10. M. M. Lipman, Emphysema takes smokers' breath away, *Consumer Reports Health Letter,* September 1990, p. 70.

11. Lipman, 1990.

12. U.S. Department of Health and Human Services, Public Health Service, *The Health Benefits of Smoking Cessation: A Report of the Surgeon General* (Washington, D.C.: Government Printing Office, 1990): 279–366.

13. American Cancer Society: *Cancer Facts and Figures—1988* (New York: American Cancer Society, 1988).

14. S. H. Zahm, P. Cocco, and A. Blair, Tobacco smoking as a risk factor for colon polyps, *American Journal of Public Health* 81 (1991): 846–849; Women at risk, *University of California, Berkeley Wellness Letter,* February 1991.

15. C. T. Orleans and coauthors, A survey of smoking and quitting patterns among black Americans, *American Journal of Public Health* 79 (1989): 176–181.

16. K. Napier, Alcohol and tobacco: A deadly duo, *Priorities for Long Life and Good Health,* Spring 1990, pp. 6–7.

17. C. B. Popescu, Cigarettes and asbestos: A tale of two industries, *ACSH News and Views,* March/April 1983, pp. 1–3; Suit looks at effects of smoking on those exposed to asbestos, *Tallahassee Democrat,* 15 June 1988.

18. Smoking and health, 1989.

19. J. Barry and coauthors, Effect of smoking on the activity of ischemic heart disease, *Journal of the American Medical Association* 261 (1989): 398–402, 438.

20. D. Model, Smoker's face: An underrated clinical sign? *British Medical Journal* 291 (1985): 1760–

1762, as cited in U.S. Department of Health and Human Services, Public Health Service, *Health Benefits of Smoking Cessation,* 1990, pp. 427–468.

21. R. F. Anda and coauthors, Smoking and the risk of peptic ulcer disease among women in the United States, *Archives of Internal Medicine* 150 (1990): 1437–1441; U.S Department of Health and Human Services, *Reducing the Health Consequences of Smoking: 25 Years of Progress, A Report of the Surgeon General* (Washington, D.C.: Government Printing Office, 1989).

22. M. J. Stjernfeldt and coauthors, Maternal smoking during pregnancy and risk of childhood cancer, *Lancet,* 14 June 1986, pp. 1350–1351; B. Haglund and S. Cnattingus, Cigarette smoking as a risk factor for sudden infant death syndrome, *American Journal of Public Health* 80 (1990): 29–32; J. Coste, N. Job-Spira, and H. Fernandez, Increased risk of ectopic pregnancy with maternal cigarette smoking, *American Journal of Public Health* 81 (1991): 199–200.

23. F. S. Anderson, I. Transbol, and C. Christiansen, Is cigarette smoking a promoter of the menopause? *Acta Medica Scandinavica* 212 (1982): 137–139; Tobacco smoke may speed bone loss, *Health and Environment Digest,* March 1989, p. 6.

24. D. J. Weeks, Do chronic cigarette smokers forget people's names? *British Medical Journal,* 22–29 December 1979, p. 1627.

25. C. R. Soldatos and coauthors, Cigarette smoking associated with sleep difficulty, *Science* 207 (1980): 551–553.

26. Note what a cigarette packs in radiation (Correspondence), *New England Journal of Medicine* 307 (1982): 309–313; Radiation, smoking and lung cancer, *Health Gazette,* October 1989.

27. H. J. Evans and coauthors, Sperm abnormalities and cigarette smoking, *Lancet,* 21 March 1981, pp. 627–629.

28. A. S. Ibrahim and A. S. Fatt-hi, Cigarette smoking and hearing loss, *World Smoking and Health,* Summer 1982, pp. 42–45.

29. A. I. Ismail, B. A. Burt, and S. A. Eklund, Epidemiologic patterns of smoking and periodontal disease in the United States, *World Smoking and Health,* Spring 1985, pp. 14–15.

30. Smoking and leukemia, *Health Gazette,* December 1988.

31. Tobacco Institute: Cigarette fires human behavior problems, *Nation's Health,* October 1981.

32. Smoking in teens fails to decrease significantly, *Nation's Health,* April 1989.

33. J. R. Palmer, L. Rosenberg, and S. Shapiro, "Low yield" cigarettes and the risk of nonfatal myocardial infarction, *New England Journal of Medicine* 37 (1989): 1569–1573.

34. K. McCusker, E. McNabb, and R. Bone, Plasma nicotine levels in pipe smokers, *Journal of the American Medical Association* 248 (1982): 577–578; T. Pechacek and coauthors, Smoke exposure in pipe and cigar smokers: Serum thiocyanate levels, *Journal of the American Medical Association* 254 (1985): 3330–3332.

35. J. K. Ockene and coauthors, Does switching from cigarettes to pipes or cigars reduce tobacco smoke exposure? *American Journal of Public Health* 77 (1987): 1412–1416.

36. Heart risk drops in women ex-smokers, *Science News* 27 (1990): 55.

37. R. Keeshan, Children and smoking, in *Smoking and Health,* proceedings of a conference commemorating the 20th anniversary of the first Surgeon General's Report on Smoking and Health, 11 January 1984 (available from the American

Council on Science and Health, 47 Maple St., Summit, NJ 07901).

38. T. Hirayama, Passive smoking and lung cancer: Consistency of association, *Lancet,* 17 December 1983, pp. 1425–1426.

39. National Academy of Sciences, National Research Council, *Environmental Tobacco Smoke: Measuring Exposure and Assessing Health Effects* (Washington, D.C.: National Academy Press, 1986), as cited in S. A. Glantz and W. W. Parmley, Passive smoking and heart disease: Epidemiology, physiology, and biochemistry, *Circulation,* January 1991, pp. 1–12.

40. Glantz and Parmley, 1991.

41. Glantz and Parmley, 1991.

42. J. F. Wisniewski, G. R. Mohl, and D. M. Shedroff, Smokeless tobacco use by high school baseball players, *Health Education,* January 1990, pp. 10–15.

43. Wisniewski, Mohl, and Shedroff, 1990.

44. G. N. Connolly and coauthors, The reemergence of smokeless tobacco, *New England Journal of Medicine* 314 (1986): 1020–1027.

45. Connolly and coauthors, 1986.

46. Wisniewski, Mohl, and Shedroff, 1990.

47. Clearing the air: Make your environment smoke-free, *Executive Fitness,* November 1989.

48. Columnist Bob Greene of the *Chicago Tribune,* as quoted by B. Popescu, Dying for a cigarette? Help may be on the way, *ACSH News and Views,* September/October 1983, pp. 10–12.

49. Psychological and behavioral consequences and correlates of smoking cessation, in U.S. Department of Health and Human Services, Public Health Service, *Health Benefits of Smoking Cessation,* 1990, pp. 519–578.

50. Smoking cessation: Tips on how to kick the habit for good, *University*

of Texas Lifetime Health Letter, September 1990, pp. 4–5.

51. R. M. Carney and A. P. Goldberg, Weight gain after cessation of cigarette smoking: A possible role for adipose-tissue lipoprotein lipase, New England Journal of Medicine 310 (1984): 614–616.

52. Don't drink and chew this gum at the same time, Tufts University Diet and Nutrition Letter, December 1990, p. 1.

53. Help wanted: No smokers need apply, ACSH News and Views, September/October 1982, p. 7.

SPOTLIGHT

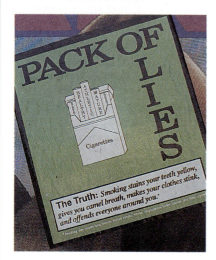

Tobacco Advertising and Ethics

Should tobacco companies be free to advertise products that are both addictive and deadly? The tobacco companies, of course, say yes—but the federal government, backed by a wide array of medical and health groups—is moving toward banning all advertising and promotion of tobacco products.

How do the opposing sides state their cases?

The tobacco companies argue that banning tobacco advertising would violate the Constitution's First Amendment—freedom of the press—which is central to the democratic way of life. They say that all viewpoints should be expressed, and that consumers should judge for themselves what may be harmful to them.

Opponents of tobacco advertising argue that the state should relieve consumers of the burden of choosing. Consumers cannot, they say, judge wisely for themselves.

The tobacco industry retorts that this smacks of totalitarianism. (In a totalitarian state, the state suppresses views it does not want its citizens to hear.)

Can the tobacco companies really demand freedom of the press for their advertisements? After all, their products harm people.

Yes they can, because freedom of the press protects the right to express opinions, and even misinformation. It withholds only the right to publish slander—that is, false information about a person that injures the person or damages the person's reputation.

Tobacco advertising is not slander; it simply implies that consumers will like the product. Tobacco ads make no health or safety claims, so they cannot be accused of telling lies. They are deceptive, because they glamorize tobacco use by portraying cigarette smokers as healthy, active people, but to deceive is not a crime. The law says, "Let the buyer beware": it is up to consumers to protect themselves against deception.

To promote its right to advertise its products, Philip Morris publishes its own magazine and also produces the *Great American Smoking Manual.* The manual provides smokers with arguing points such as this popular tobacco-industry contention: "Advertising does not induce smokers to start smoking." Philip Morris says that virtually any ban on advertising is a threat to the most basic right of Americans to exchange ideas. Philip Morris even enticed the National Archives to allow it to sponsor a

national tour for a display of the Bill of Rights as part of a sophisticated advertising campaign to improve its reputation.

But cigarette smoking is still becoming more unfashionable every day, isn't it?

Yes, and yet ironically, tobacco companies continue to thrive. They are even considered respectable businesses, because they channel some of their tremendous profits into hospitals, universities, churches, and charities, as well as into buying political influence and into "research" on tobacco's effects.

Did you say research? Are there still scientists who believe tobacco may not harm health?

Actually, no. Even the scientists who are being paid by the tobacco industry to do research agree that "smoking is an addiction that causes a wide range of serious, often fatal, diseases."[1]* The tobacco industry doesn't use their findings, but uses their activities to back the claim that research is still being done, and that conclusions as to the effects of tobacco have yet to be drawn.

How can these wily tactics be opposed?

Powerful groups are working on that. Groups such as the New York–based antitobacco activist group Doctors Ought to Care (DOC), the American Public Health Association, the American Council on Science and Health, and the American Medical Association (AMA) argue that the scientific case against cigarette smoking is firmly established.

*Reference notes are at the end of the Spotlight.

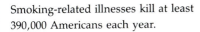

Smoking-related illnesses kill at least 390,000 Americans each year.

Is that working? Do tobacco companies admit that their products are harmful?

No, and in fact, they are still gearing their advertisements toward young people, encouraging them to smoke. As always, that strategy promotes harm to youngsters' future health, but favors the interest of the $30 billion tobacco industry that thrives on nicotine addiction.[2] In short, tobacco companies get away with murder.

Wow. One minute you're talking about deceptive advertising and the next, you're talking about murder. Is that accusation literally being debated seriously?

Yes, it is. A question that is central to the issue of tobacco advertising and ethics is, "Are tobacco companies liable for deaths caused by their products?" This question has already been put to the test in court, and the tobacco industry has lost a case. It was a product liability suit, in which the husband of a smoker who had smoked for 40 years and died of lung cancer alleged that three tobacco companies were responsible for his wife's death. The man was awarded $400,000.

That sounds like quite a victory for tobacco's opponents.

Actually, it was less of a victory than it appears. The $400,000 didn't begin to cover the nearly $3 million it cost to see the case through to a jury verdict. The case made it obvious to product liability lawyers that they cannot make money against opponents such as the tobacco industry, who have virtually unlimited resources. As a result, the number of product liability cases against tobacco companies has declined.

Is it possible to prove that smoking has caused a lung cancer death?

Not in individual cases, no. As you saw from the statistics in the chapter, smoking greatly increases the number of deaths from many kinds of diseases, so clearly it does cause individual deaths. But some nonsmokers die of these same diseases, too—so you can't tell whether a particular death was caused by smoking. The person might have died of the disease anyway.

That makes smoking deaths different from, say, accidental deaths caused by negligence in building maintenance. If an elevator cable breaks and Mr. C falls to his death, his family can sue the company for negligence. But suppose seven out of ten smokers die of lung cancer, and Mr. C is among them. Two would have died of cancer anyway, even if they had not smoked. The family cannot prove that Mr. C was one of the five whose deaths were caused by smoking; he might (though less probably) be one of the two who would have died of lung cancer anyway. This legal problem arises whenever statistical responsibility can be proved, but direct individual responsibility cannot be.

So how can tobacco's opponents keep the tobacco companies from "committing murder," as you say?

The group already mentioned, Doctors Ought to Care (DOC), is working on that. DOC first wants to convince lawmakers that smoking does cause deaths. It is conducting a campaign in which, each time a smoker dies of lung cancer, coronary artery disease, emphysema, or any other tobacco-related illness, the health care provider sends a black-bordered announcement of the death to the client's senator or representative. The announcement reads: "Dear __, I wish to inform you that one of your constituents, who was a patient of mine, has died. The death was due to the following disease: __. This person was a smoker. Tobacco smoking is the major avoidable cause of this disease." DOC even suggests that the health care provider fill in the brand name of the tobacco product used.[3]

DOC will thus have made its point that smoking does cause deaths, and it will have influenced lawmakers to at least consider banning or severely restricting tobacco advertising. A similar campaign, conducted in England in 1984, led to stringent restrictions on tobacco advertising.[4]

While the legal question is being debated, do the media have to accept tobacco ads?

No, they don't, and many magazines in fact no longer accept tobacco advertisements. This is brave, for advertising money is essential to the survival of the magazines. Among publications that refuse tobacco money are the *Reader's Digest*, the *New Yorker*, *Good Housekeeping*, *National Geographic*, and *Scientific American*. The result is that fewer people in their readerships are influenced to use tobacco, and these magazines are completely free of liability in relation to readers who are harmed by tobacco.

The Tobacco Divestment Project, a new force in the battle to end tobacco addiction, supports the simple proposition that "we should not place profits above the health and welfare of millions of citizens".[5] The Tobacco Divestment Project calls on public and nonprofit organizations to divest themselves of tobacco securities. For instance, among their victories, the City University of New York voted to sell $3.5 million of Philip Morris stock, noting that "owning stock in a company whose purpose is to addict to a lethal drug as many young people as possible calls our educational leadership into question."*

Well, at least they can't advertise tobacco on television any more.

That's true in theory, but the tobacco industry has found a way around that

*In case you missed it the first time, the telephone number of the Tobacco Divestment Project is 617–266–6130.

law. They sponsor motor races. Drivers and cars sporting logos for Marlboro, Winston, Philip Morris, Skoal, and other brands are all over the television screen throughout these popular sports programs. Millions of viewers see them, and whether they realize it consciously or not, the appearances work just as ads do, to make the products appear acceptable, to associate them with attractive people and exciting activities, and to persuade viewers to buy the products.[6] If we are serious about banning tobacco advertising from the screen, we will have to ban tobacco companies' promotions of sports events, too.

Is there any question about the way the First Amendment is being interpreted? Should it perhaps be used to forbid tobacco advertising after all?

Yes, the question is still being debated. Perhaps, if someone writes something that influences you to take action, and that *action* harms your health, the law should protect you from harming yourself. Where the harm is to the pocketbook, except in cases of slander, the courts have consistently held the position "let the buyer beware." But that position assumes that buyers are adults, supposedly capable of protecting themselves. In the case of tobacco ads, the people influenced are often children, incapable of making the necessary judgments to protect themselves. Furthermore, the harm is not only to financial well-being, but to health and life. The next few years should see some interesting new perspectives shed on this question by the courts.

■≡ Spotlight Notes

1. K. M. Cummings, R. Sciandra, A. Gingress, and R. Davis, What scientists funded by the tobacco industry believe about the hazards of cigarette smoking, *American Journal of Public Health* 81 (1991): 894–896.
2. L. C. White, The teflon coating of cigarette companies, *Priorities for Long Life and Good Health* (a publication of the American Council on Science and Health), Spring 1990, pp. 3–5.
3. Doctors Ought to Care (DOC) and Tobacco Products Liability Project (TPLP), law student essay competition (Advertisement), *The Nation* 243 (1986): 688.
4. DOC and TPLP, 1986.
5. B. S. Krevor, Tobacco divestment: A new front in the tobacco wars, *Priorities for Long Life and Good Health,* Fall 1990, pp. 37–39.
6. A. Blum, The Marlboro Grand Prix: Circumvention of the television ban on tobacco advertising, *New England Journal of Medicine* 324 (1991): 913–917.

CHAPTER 12

Intimacy, Pairing, and Commitment

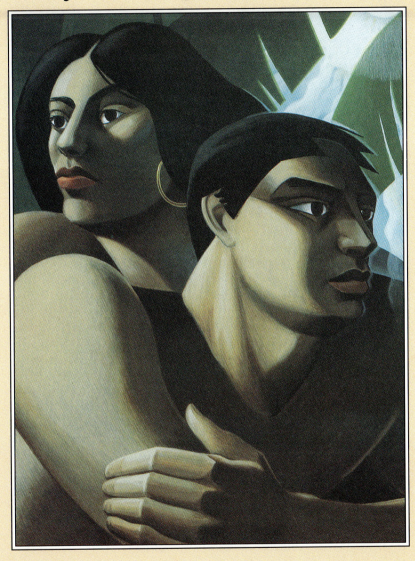

FACT OR FICTION

Just for fun, respond true or false to the following statements. If false, say what is true.

■ Having sex is being intimate. (Page 317)
■ Couples in healthy intimate relationships spend all their free time together. (Page 319)
■ Sexual activity begins early in healthy intimate relationships. (Page 321)
■ To cope with a breakup, it is beneficial to get into another relationship as soon as possible. (Page 327)

■ A man's ability to give pleasure is directly related to the size of his penis. (Page 335)
■ Good sexual technique is the most important quality in a satisfying love relationship. (Page 335)
■ Women must experience several orgasms during a lovemaking session in order to be satisfied. (Page 337)

sexuality refers to all aspects of being sexual. Sexuality involves all components of the total person: intellectual, emotional, social, spiritual and physical.

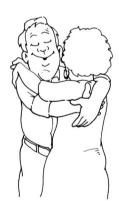

The need for physical affection may be even more basic than the need for sex.

primary sex characteristics the anatomical characteristics that distinguish the sexes at birth—primarily, the genital organs.

What comes to mind when you think of sexuality? Many people say sexual intercourse, but the sex act is only a part of sexuality. Another is physical affection, a need probably more basic than sexual intercourse.

The term **sexuality** refers to all aspects of being sexual.[1]* Sexuality includes all components of the total person—intellectual, emotional, social, and spiritual, as well as physical. Thus sexuality cannot be measured by physical attractiveness alone. Nor can sexuality be measured by the size of the penis or breasts, despite movies and advertisements that would have you believe otherwise. Your sexuality is influenced by the way you feel about yourself, so it is most accurately reflected in your self-esteem.[2] Your thoughts, feelings, values, and self-concept are all part of your sexuality.

Because human sexuality encompasses all components of the total person, it is distinctly different from animal sexuality. Sex, for most animals, is primarily biological. In contrast, sex, for most people, is not simply a pleasurable biological experience, but is meaningful because it involves a union of minds and feelings as well. Most human sexual experiences occur within special relationships between people.

This chapter begins by presenting sexual development and theories about sexual preference. It then explores sexuality in terms of intimate adult relationships and commitment. It also deals with relationship problems, discusses the physical component of sexual activity, and offers tips on how to cultivate a healthy relationship.

■ Sexual Development

Sexual development starts at conception and continues throughout life. Before birth, sexual development is controlled primarily by biological forces: a baby inherits male or female gender. The hormones of gender produced before birth govern the development of male organs in boys and of female organs in girls (the **primary sex characteristics**.) After birth, the ways people formulate their sexual roles and identity are influenced both by their biology and by outside environmental factors.

*Reference notes are at the end of the chapter.

Gender Roles

The characteristics deemed by society to be appropriate for people of each gender are **gender roles**. The characteristics that a person internalizes are that person's **gender identity**. Norms for sexual behavior are determined by society and internalized by individuals.

Gender identity develops from an interaction between biological and social forces in the first few years of life. Some people believe that a person's gender identity depends more on social factors than on biological factors. Societal training has an enormous impact on gender-related behavior.

Society responds even to its newest members in keeping with its gender roles. People can be overheard to say, when observing a newborn boy, "My, how big and strong he is!" or if the baby is a girl, "She's so tiny and delicate!" Actually, newborns are more similar than different. The differences newborns do exhibit in size, strength, and activity vary, not according to gender, but according to the individual. Older children of both genders, too, are naturally more similar than different. But toddlers begin to learn gender roles before they can even talk, and two-year-olds show real understanding of them.[3] By age 11, the patterns are deeply ingrained.

The development of gender identity continues throughout adolescence. During adolescence, rising levels of the hormones that determine gender accentuate the physical differences between males and females and make sexual reproduction possible.

In this transition, two dramatic physical changes occur: the adolescent growth spurt and the development of **secondary sex characteristics**. In addition, important psychological and social changes occur.

Adolescents face a wide variety of social demands. They must become independent from their parents, must develop skills in interacting with their peers, must devise a workable set of ethical principles, must become intellectually competent, and must acquire a sense of social and personal responsibility. At this same time, they must also cope with their sexuality. This means that they must learn how to deal with changing sexual feelings, must decide whether to participate in various types of sexual activity, must discover how to recognize love, and must learn how to prevent unwanted pregnancy and sexually transmitted disease. Adolescence is also a time when most people recognize their sexual orientation.

≡▶ *The process of sexual development includes developing gender identity and gender roles. These are shaped both by biological and social forces. Sexual development progresses through adolescence, bringing a series of social demands for the adolescent, and physical changes that make sexual reproduction possible.*

Sexual Preference

Most people are attracted to members of the opposite sex—they are **heterosexual**—while some people are attracted to members of the same sex—they are **homosexual**. People can also be **bisexual**, a term that refers to experiencing sexual desires for members of both sexes. This is not the same as feeling warm toward members of both sexes and expressing affection for them by hugging, kissing, or patting on the back; most people express such feelings and they do not imply bisexuality. Still other people are **asexual**, meaning that they are sexually attracted to neither sex.

gender roles roles assigned by society to people of each gender, an individual's outward expression of maleness or femaleness in societal settings.

gender identity the part of a person's self-image that is determined by the person's gender, an individual's personal perception of being male or female.

secondary sex characteristics anatomical sex characteristics that develop during adolescence:
In males—facial hair, deep voice, body hair.
In females—breasts, body hair.

heterosexual feeling sexual desire for persons of the other gender.

homosexual feeling sexual desire for persons of the same sex, popularly called *gay* or, in women, *lesbian*.

bisexual being sexually oriented to members of both sexes.

asexual having no sexual inclinations.

In all known societies, a heterosexual orientation is preferred for most people most of the time. However, homosexuality has existed throughout history and in some societies it is widely accepted.

In the United States, the subject of homosexuality provokes strong reactions from many people. The prevailing negative attitudes toward homosexuality stem originally from religious beliefs. Years ago, the scientific community considered homosexuality a form of poor psychological adjustment, and the American Psychiatric Association defined it as an illness. In response, homosexuals began to unite and develop strong political power, and many became outspoken about their lifestyles. As a result, tolerance for homosexuality has gradually increased in our country during the 1960s and 1970s. The American Psychiatric Association redefined homosexuality, no longer considering it an illness. It now defines homosexuals as practitioners of an alternative lifestyle, members of a new community.

In the 1980s, however, the progress toward tolerance and acceptance of homosexuality came to an abrupt halt when the disease, AIDS (discussed later in Chapter 17) began to spread, primarily among homosexual males. Homosexuals in our society today are clearly a minority faced with social, religious, and legal prejudices.

In attempting to understand homosexuality, people ask all types of questions about why people become attracted to others of the same gender. They wonder if homosexuality is a life-long condition over which a person has no control. They wonder if it is an entirely voluntary choice, consciously and deliberately made at a certain phase in life. Some people theorize that homosexuality is a response to the role models a child is exposed to at home or at school.

No one really knows what causes homosexuality just as no one fully understands how heterosexuality develops. Researchers have studied how sexual preferences arise, and have advanced many theories, each possibly accounting for a certain percentage of the homosexuality in our society. There are no definite conclusions.

Those who favor the view that homosexuality has biological origins point to genetic and hormonal factors seen in people who are homosexual. Many homosexuals claim that their sexual orientation is the result of biological forces over which they have no control or choice.

Those who see psychological and social factors as responsible for the development of homosexuality state that faulty upbringing may be its cause. They claim that male homosexuality may result from having a weak, passive father and a dominant, overprotective mother.

Others who attribute homosexuality to psychological and social influences believe that homosexuality is learned. They think sexual orientation is partly dependent on the nature of early sexual experiences. They believe that reinforcement (positive or negative) controls the early process of sexual orientation. Thus, people's early experiences may steer them toward homosexual behavior by pleasurable, gratifying same-sex encounters, or by unpleasant, dissatisfying or frightening heterosexual experiences. These people theorize that if a person has unpleasant heterosexual experiences combined with rewarding homosexual encounters, there may be a gradual shifting in the homosexual direction. The observation that some female rape victims shift to lesbianism supports this view.

In any case, growing up homosexual is not easy. A later section revisits the problems homosexuals face, but the rest of this chapter is about all relationships, most of which are heterosexual.

≡▶ *Many theories exist about the development of sexual preference; researchers continue to explore biological versus social possibilities. Homosexuality has become more tolerated in the United States, but still remains a lifestyle practiced by a minority.*

■≡ Relationships with Others

No matter who you are, you need close relationships with other people. It is important to share even ordinary life events with someone else, to reflect your life in their understanding. Sharing life's experiences with others can help you double your joy and comfort your sadness. Relationships with others are crucial for emotional health. People who live without such friendships more often suffer poor mental and physical health than do people who maintain close relationships.[4]

Besides close relationships with family and friends, most people want and need special love relationships. Having a special love relationship can enhance your life and improve your emotional health, but it is not continuously necessary for positive emotional growth. People can grow both within and outside of intimate love relationships. This chapter is for anyone who is in a love relationship, or wants to be in one.

The first step in learning how to have an intimate love relationship is learning what one is. "Am I really in love, or am I just infatuated?" If you have ever asked yourself this question, you're not alone. This section explores the differences between infatuation and love.

LYNDON WAS INFATUATED WITH SOAP OPERA QUEEN DAHLIA BOEBAY....

Infatuation is an excited state, and thrives on illusion.

Infatuation

Infatuation is often mistaken for love. **Infatuation** (sometimes called romantic or addictive love) is the state of being completely carried away by unreasoning passion or attraction. Infatuation is a passionate, all-consuming preoccupation with the object of desire. It is different from love in that it often quickly fades. It leads people to do things they ordinarily would not even consider doing. Luckily, infatuation's usually short life most often allows for recovery of reason in time to prevent disasters.

Old myths often label infatuation as love. For example, the myth that "love conquers all" may lead people to ignore a partner's real self in the belief that if love is strong enough, the partner will become the perfect mate. "You only love once, and when you meet him or her, you'll know it" leads people to ignore a rich selection of real-people partners who may not be princes or princesses but who aren't toads either. Real people become lovers; fairy tales are useful for lulling young children to sleep.

Characteristics of infatuation and love are contrasted in Table 12–1. The major distinction between the two is that infatuation occurs when people don't know each other well, and mature love can exist only when they do.

infatuation the state of being completely carried away by unreasoning passion or attraction; addictive love.

TABLE 12–1 ■ **Infatuation versus Love**

In Infatuation:	In Mature Love:
The beginning of the relationship is the most exciting.	The relationship develops gradually and becomes richer with deepening acquaintanceship.
There is intensity, sexual desire, anxiety.	There is calmness, peacefulness, empathy, support, and tolerance of partner.
Each feels excitement at being involved with a person whose character is not fully known.	Each feels deep attachment, based on extensive familiarity and knowledge of partner (both positive and negative qualities).
One or both are extremely absorbed in the other.	Both want to be together without obsession.
Sexual attraction is central.	Warm affection/friendship is central; sexual attraction is positive but not the focus.
Insecurity, distrust, lack of confidence, feelings of being threatened and unfulfilled are typical.	Security, trust, confidence, an unthreatened feeling, and a sense of fulfillment are typical.
Nagging doubts and unanswered questions exist; parts about partner remain unexamined so as not to spoil the dream.	Thorough knowledge of partner exists, with mature acceptance of imperfections.
Fantasy is the basis.	Reality is the basis.
Energy is consumed, often exhausted.	Energy is generated in a healthy way.
One or both have low self-esteem (and look to partner for validation and affirmation of self-worth).	Both have high self-esteem (each person has sense of self-worth with or without partner).
Each needs the other to feel complete.	Each can feel complete without the relationship but the relationship enhances the self.
One or both feel discomfort with individual differences (need to be the same).	Individuality is accepted.
Each often tears down or criticizes the other.	Each brings out the best in the partner; relationship is nurturing.
Fondness may not be mutual; one partner may feel strongly toward an unobtainable or unavailable person (for example: a celebrity or sports figure).	Fondness is mutual; each person is aware of the shared involvement.
The partners need to rush things, like sex, marriage, or having children; they feel an urgency not to lose the partner.	Partners are patient; feel no need to rush the events of the relationship, have a sense of security and no fear of losing partner.
One is threatened by the other's individual growth.	Each encourages the other's growth.
The relationship is not enduring because it lacks a firm foundation.	The relationship is enduring, based on a strong foundation of friendship.

It is OK and natural to feel infatuated at times, and experiencing it can be part of learning about love. Some relationships that begin with infatuation develop into love. However, relationships built solely on infatuation usually do not work out well. Sometimes they turn into unhealthy dependency relationships, and other times they end because fantasies fade.

≡▶ *Infatuation, often mistaken for love, is an all-consuming desire for the partner. It occurs between people who do not know each other well and is a poor basis for a relationship.*

Mature Love

Mature love is a strong affection for, and an enduring deep attachment to, a person whose character the partner knows well. It is a mature acceptance and tolerance of the partner's negative qualities. Mature love involves a *decision* to be devoted to a person. It also requires psychological intimacy.

Intimacy is probably the most important aspect of a love relationship.[5] Intimacy builds gradually as two people become familiar with and close to each other, and it involves private, personal sharing. Two intimate people disclose, a little at a time, the good and bad parts of themselves that they keep hidden from others. Both are vulnerable, trusting each other with the parts that can be hurt.

To be psychologically intimate, people have to feel good about revealing who they really are. Before people can become intimate, both must feel that, even with their faults honestly displayed, they are worthy of love. That is, they must be emotionally healthy and have high self-esteem.

To be intimate, you not only have to feel good about yourself, you also have to *trust* your partner. You cannot be vulnerable with someone who is not trustworthy; lack of trust can destroy relationships. Learning to develop trust will be discussed later in this chapter.

There is no such thing as "instant intimacy." There are instant hot chocolate, instant food or products, and even instant sex, but intimacy develops with time. Patience is often not familiar in fast-paced, "must have it now" societies, but only time permits relationships to develop in stages, as described in the next section.

≡▶ *Mature love is a strong attachment to someone who is well known. Mature love requires psychological intimacy.*

■≡ Healthy Relationships

No two relationships are exactly alike or develop in just the same way, but healthy relationships exhibit some common characteristics. This discussion provides some insight and suggestions for developing them. As previously mentioned, the first, most essential step to take in learning to have a healthy relationship with another person is to have a healthy relationship with yourself. Being emotionally healthy and having high self-esteem are most essential.

mature love   a strong affection for, and an enduring deep attachment to, a person whose character is well known.

intimacy   being psychologically familiar with and close to another, involving private and personal sharing.

See Chapter 2 for ideas on improving self-esteem.

■ *FACT OR FICTION:* Having sex is being intimate. *False.* Intimacy is psychological. People can have sex without being intimate.

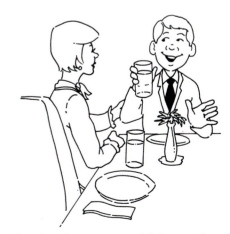

Love is an honest state and thrives on clear vision

Screening Potential Partners

A first step in developing a healthy love relationship is to make sure the person you are interested in is *available* for love. Getting involved with someone who is not available is a common mistake, and causes many unnecessary heartaches. To avoid this problem, screen people for availability. People are available when they:

■ Are unmarried and not involved in other love relationships.
■ Have been over heartaches for some time (are not recently divorced or have not just previously ended another love relationship).
■ Want to be in a relationship with you.
■ Are free of chemical or psychological addictions or are willing to undergo treatment (people with active alcoholism or other drug addictions, people who gamble, or people with eating disorders cannot function fully in love relationships).
■ Are not closely tied to families that require extensive material or emotional support (for example, adult children of people with addictions who are ensnared in their families' problems).
■ Are not so devoted to a career that they do not have the time to devote to a relationship.
■ Are physically available—they live in your city or state.[6]

You can be friends with people who lack these qualities, but you must keep their limitations in mind. Also, be sure that *you* are available for a relationship. For example, if you go to school and are also climbing a career ladder, you may be too busy at this time for a relationship.

≡▶ *People in certain situations are emotionally unavailable to be in healthy, intimate relationships. Screen potential partners carefully.*

Stages of Development of a Healthy Relationship

A healthy relationship develops in stages. The goal is to get to know the other person and gradually let yourself be known. In reading about these stages, notice that the people involved become acquainted with all aspects of each other—the relationship does not focus on one component. In a healthy relationship, all dimensions develop: intellectual, social, emotional, spiritual, and sexual. The stages include: meeting, casual friendship, close friendship, intimate friendship, and finally, intimate love friendship.

MEETING In the meeting stage, a person becomes attracted to, and acquainted with, another person on a surface level. The person feels a sense of liking for the other, and they become socially acquainted. At this stage, the social and intellectual aspects of the relationship may begin to develop.

CASUAL FRIENDSHIP In the second stage, the relationship is characterized by participation in leisure activities or projects, exploring common interests—for example, going to movies together. During this stage the social and intellectual components of the relationship begin to grow.

These early stages are a time to watch the other person's behavior carefully to determine if you want to continue growing closer. You may be feeling somewhat infatuated, but try to remain objective. Early on, both people are on their best behavior, putting their best foot forward, sort of "marketing" themselves. It takes time for people to relax and be themselves. Ask the following questions about the person:

- *Does the person have several close friends?* A person who has learned to enjoy and foster intimate relationships can put this talent to work in a love relationship.
- *Do you keep putting off introducing this person to your friends and relatives? Does the person keep postponing introducing you to family?* A hesitancy to show off a partner to the people who are most important may be a sign of uncertainty.
- *If the relationship folded, would you still want that person as a friend?* If not, the relationship may crumble during times of conflict due to a lack of friendship.
- *Are you happy with the way the person treats other people?* Watch how the person deals with employees, waitresses, maids, salesclerks, parking-lot attendants, telephone operators, and close friends. If you wouldn't want to be on the receiving end of that behavior, don't get involved. You may be an exception during courtship, but you won't be later on.[7]

During the early stages you may also mutually disclose parts of your past relationships or sexual experiences. This doesn't mean you should belabor past loves or tell of exploits, but disclosing can help the relationship to grow. For example, you and your possible partner need to know if your sexual attitudes and behaviors reflect the same value system. Other pertinent information includes whether either of you has risked contracting, or has contracted, a sexually transmitted disease.

Developing a new relationship takes time, so give it time, but don't sacrifice the balance in your life. It is wise not to focus all your attention on one relationship. Although you may be tempted, don't neglect other friends. This is unhealthy, because it results in a person's building the entire self around the other, and losing self-identity. Also, in the case of breakup, recovery is most difficult if you have built all your activities around one person. In healthy relationships, people spend time together as couples, time alone, and time with mutual and separate friends. It is a myth that healthy relationships involve a couple's spending all their free time together. Table 12–2 displays more myths and truths about healthy relationships.

CLOSE FRIENDSHIP The third stage in the development of a healthy relationship is the development of a *close* friendship. You and your partner grow more intimate as you learn each other's values and feelings. You become more compatible, and the time you spend together becomes more important than the activity you are sharing. You already know much about each other socially and intellectually; now you begin discovering your emotional and spiritual sides.

Emotional closeness arises from shared feelings. This part of intimacy is as common between good friends as it is between lovers. Each person hears and accepts the other person's feelings—all of them—thus validating the

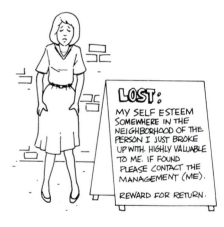

Be sure to spend time with both mutual and separate friends; maintain your identity and self-esteem.

■ *FACT OR FICTION:* Couples in healthy intimate relationships spend all their free time together. *False.* Couples in healthy relationships spend time together, time alone, and time with mutual and separate friends.

TABLE 12–2 ■ **Myths and Truths about Healthy Relationships**

MYTH:	If I am involved with you, I will lose me.
TRUTH:	Healthy relationships enhance the self and do not absorb it.
MYTH:	Being vulnerable always leads to getting hurt.
TRUTH:	Being vulnerable sometimes leads to hurt but sometimes leads to emotional rewards. It is the only route to intimacy.
MYTH:	We will never argue with or criticize each other.
TRUTH:	Couples argue from time to time and are critical of each other's behavior.
MYTH:	In order to be lovable, I must be perfect and happy all the time.
TRUTH:	Nobody is perfect. To try to appear perfect is not honest. Sometimes people are happy, and sometimes they are not.
MYTH:	We will trust each other totally, automatically, and all at once.
TRUTH:	Trust builds gradually over time.
MYTH:	My partner will meet all of my needs and will instinctively anticipate my every desire and wish.
TRUTH:	A partner will meet some of your needs, but you must meet some needs by yourself or through other friendships. People are not mind readers. If you don't communicate your needs, desires, and wishes clearly, your partner won't be able to fulfill them.
MYTH:	If we really love each other, we will stay together forever.
TRUTH:	People stay together and people separate for many reasons. You can love someone and still terminate a relationship.
MYTH:	My partner will make me happy.
TRUTH:	People who are happy before entering a relationship are most likely to be happy in a relationship.
MYTH:	Given time, I can change what I don't like about my partner.
TRUTH:	In healthy relationships, people accept the positive and negative traits of their partners. Trying to change a partner is usually unsuccessful and detrimental.

---

person disclosing those feelings. As for spiritual closeness, some people share the same religious affiliation, or they pray together, or they worship together. Others find spiritual closeness through intellectual means: they share a natural connectedness through ethical commitments, say, to the environment or to volunteer work. Still others feel destined to be together: they are soul mates. Spiritual closeness often marks a relationship moving beyond the stage of friendship.

During the third stage, you and your partner are also beginning to learn about each other's faults. Reality sets in: each partner has failings that the other can no longer ignore. Nor should you ignore them, because recognizing them is the path to mature love. If this predictable but nonetheless rocky period can be weathered, the partners can gain the security of trusting each other to be accepting, because the true self of each, complete with faults, has been seen by the other. At this point, people become intimate enough to consider making a long-term commitment. Of course, as they grow closer, the potential for conflict also increases, as does the learned ability to resolve conflict in healthy ways that strengthen the relationship. (Working through conflict is discussed later.)

INTIMATE FRIENDSHIP In this stage, there is still more self-disclosure, greater acceptance, and less threat. As the relationship develops, it meets emotional needs: to confide and to be trusted, to support, and to be encouraged. Each fully trusts the other, and therefore each can be fully vulnerable. The pair continue to develop social, intellectual, emotional, and spiritual closeness. In a healthy relationship, sexual involvement begins at this late stage of the process.[8]

The sexual involvement parallels the couple's emotional development and commitment to each other. Early sexual involvement may bring temporary immediate pleasure but actually hinders the growth of intimate love. Besides the physical risks of sexually transmitted disease, three major relationship problems can arise from becoming sexually involved too soon.

First, early involvement in sex often inhibits the growth of other parts of the relationship. This is particularly likely when the partners become so focused on sex that they neglect developing the intellectual, emotional, social, and spiritual aspects of their relationship.

Second, sexual involvement clouds objective judgment. People who are involved sexually are likely to overlook character traits or other qualities that they would be wise to acknowledge. One student asked, "Why is it that you can see that a friend is in an unhealthy, even abusive, relationship, yet the friend, who is a very bright person, cannot see this?" Another responded with the familiar saying "Love is blind," meaning that sexual infatuation can make you blind. Sexual involvement makes a person more receptive to a partner, psychologically and physiologically, than the person would be otherwise.[9] This is a benefit in a committed relationship, but a detriment when you don't know your partner well or when the relationship is unhealthy.

Third, early sexual involvement creates distrust. If you know that your partner gets sexually involved easily with any potential lover, doubts about the person's ability to be faithful arise early on. Self-control is a quality necessary even in marriages from time to time and is indispensable for the development of trust.[10] Thus, for reasons of both emotional and physical health, chastity is becoming more popular and prized than ever before in our century.

■ *FACT OR FICTION:* Sexual activity begins early in healthy intimate relationships. *False.* In healthy intimate relationships, sex begins later, as an expression of the intellectual, social, emotional, and spiritual closeness that couples have come to share.

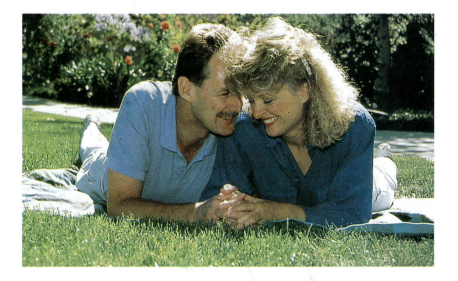

A psychologically intimate relationship is most fulfilling.

monogamy (moh-NOG-uh-mee) a term used to refer to sexual exclusivity in marriage and other relationships.

INTIMATE LOVE FRIENDSHIP The fifth stage in a healthy relationship is the development of an *intimate love* friendship. In this stage each person knows deeply all dimensions of the other. All components of the relationship are well developed and in balance. Three qualities underlie the success of an intimate love relationship: trust; exclusivity, or **monogamy**; and commitment.

≡▶ *Healthy intimate relationships evolve gradually in stages and bring people close socially, intellectually, emotionally, spiritually, and sexually. Sexual activity occurs late in healthy relationships; sexual involvement parallels emotional involvement. Healthy intimate relationships require trust, monogamy, and commitment.*

Commitment

commitment a decision to embark on a long-term monogamous relationship with another person, without a guaranteed outcome.

A **commitment** is a promise to take on a long-term obligation, made in the face of many choices, with the knowledge that all will not always go well. Some consider commitment to be the highest form of maturity in relationships.[11]

Choosing a life partner is a tricky business, and many people choose wrongly. To form a long-term, intimate bond that truly satisfies both partners involves more than simply the wish to do so. Long ago, psychologist Carl Rogers conducted a study of couples who had formed various types of bonds and attempted to define the ingredients that accounted for success. His findings still hold true today; here is what he found.[12]

It is not enough to say, "I love you" or "We love each other." We may mean what we say, but these statements easily change into "I thought I loved you" or "We thought we loved each other." It is also not enough (or it is a mistake) to say, "I commit myself wholly to you and your welfare." This can lead to a submergence of self that is fatal to the partnership. Nor is it enough to say, "We will work hard on our marriage"; work alone is insufficient. "We hold the institution of marriage sacred" or "We pledge ourselves to each other until death do us part" are also not enough; witness the statistics on divorce after such pledges. People also break up even when they feel deep biological bonds through their children.

So what *does* hold a partnership together? Psychologist Carl Rogers states:

Meanings of words in Rogers's statement:

Each—we are both doing it.

Commit—we won't back out.

Working—it takes work, and we are willing to work.

Together—it is cooperative, not one for the other, but each with the other.

Changing—we know we cannot keep it as it was in the beginning; we have to take the risks of growing and learning.

Present, currently—it is not that we promised each other long ago that we would do this; we are doing it now.

Enriching—the rewards are also present; we feel them today.

Grow—we see the process of change as necessary and desirable.

We each commit ourselves to working together on the changing process of our present relationship, because that relationship is currently enriching our love and our life and we wish it to grow.

Every word in this statement is significant; the margin shows what they mean. "When dedication and commitment are defined in [this] manner, then I believe they constitute the cradle in which a real, related partnership can begin to grow," Rogers says.[13]

These are among the rewards of a successful relationship: enjoying the other person, working out a lifestyle that suits both people, allowing the freedoms the other most needs, and meeting some of the most important needs of both people.

Independence is important, too. The person who finds ways to meet many needs outside of the paired relationship will be most successful at pairing. Recall the needs described in Maslow's scheme (Chapter 2). You cannot realistically ask your partner to provide total security—whether emo-

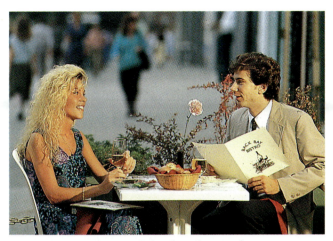

In a fantasy marriage, people live happily ever after.

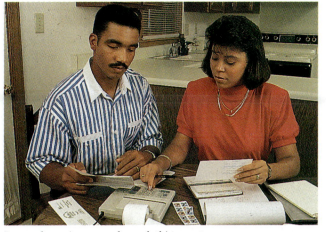

In a real marriage, people work things out.

tional, financial, or physical. You must stand on your own feet and provide your own security. You, yourself, are the only person you will never leave nor lose. The person who is most independent is best equipped to become interdependent.

≡▶ *Feeling in love is not enough for a long-term relationship. Commitment to working on the relationship by both people is necessary.*

Marriage

Did you ever wonder what happened to Cinderella and the Prince after they married? Did they really live happily ever after? Probably the most destructive concept associated with marriage is that this could possibly be the case. Marriage is never the *end* of the story, as in fairy tales. It is the beginning. The plot thickens.

The highest form of committed relationship in our society is the legal bond of **marriage**. The majority of people who get married assume that their relationship will be based on these premises:

■ The relationship is permanent, or at least permanence is something the partners are willing to work for.
■ The partners will be mutually primary to one another. No other relationship will have a higher priority.

Permanence distinguishes marriage from all other relationships. Dating and even living together usually do not possess the permanence of marriage. Married life demands conscious effort; investments of time, care, and patience; and even personal sacrifice.

Before marrying, people would do well to look honestly at their own expectations. One way to do this is to explore together the answers to the questions in this chapter's Life Choice Inventory. Clearly it is essential to establish what a potential partner means when the word *marriage* comes up.

≡▶ *Marriage is the highest form of committed relationship in our society. It is wise for people to examine their expectations of marriage before entering into it.*

marriage the legal institution that joins a man and a woman by contract for the purpose of creating and maintaining a family.

LIFE CHOICE INVENTORY

Will your marriage work? Differences of opinion will pepper an otherwise bland relationship with challenges—but they can also destroy the relationship. It helps to know ahead of time where the major differences will be. The more of these questions you and your proposed partner agree on, the more likely your marriage will work.

Money

1. Should we both work? Should one partner stop working after children come?
2. Should we keep all our money in a shared bank account? If so, who should pay the bills? If not, who should pay which bills?
3. What should the limits be on use of credit cards?
4. Who decides on "big" purchases? Should both parents decide together?
5. Should we follow a written budget? How closely?
6. If one of us wants to do something more rewarding personally than financially, will that be all right?
7. If one of our careers requires a move, will that be all right with the other?
8. How much of our income should we save, invest, spend on insurance, and give to our church or synagogue?
9. Will we own the home, car, and other property jointly? If not, who will hold the titles?

Children

1. Do we want to have children? How many? When?
2. Should children's needs be put before our needs?

3. How much money shall we save for, or spend on, children's education, recreation, and other options?
4. Who should discipline the children, and how?

In-laws

1. How close is each of us to our families (geographically and emotionally)? Will it be important to see them frequently?
2. Is each of us willing to receive advice from the other's parents?
3. Can we, or should we, accept financial help from our families? How much, for what, and from which family?
4. Where will we spend our major holidays?

Religious Traditions

1. Are our religious beliefs compatible? If not, can we each live with the other's different beliefs?
2. Does either of us feel strongly that the other must attend religious services?
3. Should children be raised with particular religious beliefs?

■ ≡ Relationship Problems

A relationship may encounter problems for many reasons. One is the stress of anger and conflict within the relationship. Another is stresses imposed by society from outside.

Conflict

Partners may think that anger and conflict have no place in a "happy" committed relationship and so may try to deny their negative feelings. In reality, every human relationship contains conflicts, and how those conflicts are handled can determine whether the relationship grows or dies.

Destructive things happen when people don't address their feelings of anger. People who keep them inside often find other, unhealthy ways of

4. Should religious practices be part of every day's routine? How will religious holidays be spent?
5. How much money, energy, or time should we spend on religious and charitable organizations?

Sexuality

1. Is sexual intercourse before marriage forbidden, permitted, or endorsed? For both of us or only one?
2. How often will each of us want to have intercourse? When, where, and under what circumstances?
3. Should each person be willing to have sex if the other wants it? Can each express desire freely to the other?
4. Is nudity acceptable around the house?
5. Is it important to either partner how the other dresses?
6. Is it acceptable to each of us if the other flirts?
7. How much of a display of affection is appropriate in public?

Miscellaneous

1. Is profanity acceptable? Under what conditions?
2. Is alcohol drinking acceptable? Is occasional drunkenness acceptable? How much of our money should be spent on alcohol?

3. Is drug use acceptable?
4. Is smoking acceptable? Under what conditions?
5. Should underage children be allowed to drink, use drugs, or smoke?
6. How should each of us behave in the home? Should we be available at all times to each other, or should we each have time alone or for projects of our own?
7. Should both of us go to bed at the same time? Who should get up first?
8. Who should do the shopping? Cook meals? See to repairs? Clean the bathroom? Tend to other household tasks (laundry, lawn, dishes, etc.)?
9. How important are reading, TV, movies, sporting events, other entertainment?
10. Should each of us be willing, if asked, to tell each other everything we think, feel, and do?
11. How will we coordinate fitness and leisure activities?
12. How should each person express anger? What verbal or physical expressions of all feelings are acceptable?

dealing with the feelings, such as engaging in compulsive behaviors (drinking, drug abuse, overeating, or gambling). Alternatively, they may talk to inappropriate others about their anger instead of telling the one who needs to know—the partner. Physical illness may develop, as may psychological problems such as depression and others already discussed in Chapter 3.

Depending on childhood experiences and societal influences, people handle emotions like anger in different ways. Instead of directing the anger inward, the person may express it inappropriately and destructively. The person who chronically criticizes, nags, or uses sarcasm is ventilating well enough to release personal tension, but is just hurting the other person, not curing the problem. More subtle forms of attack are sabotage (messing up the other's plans), anger displacement (being rude to, or angry at, in-laws or children), or verbal abuse of the mate. In some cases, spouse abuse—physical violence against the mate—occurs.

bond fighting constructive settling of differences; a mode of conflict resolution that couples can employ.

Some people believe (falsely) that mild episodes of physical aggression can help to "clear the air." Actually, partners and family members withdraw in response to such displays. Assertion, not aggression, is the path to clear air (see Chapter 3). Equally useless are tactics to evade issues, such as leaving when disagreement arises, refusing to talk, not taking the other seriously ("He's just had a hard day"/"She must be having her period"), or not giving the other time to respond. Evading quarrels by saving up hurts is useless—they come spilling out in a confusing mess at some later date.

People can handle differences constructively by learning and practicing the art of **bond fighting**. Bond fights are conflicts in which the participants have a positive goal: to build up, not tear down, each other's self-esteem. The rules for bond fighting are summarized in this chapter's Strategies.

Some conflicts are truly beyond the scope of self-help. Clues that such conflicts are occurring are inability to solve the problem, incessant hostility, the feeling that the "last straw" has threatened the relationship, an episode in which either has become physically aggressive or threatened suicide, or the emergence of an observable personality disorder. In such cases, look for a counselor who is a member of the American Association of Marriage and Family Therapists. (Others may have little training or may be self-taught, because most states have no licensing requirement.)

≡▶ *Every human relationship experiences conflicts, and how these conflicts are handled can determine whether the relationship grows or dies. Working through conflict includes clearly defining and addressing each problem. Resolving disagreements in a way that nurtures the relationship is the goal.*

Breakup

Sometimes it is best for both partners' wellness to acknowledge that a relationship should end. The breakup of a special love relationship can be one of the most difficult events to face in life. Regardless of who initiates it, it is painful. One often feels lonely, rejected, and depressed. What can be done?

Many people, upon ending a relationship, immediately seek another partner. This is common and tempting, because loneliness and pain are intense at first. But it can actually be detrimental, for two reasons.

First, remember, from Chapter 3, the emotionally ·healthy way to go through grief? You have lost a loved one, or the hope of a love, and you need to grieve. Remember the problem of carrying unresolved grief? Jumping fully into a new relationship may mask the pain for a while, but will only postpone your grief, which will have to be faced sooner or later. Also, the unresolved grief from the past relationship will interfere with the ability to form a new one. Getting involved "on the rebound" will likely result in the breakup of the new relationship. People who do this often end up with *two* relationships to grieve.

Another reason not to hurry into a new involvement is that self-esteem is low at this painful time. Even an emotionally healthy person, when going through a breakup, has lowered self-esteem immediately after a breakup. When self-esteem is low, people will likely be attracted to, and attract, new partners with low self-esteem to match. People with low self-esteem are not capable of mature love.

■ ■ ■ ■ ■ STRATEGIES: *HOW TO RESOLVE CONFLICT IN A WAY THAT BUILDS A RELATIONSHIP*

To work through conflict:

1. Be honest—say what you mean.
2. Be authentic—say what you feel.
3. Use only "I" statements ("I don't like it when . . .") rather than "you" statements ("Why don't you . . ." or "You make me . . ." or "You are a . . .").
4. Reflect—repeat your partner's grievance in your own words, to be sure you understand—and wait for affirmation. You are now facing an issue that contributes to conflict.
5. Ask what is on your partner's mind; don't answer your own questions—you don't really know the answer until you ask. Many people mistakenly believe they do know what the person thinks and feels.
6. Choose the time and place for airing grievances—some people agree on formal "gripe hours."
7. Define the territory, and stay within it—issues from other times demand their own gripe sessions. Right now, solve this one issue only.
8. Be sure that the issue at hand is the real issue and that some deeper, more personal grievance is not hiding behind the complaint. For example, someone who complains about a mate's leaving clothes on the floor may really feel that the domestic work is unfairly divided.
9. Ask for specific changes, selecting those that will lead to a resolution of the conflict. Don't request too many changes at once, for this makes compliance impossible. Ask only when necessary.
10. Be open to compromise; be willing to change yourself.
11. Don't try to win—if there's a winner, there's a loser. When a bond fight is successful, both people benefit (or win)—in terms of closeness, intimacy, and self-esteem.[14]

After a breakup, one needs time to heal emotionally. Therapists recommend a person wait six months to a year—depending on the degree of involvement—before entering into a new relationship.

Another way some people handle breakups is by "playing the field," or trying to have as much sex as possible with as many different people as possible. This is not wise, for several reasons. First, it increases risks of contracting sexually transmitted diseases. Second, people who engage in casual sex sometimes end up hurting those they are using for sex. They find they have to deal with angry sex partners who feel deceived and may threaten drastic actions. And third, people trying to recover from a breakup risk getting emotionally involved before having had enough time to heal.

Be patient, let yourself heal, and nurture yourself in healthy ways. Turn to friends for emotional support, strengthen your support network, and get involved in a balanced variety of health-promoting activities. When you are once again serene and contented with yourself, you are ready for a new relationship.

≡▶ *When coping with a breakup, it is best to avoid getting into a new love relationship right away. Instead, pass through the stages of grief and build alternative support systems. Nurture yourself in healthy ways.*

■ *FACT OR FICTION:* To cope with a breakup, it is beneficial to get into another relationship as soon as possible. *False.* To cope with a breakup, it is best to devote six months to a year to healing.

Social Stresses

Society frowns on some kinds of couples, notably homosexual couples, couples of mixed race, and couples of widely different ages, among others. Maintaining self-esteem while participating in a relationship that society frowns on is difficult. People in these relationships face more than the ordinary challenges that accepted relationships bring.

An extreme form of societal rejection is the **homophobia** that homosexuals face. Homophobia is the extreme hostility and fear that many people feel toward homosexuality. Homophobia is widespread. Some psychologists believe that homophobia is partly a defense that people use to insulate themselves from any awareness that they themselves might possess homosexual traits. Thus, in cases of brutal beatings or murders of homosexuals (the ultimate expression of homophobia), the motivation may be partly to stamp out any inherent homosexual impulses that may lurk in the attacker's heart.

Another possible reason for homophobia is the misconception that all homosexuals are alike. Yet if you tried to identify "the" homosexual lifestyle, you could not do it. Homosexual people's lifestyles differ just as lifestyles of heterosexual people do. They may be uncommitted or monogamous, secretive or open. They are lawyers, dentists, grocers, accountants, prostitutes, and everything that heterosexuals are. They are not usually recognized by their outward appearances, mannerisms, or occupations. Still, some generalizations are valid.

In general, homosexual men are more active sexually and have more sex partners than homosexual women or heterosexuals.[15] However, many gay men and women have lasting, committed same-sex relationships.

The gay world has its visible and invisible components. Today, in addition to gay bars and baths, there are also gay churches, political parties, newspapers, and—in larger cities—full-scale businesses and social communities. But homosexuality has a less pleasant side, with impersonal, hurried sex; fear of police entrapment; high rates of sexually transmitted disease; alcoholism; and personal guilt or fear of discovery. These negatives, and especially the mounting fear of AIDS, have led to changes in sexual behavior within some segments of the gay male community. Some are abstaining from sex, some are restricting their sexual activities to one partner, and some are attempting to develop a heterosexual orientation.

Homosexual couples, as well as other couples that experience social rejection, seek identity and support, as all couples do. Some fail to find it and decide to discontinue their relationships. Others find or form communities within which they are accepted. A few stay together without external support, and pay the price of societal rejection.

≡▶ *Couples that are not socially accepted face challenges beyond the ordinary in maintaining intimate relationships.*

homophobia   extreme hostility toward and fear of homosexuality.

■≡ Sexual Activity

Sexual activity is important in intimate relationships and can be a creative way to communicate tenderness, love, and a sense of unity. In healthy relationships, sexual activity is not only the expression of a physical bond, but of the intellectual, social, emotional, and spiritual bond between two people. How well a couple's sex life is doing usually reflects how well the nonsexual relationship is doing; a healthy sex life is typically embedded in a healthy relationship. This section discusses how sexual activity progresses from childhood to full maturity. Figures 12–1, 12–2, 12–3, and 12–4 provide the relevant anatomical details, and the Miniglossaries of Male and Female Terms define the related terms.

Masturbation

A person's first sexual relationship is with self. When you flirt with yourself in the mirror, appreciating your own attractiveness, you may be learning about your sexuality. Whenever you enjoy physical sensations, your sexuality is involved—it is **sensuous** to smooth lotions onto your skin, to sunbathe, to bathe, or to swim.

Children's natural playfulness and curiosity lead to exploring their **genitals**, and they learn to masturbate. **Masturbation** may continue in adulthood. Many sex therapists recommend masturbation to clients as a way to find out what sorts of stimulation please them. Later, they can communicate such information to their sex partners.

Masturbation can be useful because it does not involve other people. When partners have problems, it enables each to release sexual tension without becoming involved with someone else while they work out their differences. For people without partners, it provides a way to release sexual tension and can be a healthy strategy for avoiding contracting sexually transmitted diseases.

≡▶ *Masturbation is an activity that often begins in childhood. Masturbation may be a useful release for adults at times.*

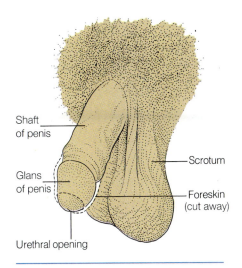

FIGURE 12–1 ■ External male organs.
The *shaft*, or cylindrical body of the *penis*, ends at the *glans* or the tip, also called the head. The glans, which is the part of the penis most sensitive to pleasure, usually retracts beneath a sheath of skin, the *foreskin*. In some males, this sheath has been cut away, revealing the glans (see *circumcision* in Chapter 14). The *scrotum* is a loose pouch that contains the testes.

sensuous related to the experience of pleasure through the senses, particularly the sense of touch.
genitals the external organs of the reproductive system— the penis and scrotum in men; the clitoris and labia in women.
masturbation stimulating one's own genitals.

FIGURE 12–2 ■ Anatomy of the male reproductive system.
Sperm cells are produced in the *testes*, or *testicles*. The testes are surrounded by a toughskinned sac, the *scrotum*, which contains muscles that contract and relax to bring the testes closer to, or farther away from, the body in order to regulate their temperature. A temperature slightly cooler than core body temperature is critical to the making of sperm.

Mature sperm travel to the *epididymus*, a storage place, where they remain until ejaculation takes place. Then the storage organ contracts and propels the sperm into a conducting tube, the *vas deferens*. This tube also contracts, propelling the sperm farther toward the *urethra*. On the way, the sperm combine with fluids from glands to form the mixture, *semen*, that leaves the penis. A single ejaculation yields approximately 3 to 4 milliliters (about a teaspoonful) of semen, containing approximately 400 million sperm.

Three glands or sets of glands contribute fluids to form semen: *cowper's glands*, the *prostate gland*, and the *seminal vesicles*.

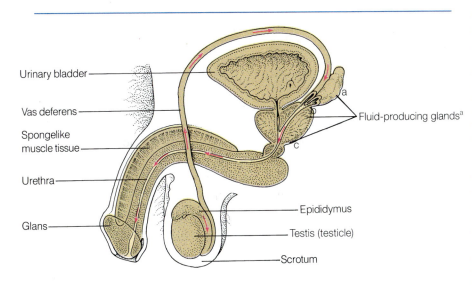

FIGURE 12–3 ■ **External female organs.**

Two sets of ridges, the *labia,* enfold the other female organs. The *labia majora* are the more external, larger ridges covered with pubic hair. The *labia minora* lie between them. The labia minora border the vaginal and urethral openings and join together over the shaft of the *clitoris,* forming its *hood.* The visible *glans* of the clitoris is just the top of a rodlike structure that is made up partly of spongelike muscle tissue that becomes erect when stimulated. The clitoris is highly sensitive because it contains a tremendous number of sensory nerve endings. In young girls, a thin, fragile membrane, the *hymen,* partly covers the vaginal opening. Once thought to be "proof of virginity," the membrane is now known to disintegrate during early life due to exercise or use of tampons, or it may rupture at the time of first sexual intercourse.

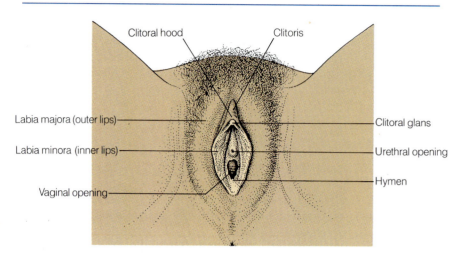

FIGURE 12–4 ■ **Anatomy of the female reproductive system.**

One of the *ovaries* releases an *ovum* in close proximity to the gently grasping "fingers," or fringe, on the end of one of the *fallopian tubes.* This fringe draws the ovum in and propels it into the fallopian tube. The tube is lined with cilia, which sweep the ovum along to the *uterus.* There, if fertilized, the ovum will implant itself in the prepared lining. If not fertilized, it will be shed through the uterine opening (*cervix*) into the *vagina,* together with the materials of the uterine lining. The *urethra* serves no reproductive function in the female, but discharges urine from the urinary bladder.

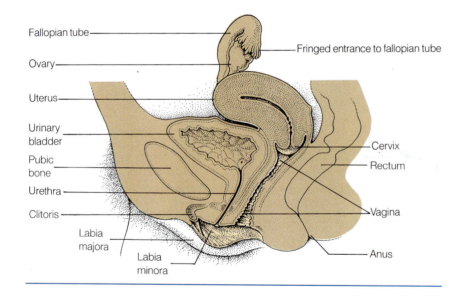

sex play   physical expression of affection and sexual desire that does not involve sexual intercourse; hugging, kissing, fondling; also called *petting.*

See Chapter 17 for more about sexually transmitted diseases.

Sex Play

One example of interpersonal sexual expression is **sex play** (commonly called *petting*). It is shared sexual stimulation that does not involve sexual intercourse. Kissing can be one form of sex play; the lips are especially sensitive receptors. Kissing styles differ, but whatever the style, almost everyone in modern societies kisses.[16] Kissing may play a role in the development of a chemical bond; it may be that special substances, different for each individual, are exchanged between people who kiss. These chemicals are thought to assist one person's recognition or acceptance of another.[17]

■ **MINIGLOSSARY**
of Male Terms

cowper's glands   glands that secrete a fluid that cleanses the urethra and enhances sperm function.

epididymus (EP-ee-DID-ih-mus)   a storage area for maturing sperm cells.

foreskin   a sleeve of skin that covers the tip of the uncircumcised penis, analogous to the hood in females. *Circumcision* is surgery to remove the foreskin of the penis, usually performed shortly after birth; it may aid cleanliness, although opinions of this point vary.

glans   the tip of the penis, analogous to the clitoris in females.

penis   the male external genital organ, including the shaft, glans, and internal structural base.

prostate gland   a gland that produces fluid to carry sperm cells along the urethra and out of the penis (part of the ejaculate).

scrotum (SCROH-tum)   the double pouch that contains the testicles.

semen (SEE-men)   the fluid ejaculated from the penis that carries sperm.

seminal vesicles   glands which produce fluid that nourishes the sperm cells (part of the ejaculate).

shaft   the cylindrical body of the penis.

sperm (cells)   the male reproductive cells.

testicle or testis (plural testes)   one of the two male gonads, which produce male hormones and sperm cells.

urethra (you-REE-thrah)   the duct which, in the male, carries both urine and semen out of the body.

vas deferens (vas DEF-er-ens)   the duct in the male through which the semen is propelled during ejaculation.

■ **MINIGLOSSARY**
of Female Terms

cervix (SER-vix)   the neck of the uterus, where it joins the vagina.

clitoris (CLIT-uh-rus)   the primary organ that receives pleasure sensations, as does the glans of the penis in men.

fallopian (fah-LOH-pe-un) **tubes**   a pair of tubes that connect the ovaries with the uterus; fertilization usually takes place within these tubes.

glans   the tip of the clitoris.

hood   a sleeve of skin that covers the tip of the clitoris.

hymen (HIGH-men)   a thin membrane that partially covers the vaginal opening in early life.

labia (LAY-bee-uh)   the liplike structures of the female external genital organs. The larger, more external ones (*labia*

majora) are covered with pubic hair; the smaller, inner ones (*labia minora*) are thin folds.

ovaries (OH-vah-reez)   the two female gonads, which produce female hormones and mature ova.

ovum (OH-vum; plural, ova)   the female reproductive cell, or egg.

uterus (YOU-ter-us)   the organ that contains and nourishes the young before birth; the *womb*.

vagina   the muscular, tube-shaped organ of the female that conducts menstrual flow from the uterus to the outside of the body, surrounds the penis in intercourse, conducts semen into the uterus, and serves as the passageway for birth of the baby.

Some kisses, of course, are not related to sex but are an expression of nonsexual affection or love.

Caressing the breasts and genital organs is another form of sex play. The word *petting* conveys the image of tenderly caressing something that is

foreplay activity in which each partner gives pleasure to the other prior to intercourse.

cunnilingus (cun-ih-LING-gus) oral stimulation of a woman's labia and clitoris.

fellatio (feh-LAY-she-oh) oral stimulation of a man's penis.

erection the state of a normally soft tissue when it fills with blood and becomes firm.

engorgement swelling. With reference to the sexual response, the sex organs' filling with blood preparatory to orgasm.

See Miniglossaries for anatomical terms.

Chapter 13 explains contraception.

sexual intercourse the physical act of inserting the penis into the vagina. The term *intercourse* means connection or communication of any kind—talking or trading, for example. Sexual intercourse between human beings is termed *coitus* (CO-ih-tus); between animals it is termed *copulation* (cop-you-LAY-shun).

cherished—and that is what sex play is. During sex play, people can enjoy the emotions of tenderness, love, and gratitude, as well as feelings of sexual pleasure. Sex play may be a part of **foreplay**, the mutual pleasure-giving that precedes intercourse. (Sex play is not always followed by intercourse, however.)

Oral stimulation of the genitals—**cunnilingus** or **fellatio**—is another form of sexual expression for some. Some use oral sex as part of foreplay, and other people use it when they want to refrain from intercourse. Having oral sex instead of intercourse can prevent pregnancy but not sexually transmitted disease.

Sex play is especially useful for learning about the sexual responses of another person and for communicating one's own sexual needs. Naturally, touching gives pleasure. The skin is rich in sensory nerve endings, which communicate pleasure to the ultimate receptor, the brain. To many people, touching, hugging, and kissing meet emotional needs for closeness, and are fulfilling in themselves, whether or not intercourse follows. An advantage of sex play is that it is not focused on the self. The focus is on the pleasure that each partner can give the other.

Sex play usually results in intense sexual stimulation, with **erection** (stiffening) of the penis, enlargement of the clitoris, and **engorgement** (swelling) of the labia. Lubricating fluids begin to flow within the vagina. Fluid moves down the man's **urethra**, neutralizing the acid left by urine and creating a safe environment for **sperm**.

During erection, a drop or so of fluid leaves the penis. It may contain live sperm. This presents a risk of pregnancy, because sperm can easily travel, even from the outside of the vagina, into the uterus. If partners are using sex play as a substitute for intercourse, they can prevent pregnancy only by preventing this fluid from touching the vagina or labia.

If sex play is continued, orgasm may occur (see the later section on the stages of sexual response). Sometimes people purposely postpone orgasm to make the pleasure last.

≡▶ *Sex play is a valuable part of the sexual experience. Emotions, tenderness, and gratitude can be shared during sex play.*

Sexual Intercourse

Sexual intercourse is a simple act in a physical sense. It becomes a complex interaction, though, because individuals bring to it their moods, expectations, self-concepts, feelings about the relationship, and everything else that makes them unique.

The act of intercourse itself consists of a man's and a woman's positioning their bodies so that the woman's vagina can receive the man's penis; the two move together in a motion that brings them sexual sensation and pleasure, usually ending with the man's orgasm. The woman's orgasm usually occurs prior to, or simultaneously with, the man's; occasionally it may occur afterward, or occasionally not at all. If a woman never achieves orgasm, there may be a problem, and the couple may decide to seek help. (More about getting help in a later section.)

People usually have intercourse in one of five basic positions: with the man on top, with the woman on top, with both lying on their sides face to face, with the man behind the woman, or with the partners sitting face to face. Each of these positions has many variations, and people may experiment to find what pleases them. Different positions offer different advantages, such as face-to-face communication, ease of clitoral stimulation or other hand contact, comfort during pregnancy, or freedom of movement. A couple needn't choose just one and use it over and over; they can use positions preferred by each on different occasions. Positions are only one aspect of intercourse among many that demand clear, accurate communication between partners. Other aspects include level of desire, preferences in foreplay, readiness for intercourse, and timing of orgasm.

≡▶ *Sexual intercourse can bring sexual pleasure. It can be performed in a variety of ways, depending on the couple's preferences.*

The Stages of Sexual Response

The mystery of sexual response lies in the complex human brain—the true master sex organ. The response involves interactions among physical, social, and psychological factors.

This description centers on the primary organs of sexual response, the clitoris and penis, but pleasurable feelings also arise from many other locations in the body. Some body parts are believed to be especially sensitive to sexual sensation, but people's entire bodies can become pleasure-receiving. The key to knowing how to give pleasure is listening to the partner's signals.

The four phases of the sexual response cycle are common to both partners: **excitement**, **plateau**, **orgasm**, and **resolution**.[18] The stages of the sexual response are listed as a sequence of events, but they may occur with different timing. The physical responses of each phase may differ from person to person and may even vary in the same person from time to time.

Excitement begins with the sex play that precedes intercourse—foreplay, already described. Each partner seeks to give pleasure by stimulating the other. The most obvious event is the man's penile erection, but a corresponding event occurs in the woman as she becomes excited: engorgement of the clitoris and labia. This is when the penis releases the drop of fluid mentioned earlier, and glands of the vagina release a smooth, slippery lubricating fluid so that the vagina can receive the erect penis easily.

If stimulation continues, the partners move into the plateau phase. This phase includes constriction of the outer third of the vagina and further enlargement of the penis. The clitoris withdraws under its foreskin as it becomes increasingly sensitive, but still responds when stroked through this protective layer of skin.

After still further stimulation, orgasm occurs. Orgasm is a reflex, an involuntary response that occurs automatically after sufficient stimulation. In women, orgasm involves involuntary rhythmic contractions of the uterus, the outer portion of the vagina, and the surrounding muscles. Orgasm usually lasts about 30 seconds and is accompanied by sensations of intense pleasure. In men, **ejaculation** of semen through rhythmic contractions of the penile muscles follows orgasm. During orgasm, the blood that has engorged the penis, clitoris, vagina, and labia flows out of the veins. Orgasms may be short or long, intense or mild; they differ more among individuals than between the sexes.

excitement as used to describe a stage of sexual response, the early stage of initial arousal.

plateau literally, a high, flat place. In sexual response, the plateau phase is the period of intense physical pleasure preceding orgasm.

orgasm the climax or peak of sexual excitement that can occur during sexual intercourse, oral sex, or masturbation.

resolution in sexual response, the stage of relaxation that follows orgasm.

ejaculation the discharge of semen from the penis during a man's orgasm. A *nocturnal emission* (or wet dream) is the emission of semen during sleep.

Orgasm is the peak of sexual pleasure; the resolution phase offers further pleasures of its own. Resolution is the reversal of the physical changes of arousal—tensed muscles relax, congested blood vessels and swollen tissues return to normal. The period is usually characterized by feelings of well-being, sometimes called the **afterglow**.

The phases of sexual response are similar in men and women, but a definite distinction exists in the stage immediately following orgasm. After orgasm, men enter a **refractory period**, a recovery time during which further orgasm or ejaculation is physiologically impossible. (The refractory period may last anywhere from a few minutes to many hours.) In contrast, women do not enter a refractory period after orgasm, therefore women are capable of having multiple orgasms. Women can have one or more additional orgasms within a short period of time without dropping below the plateau level of sexual arousal (see Figure 12–5). Thus, women have a greater physical capacity for sexual pleasure than do men.

A popular myth states that the larger the man's penis, the greater his ability to provide sexual pleasure.[19] (Other myths about sex and being a good lover are found in Table 12–3.) The fallacy of penis size makes no sense either anatomically or psychologically. Anatomically, only the outer third of

afterglow   the pleasure of the resolution phase of the sexual response.

refractory period   a recovery time after male orgasm during which further orgasm or ejaculation is physiologically impossible; in most cases erection is impossible as well.

FIGURE 12–5 ■ **The sexual response cycle in women and men.**

a) Women (3 patterns). Pattern 1 shows multiple orgasm; pattern 2 shows arousal that reaches the plateau level without going on to orgasm (note that resolution occurs very slowly); and pattern 3 shows several brief drops in the excitement phase followed by an even more rapid resolution phase.

b) Men (the typical pattern and a variation on it). The dotted line shows a second orgasm and ejaculation occurring after the refractory period is over. Numerous other variations are possible, including patterns that would match 2 and 3 of the female response cycle.

SOURCE: W. H. Marxus, V. E. Johnson, and R. C. Koloduz, *Human Sexuality,* 2nd ed. (Boston: Little, Brown and Company, 1985), p. 79.

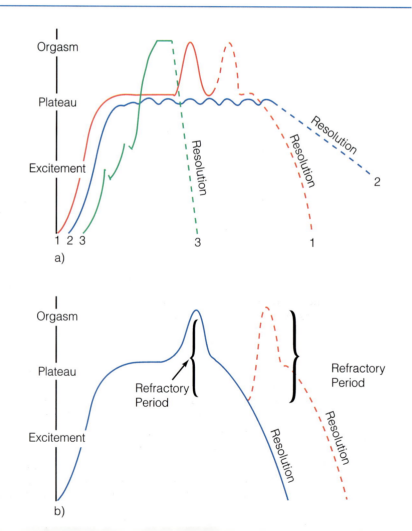

TABLE 12–3 ■ **Fallacies and Facts about Sex**

Fallcy:	A woman's sexuality is measured by the size of her breasts.
Fact:	Sexuality (for both genders) is determined by the way people feel about themselves.
Fallacy:	Physical attractiveness determines sexuality.
Fact:	Self-esteem determines sexuality.
Fallacy:	Lots of sexual experiences are necessary to learn to be a good lover.
Fact:	Having lots of sexual experiences may only mean that the person has learned bad habits and had lots of practice at performing poorly. Having the desire to please your partner and being able to be psychologically intimate are the prerequisites for being a good lover.
Fallacy:	Good technique is the most important ingredient of a satisfying sexual relationship.
Fact:	While technique is important, it is easily learned and is not the basis for a satisfying sexual relationship. Wanting to please your partner and being able to be psychologically intimate are more important qualities.
Fallacy:	It's unhealthy to become sexually aroused and then not proceed to orgasm.
Fact:	Although it may be frustrating, arousal without orgasm is not harmful and may even be useful for stimulating sexual interest.
Fallacy:	Men have a greater sexual capacity than women.
Fact:	Physically, women have an almost unlimited orgasmic potential. Men are unable to have a rapid series of orgasms because of the refractory period.
Fallacy:	A male can always tell if his female partner has had an orgasm.
Fact:	Some men are fooled by a partner who fakes orgasm by means of loud moans and groans. A woman's orgasm is less physically obvious than a man's so a man can not always tell if his partner has experienced one.

the vagina is particularly sensitive, and the organ most sensitive to sexual stimulation in women is the clitoris.[20] Many women do not achieve orgasm from vaginal stimulation alone; the clitoris must be stimulated for orgasm to occur.[21] Psychologically, sexual pleasure occurs in the mind. A letter to Ann Landers in praise of the modestly endowed male states:

There is entirely too much emphasis on a man's size these days. From my experience, lovemaking with the man who was the least endowed was by far the most fulfilling. Why? Because he was responsive, sensitive, caring, romantic, and considerate.

What too many men fail to realize is that sexual pleasure is generated in the mind . . . . That's where everything happens—or fails to happen.[22]

It is not just women who are influenced by unrealistic sexual standards. Men are also pressured to perform well sexually. While it is a healthy goal to want to sexually please each other, and a pleasing technique is necessary to do this, being a sexual acrobat is unnecessary. Having the desire to please your partner and having the ability to be psychologically intimate constitute being a good lover. Good technique is easily learned; being able to be psychologically intimate is not.

Another misconception is that all women must experience multiple orgasms in order to be sexually satisfied. Multiple orgasms are pleasurable but

■ *FACT OR FICTION:* A man's ability to give pleasure is directly related to the size of his penis. *False.* Penis size is irrelevant anatomically and psychologically to providing sexual pleasure.

■ *FACT OR FICTION:* Good sexual technique is the most important quality in a satisfying love relationship. *False.* Having the desire to please your partner and being able to be psychologically intimate are more important characteristics.

not necessary for every woman to have rewarding sexual experiences. Women's magazines suggest that multiple orgasms are crucial, and overreport the number of women achieving them. This sets up an unrealistic performance standard that can damage the self-esteem of those who fail to "measure up." Some women are content to experience single orgasms. (See this chapter's Critical Thinking for more on multiple orgasms.)

▤▶ *The stages of sexual response include excitement, plateau, orgasm, and resolution. In men, orgasm and resolution are followed by a refractory period. The sexual response is observed in the sex organs but originates in the brain. Important factors for the sexual response are responsiveness, caring, and consideration.*

Sexual Problems and Strategies

Some people experience times of inability to enjoy sex, even though they may wish to. A few have lifelong histories of such inability, and most people experience at least some difficulty at some time during their lives. Normally, it is taken in stride—it goes away by itself, but sometimes, lack of enjoyment of sex may become a problem known as **sexual dysfunction.**

Some people experience interference with arousal from no apparent physical cause. Sometimes arousal may simply take longer than usual. Other times, people may lack sexual desire or even fear sexual activity. Of course, no one need worry about occasional times of disinterest, but when involuntary disinterest is frequent or when it causes distress to the person or harms a relationship, it may be worth attention. The majority of cases are treatable.[23] Psychological therapy can help discover and treat the problems that interfere with arousal.

In men, a sexual problem may manifest itself in the inability to achieve or maintain an erection. In women, the most common complaints are lack of sexual excitement and lack of orgasm during intercourse. The causes of such complaints are varied: physical abnormalities, problems in the love relationship, lack of technique on the parts of the lovers, and others.

When the cause of the problem is physical, sexual response is usually impaired under all circumstances. A problem that occurs only with a particular person or under certain conditions is probably not physical but psychological or interpersonal. Often a person's worries about some other part of the relationship prevent enjoyment of sex, and the worries must be dealt with before the sex can return to normal. The partners need to talk the problem through and resolve it before attempting lovemaking. When such cases cannot be resolved through communication, sex therapy may be useful, but beware: sex therapy is a largely unmonitored field, and anybody can adopt the title of sex therapist. To find one of the relatively few who have adequate credentials:

■ Contact a university or hospital that provides a sex clinic.
■ Check the credentials of the therapist.*
■ Ask where the therapist received training in the specialty of sex therapy. Look for a graduate degree from a recognized university, as well as postgraduate training.[24]

*The professional organizations to look for are the Society for Sex Therapy and Research (SSTAR) or the American Association of Sex Educators, Counselors, and Therapists (AASECT).

sexual dysfunction impaired responses of sexual excitement or orgasm due to psychological, interpersonal, physical, environmental, or cultural causes; formerly called *impotence* in men and *frigidity* in women.

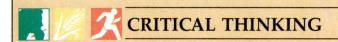 **CRITICAL THINKING**

Olympic Sex

Many studies have been conducted on the occurrence of multiple or-gasms in women. Often, questionnaires are used to collect the data. A summary of a typical study may read as follows: "In a study regarding multiple orgasms, 805 nurses answered a questionnaire. The study showed 11 percent of them had never experienced an orgasm, 47 percent experienced *only* single orgasms, and 42 percent usually experienced multiple orgasms during sexual episodes." [23]

Studies like these can provide valuable information to improve the physical aspect of sexual technique, but they are often misleading and can even be damaging. These reports can be misleading because the numbers do not accurately reflect the overall population, only the people who voluntarily responded to the surveys. Women most likely to answer a survey of this type are those who have multiple orgasms. Similarly, men who consider themselves well-endowed are most likely to complete surveys on penis size.

These reports can damage people's self-esteem and relationships. Upon reading studies like these, readers are often left feeling sexually inadequate, especially with wording such as "these women experienced *only* single orgasms." More realistically, some women are thrilled to ex-perience one orgasm and are left satisfied.

Multiple orgasms, while pleasurable, are not necessary for all women to achieve sexual fulfillment. Studies such as the one just described, along with society's emphasis on physical technique, make people feel inadequate if they are not performing like sexual acrobats competing for an Olympic event.

Emphasis on technique pushes the emotional part of love relationships out of view. Much more important is to inform people that the most sexually fulfilling experiences are those that take place within the context of healthy, psychologically intimate, exclusive, committed love relation-ships.

■ *FACT OR FICTION:* Women must experience several orgasms during a lovemaking session in order to be satisfied. *False.* While it is desirable for the woman to achieve orgasm, some women are content with one orgasm per session.

Being a sexual acrobat is not necessary for sexual fulfillment; being psychologically intimate is.

Legitimate therapists do not have sexual contact with their clients; any that suggest such contact are not ethical. (Sexual contact between a therapist and client almost always results in additional anguish and more problems.) Le-gitimate therapists do ask intimate questions about experiences to find the reasons for malfunctions, though. Honesty in answering is crucial to mak-ing progress.

Whatever a person does to resolve a sexual problem, it is unwise to turn to fad solutions, such as pills and powders sold in the marketplace. The following Critical Thinking develops this thought.

≡▶ *Sexual problems may be physical or psychological in nature. Most are treat-able.*

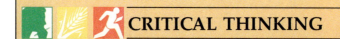

CRITICAL THINKING

Pills and Potions for Sexual Problems

People with sexual problems are often embarrassed and may be reluctant to seek help from other people. They may be tempted to turn instead to products. A warning is in order—no secret compound, no exotic ingredient, and no food or nutrient can enhance or restore sexual vitality. The substances called **aphrodisiacs** do not work, and they may be dangerous. Many are strong stimulants, hormones, or depressants. According to the Food and Drug Administration, all claims for over-the-counter aphrodisiacs are false, misleading, or unsupported by scientific evidence.[26]

Chances are that failing sexual responses, like most other messages from the body, need time, energy, and attention. Use your mind, not your money, to work on them.

aphrodisiacs (af-roh-DIZ-ee-acks)   substances reputed to excite sexual desire. Actually, no known substance does this, but many claim to do so.

When things go wrong in sex, there are no quick fixes.

Sexuality, intimate relationships, and commitment can greatly enrich life. Sexual abuse can seriously injure people's lives, as the Spotlight that follows shows. It presents the subject of rape and discusses the controversies that surround acquaintance rape. The next chapter goes on to present details of a vitally important area related to sexuality—family planning.

■≡ For Review

1. Define *sexuality*.

2. Define the terms *gender role* and *gender identity*.

3. Describe the varieties of sexual preferences: heterosexual, homosexual, bisexual, and asexual.

4. Discuss the differences between infatuation and love.

5. List conditions or situations that make people unavailable to function fully in an intimate love relationship.

6. List strategies for having a healthy intimate relationship.

7. Describe the stages of development of a healthy love relationship.

8. List reasons why early sexual involvement does not favor development of mature love.

9. Define *commitment*.

10. List constructive ways of dealing with conflict.

11. Define the terms *masturbation* and *sex play*, and describe what contributions these activities make to adult sexual activity.

12. Explain in what ways male and

female sexual organs are similar and how they differ.

13. List the four phases of the sexual response in men and women, and identify some of the characteristic physical changes that accompany them.

14. Identify the way in which a man's typical sexual response differs from a woman's.

15. Advise a person on ways to seek help for sexual problems.

■ ≡ Notes

1. Unless otherwise noted, information in this section is from W. H. Masters, V. E. Johnson, and R. C. Kolodny, *Human Sexuality,* 2nd ed. (Boston: Little, Brown and Company; 1985), p. 4.

2. S. Gordon, Sexuality education in the 1990s, *Health Education,* January/February 1990, pp. 4–5.

3. A. C. Huston, The development of sex typing: Themes from recent research, *Development Review,* March 1985, pp. 1–17.

4. Social ties: Friendships are important to your health, *University of Texas Lifetime Health Letter,* April 1990, p. 7.

5. Gordon, 1990.

6. M. Beattie, *Beyond Codependency* (New York: Harper and Row, 1989), pp. 151–164; list adapted with permission.

7. J. T. Garrity, *Total Loving: How to Love and Be Loved for the Rest of Your Life* (New York: Simon and Schuster, 1977).

8. S. Gordon, *Why Love Is not Enough* (Boston, Mass.: Bob Adams, 1988).

9. B. Nicholson, Does kissing aid human bonding by semiochemical addiction? *British Journal of Dermatology* 3 (1984): 623–627.

10. L. A. Berne and P. Wild, *Teen Sexual Behavior—A Leader's Resource of Practical Strategies with Youth* (Reston, Va.: American Alliance for Health, Physical Education, Recreation and Dance, 1988).

11. W. G. Perry, Jr., *Forms of Intellectual and Ethical Development in the College Years: A Scheme* (New York: Holt, Rinehart and Winston, 1970).

12. C. R. Rogers, *Becoming Partners: Marriage and Its Alternatives* (LaJolla, Calif.: Delta, 1972), pp. 199–202.

13. Rogers, 1972, p. 201.

14. The rules for bond fighting were adapted from M. A. Lamanna and A. Riedmann, *Marriages and Families: Making Choices throughout the Life Cycle* (Belmont, Calif.: Wadsworth, 1985), pp. 337–344.

15. Masters, Johnson, and Kolodny, 1985, p. 426.

16. I. Dierderen and L. Rorer, Do attitudes and background influence college students' sexual behavior? Paper presented at the American Psychological Association (1982), Washington, D.C.

17. Nicholson, 1984.

18. Masters, Johnson, and Kolodny, 1985, pp. 76–106.

19. The Kinsey Survey, 1990, as cited in How much do you really know about sex? *Berkeley Wellness Letter,* April 1991, pp. 4–5.

20. G. Mirkin, The real thing, *Health,* November 1984, p. 8.

21. H. Alzate, Vaginal eroticism and female orgasm: A current appraisal, *Journal of Sex and Marital Therapy,* Winter 1985, pp. 271–284.

22. A. Landers, In many cases "less is more," *Tallahassee Democrat,* 31 March 1991.

23. L. R. Schover and J. LoPiccolo, Treatment effectiveness for dysfunctions of sexual desire, *Journal of Sex and Marital Therapy* 8 (1982): 179–197.

24. Masters, Johnson, and Kolodny, 1985, pp. 524–525.

25. C. A. Darling, J. K. Davidson, and D. A. Jennings, The female sexual response revisited: Understanding the multi-orgasmic experience in women, *Archives of Sexual Behavior*, in preparation.

26. A. Hecht, Aphrodisiacs, *FDA Consumer,* December/January 1982–1983, p. 11.

SPOTLIGHT

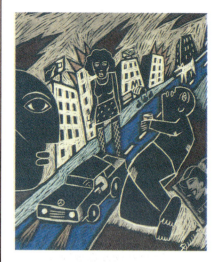

Rape and Acquaintance Rape

What do you think of when you hear the word *rape*? Most people describe a woman walking down a dark street at night and being sexually assaulted by an unknown attacker. This kind of rape (sometimes called *street rape* or *stranger rape*) does occur, but is not the most common kind of rape. In most rapes the victim knows the attacker, and the two may even be dating. This kind of rape is called *acquaintance rape,* or *date rape*. Both kinds of rape are violent crimes.

Are you saying that when a person forces sex during a date, this is a violent crime?

Yes. The *only* difference between rape by an unknown attacker and acquaintance rape is that in acquaintance rape, the attacker and victim know each other. In both instances, the

attacker forces sex, often using violence. Any form of forced sex is a crime.

Only women get raped, right?

No, although rape is most commonly an attack on women—one out of every four women will be raped in her lifetime. Men do get raped too, though—10 percent of all rape victims are men.[1]* (When men are raped, other men are usually, but not always, the attackers.) And in any case, rape is a concern for all men, because their mothers, sisters, girlfriends, or aunts can be raped. When someone close to you is raped, it affects you.

How damaging is rape?

Try to imagine how you would feel if you were raped. Someone is using violence to force you to have sex. You feel extreme fear for your safety, and even for your life. And the act is physically painful, compounding the fear. Too, you feel angry, even enraged, because you are being personally violated to an extreme. Lastly, you feel emotional pain, and this will probably last for years. A writer has said, "Rape is a crime of uniquely intimate cruelty. When the body is violated, the spirit is maimed. How long will it take, once the wounds have healed, before it is possible to share a walk on a beach, a drive home from work, or an evening's conversation without always listening for a quiet alarm to start ringing deep in the back of the memory of a terrible crime?"[2] The pain is even more extreme when the crime is incest; the violator is a person who is supposed to be a caretaker.

*Reference notes are at the end of the Spotlight.

Don't some people think that acquaintance rape is not really rape?

Yes; date rape is controversial. Consider how a date rape report reads, after the fact. Two people got together socially, and both enjoyed the early part of the evening. At the end of the evening, they went to a private place, such as the woman's or man's room or apartment. Then they had sex. The woman reports that sex was forced; the man claims it wasn't. The problem is that no one else was there; only the two people involved know exactly what happened. Cases end up being one person's word against another's.

Date rape reports present special problems for police and the courts. Attorneys prosecuting the alleged rapist hang their cases on the credibility of the victim. The outcome may seem to depend more on how well the victim wins the sympathy of the court than on the truth.

Besides, sometimes a woman behaves on a date in a way that seems to encourage sexual activity. Then, when the man becomes aroused, the woman seems to suddenly decide that she does not want to have sex. Some men do not respect the woman's right to change her mind. They claim that since she teased, she indicated her true desire for sexual intercourse. Some men think that when a woman says no, she really means yes, that she is just being coy. Rapes occur commonly under such circumstances, in our society.

Aren't date rapes equally common in all societies?

No, they are especially common in ours. Movies, television, music videos, and romance novels plant messages early on that suggest that women have rape fantasies and want to be overpowered. In the movie *Gone with the Wind*, Rhett sweeps Scarlett up the stairs despite her protests. Several soap operas show successful men overpowering protesting heroines, who then melt into their arms.

In our society, most girls learn early to be indirect about sex, to allure and resist. As women, they may say no verbally, but their body language may say yes. This confuses men. Meanwhile, many boys are taught to be aggressive—to go for what they want, with no holds barred. As men, some may take their dates' ambiguous behavior as an excuse to take what they want with power.

With all this confusion, what can men do to avoid being accused of rape?

A man must make sure that his date is fully consenting before having sex. If a woman says no verbally but her body language says yes, it is best to take her verbal no for no. Requirements for mutual consent are:

■ Both parties are fully aware—not influenced by alcohol or other drugs.
■ Both parties are equally free to act.
■ Both parties have positively and clearly communicated their intents.

Can rape occur between two people who have previously willingly had sex?

Yes. Rape can occur between lovers—if one doesn't want sex and the other forces it, that is rape. The same is true in marriage—a husband forcing himself on his unwilling wife is raping her. And a woman who has had several sex partners—even a prostitute—can also be raped, although the rapist may use her promiscuity as an excuse, saying that she has no right to refuse. Forced sex is always rape.

Is rape an act of passion?

No, it is an act of violence. The issue between rapist and victim is an issue of power, not of sexual desire.

TABLE S12–1 ■ **Rape Prevention Tips**

To Prevent Rape
Avoid feminine identification (change mailbox tag and phone listing from "Mary Jones" to "M. Jones" to conceal gender).
Draw shades of windows at night.
If you live alone and your doorbell rings, yell "I'll get it," to pretend someone else is home.
Do not open your door to strangers. Always ask who is at your door before opening it. If you are expecting a person to service something in your home, ask for identification and do not hesitate to call the company for verification.
If someone knocks on your door and asks to use your phone to call for a tow truck or other assistance, offer to make the call yourself without opening the door.
Do not go anywhere alone after dark; use an escort service.
If you run after dark, always run with a partner.
Leave word of where you plan to run (and when you will return) with family or friends.
Stay alert to suspicious-looking people.
Keep your arms free for defense.
Stay on busy, well-lit streets.
Have your keys ready before you get to your front door.
Carry your car keys or a stickpin in your hand to stab the attacker—you will not have time to fumble for them.
Carry a whistle.

If efforts fail and you are followed:
Ring the nearest doorbell.
Move away from shadowy areas into an open, well-lit area.

If you are approached:
Try to stall for time; someone may come along.
Try to attract the attention of a passing motorist.

If you are attacked:
Scream "fire" (not "police," since others are then likely to avoid becoming involved), and pull a fire alarm, if possible. Break a window; someone is likely to respond to the noise. Use your keys or a stickpin to aim decisively for the attacker's eyes, temples, Adam's apple, or ears. Stab hard without warning. Try to disgust your attacker by urinating or by gagging yourself to induce vomiting. Tell him you have a sexually transmitted disease.
These precautions are not guaranteed, but worth trying—they may save your life.

Do many cases of rape go unreported?

Yes, authorities estimate that fewer than 10 percent of rapes are reported.[3] Some rape victims do not report the crimes because they fear the police will treat them poorly. Others do not report attacks because they believe the myth that rape victims ask to be raped. Some victims fear the attacks on their character that they will undergo from the opposing attorneys. Some know that women are not likely to be believed in date rape cases.

What can I do to avoid being a rape victim?

The best protection is prevention. Do not put yourself in a position where you can be raped. Table S12–1 sums up the precautions you should take to avoid being attacked by a stranger. As for avoiding date rape, the first precaution is to get to know your potential date well before going out alone with him. Never go home with someone you do not know well. If you are interested in dating someone, socialize in groups, and watch the person's behavior for certain warning signs. Rape counselors and women who have been raped by acquaintances recommend that you stay away from anyone who displays any of these characteristics:

■ Emotionally abuses you (through insults, belittling comments, ignoring your opinion, or acting sulky or angry when you initiate an action or idea).
■ Tells you whom you may have as friends, tells you how you should dress, or tries to control other elements of your life or relationships.
■ Talks negatively about women in general.
■ Gets jealous when there is no reason.
■ Berates you for not wanting to get drunk, get high, have sex, or go with him to an isolated or personal place.
■ Refuses to let you share any of the expenses of a date and gets angry when you offer to pay.
■ Is physically violent to you or others, even if it's "just" grabbing and pushing to get his way.
■ Acts in an intimidating way toward you (sits too close, uses his body to block your way, speaks as if he knows you much better than he does, touches you when you tell him not to).
■ Is unable to handle sexual and emotional frustrations without becoming angry.
■ Doesn't view you as an equal, either because he's older or because he sees himself as smarter or socially superior.
■ Has a fascination with weapons.
■ Enjoys being cruel to animals, children, or people he can bully.[4]

Rape is a serious crime that causes serious emotional trauma. Again, the best protection is prevention.

■≡ Spotlight Notes

1. N. Gibbs, When is it rape? *Time,* 3 June 1991, pp. 48–54.
2. Gibbs, 1991, p. 53.
3. Gibbs, 1991.

4. R. Warshaw, *I Never Called It Rape* (New York: Harper and Row, 1988), p. 152.

CHAPTER 13

Conception, Fertility, and Family Planning

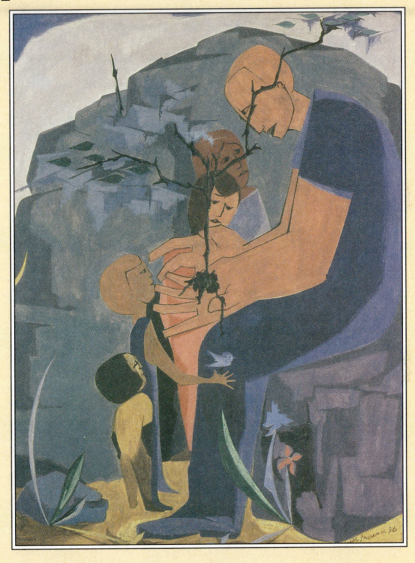

FACT OR FICTION

Just for fun, respond true or false to the following statements. If false, say what is true.

■ If a couple does not conceive in a year of trying, chances are slim that they ever will. (Page 346)
■ Contraception can help make healthy babies. (Page 348)
■ It is wise to use Vaseline as a lubricating jelly with condoms. (Page 366)

■ Withdrawal is an effective birth control method. (Page 366)
■ Sterilization operations involve lengthy, complex surgical procedures. (Page 367)

---

conception   fertilization, the union of ovum and sperm that starts a new individual.

T he event that starts a whole new human being takes place in a single moment. The event described here is **conception.**

■≡ Conception and Fertility

gamete   a cell produced for the purpose of reproduction; a sperm cell in a man, an egg cell (ovum) in a woman.

fertilization   the fusion of an ovum and a sperm.

fertility   ability to produce and expel gametes sufficient for reproduction.

Inside the woman's body, an ovum (a female **gamete,** or reproductive cell) is about the size of the period at the end of this sentence. The ovum has grown ready for **fertilization** in one of her ovaries and is traveling down one of her fallopian tubes toward her uterus. In a woman with normal **fertility,** this maturing and traveling of an ovum has occurred about once every month since she began menstruating in her teens. The man of normal fertility has been producing millions of microscopic sperm cells (male gametes) each day since puberty. Now, the man and woman have had sexual intercourse. Sperm, deposited in the vagina, swim up the uterus to the fallopian tubes, propelled by their long, whipping tails, and attach to the surface of this particular ovum. One sperm cell enters, triggering an instantaneous change in the ovum's surface so that no more sperm cells can penetrate (see Figure 13–1).

FIGURE 13–1   ■   **Fertilization.**

(1) Sperm from the penis are deposited into the vagina.
(2) Sperm travel from the vagina through the cervix, through the uterus, to the fallopian tubes.
(3) One mature ovum has been released from one of the ovaries and enters the fallopian tube. It begins to travel toward the uterus.
(4) Millions of sperm cells work together to weaken the ovum's outer layer, but only one sperm cell can enter.

(Both the sperm cells and the ovum have been greatly enlarged for illustration.)

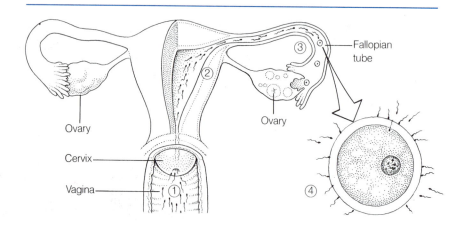

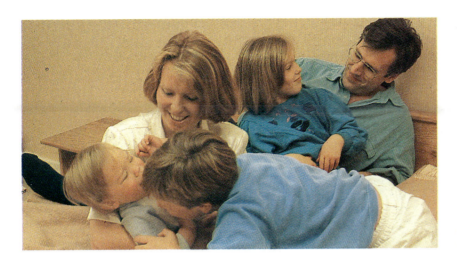

Family planning means getting the timing right.

Conception has occurred and the fertilized ovum is now called a **zygote.** The zygote continues to travel down the fallopian tube and enters the uterus where it may embed itself in the uterine wall (**implantation**). About 60 percent of all zygotes either will fail to implant or will dislodge later, to be expelled from the uterus into the vagina and lost from the body.[1]* If implantation is successful, the woman is pregnant, and some nine months hence, will give birth to a baby.

The events of pregnancy and childbirth are presented in Chapter 14. This chapter deals only with conception. Conception can be a fearsome event for people who are not ready to become parents (see box, The Power of Fertility). On the other hand, conception can be a thrilling event for people who want to have a baby. Most people have little trouble conceiving. Of sexually active couples who use no preventive measures, 90 percent conceive within one year with no conscious effort.[2] For this reason, people who do not wish to conceive must take action to avoid it. Hence, much of this chapter is about **family planning,** limiting the number of children according to the wishes of the couple.

zygote the product of the union of ovum and sperm. (After two weeks, it is called an *embryo.*)

implantation the event in which a zygote embeds itself in the wall of the uterus and continues to develop, during the first two weeks after conception.

family planning limiting the number and spacing of children according to the wishes of the couple rather than leaving them to chance. The method is called *birth control.*

≡▶ *Conception is a common event and most sexually active couples who use no method to prevent pregnancy will conceive.*

*Reference notes are at the end of the chapter.

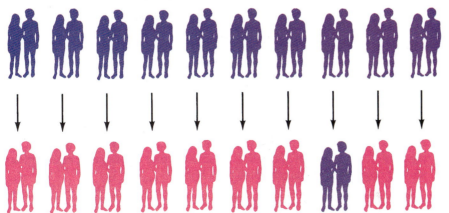

Of ten sexually active couples using no contraception,

Nine become pregnant within one year. The odds favor conception when sexually active people use no contraception.

≡◼ **Infertility**

infertility   inability to produce gametes and/or offspring.

If sexual intercourse occurs with the right timing and conception still does not take place, the problem may be **infertility.** Its causes are many and varied, and they occur with equal frequency in men and women.

Diseases can render people infertile. A cause common among women is **pelvic inflammatory disease (PID),** a dangerous infection that spreads throughout the fallopian tubes. Among the agents of PID are several sexually transmitted diseases (see Chapter 17); a result of PID sometimes is tubal pregnancy (or **ectopic pregnancy**), which can cause the fallopian tubes to rupture and can be fatal. Another cause of infertility in women is **endometriosis,** which develops when the cells of the inner lining of the uterus, the endometrium, escape into the abdominal cavity or to other parts of the reproductive system, adhere there, and grow. Endometriosis may lead to scarring of the fallopian tubes, the ovaries, and the entire abdominal cavity. In men, sexually transmitted diseases can lead to infertility.

pelvic inflammatory disease (PID)   a dangerous infection of the female reproductive tract, resulting in scarring of the fallopian tubes, temporary or permanent sterility, and possibly death. See also Chapter 17.

ectopic (ek-TOP-ick) pregnancy   a pregnancy in which the fertilized egg has implanted and begun to develop in one of the fallopian tubes or elsewhere outside the uterus, a life-threatening condition. Also called a tubal pregnancy.

Physical trauma, malnutrition, some medicines, drug abuse, reproductive tract abnormalities, inadequate production of sperm or ova, and even mild infections in both men and women also bring about temporary or permanent infertility. High testicular temperature due to fever, testicular varicose veins, or even too-tight pants may depress sperm production.

If a couple is unsuccessful in attempts to conceive for more than about a year, it may be time to seek a medical diagnosis. Even after a year, about half of all such couples succeed in conceiving with no treatment if they simply keep on trying.[3]

endometriosis (EN-doh-mee-tree-OH-sis)   invasion of the abdominal cavity or other parts of the reproductive system by the cells of the uterine lining.

The treatment of infertility depends on the cause. In the case of an anatomical problem that interferes with conception, surgery may help. A woman who produces too few ova might be treated with **fertility drugs.** These drugs induce the hormones, or are themselves the hormones, that force the ovaries to mature and release ova. No doubt you have heard of women who bore four or five children at once after taking such drugs. What happened was that the drug dose was too high and made four or five ova ready for fertilization simultaneously. (This can't be helped; the same drug dose in other women might be just right.) Multiple births of this magnitude almost never happen except when fertility drugs are used.

◼ *FACT OR FICTION:* If a couple does not conceive in a year of trying, chances are slim that they ever will. *False.* Many couples conceive without treatment if they just keep trying.

If a man produces insufficient numbers of sperm per ejaculation, the couple can be helped to conceive by **artificial insemination.** In this procedure, the man collects his semen on several occasions and takes it to a clinic to be stored until enough sperm are present to bring about conception. The woman visits the clinic at the time of ovulation, and a cup containing the semen is fitted onto her cervix to deliver the sperm.* If this fails, the couple may apply to a **sperm bank,** where stored sperm from various donors is available. The couple can choose a donor with characteristics similar to their own, as with adoption.

fertility drug   a hormone that induces the production and release of gametes, or a chemical that induces the body to synthesize such a hormone.

artificial insemination   a means of achieving pregnancy without intercourse, in which semen is mechanically introduced into the vagina.

sperm bank   a facility that stores semen for use in artificial insemination.

If the woman is infertile, the couple may elect to use a **surrogate mother.** This is a woman who agrees to be artificially inseminated with the husband's sperm, bear the baby, and surrender it to the infertile couple. Surrogate motherhood may sound good in theory, but in practice it is full of legal and emotional uncertainties; hence, couples considering this option should obtain both legal and medical advice.

surrogate mother   a woman who undertakes to bear an infant for another person.

*This is one of several procedures that may be used.

The Power of Fertility

Almost every aspect of adult life is touched by the choice of whether to reproduce. An extreme case is that of the unwed teenage mother. Just by deciding to carry an unplanned pregnancy to term, a girl may alter 50 to 90 percent of the rest of her life. She becomes isolated from her peers during her pregnancy. If she returns afterwards, they will have moved on without her. Former boyfriends probably now avoid her. Then, her educational and job opportunities shrink permanently, unless she gives the baby up for adoption. Her parents may have to take care of the baby and continue supporting her as well, or she may have to take a low–paying job to help support them. She is likely to end up with more children than her peers will ever have. Preoccupied from that time on with providing for her offspring, she is forced to neglect her own personal growth. Also, physical risks always occur with adolescent pregnancies. Both mother and infant may not be healthy.

Fertility's power touches others more subtly. People risking unwanted pregnancies can experience anxiety that pervades their lives. Surprise pregnancies are not the exception, but practically the rule, and a person who has had one or more may come to fear sexual activity itself. When unplanned pregnancies occur, careers may end, relationships may falter, and even spiritual beliefs may be compromised.

Because fertility works so well, it almost invariably produces pregnancies whenever people take no precautions to prevent them. Then, bearing children permanently alters people's lives. Time and effort spent learning about fertility and how to manage it are time and effort well spent.

An experimental measure is **in-vitro fertilization.** The name "test-tube babies" is given to children conceived this way, although only the fertilization takes place in a test tube; the fetus grows in the mother's uterus. The procedure is a complicated, expensive surgical process, and it produces pregnancy approximately one-fourth of the time, but hundreds of babies have been conceived this way.

in-vitro (in-VEE-troh) fertilization   a laboratory procedure in which fertilization takes place outside the body. *In vitro* means "in the test tube," as opposed to *in vivo* (in VEE-voh), which means "in the body."

≡▶ *Infertility can be caused by many conditions. A variety of procedures can correct most problems of infertility.*

■≡ The Choice of Family Planning

While conception is difficult for some, it is all too easy for the majority of sexually active couples. With timeless patience, nature has perfected the reproduction of living things, safeguarding the carriers of life to ensure that new generations will follow. Most people find it difficult to control their own fertility through family planning.

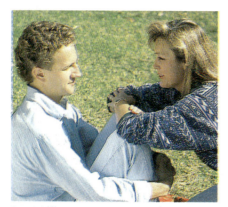

Open communication about contraception promotes both wise planning and closeness.

contraception any method of preventing conception.

■ *FACT OR FICTION:* Contraception can help make healthy babies. *True.*

Contraception and **birth control** are often used to mean the same thing, but contraception comes first. Contraception means to prevent conception. The term *birth control* means prevention of births—it includes both contraception and abortion (discussed later). This chapter distinguishes between the two terms.

birth control any method used to control the number of children born.

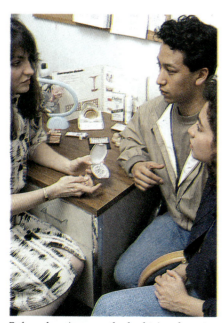

Before choosing a method, obtain adequate information.

Although it may sound preposterous, **contraception** is good for babies—for one important reason: people can use it while cultivating lifestyle practices that maximize their chances of having healthy babies. Another benefit of using contraception in family planning is that parents can choose how many children to have and when to have each one.

Contraception is a controversial subject. Some people's religious convictions forbid its use; other people would like to legislate its use for everyone who is sexually active. This chapter takes the position that the choice is personal and presents the facts people need to make choices as informed consumers.

Contraception is not for women only. It is a shared human responsibility that accompanies the personal pleasure of sexual intercourse. No one should ever assume that a partner will take care of it. Every couple should discuss the topic openly. Appropriate concern about contraception is a sign of commitment to the partner. Further, open communication about it not only helps the couple find a suitable method, but also tends to enhance their closeness, promote lasting sexual pleasure, and strengthen the relationship.

If you are now having sexual intercourse but using no means of contraception, your actions indicate that you wish to have a child. You have much to consider in committing yourself to this choice. The Spotlight that follows this chapter is dedicated to helping people make the decision whether to raise a child. Anyone who is not ready, and who is sexually active, should either abstain or opt for contraception.

Where to Get Help with Contraception

Before choosing a method of contraception, a person is wise to consult with a physician, physician's assistant, or nurse practitioner. These professionals are able to check for unsuspected health problems and provide education and, if one is needed, a prescription.

Planning centers and other resources such as student health centers or county health departments provide services much the same as those offered by private physicians, and at a reasonable cost. (Many centers use a sliding fee scale based on income.) These facilities often also provide free contraception counseling to individuals or couples, and most also have special help clinics for teenagers.

Religious organizations sometimes provide counseling services relating to sexuality, pregnancy, and other issues, as well as information on contraception. One such organization is Catholic Alternatives.

When seeking contraception assistance from one of these sources, make an advance appointment. These organizations are made up of individuals, and not every counselor is the right one for every person. If you feel uncomfortable with one counselor, ask to see someone else. If you don't get the information you are seeking from one type of center, go to another.

≡▶ *Student health centers, county health departments, private physicians, and some religious organizations offer information regarding contraception.*

Choosing a Method

No contraceptive method is perfect. The person choosing a method has to face that fact. To obtain the advantages of one method, a person has to be willing to accept disadvantages that invariably accompany it. For that reason, it is important for the person doing the choosing to decide which features are indispensable and which disadvantages are acceptable. This chapter's Life Choice Inventory asks questions to help people decide which methods they might prefer and then instructs the chooser to subject each method to a reality test based on the probable effectiveness of the method as used by that person.

First, though, a few words about **effectiveness,** sexually transmitted diseases, and side effects may help in selecting a method. A knowledgeable person may say that the effectiveness of contraceptive X is 98.5 percent. Later, an equally reliable source may say it is only 92 percent effective. Both may be giving you correct data. The difference between the two numbers reflects different approaches to research. The first person is quoting studies that answer the question, How well does this method work in 100 *couples who use it perfectly* for one year? These studies are run in controlled settings that permit no misuse and no mistakes. Under these conditions, contraceptive X prevents pregnancy 98.5 percent of the time. The second authority is quoting studies of what happens in real life: they answer the question, How

effectiveness with reference to contraception, the extent to which a contraceptive method or device succeeds in preventing pregnancy, expressed as a percentage of couples protected during a year of use.

laboratory effectiveness is the percentage of women protected from pregnancy in a year's time under ideal experimental conditions; **user effectiveness** is the percentage of typical women users who are protected.

TABLE 13–1 ■ Voluntary Risks in Perspective

Activity	Chance of Death in a Year
Risks for men and women of all ages who participate in:	
Motorcycling	1 in 1,000
Automobile driving	1 in 6,000
Power boating	1 in 6,000
Rock climbing	1 in 7,500
Playing football	1 in 25,000
Canoeing	1 in 100,000
Risks for women aged 15 to 44 years:	
Using tampons	1 in 350,000
Having sexual intercourse (PID)	1 in 50,000
Risks of preventing pregnancy:	
Using birth control pills	
nonsmoker	1 in 63,000
smoker	1 in 16,000
Using IUDs	1 in 100,000
Using diaphragm, condom, or spermicide	None
Using fertility awareness methods	None
Undergoing sterilization:	
Laparoscopic tubal ligation	1 in 67,000
Hysterectomy	1 in 1,600
Vasectomy	1 in 300,000
Risks of continuing pregnancy	1 in 14,300
Risks of terminating pregnancy:	
Illegal abortion	1 in 3,000
Legal abortion	
Before 9 weeks	1 in 500,000
Between 9 and 12 weeks	1 in 67,000
Between 13 and 15 weeks	1 in 23,000
After 15 weeks	1 in 8,700

SOURCE: R. A. Hatcher, F. Stewart, J. Trussell, D. Kowal, F. Guest, G. K. Stewart, and W. Cates, *Contraceptive Technology* (1990–1992): 146. Used with permission.

LIFE CHOICE INVENTORY

Which method of contraception is most suitable for you? The questions below point out matters to consider in sorting out your priorities. Table 13–2 will help you rate the methods according to the first nine questions; Table 13–3 will help you answer the tenth.

First turn to Table 13–2. Start by assigning 10 points to each column. (Use pencil, and write *10* at the top of each column in the blank space next to "maximum possible points.") Now, increase the point value of any column you consider especially important, and simultaneously deduct points from some other column, so that the total of all the columns remains 90. (For example, you might assign a value of "15" to column 4 and "5" to column 6.)

Next, read questions 1 through 9 below, and work your way down columns 1 through 9 in Table 13–2, scoring each method as instructed at the top of that column. Then work your way across the table, add up all the points you gave each method, and record the total in column 10.

Next, work Table 13–3, as shown on that table. Finally, return to column 11 of Table 13–2 to make a choice of method. The questions to consider are:

1. *Possible obstacles to use:*

   Do you mind using a method that requires touching your genitals?

   Are you willing (and will you remember) to use the method every time you have intercourse or to stay on a daily schedule?

   Would you find it annoying or embarrassing to interrupt foreplay to use contraception?

   Does your partner resist the idea of interrupting foreplay to use contraception? You may face a conflict in which you want to protect yourself and please your partner but find that you cannot do both.

   Do you or your partner fear or have aversions to any of the methods, or will something prevent you from using it as intended?

2. *Locus of control:*

   Have you and your partner decided together about contraception, or are you on your own? If you are on your own, choose a method that you can use on your own.

   To what extent does the method allow you to keep control? If you have to rely on your partner, is your partner reliable?

3. *Privacy and confidentiality:*

   Would you rather keep your contraception strictly your own business? If so, choose a method that does not require having devices or products on hand.

4. *Reversibility:*

   Do you feel that you have enough children? If so,

many *typical users* out of 100 become pregnant while using contraceptive X for one year? In real life, 8 women out of 100 become pregnant, because in real life mistakes and misuses occur. This chapter lists both effectiveness ratings whenever possible. Giving only one might be misleading.[4]

Only one contraceptive device offers some protection against sexually transmitted diseases: latex condoms (see Chapter 17). Therefore, couples who become sexually intimate may well need to use more than one method—for example, the Pill for contraception and condoms for partial protection against these diseases.

Be sure to consider the potential side effects of contraceptive methods, when selecting a method. Keep the risks in perspective; carrying a baby to term usually entails risks that are considerably greater than those incurred by using most contraceptive methods. Table 13–1 compares some other risks with those of contraception. With this information, you are prepared to you may wish to consider a permanent form of contraception.

Does your partner feel that you have enough children? A difference of opinion here would have to be dealt with.

5. *Frequency of intercourse:*

How often do you have intercourse? (If you are having intercourse frequently, you need a method that you can use consistently.)

6. *Noncontraceptive benefits:*

Would this method provide a health benefit, other than contraception, that would make you favor it? (For example, condom use protects against sexually transmitted diseases; birth control pills might make an irregular menstrual period regular.)

Is the method in keeping with your and your partner's religious beliefs? (If not, contact the organization of a religious group for counseling.)

7. *Cost:*

Is the method affordable? (Most county health departments provide free or low-cost contraceptive drugs and devices.)

8. *Medical side effects and risks:*

Does the method present a significant risk to you?

(Table 13–2 lists the best-known risks; in addition, follow medical advice specific to your health status.)

9. *Physical limiting factors:*

Has a pregnancy ever occurred while you were using the method? (If so, choose another method.)

Do you (if you are a woman) or does your partner (if you are a man) menstruate on a regular schedule, with the same number of days between each flow? If so, then you may consider the natural family planning methods or contraceptive pills.

Now add up the total points assigned to each method in Table 13–2, record your totals in column 10, and turn to Table 13–3.

10. *Effectiveness:*

How important is not having children at this time? (If pregnancy would be acceptable, you may choose to use a less effective method.)

How do you and your partner feel about abortion or raising a child in case your method should fail?

Circle yes or no for each method on Table 13–3, return to the last column in Table 13–2, record your answers there, and select a method.

SOURCE: Adapted from information in R. A. Hatcher and coauthors, *Contraceptive Technology* (New York: Irvington, 1990-1992).

take this chapter's Life Choice Inventory. Refer to Tables 13–2 and 13–3 as you do. The sections that follow provide more information on the individual methods.

➡▶ *No contraceptive method is perfect. Effectiveness ratings may vary depending upon how the method was studied—in the laboratory or in real life. Laboratory ratings, because they exclude the mistakes people make, are higher.*

■ The Standard Reversible Methods

This section provides a brief discussion of each of the methods listed in Table 13–2. The amount of information given here about any method does not reflect its desirability, but only its complexity.

TABLE 13–2 ■ Standard Birth Control Methods Compared According to Personal Preference

Method	1. **Possible obstacles to use.** Maximum possible points: _____ If easy for you to use, give all points; if difficult, give half. If impossible, give 0 points.	2. **Locus of control.** Maximum possible points: _____ If control lies with appropriate person, give all points; if control lies partially with wrong person, give half. If control lies entirely with wrong person, give 0 points.
Abstinence	Requires self-control and control on partner's part. Points: _____	Control is shared. Points: _____
Rhythm method	Requires self-control and partner's control, maintaining calendar, daily temperature taking, daily self-examination, record keeping. Points: _____	Control is shared. Points: _____
Oral contraceptives (combination pill and minipill)	Requires prescription, keeping schedule, willingness to take drugs. Points: _____	Control is woman's. Points: _____
Norplant	Requires willingness to have device implanted surgically. Points: _____	Control is woman's. Points: _____
Intrauterine device (IUD)	Requires professional insertion, willingness to accept initial discomfort and continuous presence of device, periodic checking of string. Points: _____	Control is woman's. Points: _____
Vaginal spermicides	Requires touching own genitals, interrupting foreplay, reapplying every 30 minutes. Points: _____	Control is mostly woman's. Points: _____
Diaphragm with spermicide	Requires initial professional fitting, prescription, touching own genitals, interrupting foreplay, reapplying spermicide every 30 minutes. Points: _____	Control is mostly woman's. Points: _____
Vaginal contraceptive sponge	Requires touching own genitals, remembering to soak sponge ahead of time, inserting ahead of time or interrupting foreplay. Points: _____	Control is mostly woman's. Points: _____
Cervical cap	Requires initial professional fitting, prescription, touching own genitals, interrupting foreplay, reapplying spermicide every 30 minutes. Points _____	Control is mostly woman's. Points: _____
Condom	Requires touching own genitals, interrupting foreplay, possible delay of male orgasm. Points: _____	Control is mostly man's. Points: _____
Condom with spermicide	Requires touching own genitals, interrupting foreplay, reapplying every 30 minutes, possible delay of male orgasm. Points: _____	Control is shared. Points: _____
Male sterilization	Requires willingness to undergo surgery, acceptance of irreversibility. Points: _____	Control is man's. Points: _____
Female sterilization	Requires willingness to undergo surgery, acceptance of irreversibility. Points: _____	Control is woman's. Points: _____

TABLE 13–2 ■ Continued

3. **Privacy and confidentiality.**
Maximum possible points:
_____ If method meets your
criteria, give all points; if method is
somewhat unsatisfactory, give half.
If method is unsatisfactory, give 0
points.

Must be shared with partner; no drugs
or devices. Points: _____

Must be shared with partner; records
and equipment are present.
Points: _____

Not necessary to tell partner; pills are
present. For minors requesting pills,
parents may be notified.
Points: _____

Not necessary to tell partner; no
evidence is present. Points: _____

Not necessary to tell partner; no
evidence is present. Points: _____

Necessary to tell partner; spermicide is
present. Points: _____

Necessary to tell partner; spermicide is
present. Points: _____

Necessary to tell partner; equipment is
present. Points: _____

Necessary to tell partner; spermicide is
present. Points: _____

Necessary to tell partner; condom is
present. Points: _____

Necessary to tell partner; equipment is
present. Points: _____

Not necessary to tell partner; no
evidence is present. Points: _____

Not necessary to tell partner; no
evidence is present. Points: _____

4. **Reversibility.** Maximum possible
points: _____ If acceptable to
you, give all points; if you prefer
reversibility and the method has a
small chance of producing sterility,
give half or 0. If unacceptable, give 0
points.

Reversible. Points: _____

Reversible. Points: _____

Reversible. On discontinuing use, user
is advised to delay conception for 3
months. Occasionally, user who
discontinues may not ovulate for
several months. Points: _____

Reversible. Points: _____

Reversible. Can cause permanent
sterility in women who develop
pelvic inflammatory disease.
Points: _____

Reversible. Points: _____

Reversible. Points: _____

Reversible. Points: _____

Reversible. Points: _____

Reversible. Points: _____

Reversible. Points: _____

Irreversible. Points: _____

Irreversible. Points: _____

5. **Frequency of intercourse.** Maximum
possible points: _____ If
continuity of protection fits your
pattern perfectly, give all points; if
imperfectly, give half. If it seriously
overprotects or underprotects, give 0
points.

Requires having no intercourse
whatever. Points: _____

Requires abstinence for about half of
every month; permits intercourse
several days in a row between times.
Points: _____

Afford continuous protection.
Points: _____

Affords continuous protection.
Points: _____

Affords continuous protection.
Points: _____

Affords protection as needed.
Points: _____

Affords protection as needed.
Points: _____

Affords protection as needed.
Points: _____

Affords protection as needed.
Points: _____

Affords protection as needed.
Points: _____

Affords protection as needed.
Points: _____

Affords continuous protection.
Points: _____

Affords continuous protection.
Points: _____

TABLE 13–2 ■ Continued

Method	6. **Noncontraceptive benefits.** Maximum possible points: _____ If benefits are significant, give all points; if somewhat significant, give half. If benefits are not significant, give 0 points.	7. **Cost.** Maximum possible points: _____ If cost is acceptable, give all points; if method is hard to afford, give half. If method is unaffordable, give 0 points. (1991 estimated prices.)
Abstinence	In harmony with certain religious beliefs; completely prevents sexually transmitted diseases (STDs) and pregnancy; shared method (promotes communication). Points: _____	Free. Points: _____
Rhythm method	In harmony with certain religious beliefs; frequent self-examination permits user to detect medical abnormalities early; shared method. Points: _____	Equipment purchases (once only), about $30 to $60. Points: _____
Oral contraceptives (combination pill and minipill)	Promotes regular menstrual cycles; reduces risk of certain cancers; can relieve acne symptoms in some users. Points: _____	Initial office visit fee of $35 to $95; $10 to $20 per month for pills. Points: _____
Norplant	Convenience. Points: _____	Depends on physicians. About $500 or more. Points: _____
Intrauterine device (IUD)	Unknown. Points: _____	Initial fee and follow-up fee; about $200 to $250 every three to five years. Points: _____
Vaginal spermicides	Unknown. Points: _____	Price varies with brand and type; about $.75 per application. Points: _____
Diaphragm with spermicide	Unknown. Points: _____	Initial office visit fee of $35 to $95; $25.00 for diaphragm; about $.75 per application for spermicide. Points: _____
Vaginal contraceptive sponge	Unknown. Points: _____	About $1.25 per application. Points: _____
Cervical cap	Unknown. Points: _____	Initial office visit fee of $35 to $95; about $30 for cervical cap; about $45 for insertion. Points: _____
Condom	Affords protection against some STDs, may delay male orgasm; shared method. Points: _____	About $.75 per condom; about $.85 for those with spermicide. Points: _____
Condom with vaginal spermicide	Affords protection against some STDs, may delay male orgasm; shared method. Points: _____	About $1.50 per application. Points: _____
Male sterilization	Slightly reduced mortality for unknown reasons. Points: _____	Depends on physician, facility, surgery; $350 or more. Points: _____
Female sterilization	Unknown. Points: _____	Typically, $1,000 or more. Points: _____

TABLE 13–2 ■ **Continued**

8. Medical side effects and risks. Maximum possible points: _____ If side effects are acceptable, give all points; if they reduce method's acceptability, give half. If unacceptable, give 0 points.	9. Physical limiting factors. Maximum possible points: _____ If no physical limiting factors would reduce effectiveness, give all points; if such a factor exists, reduce points.	10. Total score. Maximum possible points: 90. Add up the total number of points in the spaces in the previous nine columns, enter total in this column.
No side effects. Points: _____	If pregnancy has occurred with this method, do not consider it. Points: _____	TOTAL POINTS: _____
None. Points: _____	If menstrual periods are irregular, do not use this method. If pregnancy has occurred with this method, do not consider it. Points: _____	TOTAL POINTS: _____
Many are reported; most are infrequent or not serious (see text). Points: _____	If pregnancy has occurred with this method, do not consider it. Points: _____	TOTAL POINTS: _____
Relatively new. Irregular menstrual cycles during first year. Points: _____	If pregnancy has occurred with this method, do not consider it. Points: _____	TOTAL POINTS: _____
Heavy menstrual flow with anemia, ectopic pregnancy, septic abortion, pelvic inflammatory disease, puncture of uterus or cervix during insertion (see text). Points: _____	If pregnancy has occurred with this method, do not consider it. Points: _____	TOTAL POINTS: _____
Essentially none. Points: _____	If pregnancy has occurred with this method, do not consider it. Points: _____	TOTAL POINTS: _____
None. Points: _____	If pregnancy has occurred with this method, do not consider it. Points: _____	TOTAL POINTS: _____
None. Points: _____	If pregnancy has occurred with this method, do not consider it. Points: _____	TOTAL POINTS: _____
None. Points: _____	If pregnancy has occurred with this method, do not consider it. Points: _____	TOTAL POINTS: _____
None. Points: _____	If pregnancy has occurred with this method, do not consider it. Points: _____	TOTAL POINTS: _____
None. Points: _____	If pregnancy has occurred with this method, do not consider it. Points: _____	TOTAL POINTS: _____
Ordinary risks of minor surgery. Points: _____	If pregnancy has occurred with this method, do not consider it. Points: _____	TOTAL POINTS: _____
Risks of anesthesia; risks of injury to other organs, bleeding, infection. Points: _____	If pregnancy has occurred with this method, do not consider it. Points: _____	TOTAL POINTS: _____

TABLE 13–2 ■ **Continued**

---

11. **Acceptance or rejection based on effectiveness.** Use Table 13–3 to accept or reject each method; then write yes or no on each line below. Choose method with the highest score from those marked yes.

Method	Final rank list of methods
Abstinence	_____
Rhythm method	_____
Oral contraceptives (combination pill and minipill)	_____
Norplant	_____
Intrauterine device (IUD)	_____
Vaginal spermicides	_____
Diaphragm with spermicide	_____
Vaginal contraceptive sponge	_____
Cervical cap	_____
Condom	_____
Condom with vaginal spermicide	_____
Male sterilization	_____
Female sterilization	_____

---

abstinence refraining from sexual intercourse.

Abstinence effectiveness = 100%.

ABSTINENCE One method of contraception is **abstinence.** Abstinence is 100 percent guaranteed. It is the choice of many people, especially young, unmarried people. Many people share this preference because they want to avoid pregnancy and sexually transmitted diseases. Some choose this method because they desire to act consistently with their religious beliefs.

It takes courage to decide to abstain from sexual intercourse and willpower to maintain the decision in the face of social pressures to have sex. Fortunately for a person who decides to practice abstinence, this decision need not be permanent. If a person chooses not to have sex right now, this does not mean the person will never have a close sexual relationship. It does mean that the person will move at a self-selected pace and wait to have sex until the time is right.

For those with strong religious beliefs, the right time may be after they are married. For others, the right time may be when they are in a mature, committed relationship. If you are struggling with the decision, you may find it helpful to ask yourself the questions in this chapter's Strategies: How to Decide if You Are Ready for Sexual Intercourse.

Some people have already made the choice to have sex. They may feel good about it, or they may feel uncomfortable about it. Even a person who has already had sex, once or many times, can choose to say no now. The choice belongs to each individual.

The decision to have sex is strictly personal. Sex is to be enjoyed when a person decides it's right and to be less important at other times in the person's life. Remember, each person is the one in control of his or her sexuality. The best decisions are the ones that will still feel good tomorrow and a month or year from now.

TABLE 13–3 ■ Standard Birth Control Methods Accepted or Rejected on the Basis of Effectiveness[a]

Circle yes or no for each method based on the information in this table. Then return to column 11 of Table 13–2.

Method	Effectiveness if Used Perfectly (%)	Effectiveness in Typical Users (%)	Factors to Consider	Acceptability to You (circle one)	
Abstinence	100	Unknown	Chance of pregnancy within a year in a person who does not abstain is 90%.	Yes	No
Rhythm method	80 to 95	80	Ovulation is unpredictable. A high degree of training, skill, and dedication is required.	Yes	No
Oral contraceptives (combination pill and minipill)	99 99.5	95 97	Users who find it easy to take pills regularly use the method most successfully.	Yes	No
Norplant	99.96	98–99	Implant may be slightly visible. Long-term use is recommended.	Yes	No
Intrauterine device (IUD)	98.5	97	The device can be expelled without the user's awareness; pregnancy may occur with the device in place.	Yes	No
Vaginal spermicides	95 to 97	79	Users who follow directions exactly use the method most successfully.	Yes	No
Diaphragm with spermicide	98	82–86	Successful use requires proper fit and following instructions exactly.	Yes	No
Vaginal contraceptive sponge	95 to 98	76 to 83	Users who follow directions exactly use the method most successfully.	Yes	No
Cervical cap	98	73–92	Successful use requires proper fit and following instructions exactly.	Yes	No
Condom	98	88	Poor-quality condoms or leakage of sperm prior to use makes failure likely.	Yes	No
Condom with spermicide	99.5	98	Users must follow directions exactly. Poor-quality condoms or leakage of sperm prior to use makes failure likely.	Yes	No
Male sterilization	99.85	99.85	Pregnancy occurs only if the user has intercourse before sperm are absent from semen or if spontaneous repair occurs (very unlikely).	Yes	No
Female sterilization	99.7	99.7	Pregnancy is likely only if spontaneous regeneration occurs.	Yes	No

[a]Effectiveness ratings may vary depending upon how the method was studied—in the laboratory or in real life. Laboratory ratings, because they exclude the mistakes people make, are higher.

■ MINIGLOSSARY
of Female Fertility

corpus luteum (COR-pus LOO-tee-um) a mass of glandular tissue that forms from the follicle after an ovum has escaped from it.

endometrium (en-do-MEE-tree-um) the membrane lining the inner surface of the uterus.

estrogens hormones from the ovary that, in the female, regulate the ovulatory cycle. Estrogens are produced also, in lesser amounts, by the adrenal glands of people of both genders.

FSH a hormone from the brain's pituitary gland that, in women, stimulates the growth of follicles. (The abbreviation stands for *follicle-stimulating hormone*.)

LH a hormone from the brain's pituitary gland that, in women, stimulates the development of the corpus luteum. (The abbreviation stands for *luteinizing* (LOO-tin-ize-ing) *hormone*.)

progesterone (pro-JESS-tuh-rone) a female hormone secreted by the corpus luteum during that portion of the menstrual cycle in which the uterine lining builds up.

■ ■ ■ ■ ■ STRATEGIES: *HOW TO DECIDE IF YOU ARE READY FOR SEXUAL INTERCOURSE*

Are You Really Ready for Sexual Intercourse?

The way you answer the following few questions can alert you to areas of your present relationship that may need attention before you consider sexual intimacy.

1. What place does this relationship have in my life? Wishful thinking aside, does this person have the qualities I seek in a permanent partner?
2. What place does this relationship have in the life of my partner? (If you do not know the answer to this question, ask.)
3. Are you ready stop "dating" others and commit yourself wholly to this person? Can you trust your partner, also, to be monogamous? (This takes more strength that you may now suspect, becaude after the newness has worn off, other people may seem more attractive.)
4. What does having sexual intercourse mean for you? What does it mean for your partner? (If one person takes it as a sign of commitment, but the other considers it just a pleasant activity, the relationship is not a candidate for sexual intimacy until both come to some agreement.)
5. Where is the pressure to have sexual intercourse coming from? Is your internal biological drive in control of this decision, or does it seem that "everyone else is doing it?" (Sexual intercourse, while a reliever of the biological sexual drive, should be made by the conscious decision of the rational mind. It should never be a public issue. Better to find new friends than to have inappropriate sexual intercourse.)
6. Do you feel that if you do not have sexual intercourse, you will lose the affection of your partner? (Talk to your partner about this fear. If the partner rejects you because you are not ready for sexual intercourse, this is a virtual guarantee that the relationship was not as solid as you might have thought. Sexual abstinence for a time can be a test of the endurance of the love beyond sexual attraction.)
7. How does having sexual intercourse mesh with your own values and religious beliefs? (If it conflicts with these, you must resolve these issues or they could destroy your relationship.)
8. Have you both agreed on the best way to prevent pregnancy, and on the use of condoms to prevent sexually transmitted diseases? (Both are needed, especially at first.)
9. Would having sexual intercourse make me feel better about myself as a person? Would it make my partner feel better about the experience? (Sexual intercourse can bolster self-esteem when it occurs in the right context. It can also destroy self-esteem when the context is not right.)
10. Does the person make you feel loved in other, nonsexual ways? (Love should also be expressed in doing favors, giving small gifts, confiding in each other, hugging, kissing, being honest, and being sensitive to each other's needs and moods.)

Your willingness to answer these questions and to discuss them with your partner shows maturity. Mature people know that sexual intercourse is too important to just let happen on a biological whim. The sex drive can lead people into serious trouble unless they control it with willpower and make conscious choices about intercourse—when *they* are ready to make them.

---

rhythm method a method of contraception; avoiding sexual intercourse during times of fertility. It involves predicting or discerning ovulation; charting of a menstrual calendar and of body temperature; and observations of cervical mucus. Couples can use the method either to plan conception or to prevent it.

Rhythm method, laboratory rating = 80–95%

Rhythm method, user effectiveness = 80%

RHYTHM METHOD The **rhythm method** (also called *fertility awareness method,* or *calendar method*) is a method of contraception that involves limiting sexual intercourse to times of the month when the woman is not fertile.

For conception to occur, sexual intercourse must take place within a certain time span. An ovum lives for only 12 to 24 hours, and living sperm must arrive in time to fertilize it during this brief life span. Sperm can live quite well for 1 to 5 days within the female reproductive tract, so they can get there first and wait. Intercourse within this time span can result in a pregnancy.*

The female's cycle that leads to the production of one ovum each month is depicted in Figure 13–2. It is known as the **ovulatory cycle,** because it is the cycle in which **ovulation** (the production of an ovum) takes place each month. It is also known as the **menstrual cycle,** because it involves **menstruation.** The Miniglossary of Female Fertility defines the related terms.

Males produce sperm continuously, as shown in Figure 13–3. A comparison of the two figures reveals that both females and males produce and respond to some of the same hormones, but in different amounts and in different ways. The terms relating to males are defined in the Miniglossary of Male Fertility.

A couple that chooses to use the rhythm method to avoid conception avoids sexual intercourse before, during, and immediately after ovulation. Days of ovulation vary from woman to woman, so people cannot accurately estimate ovulation based on an average woman's cycle by counting days from the last menstruation. Methods to determine the time of ovulation include recording menstruation days on a calendar, measuring daily body temperature, observing changes in vaginal secretions, or a combination of these. Family planning centers offer help in learning to use these fertility awareness methods both to conceive and to prevent conception.

At-home urine-testing kits can be purchased over the counter that will show a woman when she is ovulating. They detect LH (luteinizing hormone), one of the hormones of ovulation. The tests are expensive in comparison with the standard fertility awareness methods just mentioned, but offer the advantage of predicting by a day or two the fertile time of the month so that the couple can prepare for it.

The rhythm method of contraception is available to anyone, but training by professionals is necessary for people to use it successfully. Even the most comprehensive, technically correct references warn people that merely reading about the method is insufficient to enable them to use it successfully to prevent conception.**

ORAL CONTRACEPTIVES Many women choose **oral contraceptives,** popularly known as "the Pill."[5] The Pill is the most popular nonsurgical method of contraception.[6] There are two types of oral contraceptives: the **combination pill,** which contains synthetic versions of the hormones estrogen and progesterone, taken for 21 days of each month; and the **minipill,** which contains only synthetic progesterone (**progestin**) and is taken continuously. The estrogen in the combination pills prevents pregnancy the same way as the hormones of the female cycle do, by suppressing ovulation. A woman may still ovulate during her first month on pills, and should use a backup method of contraception during this time.

*The exact life span of sperm within the female reproductive tract is not known, but is thought to be at least 24 hours, and possibly as long as five days.
**For more information about fertility awareness methods, consult the latest edition of R. A. Hatcher and coauthors, *Contraceptive Technology* (New York: Irvington). Most libraries have this book, which contains the explicit instructions needed by the person who wants to use the method.

ovulatory cycle the monthly maturing of an ovum.

ovulation (AH-vyoo-LAY-shun) the release of an ovum from one of the ovaries.

menstrual cycle the monthly fertility cycle, directed by hormones, that prepares the uterus to receive a fertilized ovum.

menstruation the monthly shedding of the uterine lining.

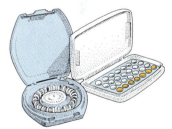

oral contraceptives pills taken by mouth, which contain synthetic hormones that prevent ovulation; used to prevent conception; often called **birth control pills.**

combination pill an oral contraceptive containing estrogens and progestin.

minipill a progestin-only oral contraceptive.

progestin synthetic progesterone, used as a contraceptive drug.

Oral contraceptive effectiveness:
Combination pills, laboratory rating = 99.5%.
Combination pills, user effectiveness = 97%.
Minipill, laboratory rating = 99%.
Minipill, user effectiveness = 95%.

FIGURE 13–2 ■ **Physiology of the female reproductive system.**

The orchestration of this cycle is as complex as that of a symphony: each musical voice is the signal for another voice to begin or end its song. Hormones are the "voices" that call forth responses with a characteristic timing and magnitude—**FSH (follicle-stimulating hormone)** and **LH (luteinizing hormone)**, **estrogens** and **progesterone**. Events occurring between day 1 of menstrual cycle (first day of flow) and ovulation. The day of ovulation varies greatly among women. It is usually the midpoint among day 1 and the last day of the cycle. Women's cycles can vary from 26 to 35 days so the days of ovulation can vary from day 12 to day 21.

Events occurring between day 1 of menstrual cycle (first day of flow) and day 14 (ovulation):

Pituitary gland releases FSH, LH.

Ovary produces estrogen.

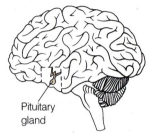
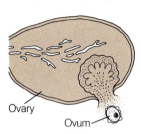
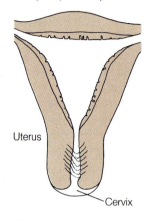

Pituitary gland

Ovary

Ovum

Uterus

Cervix

Pituitary gland monitors estrogen levels and reduces FSH and LH production when estrogen level is high enough.

Ovum matures and leaves follicle (ovulation).

Follicle becomes corpus luteum.

After shedding, endometrium begins to build up.

(a) In the first part of the monthly cycle, an ovarian follicle (an ovum with its surrounding sac of cells) begins to mature. The follicle grows. Ovulation is the bursting of this follicle, which frees the now-ripe ovum.

Events occurring between ovulation and day 1 of next menstrual cycle:

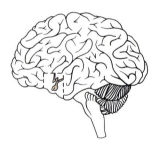
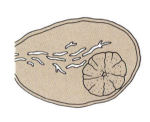
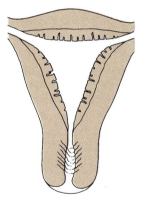

Lower FSH and LH levels.

Corpus luteum produces progesterone.

Lower estrogen production.

Thickened endometrium is maintained by progesterone.

(b) If fertilized, the ovum settles in the uterus. Simultaneously, the uterus prepares for the ovum by building up its lining (the **endometrium**), storing extra blood and glycogen in it to provide nourishment for the growth of an embryo. Meanwhile, the empty follicular sac develops into the **corpus luteum** ("yellow body"), a sort of remote control device that releases the hormone progesterone that will maintain pregnancy-favoring conditions in the uterus. (It is the corpus luteum for which the pituitary hormone, luteinizing hormone, is named.)

Events occurring on day 1 of next menstrual cycle:

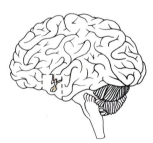
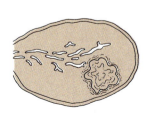
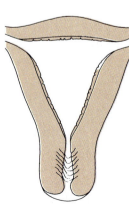

FSH and LH levels begin to rise.

Corpus lutem begins degenerating; progesterone level begins to decline; estrogen level begins to rise.

Uterine lining is shed.

(c) If fertilized and implanted, the ovum produces a factor to maintain these conditions and support pregnancy. If the ovum is shed, the conditions for pregnancy cannot be maintained. The corpus luteum withers away, the hormonal climate changes, and the cycle begins again.

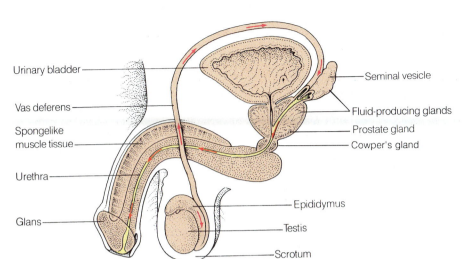

Urinary bladder

Vas deferens

Spongelike
muscle tissue

Urethra

Glans

Seminal vesicle

Fluid-producing glands

Prostate gland

Cowper's gland

Epididymus

Testis

Scrotum

**FIGURE 13–3 ■ The male's production
of sperm.**

The brain's pituitary gland starts the process
of sperm production by releasing two
hormones—**FSH** (follicle-stimulating hormone)
and **LH** (luteinizing hormone). These pituitary
compounds stimulate sperm production and
release. The testes (testicles) respond by
producing the hormone **testosterone.**
Adequate testosterone is essential for the
continuous production of sperm cells.

The minipill contains no estrogen, and most of its effects take place in the uterus itself. The progestin in the minipill makes the mucus surrounding the uterine opening (cervix) less penetrable to sperm and also may deactivate sperm cells. Progestin also interrupts the normal preparation of the uterine endometrium so that a zygote may not implant. Taking pills is not the only way to introduce progestins into the body: some contraceptive devices release the drugs directly into the uterus or vagina, and in other countries, women can receive a shot of progestins that lasts for three months.*

Some pills, the **triphasic oral contraceptives,** offer combined hormones in low doses that stop ovulation.[7] The triphasic pills deliver hormones in three levels throughout the cycle.[8] The woman takes the first type of pill for several days, then the next two types for the remainder of the cycle. This scheme prevents ovulation and promotes regular menstrual cycles.

One study reported that Pill users experienced difficulty remembering to take the Pill.[9] The effectiveness of the Pill, as of any type of contraception, depends on regular and correct use. It is imperative to ask questions of the prescribing physician or counselor to clear up any confusion about how the Pill works and how to use it. If a woman forgets to take her pill for a day or more, she should resume taking it, but also use a backup method of contraception for the remainder of that pill cycle.

All oral contraceptives present side effects, ranging from minor complaints such as breast tenderness to life-threatening conditions. The number of observed effects is impressive, but remember that most are rare and that many are known because so many millions of women have been studied. Side effects that, when they occur, warrant seeking a different method include emotional depression or fatigue, nausea or vomiting, skin conditions, weight gain or loss, stopping of menstruation, unexpected vaginal bleeding, increased frequency of vaginal yeast infections, high levels of sugar and fat in the blood, decreased sex drive, headaches, and fluid retention. The Pill may also affect the user's nutrition status as this chapter's Critical Thinking

triphasic oral contraceptives   birth control pills of low hormone content, administered in three phases over the menstrual cycle.

Report these symptoms:

Abdominal pain.

Chest pain.

Breathlessness.

Headaches.

Blurred vision or loss of vision.

Leg pain.

*Among devices that release progestin are intrauterine devices (IUDs) and vaginal rings. The shot is Depo Provera.

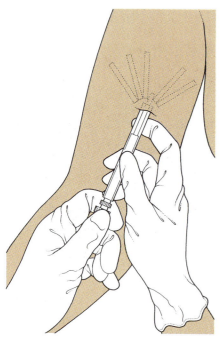

Norplant effectiveness:
Laboratory rating = 99.96%.
User effectiveness = 98–99%.

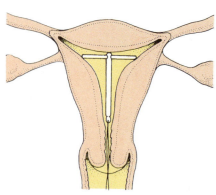

IUD effectiveness:
Laboratory rating = 98.5%.
User effectiveness = 95%.

intrauterine device (IUD) a device inserted into the uterus to prevent conception or implantation.

section explores. Among the rare conditions are diseases of the heart, kidney, liver, or gallbladder; stroke; benign tumors of the uterus; and blood clots that can lodge in vital organs and cause death. Women who take oral contraceptives should report to their physicians any of the symptoms listed in the margin. Not all side effects are negative. For example, oral contraceptives can help to regulate irregular menstrual periods.[10] They have also been associated with reduced risks of certain cancers.[11]

Some studies suggest that users of oral contraceptives have greater risk of cervical cancer.[12] Other factors make it difficult to attribute the cancer to the Pill itself. Pill users often have intercourse at young ages, have multiple sex partners, are unlikely to use condoms, and are therefore often exposed to a sexually transmitted virus that may cause cervical cancer.[13]

Women who use the Pill are strongly advised not to smoke, because smoking, together with use of the Pill, increases the risk of heart attack or stroke.

The minipill produces fewer and less severe side effects than the combination pill; hence, women sometimes switch to it. Of course, the minipill has possible side effects of its own, including menstrual disorders and, less often, headaches.

Most women who use the Pill experience no side effects at all or accept and adjust to the minor side effects they experience. Many who experience minor discomfort find that it goes away after about three months. Others need only switch from one brand of pill to another (the prescribing physician can advise about this possibility).

It is important to be aware that depression, a relatively common side effect, may take some time to develop; the user may not realize that it is associated with oral contraceptive use. When moodiness, sadness, or irritability is not brought on by explainable events and does not improve after several months, Pill users should suspect the pills and ask their physicians for another type.

A woman who believes she may be pregnant should not take the Pill, because it greatly increases the risks of defects in the fetus. In fact, a woman who decides to become pregnant and is using oral contraceptives is advised to switch to another method of contraception for at least three months (some health care providers suggest six months to a year) before attempting to conceive.

NORPLANT A relatively new contraceptive method is to surgically implant capsules of contraceptive hormones under the skin. The product's trade name is Norplant, and the implants are six thin capsules (each about the size of a matchstick) placed in the upper arm.[14] The implants work by slowly releasing the synthetic hormone progestin; they are effective for up to five years. Possible side effects of Norplant include menstrual irregularities that, for most people, are resolved after the first year. The use of Norplant has been suggested as a means to help nations around the world, whose populations are multiplying dangerously, to control their numbers.[15]

INTRAUTERINE DEVICE A method of birth control is to use the **intrauterine device,** or **IUD.** The IUD is a small plastic or plastic and metal object that is inserted into a woman's uterus by a health care provider. A thin

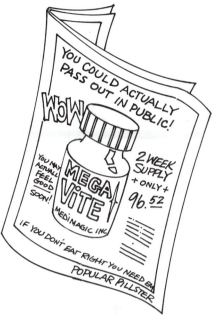

CRITICAL THINKING

Misuse of Truth

The Pill affects a woman's nutrition status, and users may wonder whether they need to take supplements to compensate. However, the Pill's effects on nutrition are not all negative: it increases blood levels of iron and copper, so that women who take it may need less of these two minerals. On the other hand, the Pill interferes with the body's use of two vitamins, folate and vitamin B_6. Deficiencies of these produce anemia or emotional depression in some users.

Vitamin companies use these findings to promote the taking (and buying) of all sorts of supplements, often recommending them instead of what the pill user needs—a balanced diet from a variety of foods. The companies may be correctly reporting the problem as an increased need for nutrients, but the solution they advocate, taking supplements, is inappropriate.

Ads may state the truth, but may misstate its implications.

nylon thread hangs from the IUD through the cervix into the vagina as an indicator that the IUD is in place and as an aid to removal.

The IUD is appropriate for long-term use; it can remain in place for 5 to 7 years. It is not appropriate for repeated insertions and removals, such as between pregnancies in a growing family. The mechanism of action of the IUD is not fully known, but one theory is that the IUD makes the uterine environment hostile to sperm or to zygotes and prevents implantation. Some IUDs slowly release the synthetic hormone progestin into the uterus, making it an even more unfavorable environment for sperm and zygotes. The IUD may be inserted up to five days *after* unprotected intercourse and still prevent pregnancy.

Many health care providers discourage the use of the IUD because of the complications that often arise from its use. Pelvic inflammatory disease (PID, discussed in Chapter 17), which can lead to sterility, can be a complication of IUD use.[16] PID is attributed to the introduction of bacteria during insertion of the IUD. IUDs also cause increased cramping and blood loss during menstruation. Women considering this method of birth control are carefully screened. The ideal candidate for an IUD is at an age where she wishes to have no more children, is in a monogamous sexual relationship, practices routine hygiene, and has mild menstrual periods with no cramping. Before inserting an IUD, her health care provider will likely have her sign a waiver claiming she's aware of the risks and willing to accept any complications that may occur.

VAGINAL SPERMICIDE Another contraceptive method involves using any of several brands of **spermicide**—sperm-killing or sperm-immobilizing products that can be inserted into the vagina just before intercourse. These are available over the counter as foams, creams, gels, sheets, or supposito-

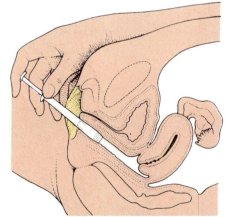

Spermicide (foams, creams, gels, sheets, and suppositories) effectiveness:
Laboratory rating = 95 to 97%.
User effectiveness = 76 to 83%.

spermicide a chemical that kills or immobilizes sperm, used in several contraceptive devices.

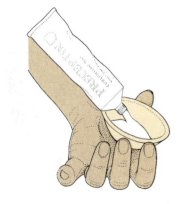

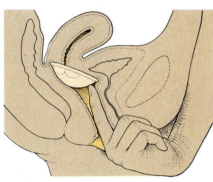

Diaphragm with spermicide effectiveness:
Laboratory rating = 98%.
User effectiveness = 82–86%.

barrier device a contraceptive device that physically obstructs the travel of sperm toward the ovum.

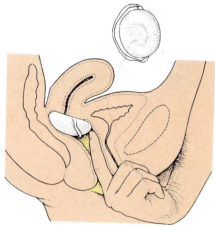

Sponge effectiveness:
Laboratory rating = 95 to 98%.
User effectiveness = 76 to 83%.

ries. These contraceptives are chemical devices—they interpose a chemical barrier between sperm and ovum at the opening of the uterus. Most do not last long—only half an hour or so—and therefore must be inserted just prior to each act of sexual intercourse. (The package will provide exact details about timing.) Some people find that spermicides act as a local anesthetic.

User effectiveness ratings for vaginal spermicides are relatively low. Vaginal spermicide appears to be most valuable when used in conjunction with other contraceptive devices such as the condom or the diaphragm.

DIAPHRAGM The **diaphragm** is a **barrier device**. (See the miniglossary of contraceptive barrier devices.) It is a circular metal spring or ring fitted with a shallow cup of thin rubber that the user fills with spermicidal cream or jelly. The device is folded for insertion into the vagina; once inside, it resumes its original shape to cover the cervix. The diaphragm holds spermicide and bars sperm from entering the uterus.

To fit a woman with a diaphragm, the health care provider measures the vaginal interior and prescribes the size that ensures the all-important proper fit. (Some people may be tempted to borrow a diaphragm "just to try it" before going in to be fitted themselves. This is a mistake, because the likelihood that a borrowed diaphragm will fit properly is slim indeed.)

The user of a diaphragm can insert it up to six hours in advance of intercourse. If the user inserts the diaphragm about two hours or more before intercourse, she should apply additional spermicide. She should leave the diaphragm in place for at least six hours after intercourse and then remove it as soon as convenient within 24 hours. The user should store her diaphragm as instructed and check it periodically for holes or other defects by holding it up to the light. It has a limited life span.

SPONGE A barrier device similar in principle to the diaphragm is the vaginal contraceptive **sponge.** The sponge is disposable and resembles a diaphragm in shape but is made of thick polyurethane and comes equipped with a woven handle for removal. The sponge contains a spermicide that becomes active when wet; the user moistens it with water before insertion. A bowl-shaped indentation in the sponge helps hold it in place over the cervix.

The user can insert the sponge several hours before sexual intercourse. It gives continuous protection for 24 hours, with nothing more to do, even for

■ MINIGLOSSARY of
Contraceptive Barrier Devices

diaphragm a barrier device consisting of a dome that fits over the cervix and holds spermicidal cream or jelly against the uterine entrance to block the passage of sperm.

sponge a barrier device similar in principle to the diaphragm that fits over the cervix and releases spermicide when moistened with water.

cervical cap a barrier device similar to, but smaller than, the diaphragm, that fits

over the cervix.

condom a barrier device consisting of a sheath worn over the penis during intercourse to contain the semen and/or reduce risk of transmission of sexually transmitted disease.

female condom a barrier device under development that lines the vagina with polyurethane and works similarly to the condom used by men.

repeated intercourse. The user must leave it in place for at least six hours after intercourse and then remove it as soon as convenient.

CERVICAL CAP Another barrier device, the **cervical cap,** is similar to the diaphragm in method of use and effectiveness. Like the diaphragm, it must fit perfectly; a health care provider chooses the size to fit the user. The cap is a flexible, cuplike device about an inch and a half in diameter that covers the woman's cervix. It differs from the diaphragm in that it is smaller and more durable. Since the cap fits tightly and rarely leaks, the reintroduction of spermicide before intercourse is unnecessary.

In a very few instances, a dangerous kind of bacterial poisoning known as *toxic shock syndrome* (TSS)* has been associated with diaphragm, sponge, and cervical cap use. (More often, toxic shock syndrome has been associated with the use of a brand of tampons that has now been removed from the market.) Because of the risk of TSS, it is wise to remove the diaphragm, sponge, or cap promptly according to directions. The early warning signs of TSS are diarrhea, fever, muscle aches (flulike), and a skin rash resembling a sunburn.

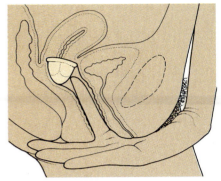

Cervical cap effectivess:
Laboratory rating = 98%.
User effectiveness = 73–92%.

CONDOM Up to this point we have discussed only female methods and devices. Use of the **condom** is the only reversible method available to men in the United States. The condom is a disposable barrier device whose effectiveness in reducing the risk of transmission of AIDS has brought it widespread attention (see Chapter 17). It consists of a thin sheath of latex (a type of rubber) or processed lamb tissue that is rolled over the erect penis before intercourse. There are many varieties, shapes, and colors, but all work the same way—they collect semen, usually in a small pouch at the tip of the condom, and retain it for disposal.

The condom offers an additional benefit to women. Because it often blocks transmission of disease organisms that cause PID, it helps protect women against tubal pregnancies.[17] For men and women, it offers some protection against sexually transmitted disease.

When applying the condom, the user should leave it rolled up as it comes from the wrapper and place it loosely on the glans of the erect penis. The rubber is gently and carefully unrolled down to the base of the penis, while the thumb and index finger of one hand hold the condom's tip to create a reservoir for the semen. The condom should not be stretched tightly over the glans—this would make it likely to break during intercourse. Some condoms are coated with lubricating jelly on the outside to reduce friction in the vagina. For maximum effectiveness in preventing pregnancy and sexually transmitted diseases, a man should use a latex (not lambskin) condom, and the woman should use a vaginal spermicide. Men can use condoms that come with spermicide already applied to them. A warning is in order here: do not use Vaseline or other petroleum-based jelly for lubrication; this can destroy the condom. Also, do not store condoms in wallets or purchase condoms from vending machines where they may undergo extended periods of time at high temperatures. This can also destroy condoms.

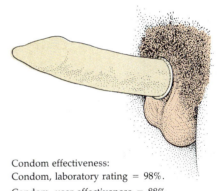

Condom effectiveness:
Condom, laboratory rating = 98%.
Condom, user effectiveness = 88%.
Condom with spermicide = more effective than condom alone.

---

*Toxic shock syndrome (TSS) is a dangerous symptom caused by a toxin produced by bacteria within the vagina and around the cervix that breed in menstrual blood that is prevented from flowing out.

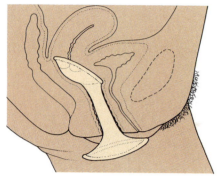

Female condom effectiveness:
Laboratory rating = 97%
(The female condom is pending approval by the Food and Drug Administration, hence user effectiveness data is not yet published.)

◼ *FACT OR FICTION:* It is wise to use Vaseline as a lubricating jelly with condoms. *False.* Vaseline makes condoms disintegrate.

The condom must be in place before any contact occurs between the penis and the vagina, because as mentioned, fluid that contains sperm is released even before intercourse begins. If the condom is applied too late, its effectiveness drops dramatically. Condoms vary in quality; some break easily, and the latex ones are recommended. (For more details about condom purchasing, storage, and use, see the Spotlight that follows Chapter 17.)

A condom will slip off a penis that is not fully erect. A man who uses one must withdraw from contact after intercourse, and a man who tends to lose his erection during intercourse should not rely on a condom for contraception.

A barrier device just being introduced is the **female condom.**[18] Available in one size, it is a disposable device made of a polyurethane sheath with a flexible ring at one end and a closed, diaphragm-like dome at the other. The closed end is inserted into the vagina and placed over the cervix like a diaphragm, while the ring at the open end remains outside the vagina. The strong material of the female condom seems less likely to tear than the man's latex condom, and some claim it may be more reliable, although effectiveness ratings have not been established. It offers better protection against sexually transmitted diseases, because there is less skin contact than with the latex condom.

Other methods of contraception are being developed. Some are available in other countries, and some are in the research stage, but none are as well researched as those just presented. Lack of government support, fear of lawsuits, and modest profits from new products slow progress in contraceptive technology.

≡▶ *A variety of birth control methods are available. The effectiveness of any contraceptive method depends on its regular and correct use.*

◼≡ Strategies Not Recommended for Contraception

Popular belief often endorses contraception strategies other than those just described. For example, some falsely believe that a couple can effectively prevent pregnancy by using a method that involves neither drugs nor devices—the **withdrawal method,** also known as **coitus interruptus.** It is just what it sounds like—the man withdraws his penis from the vagina before he ejaculates, taking care that his semen is not deposited in, at, or near the vagina.

Two built-in errors flaw the withdrawal method. The method often fails to prevent pregnancy because the man finds it difficult to withdraw his penis when he is near orgasm; he feels an urge for deeper penetration at that time. Even if he is able to withdraw before ejaculation, live sperm from the fluid at the tip of his penis will have already entered the vagina and may fertilize the ovum. Withdrawal is better than no method at all, but it still allows one woman out of four to become pregnant in one year of use. It is not recommended for individuals who are serious about preventing pregnancy.

Throughout history, women have attempted to wash out or kill sperm after unprotected intercourse by using **douches** of such preparations as lemon juice, carbonated beverages, vinegar, or even hazardous chemicals

withdrawal method (coitus interruptus) a technique in sexual intercourse of withdrawing the penis from the vagina just prior to ejaculation.

◼ *FACT OR FICTION:* Withdrawal is an effective birth control method. *False.* Withdrawal is ineffective because most men are unable to do it and because fluid that may contain sperm leaves the penis before ejaculation.

douche (doosh) a stream of fluid directed into the vagina, ineffective as a contraceptive.

such as turpentine. The repeated use of douches is associated with PID and cervical cancer.[19] Vaginal douches after sexual intercourse are not effective for preventing pregnancy. The fluid may wash sperm into the cervix as easily as it washes them out.

Women have also thought, wrongly, that as long as they breastfed their babies, they could not become pregnant. It is true that during **lactation**, the likelihood that a woman will ovulate is reduced—but unfortunately, there is no way she can know for sure. Lactation is an important means of reducing the total number of children born throughout a population, but it is unreliable as a contraceptive method for any individual woman.

≡▶ *The methods that are not effective at preventing conception are withdrawal, douching, and lactation.*

■≡ Irreversible Methods: Sterilization

In direct contrast to the approaches just discussed, **sterilization** is a highly effective contraceptive method—in most cases, irreversible. Each year, millions of people choose to be rendered permanently infertile, and the number is increasing.[20] In fact, sterilization is the leading contraceptive method in the world.

The choice to be sterilized is highly personal. No one can count on being able to reverse it later. For the person who desires temporary, reversible contraception, sterilization is not appropriate. (This does not mean, though, that sterilization is 100 percent effective; in rare cases, the ends of the tubes that are surgically severed find each other and grow back together, restoring fertility.)

The simplest and most common sterilization procedures are **vasectomy** in men and **tubal ligation** in women. The vasectomy is a safe procedure that involves making one or two tiny incisions in the scrotum and severing the vas deferens, through which the sperm travel to become part of the semen. The procedure takes about half an hour and may be performed under local anesthesia in a physician's office. The incisions are so tiny that vasectomies are called "Band-Aid surgery." The vasectomized man continues to produce sperm, but they are absorbed by the body rather than being released into the semen. Interruption of the delivery of sperm has no effect on the production of the male hormone testosterone.

Vasectomy does not affect a man's ability or desire to have intercourse, although his fear of the surgery may do so. Sometimes a man needs a brief period of adjustment after the operation before he is sure he desires and enjoys sexual intercourse as much as he did before. Thereafter, many men report increased enjoyment, because they need not fear their partners' becoming pregnant.

A man is not sterile immediately after the operation, because living sperm are still present in the tubes through which they travel. Usually it takes 6 to 8 weeks to clear them out; ejaculation removes some of them, and the others simply die. Another method of contraception must be used until tests show that no sperm are present. Once the sperm are eliminated from the semen, the chance of pregnancy is practically nil.

Vasectomy is a relatively low-cost, one-time procedure. It permits the man to resume normal activity within a day or so and sexual activity within a few

lactation the production of milk—sometimes inappropriately relied on as a contraceptive method.

sterilization the process of rendering people infertile, usually by surgically severing and sealing the vas deferens or the fallopian tubes.

vasectomy surgical severing and sealing of both of the vas deferens to sterilize men.

tubal ligation surgical severing and sealing of both of the fallopian tubes to sterilize women.

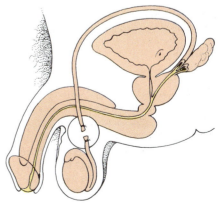

Vasectomy effectiveness:
Laboratory rating = 99.85%.
User effectiveness = 99.85%.

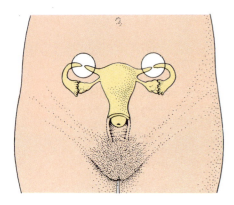

days. Ejaculation and orgasm are normal. Pain is minimal, and side effects are rare.

For a tubal ligation, a woman may require a hospital stay, although the procedure often can be performed on a walk-in basis. The operation can be performed with either a local or general anesthetic.* Commonly referred to as "tying the tubes," this permanently prevents passage of ova from the ovaries to the uterus. The procedure leaves a tiny scar on the abdomen, in the navel, or in the vagina, and the woman experiences no decline in her sexual drive or enjoyment. After the operation, the woman continues to menstruate and ovulate as before; when the ripe ovum is released, the body reabsorbs it.

≡▶ *Vasectomy for men and tubal ligation for women are safe, common, and irreversible methods of contraception.*

■≡ Contraceptive Failure

Unplanned pregnancies are not unusual, even when couples are using contraception. Any method may fail. Talking about a method's failure rate may bring impersonal statistics to mind, but in human terms it means that a couple is facing a pregnancy despite efforts to prevent it.

When you read that a certain method is 97 percent effective, think about the numbers. If the adult, fertile female population of the United States were 100 million (it's close to that number), and if all of these women were using one of the most effective methods of contraception and using it correctly, 3 million women would still become pregnant each year. Of course, in real life, the number is greater, for not all fertile women use contraception, and those who do often use it incorrectly.

Actually, over 4 million women in the United States alone face unwanted pregnancies each year. An unwanted pregnancy may result from failed contraception, rape, or sexual abuse. Each person who has an unwanted pregnancy faces the hard decision of whether or not to continue the pregnancy.

A woman who suspects that she has an unwanted pregnancy has many options as to where to go for a test. Three possible choices are a local health department, which (in some states) will offer free or low-cost tests without accompanying advice; an abortion clinic, which will assist and support a woman in obtaining an abortion if she desires one; and a religious organization that will help support a woman in carrying her pregnancy to term and assist with adoption if she chooses it.

Imagine that you are facing an unwanted pregnancy. (If you are a man, imagine that you are involved in an unplanned pregnancy). Remember from Chapter 2 ("Emotional Health") that decisions involve weighing your feelings, judgments, and values; if you are considering **abortion,** these may well conflict with one another. If you reject that choice, you face others:

abortion   a general term meaning a pregnancy that ends before the fetus is viable outside the uterus. A **spontaneous abortion** is a **miscarriage**; an **induced** or **therapeutic abortion** is one brought on by medical means.

*Several terms may be used in connection with the tubal ligation: *laparotomy* means an incision in the abdomen; the *minilaparotomy* (like the vasectomy, sometimes called "Band-Aid surgery") is a small abdominal incision; in a *laparoscopy,* the surgeon makes two smaller incisions, one to accommodate a viewing instrument and one through which the tubes are severed. (Another, different procedure, the *hysterectomy,* is the removal of the uterus. Although this major surgery produces sterility, it is usually performed for medical reasons, not for contraceptive purposes.)

whether to keep the baby or give it up for adoption, and whether to marry the father, if you are not now married. So you are under extreme stress, and in addition, pregnancy causes hormonal changes that intensify that stress. A pregnant, unmarried woman may also be experiencing guilt, anger, embarrassment, concern for feelings of parents or partner, and dread of others' reactions to the news.

Objective counseling can be a great help in deciding how to handle an unplanned pregnancy. Act promptly, for delays increase a woman's risks, whether she ultimately has an abortion or continues the pregnancy. If she chooses abortion, the longer she waits, the riskier the procedures become. If she continues the pregnancy and prenatal care is delayed, the health of her fetus, as well as her own health, may be compromised.

For those who choose abortion, most abortion clinics offer a range of services: free or low-cost pregnancy tests, preabortion counseling, examinations, standard blood tests, and abortions. Hospitals provide equally safe abortions,[21] and the hospital's personnel and equipment are better able to handle medical emergencies, should one arise.

The facility chosen should have the same degree of professionalism as any other medical facility. The physical surroundings should be clean, the staff should be courteous, and the woman should be afforded privacy. If any of these conditions is lacking, or if a woman feels uncomfortable for any reason, she should look elsewhere. Remember, walking into a medical office does not obligate you to be treated there. Feel free to leave and try another.

Abortion methods vary according to the length of the pregnancy. Abortions that take place early in pregnancy require minimal or no anesthesia; they are routine for the medical staff; and most women tolerate them well. Abortions can also be induced nonsurgically; by taking the pill RU 486 (trade name Mifepristone), pregnancies of less than seven weeks can be terminated safely and effectively. The drug blocks the action of the hormone progesterone; a follow-up dose of prostaglandin, given 48 hours later, causes uterine contractions and results in expulsion of the fetus. RU 486 has been available in France since its first clearance as a birth control method, and it may become available in the United States.[22]

In early abortions, through 13 weeks' gestation, a thin, hollow tube is inserted into the uterus, suction is applied, and the contents of the uterus are vacuumed out in a process called **vacuum aspiration.** Between 13 and about 16 weeks, suction alone cannot remove all of the uterine contents. A large-diameter vacuum tube is needed and requires that the cervix be dilated enough to accommodate it and other tools used for removal. This operation is known as a **D and E** (dilation of the cervix and evacuation of the uterus). A similar procedure, the **D and C** (dilation and curettage), involves scraping the uterus with other tools. This is most often used for medical problems, not abortion.

For abortions after 13 weeks of gestation, medical methods are an alternative to the surgical methods just described. Chemicals are administered to induce labor: prostaglandins and solutions of salt or urea may be injected directly into the sac surrounding the fetus, and a labor-inducing hormone* may be administered to the woman.

The physical risk of abortion performed by a trained medical professional is much lower today than in the past. The procedures still carry some slight

vacuum aspiration vacuuming of the uterus.

D and E dilation (alternate spelling *dilatation*) of the cervix and evacuation of the uterus.

D and C dilation of the cervix and curettage (scraping of the uterus).

*The hormone is oxytocin.

risk, however, especially late in pregnancy. Generally, abortion during the first three months poses a risk to the woman's life only slightly higher than that of contraception; and up to 16 weeks, abortion remains much less risky than pregnancy and childbirth. However, some question remains about whether late abortions have long-term effects on fertility and on the outcomes of future pregnancies.

Agencies are available to help women who choose to carry their unplanned pregnancies to term. Such agencies can usually refer women to sources of help for problems such as abandonment by family or father of the child, poor health, insufficient income, lack of emotional support, and many others.

Many such agencies are associated with organizations called pro-life or right-to-life. They hold strong moral convictions against abortion. They may be supported by religious groups and may include religious teaching in their counseling. They can be especially helpful when a woman wants to continue a pregnancy but is unable to pay for the needed services. Services vary from place to place, but they can include free pregnancy testing; group counseling; medical care before, during, and after the birth; housing; adoption services; maternity and infant clothing; and day care.

Whether a woman chooses abortion or carries her unplanned pregnancy to term, she urgently needs a reliable means of contraception thereafter, so that she can hope to avoid being faced with the same hard choice all over again—a common occurrence. Almost all clinics provide postabortion contraception information and prescriptions, and probably all should be required to do so. Most people could be spared the emotional and physical stress of abortion if they would begin, now, to use a reliable method of contraception and continue using it faithfully and correctly every time they have sexual intercourse.

≡▶　*When contraceptive failure occurs, people must choose whether to carry an unwanted pregnancy to term or to get an abortion. Most people could avoid the stress of contraceptive failure if they would consistently use a reliable means of contraception.*

People who engage in sexual activity risk pregnancy and sexually transmitted disease. This hinders full enjoyment of the closeness that, ideally, sexual activity brings. People who use the most effective methods possible to protect themselves against mishaps have a greater hope of enjoying good health and a fulfilling relationship. Then, if they choose to start a family, they start off with these advantages. The chapter that follows discusses the course of events that transpire when pregnancy does occur. When a pregnancy is planned for and desired, this can be one of life's happiest times.

■≡ For Review

1. Describe the events of conception.
2. Define the term *fertility*, and discuss its significance in people's lives.
3. Define the term *family planning*, and identify two of its benefits.
4. List some common causes of infertility and actions to correct them.
5. Describe the person who should be using contraceptives.
6. Describe the information that should be given to a person who wants to know where to get contraceptive help.

7. Describe accurately the various contraceptive methods.

8. List and describe ten elements to be considered when selecting a contraceptive method.

9. Evaluate the safety and effectiveness of several contraceptive methods.

10. Identify factors that lead to unplanned pregnancies, and list the alternatives for action.

11. Describe methods for both early and late abortions.

■≡ Notes

1. J. M. Tanner, *Foetus into Man: Physical Growth from Conception to Maturity* (London: Open Books, 1978), pp. 35–51.

2. *Contraception: Choosing a Method* (Rockville, Md.: American College Health Association, 1989).

3. J. A. Collins and coauthors, Treatment-independent pregnancy among infertile couples, *New England Journal of Medicine* 309 (1983): 1201–1206.

4. The many sources for ratings of effectiveness do not agree exactly. The ratings listed here are taken from R. A. Hatcher, F. Stewart, J. Trussell, D. Kowal, F. Guest, G. K. Stewart, W. Cates, *Contraceptive Technology* (New York: Irvington, 1990–1992).

5. R. G. Sawyer and K. H. Beck, Oral contraception: A survey of college women's concerns and experience, *Health Education,* June/July 1989, pp. 17–21.

6. W. D. Mosher and W. F. Pratt, Contraceptive use in the United States, 1973–88, Advance data from National Center for Health Statistics, *Vital and Health Statistics,* no. 182, Hyattsville, Md., 20 March 1990, as cited in W. D. Mosher and W. F. Pratt, Use of contraception and family planning services in the United States, 1988, *American Journal of Public Health* 80 (1990): 1132–1133.

7. Safety concerns, *FDA Consumer,* December 1990, p. 9; B. B. Gerstman and coauthors, Trends in the content and use of oral contraceptives in the United States, 1964–88, *American Journal of Public Health* 81 (1991): 90–96.

8. Gerstman and coauthors, 1991.

9. Sawyer and Beck, 1989.

10. Sawyer and Beck, 1989.

11. The cancer steroid hormone study of the Centers for Disease Control and the National Institute of Child Health and Human Development: The reduction in risk of ovarian cancer associated with oral-contraceptive use, *New England Journal of Medicine* 316 (1987): 650–655.

12. D. R. Mishell, Medical progress: Contraception, *New England Journal of Medicine* 320 (1989): 777–787.

13. Mishell, 1989.

14. JHU report predicts five new birth control methods by year 2000, *American Journal of Public Health* 77 (1987): 1201.

15. Skin-deep contraception, *World Watch,* September/October 1989, p. 10.

16. Mishell, 1989.

17. De-Kun Li and coauthors, Prior condom use and the risk of tubal pregnancy, *American Journal of Public Health* 80 (1990): 964–966.

18. M. Tinklenberg, New contraceptive options, *Healthline,* March 1989, pp. 1–3.

19. Douching linked to cervical cancer, *Science News,* 139 (1991): 175.

20. Mosher and Pratt, 1990.

21. J. A. Handy, Psychological and social aspects of induced abortion, *British Journal of Clinical Psychology* 21 (1982): 29–41; R. Mester, Induced abortion and psychotherapy, *Psychotherapy and Psychosomatics* 30 (1978): 98–104.

22. R. Weiss, "Abortion pill": New data, new markets, *Science News* (1990): 100.

SPOTLIGHT

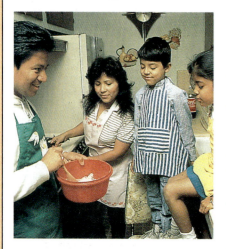

Choosing to Parent

When people become parents, they change their lives irreversibly. Most people have children without considering the amount of responsibility that being a parent brings. Few realize the amount of time, energy, work, and commitment that parenting requires.

What makes people decide to have children?

Many things—internal promptings, such as spiritual beliefs and personal needs; and outside pressures, such as spouse needs, or parents' or friends' expectations. Unconscious influences affect the decision, too: childhood memories, romantic fantasies of what families are like, the desire to live on in someone else, the need for companionship and love, and the need to demonstrate commitment to one's spouse.

If you feel these promptings, is it wise to start a family?

Not necessarily. The answers to some down-to-earth questions are relevant, too. Most are forms of a single question: How would it affect my life if I had a child to raise? After all, children are "forever," even more so than marriage partners.

To get an idea how "forever" children are, young people considering parenthood can try the following exercise. Pretend an egg is a baby, and practice being responsible for it. Carry the egg everywhere with you, even to the bathroom. Bathe it every day. Keep an eye on it at all times. Sleep with it close by. Set your alarm for 2 A.M., and check the egg. Never let it out of your sight unless you can obtain the agreement of another person to tend it as you are doing. Try this for a week, and you will get some sense of what it would be like to have a child—for a week. Multiply the week by 52 for a year, and then by about 20 for the duration of parenthood. If you find this exercise difficult, remember that this activity is only minor compared with

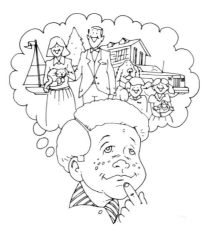

The decision whether to have a child is sometimes based on unrealistic ideas.

caring for a child. An egg does not cry or require discipline. Also, an egg does not soil diapers.

Table S13–1 highlights questions you should ask yourself before choosing to embark on the process of raising a child. If you face the trade-offs, you will be better able to answer yes or no to parenthood with realistic expectations.

Why do some people decide not to have children?

In addition to the enormous emotional and financial responsibility that parenting requires, some people have large global concerns that weigh heavily when they consider having children. Environmental concerns, particularly about the world's over-population and its limited resources, lead many people to limit their family size or to not have children at all.

Do people automatically know how to go about parenting children?

No, although they may think that they will instinctively know how to parent by doing what comes naturally. Almost everyone does have a model to follow—that of his or her own parents—but usually, the model is inadequate. And oddly enough, although schools teach young people reading, writing, and arithmetic, they do not teach them how to raise children and may not even make them aware that parenting is a skill they may need to learn.

What do parents have to do for their children?

Simply stated, parents must provide for their children's physical, emotional, social, and spiritual needs.

Physically, until the children are mature enough to meet these needs themselves and financially able to do

TABLE S13–1 ■ Are You Ready to Have a Child?

Answer these questions to explore your readiness to have a child.

1. How will having a child affect your job or career? It is difficult to work full-time and be a full-time parent, too.
2. Someone has to be aware of the child's whereabouts and needs, 24 hours a day, for 15 or so years. During the hours that you can't do it, will your partner do it? If not, who will?
3. If your partner should become unwilling or unable to continue carrying the responsibility of parenthood, are you prepared (or can you get prepared) to carry it by yourself? Accidents happen.
4. How will having a child affect your relationship with your present or future partner? Will your partner be willing to share your attention, energy, and love with another human being who will be very important to you?
5. Are you and your partner equally enthusiastic about becoming parents? A partner who is unwilling may withdraw emotionally from both you and the child.
6. Where will you be able to get help (for example, baby-sitters, parents of playmates, or relatives) when you need to get away? You cannot raise a child without help.
7. Will you be willing to give up much of your free time to devote yourself to the needs of a child? Will your partner? Children limit your freedom to play.
8. Do your finances allow for proper prenatal and newborn care? Pregnant women, new babies, and new mothers have needs that cost money in addition to the costs of the birth. Can you meet more needs on less income for a while?
9. Are you willing and able to invest your financial resources for years in the well-being of your child?
10. Do you know your chances of having a child with a hereditary disease? If not, get genetic counseling before making your decision (see Chapter 14).
11. How well would you be able to adjust to raising a less-than-perfect child? Parents always run a small risk of having a handicapped child, even if they follow all of the rules before and during pregnancy.
12. Are you willing to make a new baby the center of attention? The new family member will most certainly grab the spotlight, and you may feel neglected because the baby gets more nurturing than you do.
13. In deciding to become the parent to a second or later child, will you be able to stretch your physical, emotional, financial, and other resources that much farther? In some ways, two children are as easy to raise as one; in others, they are harder.
14. Have you vented anger and frustration on pets or children in the past? If so, wait to have children until you receive help in learning to redirect hostility—important in stopping the pattern of child abuse.
15. Have you already had one or two children? If so, you may want to limit your family size for environmental reasons.

so, parents must provide food, clothing, play activities, school equipment, the company of other children, transportation to wherever these resources are, health care, and medical care.

To foster their emotional and social development, parents need to instill trust, foster autonomy, and encourage initiative and industry. In other words, the parent should nurture and shape the child who will finally emerge from the family as an adult, ready to assume the roles of a responsible member of society.

Like adults, children have spiritual needs. Parents can help meet these needs by providing an environment conducive to spiritual growth. Children who receive spiritual guidance while growing up enter adulthood with positive values and a sense of purpose and meaning to their lives. They often have a foundation for building spiritual healing; this enhances self-esteem.

What's the most important part of parenting?

Probably the single most important thing parents can do for a child is to instill a strong sense of self-esteem. As earlier chapters showed, the feeling that ''I am OK, I am worthwhile'' helps an individual to be effective in every area of life—relationships with others, work, play, contributions to the larger society. Giving love, attention, and discipline consistently throughout the years will help instill self-esteem. To do this, it is helpful to understand a child's developmental stages and how to best provide care during each stage.

Describe what is most crucial to development in infancy.

A newborn is profoundly dependent on adults to feed it, carry it around, and protect it from the world. It needs a close, intimate bond with parents, and the infant's nervous system readily forms this connection.

Those who have bonded successfully with their mothers (or mother substitutes) learn life's first major emotional lesson: trust. On this foundation, all later emotional development builds.

Until three months of age or later, an infant is not able to cry out of anger or will. Some people think that picking up a crying baby will "spoil" the child, but researchers have found that babies who are consistently picked up and comforted at the whimpering stage turn out to cry less, be more secure, and need less physical contact as they grow older than infants who are allowed to cry.[1*] Thus parents should try to meet the young infant's needs consistently to establish trust and, later, independence. Another guideline is to interact with the infant affectionately and often, so as to begin the process of socialization and to develop intellectual capacity.

What can a parent expect at the toddler stage?

At the toddler stage, children need experiences that use each of their senses, and they need the freedom to discover what the world is like on their own. Toddlers are developing language, so listen to them and try to respond to what they are saying.

Older toddlers become willful and resist adult commands. The emergence of will has won the late toddler stage the name "terrible twos." Two ideas that can help parents weather the twos are (1) that willful behavior is normal and desirable, because it heralds the beginnings of autonomy; and (2) that the stage is short, and the two-year-old will turn three.

*Reference notes are at the end of the Spotlight.

Most parents want to provide the kinds of experiences that their children need in order to develop to their potential. In terms of competence, a young child develops best when parents:

■ Provide an environment rich in varied colors, shapes, and textures.
■ Interact with the child for a few seconds at a time, at frequent intervals, at the child's request.
■ Name objects, even before the child can speak.
■ Encourage the child to communicate.
■ Read to the child.
■ Plan activities within the child's attention span.
■ Expect to have fun when sharing activities with the child, rather than expect to see the child demonstrate academic ability.

During the years from three to six, play, in particular, facilitates development. As children climb, swing, dig, and run, their bodies develop motor skills. "Pretend" games let them try out social roles and develop creativity. Solving puzzles gives them mental work. Reading helps develop curiosity. Ideally, parents will provide a rich and varied environment full of opportunities for all these things. If parents must use child care, they should look for adults who will provide these same enrichments for their children, as well as for settings that are safe and clean.

What other things can I look for when selecting a day care center?

Of utmost importance is selecting a day care center that is clean and safe. When visiting a day care center, ask yourself the following questions.

■ Is it uncluttered?
■ Is it uncrowded?
■ Is trash and garbage removed regularly?
■ Is it free of pests?
■ Is the bathroom sanitary?
■ Is the kitchen clean and orderly?
■ Is the lunch area clean?
■ Is the nap area clean? Is the bedding fresh?
■ Is all equipment in good repair? Are the toys safe?
■ Is the wiring in good repair? Are the electrical outlets covered?
■ Are all poisons and medicines kept out of children's reach?
■ Is there a properly stocked first aid kit and a staff person trained to administer first aid?
■ Are there adequate exits and fire extinguishers?
■ Does the center hold fire drills?

Next, you will want a day care center that provides experiences to meet your child's developmental needs. Ask about the center's philosophy of parenting and its discipline strategies; be sure what they do is consistent with your views about raising children.

What are some effective means of discipline?

Discipline styles range from authoritarian to permissive. Children who were raised under strict authoritarian discipline experienced punishment as their parents' primary mode of behavioral guidance. They tend to be more moody, hostile, and vulnerable to stress than children of parents who act more positively.[2] Children raised permissively tend to internalize more guilt than do children who are simply told what to do, and it may hamper their effectiveness in later life.[3] The most effective means of child raising seems to be a style that is not extreme in either direction. A straightforward, honest, assertive approach is most effective. Parents take into account their children's feelings and offer positive reinforcement for desired behavior, but they also set no-nonsense limits without manipulation. Children raised this way tend to become self-confident, cheerful, friendly adults.[4] Table S13–2 lists some suggestions for discipline strategies and gives some guidelines for effective use of punishment.

What about parenting during the preteen and teen years?

Many parents fear the teen years and imagine them as a time when seething hormones turn life into continuous turmoil. Actually, many teenagers manage this period of life with relative ease, making adjustments as needed, experiencing and trying out new intellectual and physical capabilities.

The development of personal identity is the teenager's main task. The emerging self may contrast sharply with parental traits and so become a source of conflict with parents, but it may also set the stage for constructive parental involvement. Parents should be available when their children want to talk, and they should listen intently to what is said, without interruption or judgment. To accept the emerging identity of the teenager, the parents must themselves have self-concepts strong enough to tolerate differences. As the teen years pass and young adulthood ensues, the person who was adequately parented will have developed a firm sense of self, the ultimate goal of parenting.

TABLE S13–2 ■ **Strategies for Discipline and Guidelines for Effective Punishment**

Discipline is most effective when you:	When punishment is needed:
1. Discipline yourself first. Live by the rules you set. 2. Include the child in decisions about limits and consequences. 3. Explain the reasons for the rules. 4. Remove sources of trouble, or remove the child from trouble. 5. Redirect the child's behavior or energy in a safe direction. 6. Let natural consequences teach the child, unless it would cause injury. 7. Warn before punishing. 8. Warn only once. 9. Threaten only humane punishment that you are willing to administer. 10. Give the child a chance to answer any accusations. 11. Punish as little as possible; communicate as much as possible. 12. Love the child.	1. Be consistent about which behaviors are acceptable and which are not. 2. Punish immediately. However, if you tend to be emotional, be sure not to administer punishments while you are upset. 3. Do not use the "Wait until Father (or Mother) comes home" approach. 4. Make the punishment proportional to the misbehavior. Use the minimum amount of punishment that will successfully accomplish your goal. 5. Combine punishment with reinforcement for the correct response. This enhances the effectiveness of both. 6. Be certain to keep the lines of communication open. Overreliance on punishment impairs communication, as children become afraid to confide in adults.

■≡ **Spotlight Notes**

1. U. A. Hunziker and R. G. Barr, Increased carrying reduces infant crying: A randomized controlled trial, *Pediatrics* 77 (1986): 641–648; S. M. Bell and M. D. Ainsworth, Infant crying and maternal responsiveness, *Child Development* 43 (1972): 1171–1190.

2. J. Belsky and coauthors, *The Child in the Family* (Reading, Mass.: Addison-Wesley, 1984), as cited in B. Strong and C. DeVault, *The Marriage and Family Experience*, 3d ed. (St. Paul, Minn: West, 1986), p. 375.

3. Strong and DeVault, 1986, p. 376.

4. Strong and DeVault, 1986, p. 376.

CHAPTER 14

Reproduction and Pregnancy

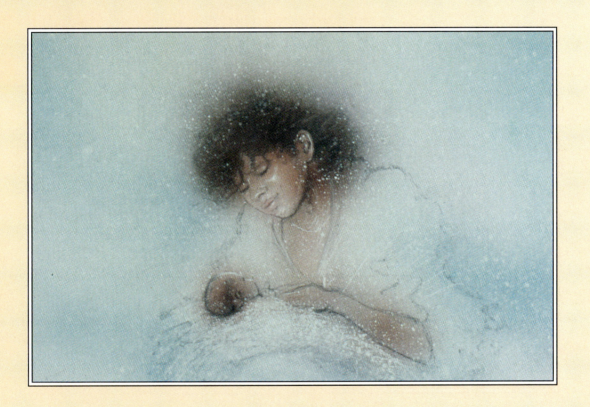

Heredity
Pregnancy
Breastfeeding and Formula Feeding

■ **SPOTLIGHT** Childbirth Choices

Review of terms from earlier chapters:

The *gonads* are the organs—the testes in men and the ovaries in women—that make the gametes.

A *gamete* is a reproductive cell—ovum or sperm.

After sexual intercourse has delivered sperm into the woman's reproductive tract, *conception* is the event that unites one gamete from each parent (a sperm with an ovum).

The *zygote* is the product of their union, so-called for the first two weeks of its life. (Thereafter, it is called an *embryo*; see later in this chapter.)

When the zygote embeds itself in the uterine wall, the event is called *implantation.*

chromosomes the bodies within each cell that contain the genetic material (deoxyribonucleic acid, or DNA).

genes the basic units of heredity, made of DNA, that are passed from parent to offspring in the chromosomes of the gametes.

R eproduction is an astonishing process. That human bodies package, into cells too small to see, entire libraries of all the information necessary to make human beings inspires wonderment. This chapter focuses on the biological and social event of reproduction, beginning with a discussion of heredity.

■ Heredity

The gametes formed in the parents' reproductive organs unite at the time of conception and then divide, becoming a new human being. Throughout these astonishing events, the transmission of billions of pieces of inherited information proceeds almost invariably without a hitch. This first section describes the wonders of normal inheritance; the next one describes the problems of inherited abnormalities and strategies to prevent or minimize them.

Normal Inheritance

A female gamete, an ovum, carries within it a set of 23 **chromosomes.** Each chromosome bears along its length thousands of **genes.** Each gene is a set of molecular instructions for making a single protein: an enzyme, a structural protein, a muscle protein, or some other body protein. Each protein will determine, or help to determine, traits for the new person, such as eye color or susceptibility to disease. Thus the ovum contains one copy of each gene— one copy of each piece of the genetic information necessary to make a human being.

A male gamete, a sperm, also contains 23 chromosomes bearing genes that govern the same characteristics. When the ovum and sperm merge at conception to form a single cell, the zygote, the chromosomes from each parent line up side by side, forming 23 *pairs*— 46 chromosomes in all (see Figure 14–1). The zygote thus contains two genes for every trait, one from the sperm and one from the ovum.

After conception the zygote splits into two new cells, and those cells split again and again. All 46 chromosomes are faithfully copied at each division

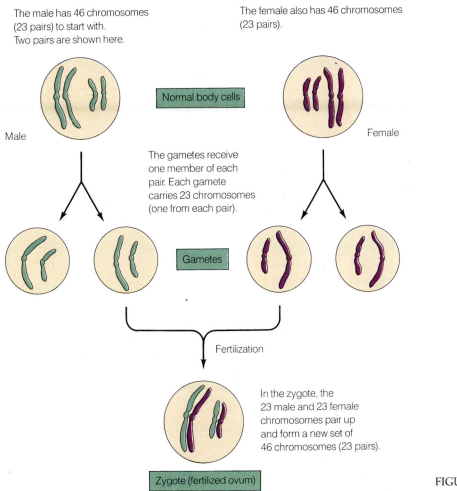

The male has 46 chromosomes (23 pairs) to start with. Two pairs are shown here.

The female also has 46 chromosomes (23 pairs).

Normal body cells

Male

Female

The gametes receive one member of each pair. Each gamete carries 23 chromosomes (one from each pair).

Gametes

Fertilization

In the zygote, the 23 male and 23 female chromosomes pair up and form a new set of 46 chromosomes (23 pairs).

Zygote (fertilized ovum)

FIGURE 14–1 ■ **Gametes and chromosomes.**

so that every new cell (with one exception) inherits the entire set of 46 chromosomes, 23 from each parent. (Only in the new individual's gonads will division produce cells with just 23 chromosomes again: these are the special reproductive cells, the gametes, through which the individual will contribute genetic information to the *next* generation.) Thus a parent passes along some chromosomes from its father, and some from its mother, to its child.

So it is that a new human being inherits two sets of genes, or instructions for making each piece of molecular machinery—one set from each parent. Some of the baby's traits may be identical to the father's, some to the mother's, and some intermediate between the two. Some brand-new traits will also emerge: for example, traits determined by genes on chromosomes donated by the grandparents—genes that were hidden but not expressed within one or the other parent. New traits may also arise from unique combinations of genetic information occurring for the first time in this new individual.

dominant gene   a gene that produces a trait or characteristic in the offspring.

recessive gene   a gene that does not express itself when a dominant gene appears in the same cell.

Whenever two genes for a single trait differ from each other, one may be **dominant** over the other, which is called **recessive.** Eye color is a trait that provides a simple example. One gene from the mother and one gene from the father govern this characteristic. The two genes may or may not be identical; the combination determines what the actual eye color will be.

Say, for example, that the father's gene specifies blue-eye pigment, and the gene from the mother codes for brown pigment. Logic might suggest that the baby would have eyes of some intermediate shade, but in this case, the eyes will be brown, because the gene for brown pigment (a dominant gene) wins out over blue pigment (a recessive gene). Thus the baby who inherits one copy of each gene will have brown eyes. If the mother's chromosome had also carried the gene for blue eyes, as the father's did, the baby's eyes would have been blue. (Remember, the mother also inherited two genes for eye color; she can pass along either one, regardless of her eye color.) The products of recessive genes become visible only when no dominant gene is present. This is why two brown-eyed parents can have a blue-eyed child. Table 14–1 shows traits that are inherited according to this simple dominant-recessive system.

The way a baby's gender is determined is a variation on this theme. One of the 23 pairs of chromosomes carries the sex-determining genes. A woman's cells always contain pairs of "X" chromosomes (named for their appearance under the microscope). The "X" chromosomes code for female

TABLE 14–1   ■   **Some Hereditary Traits in Human Beings**

Dominant	Recessive
Curly hair	Straight hair
Dark hair	Light hair
Nonred hair	Red hair
Coarse body hair	Fine body hair
Normal skin color	Albinism
Brown eyes	Blue or grey eyes
Nearsightedness or farsightedness	Normal vision
Normal hearing	Deafness
Normal color vision	Color blindness
Normal blood clotting	Hemophilia
Broad lips	Thin lips
Large eyes	Small eyes
Short stature	Tall stature
Normal muscle tone	Muscular dystrophy
Hypertension	Normal blood pressure
Diabetes (inherited)	Normal metabolism
Normal mentality	Schizophrenia
Nervous temperament	Calm temperament
Average intellect	Genius or retardation
Migraine headaches	No migraine headaches
Normal immune system	Susceptibility to disease
A or B blood factor	O blood factor
Rh positive blood factor	Rh negative blood factor

SOURCE: Adapted from G. J. Tortora and N. P. Anagnostakos, *Principles of Anatomy and Physiology,* 5th ed. (New York: Harper and Row, 1987), p. 761.

One chromosome pair governs sex inheritance. In the woman's cells, both members of this pair contain only genes for producing females (X).

In the man's cells, one of the chromosomes is for females (X), one for males (Y).

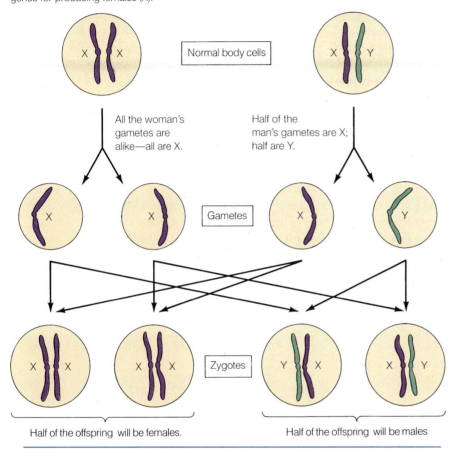

Normal body cells

All the woman's gametes are alike—all are X.

Half of the man's gametes are X; half are Y.

Gametes

Zygotes

Half of the offspring will be females.

Half of the offspring will be males

FIGURE 14–2 ■ **Sex inheritance.**

characteristics, and each of a woman's gametes always carries one "X" chromosome. As a result, she donates an "X" chromosome to every infant that she conceives. A man's cells, on the other hand, each contain one "X" and one "Y" chromosome, and each of his sperm contains only one or the other. In the race to fertilize the ovum, the sperm that swims best or that gets through the ovum's outer covering first is the winner—and is the one that determines the gender of the future baby (see Figure 14–2). If it's an "X," the baby will be a female; if a "Y," a male.

≡▶ *The merging of a female gamete (an ovum) with a male gamete (a sperm) brings together two sets of 23 chromosomes carrying thousands of genes. These genes contain all the genetic information needed to create a new human being from this union.*

As mentioned earlier, genes are normally copied with amazing accuracy. Occasionally, however, something goes wrong. The following section considers inherited abnormalities.

■ *FACT OR FICTION:* The sperm, not the ovum, always determines the gender of the baby. *True.*

Inherited Abnormalities

mutation   a change in a cell's genetic material (DNA).

mutagens   agents or events that cause genetic mutations.

congenital (con-JEN-ih-tal) **abnormalities**   abnormalities present in an individual from birth.

teratogens (teh-RAT-oh-gens)   chemical or physical agents that cause birth defects.

Every now and then—about once in every 100 million copies—a cell makes a mistake in copying its genetic material. This mistake—a **mutation**—may be transmitted to all the new cells that descend from the mutated one. Mutations are as faithfully copied as normal genes are. Mutations arise in response to **mutagens,** and they can cause cancer or **congenital abnormalities.** The special class of mutagens that can lead to congenital abnormalities are known as **teratogens**.

Chemical mutagens include the tars in tobacco; toxins produced by bacteria; many pesticides; heavy metals such as mercury and lead; toxic wastes such as PCBs and dioxin; and many drugs, including alcohol, illegal drugs of abuse, and prescription medicines. Exposure to these mutagens prior to or during pregnancy can damage the genetic material of gametes or of the developing infant. Even ordinary household chemicals, such as insecticides or cleaning fluids, can be toxic and should be avoided or used with extreme care during pregnancy. Anyone who might have been exposed to an environmental teratogen should call a hotline to find out what to do.*

Among physical mutagens are several forms of radiation, including the sun's ultraviolet rays and radioactivity. Like chemicals, radiation of certain kinds can harm cells; it penetrates them and disrupts the genetic code. One way a fetus might be exposed to such radiation is through X rays. If X rays should become necessary (even routine dental X rays), the woman who knows or suspects that she is pregnant should inform all medical personnel. They may then choose to use smaller amounts of radiation or to postpone the procedure.

Mutations that occur in the line of cells that produces the gametes, or in the gametes themselves, have a greater impact for a longer time than mutations in other body cells. Mutations carried by gametes can be particularly harmful, because such mutations will be passed on to every cell of the offspring's body *and from generation to generation.* This may present no problem if the characteristic governed by the mutated gene is not essential to life or health. Then again, it may cause a major defect known as an **inborn error of metabolism,** a spontaneous abortion, or a stillbirth.

inborn error (of metabolism)   an inherited disorder of the body's chemical workings, present from birth. (See the Miniglossary of Hereditary Diseases.)

When mutations occur in body cells other than the gametes, they are not passed on to the person's offspring. Of course, such mutations can still be devastating, because every single cell in an early stage of development multiplies to become many cells later: single cells in an embryo become whole limbs, organs, or organ systems in the adult. Thus a cell that mutates early in development may become a deformed limb or abnormal organ or organ system. Major defects that arise early in development frequently lead to **birth defects,** spontaneous abortions, or stillbirths.

birth defects   anatomical abnormalities present in an individual from birth.

The accompanying Miniglossary lists a small sampling of the more than 6,000 known inherited disorders. The odds of giving birth to a child with such an inherited disorder are relatively small. However, for people who carry the genes for inborn errors, the odds increase.

Most inborn errors are recessive, and appear only when a person inherits *two* defective genes—one from each parent. This can occur when both parents have the disorder, when one has the disorder and the other is a carrier, or when both are carriers (see Figure 14–3). Carriers are people who inherit

*The number for the Pregnancy/Environmental Hotline of the National Birth Defects Center is 1–617–787–4957; toll-free in Massachusetts: (800) 322–5014.

■ MINIGLOSSARY
of Hereditary Diseases

cystic fibrosis   a hereditary disease of the glands that secrete mucus, sweat, and digestive juices; leads to severe digestive disturbances, liver damage, chronic lung disease, and early death.

diabetes   a group of diseases characterized by an abnormality in carbohydrate metabolism, at least one of which is inherited. (See the Spotlight following Chapter 18.)

Down's syndrome (or **Down syndrome**) a hereditary combination of physical deformities and mental retardation caused by the inheritance of an extra chromosome so that instead of two members of pair 21, the individual has three. An alternative name, no longer favored because of its negative connotations, is *mongolism* (MONG-oh-lism).

hemophilia (he-mo-FIL-ee-uh)   a hereditary disease characterized by a greatly prolonged blood-clotting time and therefore an abnormal tendency to bleed, caused by the lack of a protein factor involved in the clotting process.

mongolism   see *Down's syndrome.*

muscular dystrophy   a hereditary disease of increasing loss of muscle control, with muscle tissue destruction.

phenylketonuria (PKU) (FEN-il-kee-tone-YOUR-ee-uh)   a hereditary disease characterized by abnormal use of amino acids by the body, with resulting mental retardation. PKU need not cause mental retardation if the mother consumes a special diet during pregnancy and the infant consumes a special diet beginning immediately after birth.

sickle-cell anemia   a hereditary disease that occurs almost exclusively in blacks, characterized by red blood cells that assume a sickle shape. The sickle-shaped blood cells are protective against malaria but also cause anemia symptoms, such as tiredness and apathy.

Tay-Sachs syndrome   a hereditary disease characterized by deterioration of the nervous system. The rate of occurrence in Jewish children is about 100 times that in others.

one defective gene and one normal gene. They may be unaware that they carry a defective gene, for their normal genes are dominant, and so symptoms are usually mild or absent.

Many inborn errors impair an infant's brain development, leading to mental retardation. In many cases, such damage can be prevented or controlled with early detection and treatment with special diets or drugs. For this reason, newborns are routinely tested for some genetic disorders such as phenylketonuria (PKU) and sickle-cell anemia.

People with inherited disorders who want children can benefit from genetic and medical counseling. They must consider the possible consequences of bearing their own children and the option of adoption. A **genetic counselor** can advise prospective parents, using laboratory tests and family medical histories. Even so, all prospective parents need to understand that genetic disorders can occur unexpectedly among children of apparently healthy parents.[1]*

genetic counselor   an advisor who is qualified in several medical specialties (such as internal medicine, pediatrics, and genetics) to predict and advise on the likelihood that genetic defects will occur in a family.

≡▶   *Just as genes can pass on the trait of blue eyes, they can pass on disorders that lead to major health problems. Whether the disorders will affect future generations depends on whether the mutations occurred in the body cells of an individual or in the reproductive cells (the gametes).*

*Reference notes are at the end of the chapter.

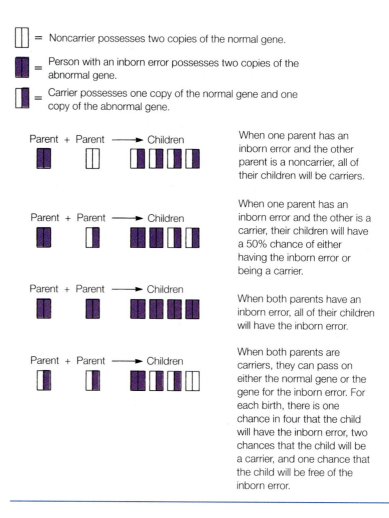

When one parent has an inborn error and the other parent is a noncarrier, all of their children will be carriers.

When one parent has an inborn error and the other is a carrier, their children will have a 50% chance of either having the inborn error or being a carrier.

When both parents have an inborn error, all of their children will have the inborn error.

When both parents are carriers, they can pass on either the normal gene or the gene for the inborn error. For each birth, there is one chance in four that the child will have the inborn error, two chances that the child will be a carrier, and one chance that the child will be free of the inborn error.

FIGURE 14–3 ■ **The inheritance of an inborn error.**

■ ≡ Pregnancy

Preparation for a healthy pregnancy ideally begins far in advance of the actual conception. Advance planning puts prospective parents in an excellent position to make choices that will give the baby-to-be every possible advantage.

Prior to Conception

During the reproductive years, people nourish and care for their bodies not only for their own sakes, but also for future generations. The better they care for themselves, the better the chances of having a healthy pregnancy and baby. For example, for at least three months before conception, *both* prospective parents should abstain from drugs of all kinds—alcohol, illegal drugs of abuse, and over-the-counter medications. They should even minimize their use of prescription medications (under medical supervision).[2] During those three months, the gamete cells—the ovum of the mother and the sperm of the father—mature and divide. Any substance that interferes with cell division or prevents the full and normal expression of the genes can impair the development of those new cells during this vulnerable stage.

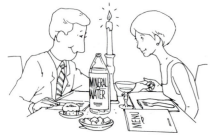

Both prospective parents can prepare in advance for a healthy pregnancy.

Clearly, both a man's and a woman's health habits *before conception* are important.

Both prospective parents should also be well nourished. It has long been known and is well documented that malnutrition and food deprivation can reduce fertility: studies from as far back as the second world war show that malnourished women may stop menstruating and produce no ova, and that men may lose the ability to produce viable sperm.[3] A diet that follows the guidelines presented in Chapter 5 would well cover the nutrient needs of the prospective parents (diet for a woman during pregnancy is discussed later).

When a malnourished woman becomes pregnant, she faces the challenge of supporting both the growth of a baby and her own health with inadequate nutrient stores. One of the first tasks a woman's body performs at the start of pregnancy is to develop a **placenta,** the organ that delivers food to the developing fetus (more about the placenta later). When malnutrition occurs prior to and around conception, the placenta fails to develop fully.[4] A poorly developed placenta cannot provide nourishment, even if the mother is able to eat well throughout the remainder of the pregnancy. Historical records show that when women conceive and go through their early pregnancies during times of famine, their infants develop congenital malformations.[5] This demonstrates that full nutrient stores *before* pregnancy are essential not only to conception but to development of a healthy infant *during* pregnancy.

Both underweight and overweight women have higher rates of complications during pregnancy and give birth to babies who develop more medical problems than do women of normal weight. To prevent these problems, women are advised to achieve healthy body weights before becoming pregnant. If a woman is following a weight-loss diet, she should postpone pregnancy; if she is pregnant, she should postpone weight-loss dieting. Any woman wanting to do all that she can to make a future pregnancy healthy should develop healthy eating habits prior to conception and maintain them thereafter. She should also be physically active, so that she can continue her activities throughout her pregnancy.

Many health problems, such as diabetes, can adversely affect both a pregnant woman and her developing infant. A woman must seek medical help for such conditions to be sure that they are well under control before she becomes pregnant. A woman must also take precautions against communicable diseases, such as **rubella,** or German measles. If contracted during early pregnancy, rubella causes fetal malformations, especially cataracts that cause blindness. Rubella does not yield to medical drugs; it has to be prevented in advance, by vaccination. The vaccine contains active viruses, theoretically able to infect a fetus, so women are advised to wait at least three months after being vaccinated before getting pregnant.[6]

≡▶ *When prospective parents adopt healthy lifestyle habits before conception, they help to provide the developing fetus with a nurturing environment in which to grow.*

Detecting Pregnancy

Long before any tests are taken, a woman may suspect that she is pregnant. Typically she notices a missed menstrual period, but that is not always an

■ *FACT OR FICTION:* The lifestyle choices a man makes up to three months before he impregnates a woman can affect the development of his baby-to-be. *True.*

placenta (plah-SEN-tuh)   an organ that develops during pregnancy, in which maternal and fetal blood circulate in close proximity so that materials can be exchanged between them. See Figure 14–5.

rubella   an infectious disease, especially dangerous to pregnant women because it can cause congenital cataracts and other malformations in their unborn infants; also called *German measles* or *three-day measles.*

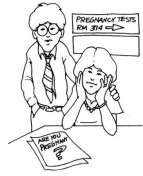

Only an accurate test can resolve immense suspense.

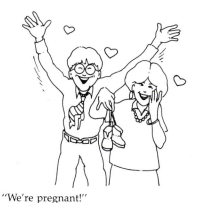

"We're pregnant!"

■ *FACT OR FICTION:* An enlarging abdomen is one of the first clues that a woman is pregnant. *False.* Subtle changes in the cervix, outer genital area, and breasts are the first signs of pregnancy.

human chorionic (CORE-ee-AHN-ick) **gonadotropin** (go-NAD-oh-TROPE-in), or **HCG**   a hormone produced immediately after implantation by the zygote and the tissues surrounding it; the hormone detected in pregnancy tests.

identical twins   twins produced from a single fertilized ovum when the two cells produced by the first division separate and develop into two individuals instead of remaining together and producing one individual, as they normally do.

fraternal twins   twins formed by the fertilization of two different ova by two different sperm.

FIGURE 14–4 ■ **Development of the zygote.**

accurate indicator. A woman can miss a period because of any kind of stress—a move, extreme weight loss, or an emotional upset—or may continue to experience some menstrual flow on schedule during the first couple of months of pregnancy.

A more accurate indicator is subtle color changes in the tip of the uterus (the cervix) and outer genital area, which darken with a bluish cast. The breasts may become tender and full, and the nipples may darken. A health care provider who examines the woman can identify these signs.

A chemical test can confirm that a woman is pregnant. Some tests use urine and some use blood, but they all rely on detecting one of the many hormones present during pregnancy, **human horionic gonadotropin (HCG).** HCG is produced by the zygote and the tissues that surround it almost immediately upon implantation, and then rapidly increases in concentration. In the first days of pregnancy, blood tests can discern the minute amounts of HCG being produced; later, when HCG is plentiful, urine tests can be used.

Home pregnancy test kits offer the advantages of immediacy and privacy, but they also present serious problems.[7] Women frequently have difficulty using the home test kits and interpreting the results; the tests also have an unacceptably high error rate; they are accurate only about 50 to 90 percent of the time.[8] If a woman gets a negative reading and she really is pregnant, she may delay obtaining prenatal care. If she gets a positive reading and she really is not pregnant, she may experience unfounded joy or unnecessary anguish. Tests conducted by health care providers, although more expensive, are recommended for accuracy's sake.

≡▶   *Physical and biochemical changes in the woman's body signal the onset of pregnancy. Most pregnancy tests are based on the detection of the hormone HCG in blood or urine.*

Fetal Development

The zygote begins the process of dividing within a day after fertilization, even as it travels toward the uterus through the fallopian tube. (Sometimes the two new cells become detached at this stage and produce **identical twins.** In contrast, if two eggs had been released and fertilized at the same time, the result would have been **fraternal twins.**) Figure 14–4 shows how the cells divide. Within the next few days, the zygote embeds itself in the uterine wall. Cell division continues, with each new set of cells dividing

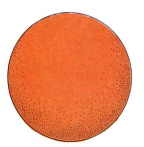

Fertilized ovum (1-cell stage)

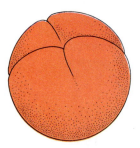

4-cell stage

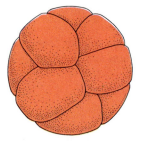

16-cell stage

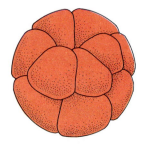

Many-cell stage

again to create many smaller cells. These cells sort themselves into three layers that, later in **gestation,** form the various body systems. As development proceeds, the zygote becomes an **embryo,** then a **fetus.**

During this same time, the placenta grows within the uterus as shown in Figure 14–5. Two associated structures also form. One is the **amniotic sac,** a sort of fluid-filled balloon that houses the developing fetus. The other is the **umbilical cord,** a ropelike structure containing fetal blood vessels that extends from the fetus's "belly button" to the placenta.

The placenta is an organ composed of spongy tissue in which fetal and maternal blood flow side by side, each in its own vessels. The placenta transfers oxygen and nutrients to the fetus and returns fetal waste products to the mother, thus performing the respiratory, absorptive, and excretory functions that the fetus's lungs, digestive system, and kidneys will provide after birth. The placenta is a versatile, metabolically active organ. Much like muscles and other body tissues, it uses energy fuels to support its work. It produces an array of hormones that maintain pregnancy and prepare the mother's breasts for lactation, the making of milk. It shields the fetus from its mother's immune system, which would otherwise perceive the fetus's blood as foreign and would attack it. As mentioned earlier, normal development of the placenta is essential for the developing fetus to attain its full genetic potential.

The embryo accomplishes amazing developmental feats. The number of cells in the embryo doubles approximately every 24 hours; later the rate slows gradually, and during the final 10 weeks of pregnancy only one doubling occurs. The embryo's size changes very little up to the eighth week of pregnancy, but the events taking place during that time are momentous. From the outermost of the three layers of cells, the nervous system and skin begin

gestation (jes-TAY-shun) the period from conception to birth; for human beings, gestation lasts from 38 to 42 weeks. The term of pregnancy itself is often divided into thirds, called *trimesters.*

embryo (EM-bree-oh) the name given to the developing infant from 14 days to eight weeks after conception. (After that, it is called a *fetus.*)

fetus (FEET-us) the developing infant from the ninth week after conception until birth.

amniotic (am-nee-OTT-ic) **sac** the "bag of waters" in the uterus, in which the fetus floats.

umbilical (um-BIL-ih-cul) **cord** the ropelike structure through which the fetus's veins and arteries reach the placenta; the route of nourishment and oxygen into the fetus and the route of waste disposal from the fetus.

FIGURE 14–5 ■ **The placenta.**

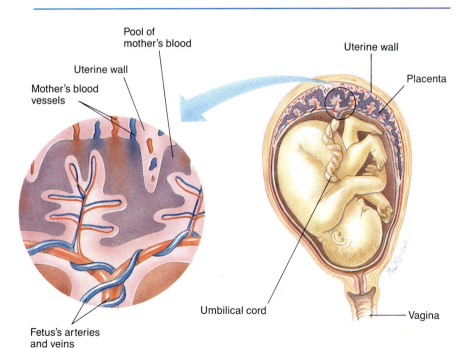

Pool of mother's blood

Uterine wall

Mother's blood vessels

Uterine wall

Placenta

Umbilical cord

Vagina

Fetus's arteries and veins

to develop; from the middle layer, the muscles and internal organ systems; and from the innermost layer, the glands and linings of the digestive, respiratory, and excretory systems. At eight weeks, the 1¼-inch-long embryo has a complete central nervous system, a beating heart, a digestive system, well-defined fingers and toes, and the beginnings of facial features.

Thereafter, during the seven months of fetal development, each organ grows to maturity according to its own characteristic schedule, with greater intensity at some times than at others. As Figure 14–6 shows, the growth of the fetus is phenomenal, with weight increasing from less than a gram to about 3,500 grams (7½ pounds).

Times of intense development and rapid cell division are **critical periods**—critical in the sense that the events taking place during those times can occur only then and not later. If cell division and the final cell number achieved in an organ are limited during a critical period, recovery is impossible. Each organ and tissue is most vulnerable to an insult (such as a toxin or a nutrient deficiency) during its own critical period. For example, the heart is well developed at 16 weeks; the lungs are still immature 10 weeks later. Therefore, early malnutrition affects the heart most severely, while later malnutrition especially affects the lungs. Pregnancy, then, is a time for a woman to take especially good care of her health.

> ■▶ *A zygote develops into an embryo, and an embryo into a fetus. A placenta, umbilical cord, and amniotic sac develop to help support the growth and development of the baby-to-be. Many critical periods occur between conception and birth.*

Ectopic Pregnancy and Spontaneous Abortion

Approximately 10 percent of all zygotes fail to implant in the uterus. In **ectopic pregnancy,** the zygote implants in the fallopian tube or in the abdominal cavity instead of in the uterus. This can happen when the ovum

critical periods   finite periods during development in which certain events occur that will have irreversible effects on later developmental stages. In a body organ, a critical period is usually a period of cell division.

The brain and central nervous system are first to reach maturity. The fetal brain increases by 100,000 cells every minute.

ectopic (ek-TOP-ick) **pregnancy**   a pregnancy in which the zygote has implanted and begun to develop in one of the fallopian tubes or elsewhere outside the uterus, a dangerous situation.

FIGURE 14–6 ■ **Stages of embryonic and fetal development.**

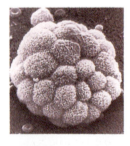

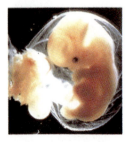

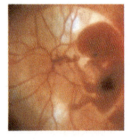

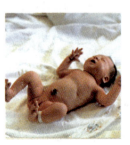

1. A newly fertilized ovum is about the size of the period at the end of this sentence. This zygote, less than one week after fertilization, is not much bigger and is ready for implantation.

2. An embryo 5 weeks after fertilization is about the size of the capital A that began this sentence; after implantation, the placenta develops and begins to provide nourishment to the developing embryo.

3. A fetus after 11 weeks of development is just over an inch long; notice the umbilical cord and blood vessels connecting the fetus with the placenta.

4. A newborn infant after nine months of development measures close to 20 inches in length. From eight weeks to term, this infant grew 20 times longer and 50 times heavier.

cannot pass to the uterus, most commonly because inflammation or scar tissue that has developed during the course of a sexually transmitted disease has blocked the tube. Ectopic pregnancies cannot support the fetus's growth and threaten the mother's life; surgery is required to terminate such pregnancies.

Of zygotes that do implant in the uterus, 50 percent are shed in spontaneous abortion or miscarriage.[9] Spontaneous abortion is a natural and expected part of fertility; it prevents imperfect embryos from becoming full-term infants or occurs when a woman's uterus is unable to support a pregnancy.

Most spontaneous abortions take place early, even before a woman knows she is pregnant, with no more sign than a heavy menstrual flow. The hormonal transition from pregnancy back to the nonpregnant state may alter a woman's mood, and she may not even know why.

Spontaneous abortions late in pregnancy resemble the experience of birth and may cause hazardous complications. Among the hazards: bleeding may be excessive, or infection may start in the uterus and spread through the fallopian tubes into the abdominal cavity, leading to a dangerous generalized body infection (septic abortion).

The premature termination of a pregnancy often corrects an abnormality that needs correcting. Even so, a woman may feel grief as intense as if an already-born child had died.

▶ *From time to time, a pregnancy does not follow the normal course. In an ectopic pregnancy, surgery must terminate the pregnancy. At other times, the body, in its wisdom, spontaneously aborts an unhealthy pregnancy.*

The Woman's Experience

While the momentous events of pregnancy proceed within her, a woman's life continues outwardly, seemingly as before—but she experiences it differently. Gina doesn't want to go out after work any more. Her pregnancy barely shows, yet she's always tired. Paul, the young father-to-be, wonders if she is overreacting. (Paul is used as an example, here, of Gina's chief support person; sometimes a person other than the father may be in that position.) He doesn't realize that the external changes are trivial compared with the dramatic internal events taking place in Gina's body. She is producing more blood; her uterus and its supporting muscles are increasing in size and strength; her joints are becoming more flexible in preparation for childbirth; and her breasts are growing and changing in preparation for lactation. The hormones that mediate all these changes may influence Gina's brain and mood. She may be having problems with constipation, shortness of breath, frequent urination, morning sickness, or backaches.

The nausea of "morning" sickness (which actually comes at any time of day) may be a healthy sign, because it shows that the hormones needed for pregnancy are abundant. Contending with it, though, is wearing. Sometimes, nibbling on small meals throughout the day helps.

Gina needs to be fit now, just as she did before, and exercise will help to reduce some of her discomforts. If she was not physically active prior to pregnancy, Gina may benefit from exercise that progresses from mild to moderate in small increments. If she was physically active, she can continue exercising throughout the pregnancy, adjusting the intensity and duration as she goes along. She will want to avoid sports in which she might fall or be hit by other people or objects. For example, a game of tennis played by one

See Chapter 17 for more about sexually transmitted diseases.

Warning signs of septic abortion to report to the health care provider:

Discharge of water or blood from the vagina.

Severe headaches.

Uncontrollable vomiting.

Loss of consciousness.

Sudden swelling of feet, hands, or ankles.

Chills or fever.

Abdominal pain.

Frequent, burning urination.

Failure to urinate.

Blurred vision or other vision disturbances.

■ *FACT OR FICTION:* The nausea associated with early pregnancy is gone each day by noon. *False.* So-called morning sickness actually can occur at any time of day.

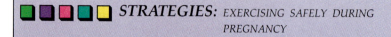

■ ■ ■ ■ ■ *STRATEGIES:* EXERCISING SAFELY DURING
PREGNANCY

To exercise safely during pregnancy:

1. Request a go-ahead from the physician or midwife before beginning.
2. Do not exceed 15 minutes of strenuous activity.
3. Drink plenty of fluids before and after exercise.
4. Avoid overheating. Do not exercise in hot, humid weather, exercise strenuously, or spend time in saunas, steam rooms, or hot whirlpools.
5. Discontinue any exercise that causes discomfort.
6. Do not exercise while lying on your back after about the fourth month of pregnancy.
7. Eat enough to support the additional needs of pregnancy plus the exercise performed.
8. Do not allow your heart rate to exceed 140 beats per minute.

partner on each side of the net is safer than a fast-moving game of racquetball. Swimming is ideal, because it allows the body to remain cool and move freely, with the water supporting its weight. This chapter's Strategies list safety guidelines for exercise during pregnancy. Several of them guard against raising the body temperature and inducing dehydration, both problems that interfere with normal fetal development.

Just as Gina needs exercise, she also needs plenty of rest. Paul might find that Gina would like to go out in the evenings after an hour's nap. Perhaps he can encourage her to rest while he takes care of some of the household chores.

Sexual activity can continue during pregnancy. Partners have no worries about birth control, and they may feel extra close. Orgasm is not harmful, and will not induce labor.

Late in pregnancy, the skin over a woman's abdomen, buttocks, and breasts may stretch, forming scars. The tendency to develop these "stretch marks" runs in families. Perhaps the most a woman can do to control them is to keep her weight gain within the recommended limits. Magic lotions just don't work, as the accompanying Critical Thinking explains.

The subject of stretch marks leads to one of the most important elements of a woman's pregnancy—namely, her feelings about it. Most pregnant women today enjoy their changing bodies. They feel strong. They willingly adopt sound eating habits and conscientious self-care. A few may fear the weight gain of pregnancy and need to remember that a gain of lean tissue is necessary. They are growing a baby and not just getting fat; this lean tissue will be shed.

Advice to Paul: Treat Gina with respect for the monumental physical and emotional adjustments she is making. Give her extra love and understanding to bolster her in making them. And Gina, keep Paul informed, and encourage him to share his feelings, too. Sensitive communication and understanding on both parts during this time of transition will help to lay a strong foundation for the shared parenthood ahead.

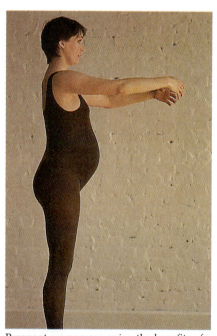

Pregnant women can enjoy the benefits of exercise.

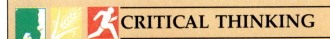

CRITICAL THINKING

Stretching the Truth

Stretch marks are permanent. No legitimate preventive measures or cures for them exist, although they can be minimized by gaining only the weight required. Spreading a product on the skin won't prevent the damage, even if the product contains vitamin E or other nutrients. Labels cannot directly claim that a product prevents stretch marks because such claims on labels are illegal, but products may imply this claim by using a name like Mother's Helper. Perhaps the best sales gimmick is a price low enough so that even though a woman may be skeptical, she'll buy it just in case it might help a little. Even at a low price, the manufacturer can make millions if enough women try the product.

Many con games work this way. Identify them by their key components: no legitimate treatments exist (a call to your pharmacist or health care provider can clarify that point), a label implies more than it says, and a low price entices you.

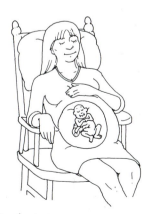

Identify fraudulent products by three clues: no legitimate treatments exist, label claims suggest more than they say, and price is tempting.

≡ ▶ *From the beginning of pregnancy, a woman experiences a multitude of physiological and hormonal changes. She will be best prepared to handle these changes with the support of a nutritious diet, regular physical activity, plenty of rest, and loving companions.*

Nutrition during Pregnancy

Earlier parts of this chapter described how malnutrition prior to pregnancy can impair fertility, placental development and, during critical periods, fetal development. This section highlights nutrition recommendations during pregnancy.

Nutrient needs during pregnancy are higher than at any other time in life. When the baby is born, its body will contain bones, muscles, blood, and other tissues made from nutrients the mother has eaten. A diet that includes a variety of foods is the best source of all the needed nutrients. Proper food choices can meet most nutrient needs, with the exception of iron.[10] Iron supplements are recommended for most women during pregnancy; a healthcare provider should evaluate the need for them. Health care providers usually prescribe multivitamin-mineral supplements that contain a wide range of vitamins and minerals.[11] This is especially important if overall nutrition is suspected to be poor.

The dietary challenge during pregnancy is to meet nutrient needs without overconsuming calories; energy needs during pregnancy increase, but less than nutrient needs do. A pregnant woman should not "eat for two," or she will gain unneeded fat and bear a fat baby. A pregnant woman must choose foods whose nutrient contributions are high relative to their calorie amounts—that is, nutrient-dense foods, the same ones that dieters are advised to select. A balance similar to that suggested in Chapter 5

Relaxing for two.

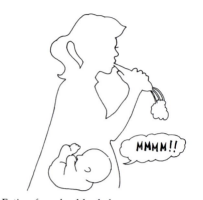

Eating for a healthy baby.

is recommended, but with an additional serving of meat or meat alternates and two additional servings of milk.

Most women should gain about 25 to 35 pounds, mostly of lean tissue, during pregnancy.[12] This weight gain supports normal growth and development of the placenta, uterus, blood, fluid, and breasts, and of the 7½-pound baby. Some women should strive for gains at the upper end of this range, notably adolescents, who are still growing themselves; and women who have been underweight or otherwise poorly nourished prior to pregnancy. Short women (5 feet 2 inches and under) should strive for gains at the lower end of the range. Obese women should gain less—from 15 to 25 pounds—and should be equally careful to eat nutrient-dense foods so that their gains will be mostly of lean, not fat, tissue. Some of their own body fat can supply energy to support the pregnancy.

≡▶ *Pregnancy demands that a woman increase her energy intake somewhat, and her nutrient intakes even more. Careful food choices can ensure optimal nutrition and appropriate weight gain during pregnancy.*

High-Risk and Low-Risk Pregnancies

Most babies are born normal, but some are not, and some pregnancies present more risks to the life and health of the mother and baby than others. Many of the factors that threaten pregnancy can be controlled once they are discovered, an argument for early prenatal examination and care. Table 14–2 identifies those characteristics identifying ''high-risk'' pregnancies that have to do with socioeconomic status, age, and maternal diseases. (Earlier sections described how appropriate maternal weight gain and adequate nutrition support the health of the mother and growth of the infant; later sections will identify problems associated with harmful lifestyle habits.)

A woman who has none of the risk factors listed in Table 14–2 is characterized as having a **low-risk pregnancy.** The more factors that apply, the higher the risk. Even a **high-risk pregnancy,** once identified, can be managed to minimize risks. For example, a woman known to have diabetes can be closely monitored to ensure that the disease is under control throughout the pregnancy; a woman who develops **pregnancy-induced hypertension** should be similarly treated. To see if your pregnancy is likely to be at risk, answer the questions in the Life Choice Inventory.

The most common outcome of a high-risk pregnancy is an infant of **low birthweight.** Infant birthweight is a potent indicator of the infant's future survival and health. Low-birthweight infants most often face illnesses and death early in life; about two-thirds of the infants who die before their first birthdays are low-birthweight infants.[13] They may be too weak to suck effectively or to cry to win their caretakers' attention. They can therefore become apathetic and neglected, compounding the original problems.

Low-birthweight infants, defined as infants who weigh 5½ pounds or less, are classified by the extent of their development at birth. Those called **premature** are born before their gestational development is complete; they may be small, but if they are appropriate in size and weight for their age, they do catch up in growth given adequate nutritional support. In contrast, **small-for-date** infants are underdeveloped; they have suffered growth failure in the uterus and do not catch up as well.

low-risk pregnancy a pregnancy characterized by indicators that make a normal outcome likely.

high-risk pregnancy a pregnancy characterized by indicators that make problems surrounding the birth likely—problems such as premature delivery, a collapsed umbilical cord, difficult birth, low birthweight, retarded growth, mental retardation, birth defects, and early infant death.

pregnancy-induced hypertension a medical problem in pregnancy that occurs in two stages. The first stage, **preeclampsia** (pree-ee-CLAMP-see-ah), is characterized by increasing edema (fluid retention), hypertension (high blood pressure), and protein in the urine. The second stage, **eclampsia** (ee-CLAMP-see-ah), is characterized by convulsions and coma. Pregnancy-induced hypertension was formerly called *toxemia* (tox-EEM-ee-ah).

low birthweight a birthweight of 5½ lb (2,500 g) or less; used as a predictor of poor health in the newborn and as a probable indicator that the mother was in poor nutrition status during and/or before pregnancy. Normal birthweight for a full-term baby is 6½ lb (3,000 g) or more.

premature born before the 38th week of gestation; also referred to as *preterm.*

small-for-date a term describing premature infants that are underdeveloped in comparison with others of the same gestational age, a characteristic that often reflects malnutrition.

TABLE 14–2 ■ **Factors Affecting Pregnancy Outcome**

Factor	Effect on Risk[a]
Maternal weight	Too low and too high increase risk.
Maternal malnutrition	Nutrient deficiencies and overdoses increase risk. Food faddism increases risk.
Socioeconomic status	Poverty, lack of family support, and low level of education increase risk.
Lifestyle habits	Smoking and drug and alcohol abuse increase risk.
Age	The youngest and oldest mothers have the greatest risk.
Pregnancies	
Number	The more previous pregnancies, the greater the risk.
Interval	The shorter the interval between pregnancies, the greater the risk.
Outcomes	Previous problems predict risk.
Multiple births	Twins or triplets increase risk.
Maternal health factors	
High blood pressure	A condition known as *pregnancy-induced hypertension*—formerly known as *toxemia*—increases risk.
Rh factor in blood	Lack of Rh factor in mother's blood increases risk. (See text.)
Chronic diseases	Diabetes; heart, respiratory, and kidney disease; certain genetic disorders; and others increase risk.

[a]Among the risks are low birthweight, mental retardation, a collapsed umbilical cord, and others.

Mothers who suffer social and economic disadvantages are most likely to bear low-birthweight infants. Low socioeconomic status limits a mother's access to medical care, restricts her choices of nutritious foods, and produces additional stress during pregnancy.[14] Furthermore, low income and status often lead to teen pregnancies and maladaptive behaviors such as tobacco, alcohol, and drug abuse—all predictive of low birthweight.

A pregnant teen faces special problems. The demands of pregnancy compete with those of her own growth, placing both mother and baby at risk. When their combined needs cannot be met, both mother and baby suffer. Maternal illness is especially common in pregnant teens, and they suffer more often from pregnancy-induced hypertension than do older women. A pregnant teen is likely to become anemic from iron deficiency (because of poor diet and inadequate medical care), and to experience prolonged labor (because of the mother's physical immaturity). Perhaps the greatest risk of teenage pregnancy, though, is death of the infant. Teenage mothers are more likely than any other age group to bear low-birthweight infants very likely to die during early infancy.[15]

Older women (over 35) face fewer problems than once believed, primarily because women and medicine have changed dramatically over the years. Today's typical older mother tends to be well-educated, financially secure, and medically cared for. Today's medical care offers management of chronic illnesses during pregnancy, early detection of fetal defects, and sophisticated care for newborns. Given these protective measures, older women's

■ ════════════════ ■ ════════════════ ■

LIFE CHOICE INVENTORY

Answer the following questions to determine if your or your prospective partner's pregnancy will be at risk. For women, answer the questions in this section about yourself. For men, answer the questions in this section about your prospective partner.

1. Do you have high blood pressure?   Yes No
2. Do you have chronic diseases such as diabetes or heart, kidney, lung, or liver disorders?   Yes No
3. Have you ever had a sexually transmitted disease?   Yes No
4. Is your blood Rh negative?   Yes No
5. Do you have severe anemia or other symptoms of nutrient deficiencies?   Yes No
6. Do you have convulsive diseases, such as epilepsy?   Yes No
7. Have you been pregnant within the last year, or have you had problems in previous pregnancies?   Yes No
8. Are you under 15 or over 35?   Yes No
9. Have you ever had twins or triplets?   Yes No
10. Do you smoke cigarettes?   Yes No
11. Do you drink alcohol?   Yes No
12. Do you take any drugs, including medicines prescribed by a physician, drugs of abuse, or over-the-counter drugs?   Yes No

13. Are you underweight, overweight, or otherwise poorly nourished?   Yes No
14. Do you lack the financial support needed for prenatal care?   Yes No
15. Do you have multiple sex partners?   Yes No

For men, answer the questions in this section about yourself. For women, answer the questions in this section about your prospective partner.

1. Do you have an active sexually transmitted disease?   Yes No
2. Do you drink more than two alcoholic drinks per day or more than five alcoholic drinks on any occasion?   Yes No
3. Do you take any drugs, including medicines prescribed by a physician, drugs of abuse, or over-the-counter drugs?   Yes No
4. Do you have multiple sex partners?   Yes No

Scoring
The more "yes" answers, the higher your pregnancy risk.

infants are as healthy as those of younger women.[16] The complications older women face include diminished fertility, early spontaneous abortions, and cesarean section delivery.

One risk associated with delaying a pregnancy until the age of 35 or older is that of bearing a child with Down's syndrome. Down's syndrome is caused by a genetic error: the fertilized ovum contains an extra chromosome (for a total of 47) and passes the defect on to the child's body cells. This mistake causes a host of physical and mental abnormalities. Factors that may raise the risk of Down's syndrome include:

■ Maternal age over 35.
■ Paternal age (it is thought that up to 20 percent of cases are due to a sperm-donated extra chromosome arising in an older male).
■ Radiation exposure.
■ Previous Down's conception.
■ Maternal inability to spontaneously abort imperfect zygotes and embryos.[17]

Of these factors, maternal age presents the highest risk.

Prenatal care supplied by health care providers is important to pregnant women, partly because it affords the opportunity to test for these and other problems. Many clues to abnormalities are present in samples of maternal blood or urine, in amniotic fluid, and in samples of placental or fetal tissue. Prenatal tests that sample these fluids and tissues and use other techniques can uncover numerous abnormalities.

A blood test, performed early in pregnancy, will establish whether or not the woman's blood contains a factor known as the **Rh factor.** If the factor is present, she is said to have Rh-positive blood; if the factor is absent, she is said to have Rh-negative blood. A person in whose blood the factor is present will not make antibodies against it, but if the Rh factor suddenly appears in the blood of someone who doesn't have it (for example, by way of blood transfusion), the person's immune system will attack it as if it were a virus or other foreign substance. A massive, whole-body immune reaction can disable the host as well as the "enemy."

If a woman with Rh-negative blood conceives a child with Rh-positive blood (inherited from the father), her body may detect the Rh factor's presence in the fetus and develop antibodies against it. The formation of antibodies causes no problems during the first pregnancy, but in subsequent pregnancies with Rh-positive infants, the Rh antibodies may cross the placenta and destroy fetal blood cells. The pregnancy may end in spontaneous abortion or miscarriage. At best, the baby may be born with Rh disease,* in which pigment leaks from the red blood cells, causing yellowing of the skin and eyes; anemia is likely; and heart, liver, or brain damage may occur. Many Rh babies die. Rh disease rarely occurs anymore; each Rh-negative mother receives an injection following the birth of her first Rh-positive baby to inhibit the formation of the potentially dangerous antibodies.**

The Rh test and others, which can lead to the detection and, sometimes, reversal of dangerous abnormalities, are listed in Table 14–3. Health care providers elect to perform these tests with different frequencies. Some tests, such as the test for Rh factor and for maternal diabetes, require only the taking of blood samples and are routine. Others are more invasive; they may be uncomfortable or painful and may entail risks of infection or even abortion.

Medical science has improved the odds so that today, with appropriate prenatal testing and care, the overwhelming majority of babies born to women of any age are normal. If a pregnancy is to be problematic, the woman who seeks prenatal care and testing early can, at best, protect herself and her unborn child from many preventable risks. And if prevention is not possible—if, for example, a test shows that a fetus is defective and spontaneous abortion is likely to occur—at least she can be prepared.

≡▶ *Several factors (such as age, socioeconomic status, and illness) can identify "high-risk" women who are more likely than others to deliver infants who face illnesses and an early death. Samples of maternal blood, urine, amniotic fluid, and placental and fetal tissue provide valuable information about the mother's health and the fetus's genetic makeup and development.*

Rh factor the factor produced on the surface of the blood cells of an Rh-positive individual, against which an Rh-negative individual produces antibodies. About 85% of the population is Rh positive.

Rh disease the disease produced in a fetus when it has inherited Rh-positive blood from its father and developed in an Rh-negative mother who produced antibodies against it.

*Other names for Rh disease are *hemolytic anemia* and *erythroblastosis fetalis.* The yellowing of the skin is *hyperbilirubinemia* or *jaundice.*
**The drug's brand name is RhoGAM (ROH-gam).

TABLE 14–3   ■   **Tests during Pregnancy**

Test	How Performed	Conditions Detected/Prevented
Alpha fetoprotein	Blood test	Detects a protein in the blood that indicates brain and spinal cord abnormalities in fetus
Amniocentesis	Amniotic fluid is collected and fetal cells are examined for chromosomal abnormalities	Detects gender and age of fetus along with about 70 inherited abnormalities, including Down's syndrome
Blood/urine glucose	Blood/urine test	Detects gestational diabetes[a] in time to prevent fetal damage caused by abnormal blood glucose concentration during development
Chorionic villus sampling	Placental cells are collected and tested	(Same as for amniocentesis, above)
Fetoscope	Viewing device is inserted surgically into uterus to observe fetus or collect blood or tissue samples	Risky procedure, used only when serious disorders are strongly suspected.
HIV test	Blood test	Detects presence of HIV antibodies, indicating that the sexually transmitted disease AIDS is developing
Other blood tests	Blood tests	Detect other sexually transmitted diseases
Rh factor	Blood test	Detects Rh compatibility of parents/prevents Rh disease in infants
Ultrasound	High-frequency waves produce an image of the fetus on a monitor similar to a television set	Determines age and (sometimes) gender of fetus, and can detect some physical abnormalities

SOURCES: G. H. Lowrey, *Growth and Development of Children* (Chicago: Year Book Medical, 1986), p. 60; M. T. Mennuti, Prenatal diagnosis— Advances bring new challenges, *New England Journal of Medicine* 320 (1989): 661–663; G. G. Rhoads and coauthors, The safety and efficacy of chorionic villus sampling for early prenatal diagnosis of cytogenetic abnormalities, *New England Journal of Medicine* 320 (1989): 609–617;

and I. Peterson, Ultrasound safety and collapsing bubbles, *Science News* 130 (1986): 372; Adult immunization: Recommendations of Immunization Practices Advisory Committee, *Morbidity and Mortality Weekly Report* 33 (Supplement, 1984): 17s.
[a]Gestational diabetes is a transient diabetes that may arise during pregnancy in susceptible women. (See Spotlight 18.)

Alcohol Use and Other Practices to Avoid during Pregnancy

A woman's daily choices, her lifestyle habits, may normally affect her only slightly, but these same choices can take on enormous importance when she is pregnant. Many substances can adversely influence a pregnancy. Forewarned, pregnant women can choose to avoid exposure to them or abstain from them. Table 14–4 presents some of the vast array of substances known to be harmful.

Alcohol consumed during pregnancy can retard fetal growth, impair development of the nervous system, and cause physical malformations—the abnormalities that define **fetal alcohol syndrome (FAS)**. The potential for fetal damage arises when the mother's liver receives more alcohol than it can detoxify. Alcohol-laden blood then circulates to all parts of the mother's body and freely crosses the placenta to impair fetal development. Alcohol also interferes with placental transport of nutrients to the fetus.[18]

fetal alcohol syndrome (FAS)   the cluster of symptoms seen in a person whose mother consumed excess alcohol during her pregnancy; includes mental and physical retardation with facial and other body deformities.

TABLE 14–4 ■ **Effects of Potentially Harmful Substances on the Fetus**

Substance	Effects on Fetus
Alcohol	Subclinical fetal alcohol syndrome; fetal alcohol syndrome (see text)
Caffeine	Central nervous system stimulation; increased incidence of spontaneous abortion; fetal growth retardation
Cigarette smoke	Low birthweight; increased incidence of spontaneous abortion; nervous system disturbances; increased incidence of sudden infant death syndrome (SIDS); fetal death
Heavy metals	
Lead	Spontaneous abortion; stillbirth; low birthweight; neurobehavioral deficits
Mercury	Central nervous system damage
Illegal drugs	
Cocaine	Increased incidence of spontaneous abortion; uncontrolled jerking motions; paralysis; depressed interactive behavior; poor organizational responses to environmental stimuli
Heroin, methadone	Drug addiction and acute narcotic withdrawal symptoms (tremors; excessive, high-pitched crying; and disturbed sleep); low birthweight
Marijuana	Short-term irritability at birth
Phencyclidine (PCP)	Facial malformations; tremors; low birthweight
Medications	
Aspirin and its relatives (large doses)	High blood pressure in lungs; bleeding at birth
Diethylstilbestrol (DES, now no longer prescribed)	Congenital abnormalities of the reproductive organs (see text)
Oral contraceptives or androgenic steroids	Abnormal sexual development; masculination; advanced bone age
Tetracyclines (antibiotics)	Inhibition of bone growth; discoloration of teeth
Thalidomide (now no longer prescribed)	Missing limbs (see text)
Tylenol (acetaminophen)	Renal failure
Nutrient overdoses	
Vitamin A	Small, underdeveloped brain; oversized brain with abnormal function; spontaneous abortion
Vitamin D	Bone abnormalities; calcium deposits in blood vessels; heart damage
Iodine	Damaged thyroid gland, abnormal metabolism

SOURCE: Partially adapted from S. R. Rolfes, L. K. DeBruyne, and E. N. Whitney, *Life Span Nutrition: Conception through Life* (St. Paul: West, 1990), p. 96.

At its most severe, FAS involves:

■ Prenatal and postnatal growth retardation.
■ Impairment of the brain and nerves, with consequent mental retardation, poor coordination, and hyperactivity.
■ Abnormalities of the face and skull, and other birth defects.

Perhaps most important and tragic, the damage evident at birth remains—children with FAS never fully recover.

About 1 to 3 in every 1,000 children born in the United States is a victim of FAS.[19] Moreover, for every baby born with these symptoms, several others are born with **subclinical FAS**. The mothers of these children drank alcohol, but not enough to cause visible effects immediately. These children may go undiagnosed until problems develop in the early school years.[20]

subclinical FAS   a subtle version of FAS, with hidden defects including learning disabilities, behavioral abnormalities, and motor impairments.

The many abnormalities associated with subclinical FAS are subtle, hidden under a normal-looking exterior. Without the clue from the classic facial abnormalities to alert them to the condition's presence, parents may not suspect the presence of defects. Yet they may exist, and they can be devastating: learning disabilities, behavioral abnormalities, motor impairments, and more.

The type and extent of abnormality observed in an FAS infant depends on the developmental events that occurred at the time of alcohol exposure.[21] During the first trimester, developing organs such as the brain, heart, and kidneys may be malformed. During the second trimester, the risk of spontaneous abortion increases. During the third trimester, when the fetus is fully formed and rapidly growing, body and brain growth may be retarded.

The extent of fetal damage correlates directly with the quantity of alcohol the mother consumes.[22] A pregnant woman need not be alcohol-addicted in order to give birth to a baby with FAS characteristics. She only needs to drink alcohol in excess of the liver's ability to detoxify it. Because a safe level of alcohol consumption cannot be defined, health care providers recommend that women who are planning pregnancy should refrain from drinking alcohol altogether, or at least reduce drinking to a minimum.[23] The mother who chooses to drink during pregnancy, even moderately, places her infant at greater risk than the mother who abstains completely.

All this discussion is not intended to worry a woman who is usually careful about her health but who had a cocktail during the first month of her pregnancy, before she even knew she was pregnant. Chances are that such small quantities of alcohol have not harmed the developing infant. Anyway, the episode is in the past; she should emphasize what can be done now and in the future to ensure the best possible outcome.

At the other extreme is the woman who drinks heavily or who is addicted to alcohol. Health care providers must focus their prevention efforts on reaching these women before pregnancy.[24] Women addicted to alcohol who are sexually active urgently need treatment for their alcoholism and effective methods of contraception to prevent the bearing of FAS infants.

Of the leading causes of mental retardation, FAS is the only one that is totally *preventable*.[25] The surgeon general has issued a statement that pregnant women should drink absolutely no alcohol. All containers of beer, wine, and liquor now must carry the warning: Women should not drink

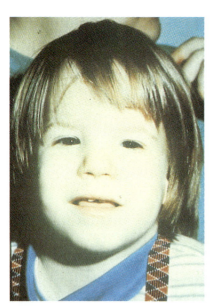

These facial traits reflect fetal alcohol syndrome, caused by maternal drinking in early pregnancy. Irreversible abnormalities of the brain and internal organs accompany these surface features.

alcoholic beverages during pregnancy because of the risk of birth defects. Everyone should hear the message loud and clear: Don't drink alcohol prior to or during pregnancy. Once present, FAS has no cure.

Drugs other than alcohol can also cause complications during pregnancy, problems in labor, and serious congenital malformations. Even aspirin, if taken late in pregnancy, adversely affects fetal circulation and uterine contractions.[26] The damage of drug use during pregnancy was tragically illustrated in the early 1960s in the case of the sedative **thalidomide.** This drug found its way from Europe to the United States and, although it had not been approved by the FDA for the U.S. market, was given to thousands of women to relieve nausea in the early critical weeks of pregnancy. Thalidomide had been found safe for animals, but in human beings, it damaged the fetal limbs just as they were budding. Almost 6,000 babies, most of them in Europe, were born with missing arms and other deformities before thalidomide was banned.[27] Another prescription drug, **diethylstilbestrol (DES),** intended to prevent miscarriage, was discovered later to produce many benign tumors and a rare cancer of the vagina or cervix in girls born to mothers who had taken DES. In sons of these women, the risk of testicular cancer was also increased.

For reasons like these, women are advised to take medicines only on their physicians' advice. Drug labels warn: "As with any drug, if you are pregnant or nursing a baby, seek the advice of a health professional before using this product." For aspirin and ibuprofen, an additional warning immediately follows: "It is especially important not to use aspirin [or ibuprofen] during the last three months of pregnancy unless specifically directed to do so by a doctor because it may cause problems in the unborn child or [excessive bleeding] during delivery."

The recommendation to avoid drug use during pregnancy includes drugs of abuse, of course. Because drugs of abuse pass easily through the placenta, their use brings a multitude of problems for infants.[28] Infants face low birthweight, developmental problems, and an increased risk of death. If they survive, their behavior at birth is abnormal. They may suffer the pain of withdrawal from the drugs—the same dysphoria that drives the addict to seek repeated doses. They may be hypersensitive and irritable, may tremble or jerk, and may cry inconsolably for hours. They may fail to bond normally to their parents early in life as normal infants do, and they may be unable throughout life to form normal, loyal relationships.

Smoking is also ill-advised. Pregnancy magnifies the harmful effects of smoking many-fold. Just two cigarettes smoked in succession reduce the chest breathing movements of the fetus. Smoking restricts the fetal blood supply and so limits the delivery of oxygen and nutrients and the removal of wastes. In addition, smokers tend to eat less nutritious foods during their pregnancies than do nonsmokers.[29] Of all *preventable* causes of low birthweight in the United States, smoking has the greatest impact; the more a mother smokes, the smaller her baby will be. The risks of spontaneous abortion and early infant death also increase directly with increasing levels of maternal smoking.[30] The same is true of chewing tobacco—infants of mothers who chew have lower birthweights and higher risks of early deaths than do other infants. Smoking during pregnancy may affect a child's mental, physical, and behavioral development at least up to the age of 11 years.

■ *FACT OR FICTION:* A pregnant woman should drink no more than two alcohol drinks per day. *False.* The surgeon general recommends that women drink no alcohol during pregnancy because of the risks of birth defects.

thalidomide (tha-LID-oh-mide) a drug given to pregnant women to relieve morning sickness—found to produce birth defects and no longer on the market.

diethylstilbestrol (DYE-eth-il-STILL-bes-trahl), or **DES** a synthetic hormone preparation possessing the characteristics of estrogen; used in pregnancy to prevent miscarriage only when the benefit is deemed to outweigh the risk of subsequent vaginal abnormalities in a girl born of that pregnancy.

sudden infant death syndrome (SIDS) the unexpected and unexplained death of an apparently well infant, the most common cause of death of infants between the second week and the end of the first year of life; also called *crib death*.

One study even suggests that smoking during pregnancy increases the risk of childhood cancer.[31]

In addition, **sudden infant death syndrome (SIDS)**, the sudden, unexplained death of an infant, has been positively linked to the mother's cigarette smoking during pregnancy,[32] and even to postnatal exposure to smoke in the household.[33] The surgeon general has concluded that maternal cigarette smoking during pregnancy can kill otherwise healthy fetuses and newborns.[34]

Pregnant women may wonder whether they should give up the caffeine in coffee, tea, and colas. Research studies have not proved that coffee or caffeine causes birth defects in human babies; limited evidence suggests that moderate to heavy use may lower infant birthweight and cause fetal growth retardation.[35] All things considered, it might be most sensible to limit caffeine consumption to the equivalent of a cup or two of coffee or tea a day.[36] Some questions have been raised about the overuse of saccharin, too—but too much attention given to these relatively safe practices might distract from what is really important. There would be little point in a woman's giving up saccharin and continuing to smoke two packs of cigarettes a day.

Pregnancy is a vulnerable time, and the effects of many lifestyle habits are compounded for the developing fetus. A woman considering a pregnancy would do well to take a look at her own habits and decide which would support a healthy pregnancy and which need improving.

≡▶ *Lifestyle habits such as alcohol use, drug use, and smoking have profound adverse effects on pregnancy and can cause irreversible fetal damage.*

■≡ Breastfeeding and Formula Feeding

Before the end of her pregnancy, a woman will need to consider whether to feed her infant breast milk, infant formula, or both. These options are the only recommended sources of nutrients for an infant during the first four to six months of life.

Most experts on infant feeding recommend breast milk as the preferred choice.[37] Breast milk's unique nutrient composition promotes optimal infant health and development. Breastfeeding benefits the mother, the infant, and the mother-infant pair in many ways. It benefits the mother by stimulating a reflex that causes uterine contractions, thus promoting return of the uterus to its normal size. It also draws, for energy, on the few pounds of maternal fat that the mother's body stored to support lactation. It benefits the infant, for breast milk's unique nutrient composition supports optimal infant growth. Human breast milk also contains antibodies, white blood cells, and other factors that protect the infant against diseases; factors to promote the absorption of iron and zinc; a factor that stimulates the development of the infant's digestive tract; and probably many others that support the infant's development. Also, the act of breastfeeding promotes bonding, which stimulates healthy emotional growth in the infant. Experts quickly add, though, that formula is an excellent alternative to breast milk, for it imitates breast milk's composition closely. And all mothers who spend time being close to their infants can bond with them.

Most healthy women who want to breastfeed can do so if they prepare ahead of time by learning what is involved. To learn about infant-feeding practices, a pregnant woman can read one of the many books available or take a class on the topic. Other good sources of information are health care providers and mothers who have successfully breastfed their infants. Successful breastfeeding requires adequate nutrition, fluid intake, and rest. Emotional support from family and friends also helps to enhance the well-being of mother and infant.

A woman who breastfeeds for the better part of a year can wean her infant to cow's milk, bypassing the need for infant formula. A woman can freely decide to use formula, either alone or in addition to breastfeeding. Both formula and breast milk support infant growth. However, some circumstances warrant the selection of one over the other. For example, breast milk best meets the specific needs of a premature infant. For another example, formula best protects the infant of a woman who tests positive for the AIDS virus, because the AIDS virus can be transmitted through breast milk.[38]

If a woman must take medication that is known to harm the infant and that will be secreted in breast milk, she must opt for formula feeding, at least temporarily. Many prescription drugs do not reach nursing infants in sufficient quantities to harm them; some, however, do.[39] People addicted to drugs, including alcohol, are capable of consuming such high doses that their infants become intoxicated by way of breast milk.[40] Infants might experience drowsiness, weakness, and slowed growth.[41] In these cases, formula feeding is preferred.

≡▶ *Breastfeeding offers many benefits to both mother and infant. Still, there are many valid reasons for not breastfeeding, and formula-fed infants can grow and develop into healthy children.*

The way a woman goes about making choices during her pregnancy can help to provide for a happy ending—the birth of a healthy baby. The Spotlight that follows describes the fetus's world inside the mother and the journey to the outside—childbirth. The next chapter goes on to explore later times in life.

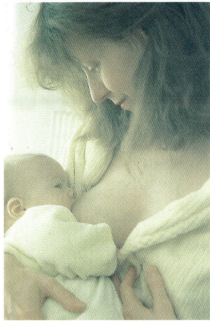

Breastfeeding goes most smoothly for the woman who prepares.

■≡ For Review

1. Explain, in simple terms, how inheritance works, and in particular why each new individual differs from both parents.

2. Define the term *teratogen*.

3. Advise a couple considering starting a pregnancy on health habits they should adopt or maintain beforehand.

4. Characterize the kinds of problems on which genetic counselors can advise.

5. Describe the normal events of healthy placental and fetal development.

6. Define the term *critical period*.

7. Explain the significance to later life and health of environmental and nutritional influences on critical periods.

8. Explain what makes a pregnant woman feel different during pregnancy.

9. Indicate what a pregnant woman needs to know about exercise.

10. Give an example of how malnutrition impairs fetal development.

11. State the special nutritional needs of pregnancy, and describe wise food choices for the pregnant woman.

12. Define low-risk and high-risk pregnancies.

13. Describe some of the special problems of the pregnant teenage girl.

14. Describe how Rh disease develops.

15. Name two common tests performed during pregnancy, and state which conditions they are designed to detect.

16. State some effects of alcohol, other drugs, tobacco smoke, and chemicals on the outcome of pregnancy.

17. List some of the advantages of breastfeeding.

▣ ≡ Notes

1. K. Nelson and L. B. Holmes, Malformations due to presumed spontaneous mutations in newborn infants, *New England Journal of Medicine* 320 (1989): 19–23.

2. R. E. Little and C. F. Sing, Father's drinking and infant birthweight, *Teratology* 36 (1987): 59–65; M. H. Kaufman, Ethanol-induced chromosomal abnormalities at conception, *Nature* 302 (1983): 258–260; R. E. Little and coauthors, Decreased birth weight in infants of alcoholic women who abstained during pregnancy, *Journal of Pediatrics* 96 (1980): 974–977; L. F. Soyka and J. M. Joffe, Male mediated drug effects on offspring, *Progress in Clinical and Biological Research* 36 (1980): 49–66; L. M. Hill and F. Kleinburg, Effects of drugs and chemicals on the fetus and newborn, *Mayo Clinic Proceedings* 59 (1984): 707–716.

3. Z. Stein and coauthors, *Famine and Human Development: The Dutch Hunger Winter of 1944/1945* (New York: Oxford University Press, 1975).

4. P. Rosso, Placental growth, development, and function in relation to maternal nutrition, *Federation Proceedings* 39 (1980): 250–254.

5. C. A. Smith, Effects of maternal undernutrition upon the newborn infant in Holland (1944–1945), *Journal of Pediatrics* 30 (1947): 229–243.

6. Rubella vaccination during pregnancy—United States, 1971–1975, *Morbidity and Mortality Weekly Report* 35 (May 1986): 275–284, as cited in Rubella vaccination during pregnancy: New CDC advisory,

Modern Medicine, November 1986, p. 168.

7. J. M. Hicks and M. Iosefsohn, Reliability of home pregnancy-test kits in the hands of laypersons, *New England Journal of Medicine* 320 (1989): 320–321.

8. Hicks and Iosefsohn, 1989; M. L. Doshi, Accuracy of consumer performed in-home tests for early pregnancy detection, *American Journal of Public Health* 76 (1986): 512–514.

9. J. M. Tanner, *Foetus into Man: Physical Growth from Conception to Maturity* (London: Open Books, 1978), p. 38.

10. National Academy of Sciences, National Research Council, Food and Nutrition Board, *Nutrition during Pregnancy: 1. Weight Gain; 2. Nutrient Supplements* (Washington, D.C.: National Academy Press, 1990).

11. V. Newman, R. B. Lyon, and P. O. Anderson, Evaluation of prenatal vitamin-mineral supplements, *Clinical Pharmacy* 6 (1987): 770–777.

12. National Academy, 1990.

13. *Facts about Premature Birth* (a pamphlet available from the National Institute of Child Health and Human Development; Washington, D.C.: Government Printing Office, 1985).

14. J. B. Gould and S. LeRoy, Socioeconomic status and low birth weight: A racial comparison, *Pediatrics* 82 (1988): 896–904.

15. J. Menken, The health and demographic consequences of adolescent pregnancy and childbearing, in *Adolescent Pregnancy and Childbearing,* ed. C. S. Chilman, NIH publi-

cation no. 81-2077 (Washington, D.C.: Government Printing Office, 1981), pp. 177–205.

16. G. S. Berkowitz and coauthors, Delayed childbearing and the outcome of pregnancy, *New England Journal of Medicine* 322 (1990): 659–664; D. S. Kriz, W. Dorchester, and R. K. Freeman, Advanced maternal age: The mature gravida, *American Journal of Obstetrics and Gynecology,* 1 May 1985, pp. 7–12.

17. Z. A. Stein, A woman's age: Childbearing and child rearing, *American Journal of Epidemiology* 121 (1985): 327–343.

18. S. Fisher and P. Karl, Maternal ethanol use and selective fetal malnutrition, *Alcoholism* (New York: Plenum Press, 1988), pp. 277–289.

19. K. R. Warren and R. J. Bast, Alcohol-related birth defects: An update, *Public Health Reports* 103 (1988): 772–778.

20. J. M. Graham and coauthors, Independent dysmorphology evaluations at birth and 14 years of age for children exposed to varying amounts of alcohol in utero, *Pediatrics* 81 (1988): 772–778.

21. H. L. Rosett and L. Weiner, Alcohol and pregnancy: A clinical perspective, *Annual Review of Medicine* 36 (1985): 73–80.

22. W. S. Beagle, Fetal alcohol syndrome: A review, *Journal of the American Dietetic Association* 79 (1981): 274–276.

23. C. B. Ernhart and coauthors, Alcohol teratogenicity in the human: A detailed assessment of specificity, critical period, and threshold,

American Journal of Obstetrics and Gynecology 156 (1987): 33–39.

24. C. A. Raymond, Birth defects linked with specific level of maternal alcohol use, but abstinence still is the best policy, *Journal of the American Medical Association* 258 (1987): 177–178.

25. K. R. Warren and R. J. Bast, Alcohol-related birth defects: An update, *Public Health Reports* 103 (1988): 638–642.

26. New pregnancy warning on aspirin, *FDA Consumer,* September 1990, p. 2.

27. E. Zamula, Drugs and pregnancy: Often the two don't mix, *FDA Consumer,* June 1989, pp. 7–10.

28. D. B. Petitti and C. Coleman, Cocaine and the risk of low birth weight, *American Journal of Public Health* 80 (1990): 25–28; S. Parker and coauthors, Jitteriness in full-term neonates: Prevalence and correlates, *Pediatrics* 85 (1990): 17–23; M. van de Bor, F. J. Walther, and M. Ebrahimi, Decreased cardiac output in infants of mothers who abused cocaine, *Pediatrics* 85 (1990): 30–32; B. Zuckerman and coauthors, Effects of maternal marijuana and cocaine use on fetal growth, *New England Journal of Medicine* 320 (1989): 762–768; I. J. Chasnoff and coauthors, Cocaine use in pregnancy, *New England Journal of Medicine* 313 (1985): 666–669; C. N. Chiang and C. C. Lee, *Prenatal Drug Exposure: Kinetics and Dynamics,* NIDA research monograph 60 (Washington, D.C.: Government Printing Office, 1985); T. M. Pinkert, *Current Research on the Consequences of Maternal Drug Abuse,* NIDA research monograph 59 (Washington, D.C.: Government Printing Office, 1985).

29. F. M. Haste and coauthors, Nutrient intakes during pregnancy: Observations on the influence of smoking and social class, *American Journal of Clinical Nutrition* 51 (1990): 29–36.

30. U.S. Department of Health and Human Services, Public Health Service, *The Health Benefits of Smoking Cessation: A Report of the Surgeon General, 1990* (Washington, D.C.: Government Printing Office, 1990).

31. M. Stjernfeldt and coauthors, Maternal smoking during pregnancy and risk of childhood cancer, *Lancet,* 14 June 1986, p. 1350.

32. B. Haglund and S. Cnattingius, Cigarette smoking as a risk factor for sudden infant death syndrome: A population-based study, *American Journal of Public Health* 80 (1990): 29–32; National Institute of Child Health and Human Development, *Smoking and Health: A Report of the Surgeon General,* HHS publication no. (PHS) 79-50066, 1979, pp. 8–1 through 8–93.

33. National Institute of Child Health and Human Development, 1979.

34. National Institute of Child Health and Human Development, 1979.

35. National Academy, 1990, pp. 397–399; L. Fenster, B. Eskenazi, G. C. Windham, and S. H. Swan, Caffeine consumption during pregnancy and fetal growth, *American Journal of Public Health* 81 (1991): 458–461.

36. National Academy of Science, National Research Council, Food and Nutrition Board, Committee of the Mother and Preschool Child, *Alternative Dietary Practices and Nutritional Abuses in Pregnancy* (Washington, D.C.: National Academy Press, 1982), pp. 10–12.

37. American Dietetic Association, Position of the American Dietetic Association: Promotion of breast-feeding, *Journal of the American Dietetic Association* 86 (1986): 1580–1585.

38. S. Logan, M. L. Newell, T. Ades, and C. S. Peckham, Breast feeding and HIV infection, *Lancet* 1 (1988): 1346; S. J. Heymann, Modeling the impact of breast-feeding by HIV-infected women on child survival, *American Journal of Public Health* 80 (1990): 1305–1309.

39. American Academy of Pediatrics, Committee on Drugs, The transfer of drugs and other chemicals into human breast milk, *Pediatrics* 72 (1983): 375–381.

40. I. J. Chasnoff, D. E. Lewis, and L. Squires, Cocaine intoxication in a breast-fed infant, *Pediatrics* 80 (1987): 836–838.

41. R. E. Little and coauthors, maternal alcohol use during breast-feeding and infant mental and motor development at one year, *New England Journal of Medicine* 321 (1989): 425–430; American Academy of Pediatrics, 1983.

SPOTLIGHT

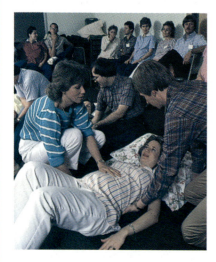

Childbirth Choices

So you are pregnant, you say. Congratulations! Where do you plan to give birth?

I don't know, yet. I'm just beginning to explore my options. What do you recommend?

The two options most people consider are hospitals and **birth centers** (see the Miniglossary of Childbirth Terms). A high-risk pregnancy may necessitate a hospital delivery, but if your pregnancy is progressing normally, you may choose to deliver at a birth center. For the many cases in which the birth is normal, a birth center provides a more homelike atmosphere. Most birth centers allow family members and friends to attend the birth if the mother wishes; in contrast, most hospitals limit attendance during labor and delivery to one or two support people. Birth centers generally employ profes-

sionally trained **midwives,** use few invasive or restrictive procedures, and provide a homelike atmosphere and attentive care. Their costs per delivery are significantly lower than the costs in hospitals. They perform **cesarean sections** in fewer than 5 percent of births, while in hospitals, the rate is almost 25 percent.[1*] This difference reflects both their noninterventive approach and their policy of accepting only low-risk pregnancies.

Perhaps the greatest disadvantage of a birth center is that lifesaving equipment and expertise may not be available quickly enough in an emergency; crucial time might be lost traveling to the hospital. Emergency transfers are necessary for about 3 percent of women admitted for labor and delivery at birth centers in the United States.[2] On the other hand, over 70 percent of all women have only minor complications or none. Perhaps the best alternative is a hospital-based birth center that offers the atmosphere of a birth center and the safety of a hospital.[3]

Can people choose whom to have in attendance at the birth?

Yes. Some people feel most secure with a nurse present during labor and a physician attending the delivery; others feel most secure with a midwife in attendance throughout labor and delivery. Possibly the most important ingredient in the relationship between family and health care provider is trust. Determine early on how willing your physician or midwife is to develop an individualized plan with you for your pregnancy and childbirth. With forethought, the birth experience can be one of the high points of your life.

*Reference notes are at the end of the Spotlight.

Each birth attendant has a philosophy on childbirth, and this dictates the procedures that will accompany the births. For example, the style of the attending physician greatly influences the rate of cesarean sections.[4] Also, some physicians administer a drug (a synthetic version of the hormone **oxytocin**) to speed labor by enhancing the contractions' strength and frequency. Other physicians and most midwives allow labors to gather momentum at their own pace. Another example: many physicians routinely perform a small surgical incision called an **episiotomy** to widen the vaginal opening to prevent tearing of tissue. They do this to ensure that the birth is timely, but a different strategy, widely used in other countries and by midwives in this country, is possible. Birth attendants can massage the tissues surrounding the vaginal opening during late pregnancy and birth. This relaxes the opening enough to permit birth without the tissues' being torn or cut, although labor may be somewhat longer.

Whatever the choice of medical attendant, most women will also want to have at least one special someone (a "labor coach") with them during labor and delivery to share the experience and help them in ways that medical attendants can't duplicate. Even speaking may become hard for a woman when labor is under way, and a partner may sense changing needs better than a stranger at that time. Labor requires rapid breathing and creates thirst; a constant supply of ice and lollipops are a comfort. Also comforting is the knowledge that someone is near who cares and who can communicate changes, as they occur, to busy medical personnel.

■ MINIGLOSSARY
of Childbirth Terms

anoxia (an-OX-ee-uh) a general term for oxygen deprivation, a particular hazard during pregnancy and delivery because of the fetal nervous system's vulnerability; it is damaged by even short-term oxygen lack.

Apgar score a system of scoring an infant's physical condition right after birth, based on responses to stimulation, respiration rate, heart rate, movement, color, and muscle tone.

birth centers nonhospital facilities that provide maternity care for women judged to be at low risk of obstetrical complications; most birth centers are regulated by state licensure, have an established program of accreditation, and are covered by insurance plans.

cesarean (sih-ZEHR-ee-un) **sections** surgical childbirths, often called simply *cesareans.* In a cesarean, the infant is taken through an incision in the woman's abdomen. (Alternative spellings: *cesarian, caesarean.*)

circumcision surgical removal of the end of the foreskin of the penis.

crowning the moment during childbirth in which the top (crown) of the baby's head is first seen.

dilation stage the stage of childbirth during which the cervix is opening, before expulsion of the infant begins.

episiotomy (eh-PEEZ-ee-OT-oh-me) a surgical incision made to prevent tearing

of the vagina when it becomes apparent that the vagina cannot stretch enough to accommodate an impending birth.

expulsion stage the stage of childbirth during which the uterine contractions are actively pushing the infant through the birth canal.

Lamaze (lah-MAHZ) **method** a method of childbirth in which the woman uses rhythmic breathing, relaxation techniques, and the help of a coach while giving birth.

midwives birth attendants. A **certified nurse midwife (CNM)** is a trained, credentialed health care professional who is part of the team that cares for mothers and their infants during normal pregnancy, labor, and childbirth. See also Chapter 20.

oxytocin (ox-ee-TOCE-in) a pituitary hormone that stimulates the uterus to contract, thus initiating the birth process. It also acts on the mammary gland to stimulate the release of milk.

placental stage the final stage of childbirth, after the infant has been born, in which the placenta is expelled.

postpartum depression the emotional depression a woman may experience after the birth of her infant, ascribed to changes in hormone levels. When a man experiences depression after the birth of his child, it is usually ascribed to changed life conditions.

Are cesarean sections ever really necessary?

Yes, cesareans offer a lifesaving alternative when things go wrong during labor. For example, if the umbilical cord is pinched or if the placenta detaches from the uterine wall before birth, the infant will be deprived of oxygen **(anoxia).** In such a case, an emergency cesarean could prevent permanent brain damage or death.

Sometimes, though, cesareans are performed unnecessarily. Health care providers become anxious when labor and delivery vary from the "ideal." They face not only the threat of infant death but also the threat of a possible lawsuit should they judge wrong, so they tend to judge too conservatively, sometimes performing unnecessary cesareans.[5]

In the last two decades, the rate of

cesarean sections in the United States has quadrupled. Approximately one out of every four deliveries is by cesarean section.[6] Experts argue about why the rates are so high; some think the reason is economic. On the average, the hospital receives an additional $3,000 and the physician, an additional $500, above the fee for a normal birth. One study reported that the rate of cesarean sections rises and falls with the income of the family, a finding opposite to what you would expect.[7] After all, it is poor women who cannot afford prenatal care, face more complications, and need more cesareans than affluent women. It would be unfair, though, to ascribe the use of cesarean sections only to greed. Most low-income women do not see private physicians, and some who need cesareans may not receive them for that reason.

Should women expect to feel much pain during childbirth?

Yes, most women experience pain during some part of labor or delivery, and they must make some choices ahead of time about how to control the pain. Like most prescription drugs, drugs for pain relief have drawbacks. Narcotics may slow labor; barbiturates can cause breathing difficulty in the infant; local anesthetics may slow the infant's heart rate; and all drugs used during delivery cause after-effects such as grogginess, nausea, or dizziness. Most women and their attendants strive to keep the use of drugs to a minimum.

Parents-to-be can take classes to prepare for childbirth, and these may help minimize the need for drugs. Several methods, including the **Lamaze method,** help women take charge of the birthing experience. They give women the tools they

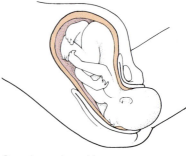

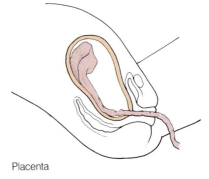

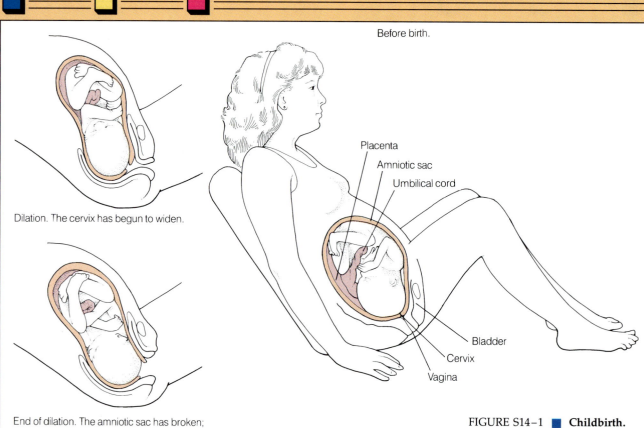

Before birth.

Placenta

Amniotic sac

Umbilical cord

Bladder

Cervix

Vagina

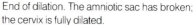

Dilation. The cervix has begun to widen.

End of dilation. The amniotic sac has broken; the cervix is fully dilated.

Crowning and expulsion.

Placenta

FIGURE S14–1 ■ **Childbirth.**

need—knowledge, relaxation techniques, and breathing control—to reduce tension and pain and to speed the labor along. These classes also teach those who will be attending the birth how to assist the laboring woman. Childbirth preparation takes practice, and not all pregnancies last the full nine months, so classes should be started at about the seventh month to ensure readiness at delivery.

What is the actual process of childbirth like?

Labor begins as the woman's hormones, including oxytocin, cause the muscles of her uterus to contract powerfully and rhythmically. Thereafter, labor proceeds by stages (Figure S14–1). In the first one, the **dilation stage,** the cervix dilates until the baby's head can pass through it,

while the contractions become more and more powerful and closer and closer together. Then a transition occurs, bringing on the still more powerful contractions of the **expulsion stage,** in which the baby's head starts to emerge from the birth canal **(crowning),** the amniotic sac breaks (if it has not broken already), and the baby is born. The final stage, the **placental stage,** consists of several final contractions that expel the placenta.

Of course, childbirth is more than just a series of terms; it is an experience like no other. Labor bears an appropriate name—it is the hardest of all physical work, and the woman cannot rest until it is finished. She feels the wavelike contractions and pain that begin at the top of the uterus and sweep downward, pulling and stretching the opening of the cervix. Full dilation of the cervix may take just a couple of hours or more than a day. When the amniotic sac breaks, the woman feels the warm fluid escaping. During the expulsion, the woman experiences a sensation she has at no other time—the urge to bear down and push the baby out.

What happens right after the baby is born?

The attendant "catches" the baby and uses a gentle suctioning device to remove fluid from the nose to help the baby start breathing. The baby usually signals its first breath by a small cry.

Immediately following the birth, the medical staff may pause to treat the eyes with a drug to prevent infection, and give a dose of vitamin K to promote normal blood clotting.[8] They also may test the baby's responses to stimulation, respiration rate, heart rate, movement, color, and muscle tone. The result of such testing is the **Apgar score,** and it helps predict the baby's future health. Right after the testing, even before leaving the birthing room, the woman may begin to feed the baby at her breast.

Within a few days after birth, all newborns receive a test to screen for specific genetic disorders such as

phenylketonuria (PKU) and sickle-cell anemia. These procedures are required by law in most states. Also, if the baby is a boy, the parents are called upon within the first two weeks of his life to decide whether he should be circumcised. Circumcision is a routine surgical procedure that involves the removal of the foreskin that covers the head of the penis.

What is the best choice—to circumcise or not?

In making their decision, most parents consider aesthetics, religion, cultural attitudes, social pressures, and tradition. In addition, they need to fully consider the possible benefits and potential risks of circumcision.[9] Most male infants in the United States are circumcised as newborns; boys who are circumcised later generally fall into two categories— those who were sick as newborns and those who developed problems.[10] Circumcision after the newborn period presents complications.

Uncircumcised boys must practice thorough genital hygiene to prevent urinary tract and other genital infections, and to reduce the risk of cancer of the penis. Some physicians liken circumcisions to immunizations—their long-term advantages (protection against future disease) outweigh their

short-term disadvantages (possible infections, and temporary pain).[11] Other physicians suggest that circumcision should be performed at the parents' discretion and not as part of routine medical care.[12]

How soon can a woman expect to recover from childbirth?

Recovery begins right away. As the infant nurses, the hormone of labor, oxytocin, stimulates both the flow of milk and the contractions that shrink the uterus from a pregnancy weight of over 2 pounds to the prepregnancy weight of about 3 ounces. Blood and fluid continue flowing for several weeks in what is similar to a long menstrual period. A woman may have sexual intercourse after she has stopped bleeding, the incisions have healed, and her health care provider has said she may safely do so (usually at her six-week checkup).

When can women resume physical activity after childbirth?

A woman can resume her activities as soon as she is comfortable with them, usually within two to three weeks after delivery. Physical activity may actually speed recovery. She can begin exercising at the level maintained during pregnancy for the first four weeks or so, gradually increasing the level, if desired. A few special guidelines are listed in Table S14–1.

I've heard that the weight a woman gains during pregnancy may be hard to lose.

At delivery, the mother loses the weight associated with the fetus and the placenta, but she retains some of the fluid and the fat she necessarily gained during pregnancy. Breast-feeding draws on these fat stores and can help the woman lose weight. Even without breastfeeding, many women lose these pounds within a few months, but it may take some effort to do so.

What about depression? I've heard it is inevitable after childbirth.

Depression is not inevitable, but it is not unusual, either. Women may feel depressed to various extents after giving birth. Some may just feel like crying or may be unable to sleep. Others may become severely

---

TABLE S14–1 ■ **Post-Pregnancy Exercise Guidelines**

1. Exercise regularly, at least 3 times a week.
2. Don't compete in sports.
3. Avoid outdoor activities in hot, humid weather.
4. Use smooth stretches, not jerky motions (joints and ligaments are softened by the hormones of pregnancy).
5. Avoid deep stretches—don't push yourself too far. Warm up well before each session, and cool down afterward with gentle stretches.
6. Avoid jarring motions or fast-reaction activities (again, because joints are vulnerable to injury).

---

depressed, if the transition to parenthood adds a "last straw" to a host of other unresolved problems. The milder forms of **postpartum depression,** or "postpartum blues," which may pass easily, may result from the sharp changes in hormone levels after birth or from simple exhaustion caused by taking care of the baby, who doesn't yet sleep for long stretches. The more severe forms of depression may be a sign that psychological help is needed (see Chapter 3).

New fathers, too, sometimes experience postpartum depression. For both parents, cutting back on all but essential activities and spending time alone or with family sometimes helps to ease the adjustments.

Childbirth is a major transition time. The better you know what to expect, and the more thoughtfully you plan for it, the more smoothly it will go. Best wishes for a highly successful childbirth experience, and—happy parenting!

■≡ Spotlight Notes

1. J. P. Rooks and coauthors, Outcomes of care in birth centers: The national birth center study, *New England Journal of Medicine* 321 (1989): 1804–1811; P. J. Placek, S. M. Taffel, and M. Moien, 1986 C-sections rise; VBACs inch upward, *American Journal of Public Health* 78 (1988): 562–563; S. M. Taffel, P. J. Placek, and M. Moien, 1988 U.S. cesarean-section rate at 24.7 per 100 births—A plateau? *New England Journal of Medicine* 323 (1990): 199–200.

2. Rooks and coauthors, 1989.

3. E. Lieberman and K. J. Ryan, Birth-day choices, *New England Journal of Medicine* 321 (1989): 1824–1825.

4. G. L. Goyert and coauthors, The physician factor in cesarean birth rates, *New England Journal of Medicine* 320 (1989): 706–709.

5. C. M. Peterson, Socioeconomic differences in rates of cesarean section, *New England Journal of Medicine* 322 (1990): 268–269.

6. Placek, Taffel, and Moien, 1988.

7. J. B. Gould, B. Davey, and R. S. Stafford, Socioeconomic differences in rates of cesarean section, *New England Journal of Medicine* 321 (1989): 233–239.

8. American Academy of Pediatrics, Committee on Nutrition, *Pediatric Nutrition Handbook*, 2d ed. (Elk Grove Village, Ill.: American Academy of Pediatrics, 1985), p. 40.

9. American Academy of Pediatrics, Task Force on Circumcision, Report of the Task Force on Circumcision, *Pediatrics* 84 (1989): 388–391.

10. G. L. Larsen and S. D. Williams, Postneonatal circumcision: Population profile, *Pediatrics* 85 (1990): 808–812.

11. E. J. Schoen, The status of circumcision of newborns, *New England Journal of Medicine* 322 (1990): 1308–1312.

12. R. L. Poland, The question of routine neonatal circumcision, *New England Journal of Medicine* 322 (1990): 1312–1315.

CHAPTER 15

Mature Life and Aging

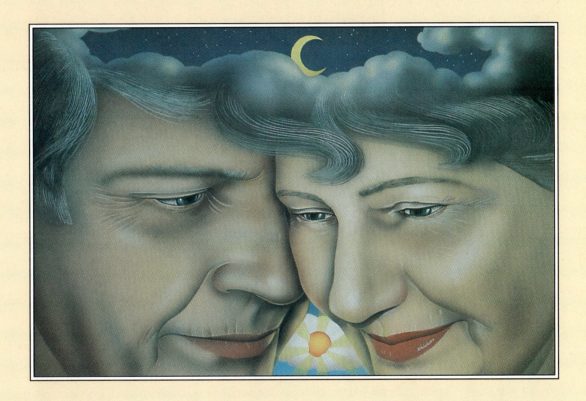

A 90-year-old man visited his physician, seeking relief from the pain in his left knee. Unable to find an obvious cause for the ache, the physician said, "For heaven's sake, at your age, you should expect such aches and pains." The mature man replied, "Look here, Doc, my right knee is also 90, and it doesn't hurt."

The physician's attitude reflects how most people view growing old: they think disability and disease are inevitable consequences of aging. In contrast, the older man's remark suggests that the advanced years can be lively. A mature life doesn't have to be one of illness, impotence, or immobility; it can be healthy, sexy, and active.

■ ≡ Expectations and Misconceptions

The quality of life in the advancing years depends largely on what people expect. Physical health matters; financial success makes a difference; but people's expectations make an equal contribution to their future.

Are you aware of your expectations of later life? Without realizing it, most people are guilty of **ageism:** they carry an internal, unconscious stereotype,

ageism a prejudice against older people; prejudging them as incompetent, infirm, and uninteresting.

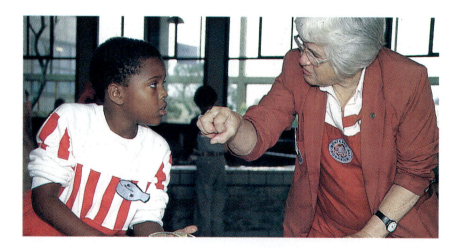

A mature life can be one of continuing productive activity.

LIFE CHOICE INVENTORY

What will aging be like for you? For each of the following questions, choose the answer that most nearly describes your expectations.

1. In what ways do you expect your appearance to change as you grow older?
   a. I expect to grow more and more wrinkled, lame, and unattractive.
   b. I expect to grow more and more radiant, confident, and attractive.

2. How fit do you expect to be at 70?
   a. I expect to be less fit than I am now.
   b. I expect to be very fit for my age.

3. What will be your financial status?
   a. I expect to be financially dependent on my family or the state.
   b. I expect to be financially independent.

4. What will your sex life be like? Will others see you as sexy?
   a. I expect my sex life to decline; other people will not see me as sexy.
   b. I expect to continue to be interested in sex; other people will see me as sexy.

5. Will you have many friends, only a few, or none?
   a. I will have only a few or no friends.
   b. I will have many friends.

6. What sorts of things will you do with your friends?
   a. I won't do much of anything with my friends.
   b. I expect to enjoy many, varied activities with my friends.

7. Will you be happy? Cheerful? Curious? Or will you be set in your ways?
   a. I will be set in my ways.
   b. I will be happy, cheerful, and curious.

Scoring: Your answers reveal not only what will probably become of you, but also what you think of older people. Count only your *b* answers:

7 *b* answers: Your attitudes are consistent with a rewarding and fulfilling later life.

5 or 6 *b* answers: You will be a happy older person, for the most part, but could be preparing better for old age in the areas in which you answered *a*.

4 or fewer *b* answers: Unfortunately, you hold some ageist prejudices, and they may adversely affect the quality of your own later life.

largely negative, of what it is like to be old—and then they become that way. To see what your life might be like as you age, answer the questions in this chapter's Life Choice Inventory.

Most people hope to age successfully. Some say they want to be like those who have made great intellectual and artistic achievements in their 70s and 80s. They claim they want to model themselves after older people they admire—people who are vibrant and happy. Those people, who have experienced more life than anyone else, can offer unique wisdom and perspective.

≡▶ *The ageist stereotype suggests that aging is negative, but it need not be. It is possible to age successfully.*

■≡ People Who Age Successfully

People who are satisfied with their later years are self-sufficient, physically active, socially involved, mentally lucid, fully participating members of society who report themselves to be happy and healthy.[1]* Such people tend to think positively throughout their lives. They do not subscribe to a rigid definition of success. Rather, they define success in light of their values and live accordingly. They work not toward power and wealth but toward meaningful goals; they feel that their lives have purpose.

Those who age successfully display these characteristics:

■ Their lives have meaning and direction.
■ They handle life events in their own, sometimes unusual, ways.
■ They rarely feel cheated by life.
■ They have attained several long-term goals.
■ They are pleased with their own growth and development.
■ They love and are loved by others.
■ They have many friends.
■ They are cheerful.
■ They can take criticism.
■ They have no major fears.

What is more, people who are enjoying life most are likely to be beyond their 20s, and have lived through the fears and anxieties of youth. Being well educated is a factor in their happiness, as is having enough money to cover life's basic needs.[2] They also know how to balance spontaneity with planning, so that their lives are neither rigid nor aimless. They strike a balance between their involvement in helping others and a healthy dedication to meeting their own needs. All of these traits taken together define successful aging.

You may think that these people were born lucky, but most were not; many of the happiest people have lived through at least one major life tragedy. They grew into their happiness, striving for it through their daily thoughts and actions. They faced up to the tasks of adult development as described in Chapter 2.

*Reference notes are at the end of the chapter.

■ *FACT OR FICTION:* People beyond their 20s generally enjoy life more than people in their 20s. *True.*

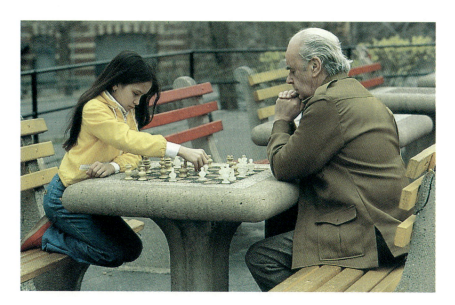

People who stay involved tend to stay happy.

In short, to be happy when you are old, you need to begin cultivating happiness when you are young. A healthy person strives for a long life, and a wise person will preserve health to support it. And it can be done: more people than ever before are living full, healthy lives in their advanced years.[3]* Successful aging is a healthy goal, and is necessary to a full life in the later years.[4] This chapter describes the aging process and offers insight into how to grow old gracefully.

≡▶ *Successful aging involves, not being free of troubles, but rising above them. Successful aging begins in youth.*

■≡ The Aging Process

Although people believe that aging starts around 40 or 45, in reality, aging begins at birth. Until about age 20, aging takes the form of growth and maturing; after growth is completed, aging brings with it the gradual loss of physical function. Everyone ages, and many people are apprehensive about it. What is happening inside your body as you age? Research provides some answers.

Of course, all body organs age at the same rate chronologically. But do they lose function at the same rate physiologically, too? Scientists have determined that the organs grow old together. Barring the onset of a disease in one organ, this means that when your heart has reached a certain physiological age, your other organs will be at the same stage of aging.[5] By implication, if you live so as to slow the aging rate of one organ, such as your heart, lungs, or brain, all other parts of your body will benefit.

Within the different body organs, though, the cells have different aging patterns and life spans. Some blood cells live only three days or so; most nerve cells last for the person's lifetime. In a healthy older person, each cell lives out its life span much as in a younger person. As the person ages, though, the cells do change in other ways: they function less efficiently, they accumulate products not found in younger people's cells, and they lose some of their ability to reproduce.[6]

The human **life span** is the *maximum* possible length of life that a member of the human species can reach, conditions being ideal. A person's **life expectancy** is the *average*, statistically predicted, length of life for that type of person. The human life span is in the neighborhood of 100 years or more. Many people, however, do not live out their full life spans, owing to disease or accidents. Today, the life expectancy for the majority of men in developed countries is about 71 years; for women, about 78 years.

You may have had the impression that people's life spans were increasing, because people are living longer today than in previous generations. The life span has not changed, however: the species' maximum length of life is the same as it has always been. What has changed is the life expectancy (the average number of years people actually live), primarily for two reasons. First, the rate of deaths from disease and accidents among the very young has declined: there are fewer young deaths to bring the average

life span the maximum years of life genetically attainable.

life expectancy the number of years an individual can realistically expect to live based on hereditary life span and environmental factors.

■ *FACT OR FICTION:* The human life span has increased steadily over the past 100 years. *False.* The maximum human life span has not changed, but the life expectancy has increased steadily over the past 100 years.

---

*The elderly are the fastest growing segment of today's society, and if predictions are accurate, their numbers will continue to increase throughout this century and well into the next.

TABLE 15–1 ■   **Examples of Unproved Anti-aging Products and Regimens**

Name of Product or Regimen	Claim Made by Product or Regimen	Comments
Amino acid L-cysteine	Protects against agents that damage the genetic material, DNA	This is an unfounded claim.
Amino acids (arginine and ornithine)	Improve immune function	This is an unfounded claim.
Antiwrinkle cream	Removes wrinkles	This is a transient effect at best, and can injure and disfigure people.
Barley juice	Retards or reverses aging	This is an unfounded claim.
Coenzyme Q	Stimulates the immune system	This is an unfounded claim.
Dimethylaminoethanol (DMAE) with para-aminobenzoic acid (PABA)	Stimulate the brain	This is an unfounded claim.
Drugs (names are Centrophenoxine, meclofenoxate, Clofenoxine, Lucidril, Helfergin, ANP 235)	Arrest deposition of aging pigment (brown spots)	This is an unfounded claim.
Gerovital H-3 (GH-3)	Stimulates vitality and youthfulness	This contains the anesthetic procaine hydrochloride (Novocaine) and various pseudonutrients.
Levodopa	Alters neurotransmitter levels and relieves senility	This is an unfounded claim. (Levodopa is, however, used legitimately in therapy for a brain disease known as Parkinson's disease.)
Live Cell Therapy	Retards or reverses aging	Cell suspensions from fetal animals are injected into clients, an extremely expensive procedure. No research supports its efficacy.
Maxilife supplements	Halt or reverses aging by destroying free radicals that attack body tissues	This product contains vitamins E and B_6, the amino acid methionine, and the trace mineral selenium. These have no anti-aging effect and vitamin B_6 is toxic in large doses.
Megadophilus	Retards or reverses aging	This is a culture of the bacterium *Lactobacillus acidophilus*, a normal inhabitant of the human digestive tract. It's not harmful, but it has no anti-aging effect.
Superoxide dismutase	Halts or reverses aging by destroying free radicals that attack body tissues	This is a totally useless product. SOD supplements are digested by the body and never reach body cells.
Youth steroid (DHEA, or dehydroepiandrosterone)	Restores lost youthfulness	This is an unfounded claim.

SOURCE: Adapted in part from J. A. Lowell, *Quackery and the Elderly* (a booklet available from The American Council on Science and Health, 1995 Broadway, 16th Floor, New York, NY 10023-5860). Reprinted with permission.

longevity   an individual's length of life.

down. Second, medical advances are prolonging adults' lives so that they more nearly reach their maximum.

Another term referring to length of life is **longevity**—the actual length of life observed in a person. Some people are blessed with extraordinary longevity, perhaps for a combination of hereditary and environmental reasons.

Many strategies have been proposed to extend human longevity—popularly known as life extension strategies. They do not work. A scientific review of some 200 research studies concluded that none of them had any

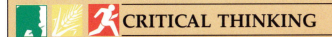

CRITICAL THINKING

Longevity Frauds

In the quest for the legendary "Fountain of Youth," people have tried everything imaginable to delay or reverse aging. Years ago, the Spaniards sailed to the New World in search of the Fountain of Youth; today, people rush to buy products, based on "new scientific breakthroughs," that promise to restore youth. Their motivation is the same: they want a miracle. Whenever many people desire something that is unobtainable, someone steps in with empty promises and useless products and wins a growing bank account for the effort.

Frauds that plague the elderly are not limited to the longevity hypes; old people are targets of many other schemes. Why are the elderly the targets for such deception? First, many of them have ready access to money—retirement funds, pensions, insurance policies, paid-up mortgages. Second, as people age, they experience more symptoms and may be frustrated by the medical profession's inability to help or unwillingness to take them seriously. They seek help where it is offered, proved or not. And as people get older, they may develop a "what have I got to lose" attitude about trying products that claim to prolong life or improve health. Money seems less important than even the slightest chance of such rewards, and even educated people let themselves be taken advantage of.

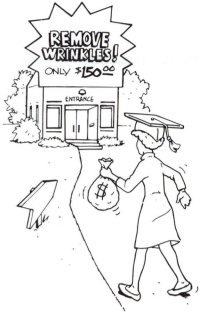

The combination of ready money and the chance for a miracle empties many people's pockets—even if the cost is high, the chance small, and the people smart.

life-extending effect.[7] Some *strategies* help retard aging, but they have to do with lifestyle, not with pills and shots. Table 15–1 exposes more antiaging myths, and the accompanying Critical Thinking helps identify them.

≡▶ *Aging alters body organs, but not all changes attributed to aging are inevitable. The human life span has not changed, but life expectancy has increased, thanks to reduced mortality among the young and to medical advances. Longevity frauds abound.*

■≡ How to Age Gracefully

No magic can keep a person young forever. No matter what you do to prevent it, your body will age. You can, however, do quite a bit to slow the process of aging and maximize your wellness and enjoyment of life. The next two sections review, first, ways to deal with physical aspects of aging; and second, ways to prepare socially and emotionally for later life. The Strategies, later, sum up these pointers.

Dealing with Physical Changes

One of the most important things to do, according to research, is to maintain appropriate body weight: obesity shortens life.[8] Aside from that, maintaining wellness in the later years is best achieved through the principles emphasized in this book—sound nutrition, including an ample water intake;

adequate sleep; regular physical activity, and managing stress; consuming alcohol in moderation (if at all); and abstaining from tobacco use.[9]

Much of the quality of the later years depends on the daily choices a person makes in youth and on the habits that become fixed as a result of those choices. People have some control over the fate of their later years; studies show that people who understand this care for themselves in later life and are more active and energetic than others of their age.[10] Table 15–2 shows a sampling of the age-related changes that are inevitable, and those that can be prevented by continued exercise and other health-supporting habits.

Some negative changes of aging are often accompanied by positive ones that seem to help compensate. For example, although older people are less able to recover physically from stress,[11] they seem to be more resilient psychologically—perhaps because they have seen more of life and have learned to adjust to unexpected turns of events.[12] Another example: the immune system becomes less efficient at fighting off disease once it takes hold, but older people get infections less often than younger people do. Perhaps this is because they have developed immunity against many diseases.

People's skin changes with age. As people grow older, the skin becomes thinner, looser, dryer, less elastic, and more wrinkled.[13] To a certain degree, this is inevitable, but much premature skin aging can be prevented. Those who spend time outdoors without sunscreen lose their skin's beauty and health at much younger ages than those who avoid the sun or screen their skin from its rays. Also, smoking, excessive alcohol consumption, and other drug abuse age the skin. Cosmetic skin preparations are limited in their usefulness, but people can adopt the opposites of the habits just mentioned to prolong their skin's youth and health.[14] According to the FDA, silicone; collagen; and the drug Retin-A, which is used in acne treatment are ineffective and dangerous as wrinkle removers. The result of their improper use is often illness and disfigurement.

In women, the later years bring **menopause,** in which monthly ovulation becomes irregular and finally ceases, as does menstruation, owing largely to diminished secretion of the hormone estrogen. Reduced estrogen secretion also causes the periodic perception of warmth some women call hot flashes. A major surge of bone loss takes place at the onset of menopause. Women whose calcium intakes and physical activity have been inadequate to build sufficient skeletal reserves before menopause may lose so much bone material as to become crippled with **osteoporosis** within a few years after menopause. Figure 15–1 shows the effect of the loss of spinal bone on a woman's height and posture. It is not inevitable that people "grow shorter" as they age, but it does happen if they experience bone loss.

In the younger years, the best strategies for osteoporosis prevention are regular physical activity; adequate calcium intakes, particularly in the late teens; adequate fluoride and vitamin D intakes; abstinence from alcohol and other drugs; moderation in caffeine use; minimal prescription drug use; control of stress; and abstinence from tobacco use. Chapter 11 gave abundant reasons for abstaining from smoking; add this one to them.

Later in life, to prevent the depletion of bone material, as well as to counter some of the other effects of menopause, physicians often prescribe estrogen replacement therapy. This therapy has been associated with possible cancer risks, but many researchers agree that the benefits far outweigh the risks.[15]

Take kindly the counsel of the years, gracefully surrendering the things of youth. . . . Beyond a wholesome discipline, be gentle with yourself. . . . Be careful, strive to be happy.

Desiderata, found in Old St. Paul's Church, Baltimore, dated 1692, author unknown.

Sun exposure can cause skin cancer. See Chapter 19 for information about skin cancer.

menopause cessation of ovulation and menstruation in a woman, due to advancing age.

osteoporosis a disease characterized by excessive adult bone loss.

TABLE 15–2 ■ **Changes with Age: Preventable versus Unavoidable**

	You probably cannot change these:	You probably can slow or prevent these changes by exercising, maintaining other good health habits, and planning ahead.
Appearance		
Greying of hair	√	
Balding	√	
Drying and wrinkling of skin		√
Nervous System		
Impairment of near vision	√	
Some loss of hearing	√	
Reduced taste and smell	√	
Reduced touch sensitivity	√	
Slowed reactions (reflexes)	√	
Slowed mental function	√	
Mental confusion		√
Cardiovascular System		
Increased blood pressure		√
Increased resting heart rate		√
Decreased oxygen consumption		√
Body Composition/Metabolism		
Increased body fatness		√
Raised blood cholesterol		√
Slowed energy metabolism		√
Other Physical Characteristics		
Menopause (women)	√	
Loss of fertility (men)	√	
Joints: loss of flexibility		√
Loss of teeth; gum disease		√
Bone loss		√
Accident/Disease Proneness		
Accidents		√
Inherited diseases	√	
Lifestyle diseases		√
Psychological/Other		
Reduced self-esteem		√
Loss of sex drive		√
Loss of interest in work		√
Depression, loneliness		√
Reduced financial status		√

Estrogen not only retards bone loss but improves the serum lipid profile and reduces cardiovascular disease risk.[16] It also helps control symptoms of menopause: hot flashes, insomnia, mood swings, and vaginal dryness.[17]

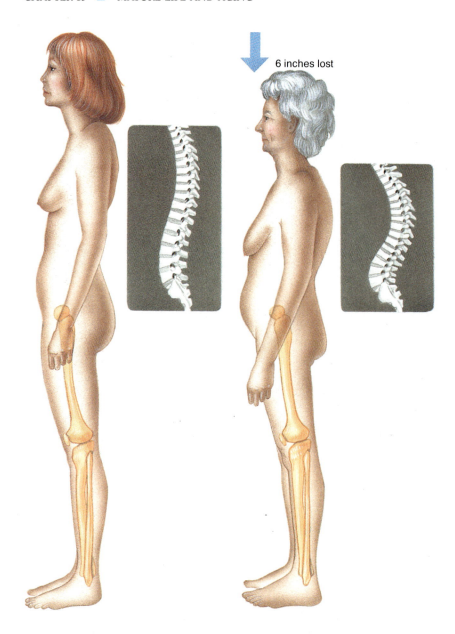

6 inches lost

Effects of osteoporosis on a woman's height. On the left is a woman at menopause and on the right, the same woman 30 years later. Notice that collapse of her vertebrae has shortened her back; the length of her legs has not changed.

FIGURE 15–1 ■ **The effect of adult bone loss on the height of an older woman.**

male menopause   the gradual decline in fertility and sexual desire due to advancing age.

■ *FACT OR FICTION:* People should expect to lose their sex drives at around 50 years of age. *False.* People can expect to remain sexual beings until they die.

Men experience a **male menopause,** but it is characterized by a gradual decline of fertility rather than the abrupt cessation experienced by women. Testosterone production gradually decreases, as does sperm production. The desire for sexual activity may decline, but complete loss of fertility is unlikely. Some men retain fertility into their 80s.

Although people fear their sex lives will wane, most remain sexual beings until they die. The sex life changes, but it need not become less satisfying. Physically, the reproductive organs diminish in size and function, but sexual activity itself helps to maintain a normal sexual response. For some, sexual desire remains unchanged. "The only thing age has to do with sex performance is that the longer you live, the more you learn," says one happy older person. An older couple may actually enjoy sex more, because the later years bring more time to relax, without worries of pregnancy.[18] Less responsibility in the later years lends itself to more time for play and affection.

Muscles also age, and as they do, they need exercise more than when they were young. Older muscles build up less quickly in response to exercise than younger ones do, so it takes longer and harder work to gain condition. Balanced against that, older muscles lose condition at a slower rate than young muscles do. Once fit, an older person who takes a break from exercise will maintain condition longer, although he or she still should resume exercising as soon as possible. The more activity people engage in, the less likely they are to die of heart and lung diseases. Physical activity may prolong life, as well as enhance the quality of life, so older people are wise to maintain physical activity throughout their lives.

To maintain muscle strength and fitness, as well as high energy and general good health, older people should be especially sure to meet the exercise recommendations of Chapter 7: 20 minutes of aerobic exercise three or four days a week—at their own target heart rates, adjusted for age as described there. Many older people believe that strenuous exercise is out of reach for them, but studies have shown that they can do more than they think they can. Even frail, institutionalized people in their 90s have been able to gain muscle bulk and strength and to put some pep in their walking steps after just eight weeks of weight training.[19] Any activity—even a ten-minute walk a day—is better than none. Training not only improves muscles but also increases the blood flow to the brain. Additionally, a person spending energy in physical activity can afford to eat more food, and with it comes more nutrients.

A common complaint in the mature population is joint pain, often due to **arthritis.** During movement, the ends of bones are normally protected from wear by cartilage and by small sacs of fluid that act as a lubricant; with age, however, the protective padding materials disintegrate. Then the joints wear and become malformed, and movement may be painful. Arthritis can arise from many causes, some of which are unknown. It afflicts millions around the world and is a major problem of the elderly.

Arthritis has for centuries been ascribed to poor diet, oftentimes by the promoters of quack remedies, including many bizarre diets advertised as arthritis cures. Two or three popular new books on diet for arthritis come out every year, urging people to eat no meat, or to drink no milk, or to eat all their food raw, or to eat only "natural" food, or to avoid all additives, or—who knows what will be next? Actually, no known diet prevents, relieves, or cures arthritis.[20] As long as people keep buying the books that make these claims, however, the law of supply and demand dictates that they will keep coming out.

Weight control is important for overweight people with arthritis, because weight-bearing joints are stressed by having to carry excess poundage. Weight-loss diets alone often relieve the worst of the pain in overweight people with arthritis.

Some people falsely attribute joint pain to arthritis. People with genuine cases of arthritis experience pain from degenerative wearing down of joints. Out-of-condition older people, however, experience discomfort from years

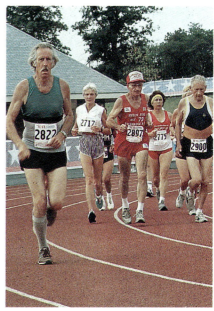

Physical activity benefits older people, and many find they can do more than they think they can.

arthritis   inflammation of a joint caused by many conditions, including infections or injuries; joint structure is usually altered, with loss of function; usually painful.

Not effective against arthritis:

Alfalfa tea.
Aloe vera liquid.
Any of the amino acids.
Burdock root.
Calcium.
Celery juice.
Copper or copper complexes.
Dimethyl sulfoxide (DMSO).
Fasting.
Fresh fruit.
Honey.
Inositol.
Kelp.
Lecithin.
Para-aminobenzoic acid (PABA).
Raw liver.
Selenium.
Superoxide dismutase (SOD).
Vitamin D, E, or C, or any B vitamin
  supplements.
Watercress.
Yeast.
Zinc.
100 other substances.

cataracts (CAT-uh-racts) thickening of the lenses of the eyes that can lead to blindness. Cataracts can be caused by injury, viral infection, toxic substances, radiation, genetic disorders—and possibly by some nutrient deficiencies or imbalances.

of inactivity. This is another reason why physical activity is especially important for people in their advanced years; it strengthens muscles and minimizes joint pain.

An age-related change in the lenses of the eyes, **cataracts,** is a thickening of the lenses that impairs vision and ultimately leads to blindness. Cataracts are brought on by injury; viral infections; toxic substances; radiation, such as that from sunlight; and genetic disorders. Most cataracts, however, are vaguely called senile cataracts, meaning ''caused by aging.''

Radiation from sunlight and tanning booths is a preventable cause of cataracts. To avoid this source of damage, wear sunglasses that filter out the sun's ultraviolet radiation and avoid tanning parlors, or at least protect your eyes if you do use them. Aside from these, no measures to avoid cataracts have proved effective. Cataracts are treatable by surgery.

The brain and nervous system also age, but the decline in mental function in older age need not be severe. Research has documented declines in five areas: reasoning skill, recall (memory), spatial sense, speed of reactions, and senses, but as these declines take place, compensatory gains are also occurring, such as improvements in wisdom and judgment.[21] People can adopt strategies to deal with these declines, too, such as learning to write things down so that they will not forget, or allowing extra time for certain tasks. One strategy is particularly important in this connection: to adjust driving habits so as to compensate for slowed reaction time. The accompanying box, Safety Tips for Older Drivers, offers suggestions.

Although people's mental function can remain sharp into old age, the ageist prejudice tends to brand many older people as ''senile,'' just because they have white hair. True **senility** is rare, however. Causes of apparent senility in older people are diverse—and most are preventable; only one (brain disease) is not. The preventable causes of senility are:

senility mental confusion that occurs as the result of deterioration of the brain, a term unjustly applied to many older people who may suffer from other, reversible causes of confusion.

■ *Abuse of drugs.* The abuse includes both alcohol abuse and misuse or incompatibility of prescription drugs. The effects of these drugs can sometimes resemble those of strokes and seizures.

■ *Accidents.* Falls can cause concussions or bleeding that put pressure on the brain, which surgery can relieve.

■ *Poor vision and hearing.* Both can cause confusion; both can be corrected or compensated for.

■ *Malnutrition.* Taste acuity, digestive secretions, and appetite diminish, causing people to eat less, yet their nutrient needs remain the same. Low blood glucose can cause light-headedness and confusion. (More about nutrition and aging in the Spotlight following this chapter.)

■ *Disease states.* Diseases present different symptoms in older people than in younger ones. Tuberculosis, diabetes, meningitis, encephalitis, and even heart attacks can all begin with confusion, rather than with obvious fever or pain. Many remediable brain problems—including nonmalignant tumors, small strokes, and seizures from epilepsy—can cause confusion.

■ *Depression.* Depression can slow down the mind in old people, as in young people. The distractedness that results may appear similar to senility, but the cause may be external—loss of family, friends, status, or income; or anxiety about anything.

■ *Dehydration.* The thirst signal may become faint, so an older person may not drink enough to meet physical needs for fluids. Drugs for high blood pressure can also cause dehydration. One of its major symptoms is confusion.

Safety Tips for Drivers Over 55

Fine wine and cheeses may improve with age, but drivers don't. Older drivers do have fewer accidents and fatalities per capita than younger drivers, often because they opt not to drive during rush hour, at night, or in bad weather. But in terms of accidents and deaths per mile driven, people over age 65 rank second only to high-risk 16- to 24-year-olds.

Driving skills and dexterity often begin to decline after age 55, partly because of hearing and vision deficits, stiffening joints and slowed reaction times. Fortunately, safety experts have come up with numerous tips to help older drivers stay in the driver's seat. Here are some pointers that can help keep older drivers safe:

■ Have regular eye exams. Aging-related declines in visual acuity, depth perception, peripheral vision and focussing ability make driving hazardous.
■ Avoid twilight and night driving whenever possible and remove sunglasses as the sun begins to set.
■ Don't drink and drive—no matter what your age. Alcohol tolerance changes with age, and even one drink can alter the older driver's already-compromised reaction time.

■ Know the side effects of medications. Pain relievers, antihistamines, blood pressure medications, and a host of other drugs can cause drowsiness, delayed reaction times, or blurred vision.
■ Compensate for slower reaction time. Allow more distance between cars, avoid rush-hour traffic, and whenever possible, take someone along to help navigate.
■ Pay attention to the task at hand. Focus on the road and on the "big picture," rather than on individual cars, billboards or other distractions.
■ Be extra vigilant in hazardous situations, such as approaching a busy intersection, making a left-hand turn, merging onto a highway, or changing lanes.

The nonprofit AAA Foundation for Traffic Safety offers several excellent brochures on keeping older drivers safe, including: *The Older Person's Guide to Safe Driving; Concerned About an Older Driver?: A Guide for Families and Friends*; and *Drivers 55 Plus: Test Your Own Performance*. Write to the foundation at 1730 M Street NW, Suite 401, Washington, DC 20036.

SOURCE: AAA Foundation, as cited in Health notes, *University of Texas Lifetime Health Letter*, May 1991, p. 2.

■ *Disuse of mental abilities.* People do lose what they don't use. Practicing reinstates mental skills.[22]

If an older person becomes confused, it is imperative to see that these possible causes are corrected before jumping to the conclusion that senility has set in.

Mental confusion, among other problems, is often caused by overmedication. Many older people take several types of long-term medications, and some use even more than 12 different drugs.[23] Interactions among drugs, as

■ *FACT OR FICTION:* Mental confusion in older people is more often preventable than not. *True.*

well as overdoses of some drugs, can cause a host of complications, including mental confusion, often mistaken for senility. People in their advanced years should request that their health care providers monitor their use of mixtures of prescription drugs.

Depression causes the symptoms of senility so commonly that an example is worth noting. A woman invited her mother-in-law to live with her while the older woman waited for a place in a nursing home. The mother-in-law had exhibited the classic signs of senility—mental confusion, inability to make decisions, forgetting to perform important tasks such as turning off a stove burner—so the family had decided she needed institutional care. After several weeks in the daughter-in-law's home—eating meals with the family and enjoying social stimulation—she became her old self again and returned to her home. This story has been repeated with many variations and serves to remind us to seek an accurate medical diagnosis from a professional who respects older people before concluding that a person needs institutional care. What harm could there be in first trying home life, regular meals, and plenty of tender, loving care?

One presently incurable cause of confusion is **Alzheimer's disease.** The condition appears most often in people over 65 and is a major cause of death in that age group. It is a progressive brain syndrome that afflicts 5 percent of the population by the age of 65 years and 20 percent of those over 80 years.[24] The symptoms of Alzheimer's disease are gradual losses of memory and reasoning, of ability to communicate, of physical capabilities, and eventually, loss of life. To date, causes are still elusive, and no cure is known. Treatment involves providing relief and support to both the clients and their families. The person with Alzheimer's disease usually requires a level of care beyond that which can be provided by family members, and obtaining quality care is often difficult.[25]

Most have heard that aluminum may have something to do with Alzheimer's disease. Brain concentrations of aluminum in people with Alzheimer's

Alzheimer's disease   a relentless, irreversible brain disease that occurs in some people with increasing age; the final stage is complete helplessness and death.

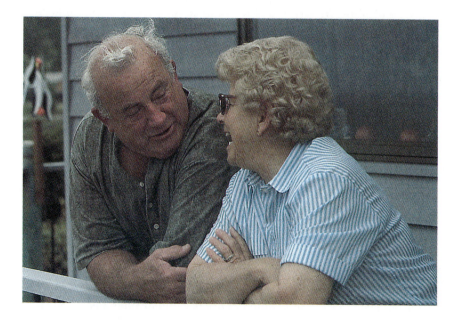

Mature life can bring enhanced intimacy and sexuality.

disease exceed normal brain concentrations by some 10 to 30 times. But blood and hair concentrations remain normal, indicating that the body has not been exposed to excess aluminum. The brain itself must be abnormal in accumulating the metal as it does. Still, environmental aluminum may play some role as yet unknown.[26]

≡▶ *Successful aging involves distinguishing between changes that can and cannot be prevented, then adopting strategies to deal with each. Lifestyle choices have increasing impact over years; nutrition, exercise, and abstinence from drug abuse help keep people physiologically young. People can learn to compensate for nervous system changes; a good mental attitude helps.*

Preparation for Later Life

Aging often brings financial and social losses with it. Being aware of this and preparing for it can help enable you to weather losses successfully. Financial planning is essential. Nearly everyone suffers a considerable loss of income in the retirement years, aggravated by inflation. It is important to have set aside enough money for retirement—to have the home paid for or adequate income to pay the rent—and to have insurance to cover unexpected medical and other expenses.

Another way to prepare is to plan an alternative living arrangement, should the responsibility for the present home become burdensome. A nursing home is not the only choice, and usually not the best one. Fewer than a third of older adults spend time in nursing homes, and those who do spend only a year there, on the average.[27] There are many alternatives. Rather than leave it to their children to decide for them where they will live, older adults can decide for themselves.

Financial preparation will not ward off the losses that take place in the emotional and social realms. These may be multiple. Old friends are lost because they die or move away; offspring move away also and may be too busy to write; income is lost upon retiring, as is status in the community. Loss of control of the environment also occurs, such as finding that the home that was to be a haven in retirement now sits in the middle of a high-crime area, or that the familiar shops and fruit stands have closed. A person can develop a feeling of deep loneliness as the familiar environment shifts. A loss of identity may accompany retirement or the death of a spouse. A working person can say, "I'm a farmer, a nurse, a manager," but after retirement, that part of the self is gone. A married person might say, "My spouse is a golfer, an artist, a bird-watcher," but when the spouse dies, that part of the self is gone. How can an older person meet new friends or find a new spouse?

The person who does not take positive steps to replace each loss can gradually become overwhelmed with loneliness. Depression is common in the elderly and can be severe.[28] Try to imagine how it would be to wake up tomorrow with all these changes having taken place at once. You have no one to report to, no deadlines, no place in particular to go. It might be wonderful to lie in bed for a day, or two, or three. But imagine that the days stretch into weeks or months, and still, nothing pushes you to do your best, expand your mind, or accomplish things. Add to this your lack of friends, your physical inability to pursue your favorite activities, and the strangeness

■ *FACT OR FICTION:* Most people's incomes are considerably reduced at retirement. *True.*

■ *FACT OR FICTION:* Most people can expect to spend their later years in nursing homes. *False.* Fewer than 1 out of 3 old people end up in nursing homes.

■■■■■ *STRATEGIES:* GROWING OLD GRACEFULLY

To maximize the quality of your later years:

1. Eat nutritious meals regularly; maintain appropriate body weight.
2. Drink eight glasses a day of water or other liquids, even if you aren't thirsty.
3. Maintain physical fitness, and change activities to suit changing abilities and tastes.
4. Obtain regular and adequate sleep throughout life.
5. Consciously practice your stress-management skills.
6. Limit your time in the sun, or use sunscreen protection.
7. For women, see your physician about estrogen replacement therapy for osteoporosis prevention.
8. Use medicines only as prescribed. Ask your physician about potential drug interactions.
9. Use alcohol only moderately, if at all.
10. Do not smoke or otherwise use tobacco; if you do, quit.
11. Expect to enjoy sex, and learn new ways of enhancing it.
12. Protect your eyes against excessive sunlight.
13. Be aware of changing nervous system function; plan to compensate.
14. Take care to prevent accidents; seek medical attention if recovery seems slow.
15. Expect good vision and hearing throughout life; obtain glasses and hearing aids if necessary.
16. Be alert to confusion as a disease symptom, and seek diagnosis. Do not live with an unidentified disease.
17. Stay interested in life, make new friends, adopt new activities—control depression.
18. Practice your mental skills. Keep on solving math problems, reading, following directions, writing, imagining, and creating.
19. For adult children of aging parents: provide or obtain the needed care and stimulation.
20. Make financial plans early to ensure your security.
21. Accept change. Work at recovering from losses; make new friends.
22. Pursue your education forever. Take classes to learn new skills and study new subject areas.
23. Cultivate spiritual wellness. Consult your values, and make your life meaningful.

of your environment. Changes creep up gradually on people as they age; it takes effort to remain aware of them and take measures to counter them.

You may think it unnecessary for a person of 18 or 28 to confront problems of loneliness and loss that will come so much later, but such is not the case. Emotional and social health in the later years is built upon a foundation established in youth. To be happy when you are old, you need to practice happiness when you are young. Losses occur then, too. Learn to grieve over them and move on. Refill your life with new loves, new activities, new enthusiasms. Keep reaching out; create a web of support so that as relationships are lost, others are gained.

Pursue your education forever.[29] Lifelong learning institutions are available in many locales. There are colleges for seniors, leadership programs,

programs that involve seniors in the school system, art and writing classes, and many more. Find one you like and join up.

Cultivate spiritual wellness, too. Delve into the meaning of life and how you can make it meaningful for others. Instead of looking back longingly to former years, joyfully take each season of life as it comes. Find ways to contribute your gifts, to leave something of value to those you care for. Keep working at projects that are meaningful to you. Growing is not for children only; it is a lifelong enterprise.

≡▶ *Wise adults will start planning early for their later years. Financial planning is important, and continued growth emotionally, socially, intellectually, and spiritually is vital to well-being in later life.*

"I've spent my whole life becoming who I am. Was it worth it?" A major message of this chapter has been that what a person becomes in later life is, to a large extent, whatever that person chooses to become. In the same way, the way a person encounters life's final challenge, death, is often also a matter of choice, as the next chapter shows.

■≡ For Review

1. Describe how people's expectations of the aging process can influence the way they will age.
2. Identify the characteristics of people who are happy in later life.

3. Distinguish what is inevitable about the aging process from what is not.
4. List some preventable, reversible, and controllable causes of mental confusion in older people.

5. Describe strategies to maintain a high quality of life into the later years.

■≡ Notes

1. S. M. Golant, *A Place to Grow Old: The Meaning of Environment in Old Age* (New York: Columbia University Press, 1984), pp. 137, 316.
2. G. Sheehy, *Pathfinders* (New York: Bantam, 1982), as summarized in J. M. Elston, G. G. Koch, and W. G. Weissert, Regression-adjusted small area estimates of functional dependency in the noninstitutionalized American population age 65 and over, *American Journal of Public Health* 81 (1991): 335–343.
3. J. A. Brody, D. B. Brock, and T. F. Williams, Trends in the health of the elderly population, *Annual Review of Public Health* 8 (1987): 211–234, as

cited in J. A. Brody, Toward quantifying the health of the elderly, *American Journal of Public Health* 79 (1989): 685–686; U.S Bureau of the Census, Projections of the population of the United States, by age, sex, and race: 1989–2010, *Current Population Reports,* series P25, no. 1053 (Washington, D.C.: Government Printing Office, 1990), as cited in M. G. Kovar and M. Feinleib, Older Americans present a double challenge: Preventing disability and providing care, *American Journal of Public Health* 81 (1991): 287–288.
4. N. P. Roos and B. Havens, Predictors of successful aging: A

twelve year study of Manitoba elderly, *American Journal of Public Health* 81 (1991): 63–68.
5. J. R. Bianchine, N. Gerber, and B. D. Andersen, Geriatric medicine, in *Current Concepts* (Kalamazoo, Mich.: Upjohn, 1981), pp. 6–8.
6. E. L. Schneider, *Cells and Aging,* NIH publication no. 74-1860 (Washington, D.C.: Government Printing Office, 1979).
7. E. L. Schneider and J. D. Reid, Jr., Life extension, *New England Journal of Medicine* 312 (1985): 1159–1168.
8. T. Harris, M. G. Kovar, R. Suzman, and coauthors, Longitudinal

study of physical ability in the oldest-old, *American Journal of Public Health* 79 (1989): 698–702.

9. J. M. Guralnik and G. A. Kaplan, Predictors of healthy aging: Prospective evidence from the Alameda County study, *American Journal of Public Health* 79 (1989): 703–708.

10. M. E. Taylor-Nicholson, D. Brannon, B. Mahoney, and coauthor, Assessing the need for health promotion programs in nursing homes, *Health Education* 21 (1990): 23–28.

11. R. M. Sapolsky, L. C. Krey, and B. S. McEwen, The adrenocortical stress-response in the aged male rat: Impairment of recovery from stress, *Experimental Gerontology* 18 (1983): 55–64; R. M. Sapolsky, L. C. Krey, and B. S. McEwen, Corticosterone receptors decline in a site-specific manner in the aged rat brain, *Brain Research* 289 (1983): 235–240.

12. D. Blazer, Life events, mental health functioning and the use of health care services by the elderly, *American Journal of Public Health* 70 (1980): 1174–1179.

13. A. K. Balin and L. A. Pratt, Physiological consequences of human skin aging, *Cutis* 43 (1989): 431–436.

14. Wrinkles, *Health Gazette*, October 1990, p. 3.

15. *Lancet* 336 (1990): 1121, as cited in Safety of estrogen after the menopause, *Health Gazette*, January 1991, p. 4.

16. P. C. MacDonald, Estrogen plus progestin in postmenopausal women—Act II, *New England Journal of Medicine* 315 (1986): 959–961; R. B. Harris, A. Laws, V. M. Reddy, and coauthors, Are women using postmenopausal estrogens? A community survey, *American Journal of Public Health* 80 (1990): 1266–1268.

17. Hormone-replacement therapy: Should every older woman have it? *University of Texas Lifetime Health Letter,* September 1989, pp. 7–8.

18. Sex and aging: Relationships change, but often for the better, *The University of Texas Lifetime Health Letter* 2 (1990): 1, 6.

19. M. A. Fiatrone and coauthors, High-intensity strength training in nonagenarians, *Journal of the American Medical Association* 263 (1990): 3029–3034.

20. K. A. Meister, Can diet cure arthritis? *ACSH News and Views,* September/October 1980, p. 10; and Morsels and tidbits, *Nutrition and the MD,* January 1982.

21. T. A. Salthours, *Adult Cognition: An Experimental Psychology of Human Aging* (New York: Springer-Verlag, 1982), pp. 199–202.

22. Mental skills of the elderly: Lost and found, *Science News* 129 (1986): 244.

23. L. D. Reid, D. B. Christensen, and A. Stergachis, Medical and psychosocial factors predictive of psychotropic drug use in elderly patients, *American Journal of Public Health* 80 (1990): 1349–1353.

24. Much of the discussion of Alzheimer's disease is based on M. S. Claggett, Nutritional factors relevant to Alzheimer's disease, *Journal of the American Dietetic Association* 89 (1989): 392–396.

25. P. G. Weiler, The public health impact of Alzheimer's disease, *American Journal of Public Health* 77 (1987): 1157–1158.

26. C. N. Martyn and coauthors, Geographical relation between Alzheimer's disease and aluminum in drinking water, *Lancet* 1 (1989): 59–62.

27. P. Kemper and C. M. Murtaugh, Lifetime use of nursing home care, *New England Journal of Medicine* 324 (1991): 595–600.

28. D. Blazer, Depression in the elderly, *New England Journal of Medicine* 320 (1989): 164–166.

29. Learning opportunities are documented in S. B. Merriam and R. S. Cafforella, *Learning in Adulthood* (San Francisco, Calif.: Jossey-Bass, 1991), pp. 140–159.

SPOTLIGHT

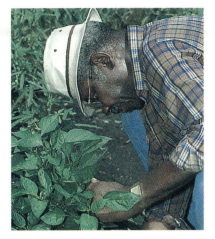

Can Nutrition Influence Aging?

People have tried everything to delay or reverse aging. Charlatans who sell to the elderly nibble away retirement funds in exchange for vitamins, "nutrients," or "essences" falsely promoted as aging remedies. With advancing age, people experience more aches and pains, and if health care providers cannot provide cures, older people tend to fall victim to quacks who promise unlimited help. To a person who experiences painful symptoms, saving money may seem less important than even the slightest chance of a miracle; and even brilliant, sophisticated people let themselves be bamboozled.

In contrast to the claims of quacks, the legitimate study of aging is a young science, not nearly ready to offer potions, regimens, or gadgets to bestow longevity or restored health

on anyone.[1*] Instead, researchers are asking how and why human beings age, including what roles nutrition plays in longevity and in aging of the mind, and what roles it can play in retarding such aging. This Spotlight takes up these questions and presents research results.

What do studies show about nutrition and longevity?

Remember the study of nearly 7,000 adults in California, mentioned in Chapter 1? Some were young for their ages, others old for their ages.[2] The researchers found that among the factors affecting physiological age, several were related to nutrition: abstinence from, or moderation in, alcohol consumption; eating regular meals, including breakfast, rather than snacking; and weight control. (The others were related to sleep, smoking, and exercise habits.) In this study, overweight, especially high degrees of overweight, correlated with poor health. Irregular eating habits also seemed detrimental to health. The effects of all these factors were cumulative; that is, those who followed all of the recommended health practices remained in better health, even if older in calendar years, than people who failed to do so. In fact, the physical health of those who reported all positive health practices was comparable to that of people *30 years younger* who followed few of them. These findings demonstrate that although you cannot alter the year of your birth, you can, by making appropriate lifestyle choices, alter the probable length of your life.

*Reference notes are at the end of the Spotlight.

Insurance companies have compiled many years of data on mortality in relation to people's weights and heights. Generally their findings indicate that the more overweight an individual is, the greater the risk of mortality.[3] The same is true for severely underweight individuals.

If overweight individuals have an increased mortality risk, why, then, do many live long, healthy lives?

No one knows, but the question shows that body weight alone is not responsible for the increased mortality of obese people. Many other factors enter in—genetics, disease state, and medical care, just to name a few. Nevertheless, data confirm that most people who live to advanced ages are leaner than most people who die younger.[4]

Do any individual nutrients affect longevity?

In none of the studies do individual nutrients affect longevity. No supplement, nutrient, food, or any other product has been shown to extend life or to have antiaging effects, regardless of the many claims by quacks that they do. Furthermore, many "life-extending" regimens can be dangerous. Many popular books on the topic cite scientific references but misinterpret them and twist the facts to support their claims. Nutrient supplements do not improve mental functioning or cure mental illnesses of old age, as many quacks claim.

What about mental acuity? Can aging of the brain be controlled?

The brain ages in some characteristic ways, some due to disease and some the result of cumulative, extrinsic factors such as diet. The number of neurons decreases as people age, and so does blood flow to the brain. When the number of nerve cells in one part of the cerebral cortex diminishes, hearing and speech are affected. Losses of neurons in other parts of the cortex can impair memory and cognitive function. When the numbers of neurons in lower brain centers diminish, balance and posture are affected. Losses of neurons in other parts of the brain affect still other functions.

Clinicians now recognize that much of the cognitive loss and forgetfulness generally attributed to aging is due in part to extrinsic, and therefore controllable, factors. In some instances, cognitive loss is attributable to a specific disorder. In other instances, the loss of memory and cognition is attributable to moderate, long-term nutrient deficiencies. And in some cases, deterioration of the brain is genetically determined and will not yield to external approaches.

How do nutrient deficiencies affect brain function?

General poor nutrition affects the brain in several ways. The enzymes involved in neurotransmitter synthesis require vitamins and minerals to function properly.[5] Research on animals and human beings clearly shows that severe dietary deficiencies of thiamin, niacin, vitamin B_6, vitamin B_{12}, folate, and vitamin C impair mental ability, including memory.[6] Trace elements such as iodine, iron, copper, and zinc also support normal brain function.[7] Memory impairments are observed in people and animals with severe nutrient deficiencies and could develop

in some older adults because they have experienced moderate (subclinical) deficiencies for long times.

One group of researchers studied the relationship between nutrition status and cognitive functioning in older, healthy adults and found that subjects with low blood concentrations of vitamin C or vitamin B_{12} scored worse in short-term memory and problem solving than better-nourished participants. Those with low blood concentrations of riboflavin or folate also scored worse on the problem-solving test.[8]

It is important to note that even the lowest scores in this study were still within the normal range for men and women of the same age. Also, the relationship between poor cognition and poor nutrition might be compared with the question of whether the chicken or the egg came first. Poor cognition is itself a risk factor for poor nutrition, because people with impaired thinking ability might be less adept at meal preparation. However, the participants in this study had no history of dementia or impaired mental status, and so the researchers concluded that poor nutrition status might contribute to poor cognitive functioning in healthy, elderly people.

Evidence that vitamin B_{12} deficiency accounts for some cognitive deficits in older people comes from a study that revealed abnormal short-term memory in more than two-thirds of clients with the vitamin B_{12}–deficiency disease (known as pernicious anemia).[9] Treatment with vitamin B_{12} restored memory within one month in three-fourths of the clients. The researchers recommend that physicians never diagnose senile dementia,

even in the absence of obvious anemia, without first determining vitamin B_{12} status biochemically.

Rats fed diets low in copper and vitamin B_6 develop brain changes that resemble the degenerative changes that occur in the brains of human beings as they age.[10] The rats' diets were extremely deficient in vitamin B_6, an unlikely situation for human beings. Vitamin B_6 intakes of many older adults vary, however, and many people are ingesting amounts well below recommendations.[11]

A study in England showed that people with senile dementia had much lower blood concentrations of zinc than those without dementia.[12] Among older women in the United States, as many as 25 percent take in less than half of their recommended allowance.[13]

What about other minerals? I've heard that iron deficiencies cause a common anemia—do they also impair brain function?

Iron deficiency is well known to impair mental function. Research on children shows an especially dramatic effect on cognitive function.[14] Also in college students, researchers have found a relationship between body iron stores and cognition.[15] The effect is not fully understood, but research on animals also supports a relationship between iron deficiency and cognition.[16] The offspring of rats fed an iron-deficient diet were less responsive to adverse stimuli than were the offspring of iron-sufficient rats. In view of the widespread occurrence of iron deficiency, the role of lifelong deficiencies on mental function in the aged deserves further research.

Does this mean that I should buy a vitamin-mineral supplement?

As discussed in the Spotlight following Chapter 5, the only way to be sure to get the needed assortment of nutrients is to construct a balanced diet from a variety of foods. No supplement can match a balanced diet, and no combination of supplements can, either.

Beware of charlatans selling nutrients, especially large doses of nutrients, as "megavitamin therapy" to correct mental illness. When any "therapy" includes nutrient megadoses, this should sound an alarm in your mind to warn you of the possibility that you are dealing with quackery.[17]

Do people's nutrient needs change as they grow older?

Yes, they do, and nutrient needs change differently for different people. For example, one individual may need more iron because that person's stomach acid secretion has declined (stomach acid helps in iron absorption). Another person may excrete more folate (and thus need to obtain more), due to past liver disease. Unfortunately, though, there is no way to make distinct recommendations for different older individuals—everyone over 50 years of age is grouped together in the RDA (Recommended Dietary Allowance) tables (see Appendix B).[18]

How do nutrient needs change with age?

First and foremost, energy needs decline. For one thing, the number of active cells in each organ decreases, reducing the body's overall metabolic rate (although this is not inevitable). For another, older people usually reduce their physical activity (although they need not do so). After about the age of 50 years, the RDA for energy assumes about a 5 percent per decade reduction in energy output. The variation is great, so the ranges are wide (see inside front cover). On such a limited energy allowance, there is little leeway for low-nutrient-density foods, and older people must limit their intakes of sugars, fats, oils, and of course, alcohol.

Second, among carbohydrates, fiber takes on extra importance for its role against constipation—a common complaint among older adults and especially among nursing home residents. Few older adults obtain currently recommended fiber intakes.[19] When low fiber intakes are combined with low fluid intakes, inadequate exercise, and constipating medications, constipation becomes almost inevitable.

Third, fat needs decline. Fats should be limited in the diet of older adults for many reasons. Foods low in fat are often rich in needed vitamins and minerals and may also help retard the development of cancer, atherosclerosis, obesity, and many other diseases.

Do vitamin and mineral needs change, too?

Apparently not much, although there are two exceptions. One is vitamin A: its absorption appears to increase with aging.[20] For this reason researchers have proposed lowering the RDA for vitamin A in aged populations. Some resist such a change, though, citing research that shows the vitamin A compound beta-carotene to be active in cancer prevention.

The other exception is vitamin D. Older adults face a greater risk of vitamin D deficiency than younger people do. Many older adults drink little or no vitamin D–fortified milk, and many go day after day with no exposure to sunlight, especially if they reside in nursing homes.[21] Also, vitamin D synthesis declines with age, setting the stage for deficiency. These age-related changes have inspired the suggestion that the RDA for vitamin D be raised for the elderly, but a more effective approach would be to ensure that elderly people drink more vitamin D–fortified milk and get outside more often, or even just sit by a sunny window some of the time.

How can older people get enough vitamins and minerals?

Adequate vitamin and mineral intakes can be ensured by including foods from all food groups in daily meals. Studies have shown that the elderly most often omit foods of the vegetable group, either to save money or because their preferences have changed.[22] About 18 percent of older people are reported to eat no vegetables at all. Fruit is also lacking in many diets, and people who omit foods of both groups are almost sure to become nutrient deficient. Some older adults do not eat whole-grain breads and cereals, a significant source of many B vitamins.

I have older family members that I care about, but I don't live with them. How can I make sure they get good meals?

Assistance programs are useful when older people have problems obtaining proper, nourishing meals for financial or other reasons. Three major federal programs can help with money problems, at least a little. Under Social Security, employees and employers pay into a fund from which the employees collect benefits at retirement. The Food Stamp program enables people who qualify to obtain stamps with which to buy food. The Supplemental Security Income program is aimed at directly improving the financial plight of the very poor by increasing a person's or a family's income to the defined poverty level.

Another program to benefit the elderly is the part of the Older Americans Act called the "Nutrition Program for the Elderly." The major goals of this program are to provide:

■ Low-cost, nutritious meals.
■ Opportunities for social interaction.
■ Homemaker education and shopping assistance.
■ Counseling and referral to other social services.
■ Transportation services.

The program is intended to improve older people's nutrition status and enable them to avoid medical problems, continue living in communities of their own choice, and stay out of institutions.

Under this program, congregate meals are provided at sites accessible to most of the target population. Volunteers may also deliver meals to those who are homebound either permanently or temporarily; these efforts are known as Meals on Wheels. Food banks have been estab-

lished in several areas to help older people stretch their food dollars. A food bank project buys industry's "irregulars"—good products that have been mislabeled, under-weighted, redesigned, or mispackaged and would ordinarily therefore be thrown away. Whenever government money dwindles, the nutrition status of low-income people of all ages depends more and more on private efforts such as food banking.

What if an older person is given good meals, but doesn't eat them?

That's a crucial question. Studies that focus on foods and nutrients tend to forget the most important facet of eating—the psychological well-being of the individual. Dr. Jack Weinberg, professor of psychiatry at the University of Illinois, wrote perceptively:

It is not *what* the older person eats but *with whom* that will be the deciding factor in proper care for him. The oft-repeated complaint of the older patient that he has little incentive to prepare food for only himself is not merely a statement of fact but also a rebuke to the questioner for failing to perceive his isolation and aloneness and to realize that food . . . for one's self lacks the condiment of another's presence which can transform the simplest fare to the ceremonial act with all its shared meaning.[23]

Of all the problems affecting nutrition of older people, that of loneliness has

the most impact. To make sure people eat well, make sure they eat in the company of other people they enjoy.

What about the preparing of meals? Doesn't that sometimes become difficult for older people, too?

Yes. Many older people, even able-bodied ones with financial resources, find themselves unable to perform the tasks of cooking, cleaning, and shopping. The following story illustrates this point. A man who had never prepared food for himself became a widower and suddenly became responsible for planning and preparing his own meals. During the year following his wife's death, he subsisted on a diet of black coffee, hamburgers, martinis, and steaks. He developed symptoms, and his health care providers treated him for many ailments. Finally, a registered dietitian made the correct diagnosis: scurvy from vitamin C deficiency. Even an occasional baked potato with his steak would have improved his vitamin C status, but without knowledge he was at a loss to select it, and baking it was beyond his skill. Furthermore, his loneliness robbed him of self-concern. With no one to share his meals, self-care became unimportant, and food lost its appeal.

For anyone living alone and for those of advanced age especially, it is important to work through the problems food preparation and mealtimes present. Wise adults will plan ahead to maximize their enjoyment of the later years.[24]

■≡ Spotlight Notes

1. E. L. Schneider and J. D. Reed, Life extension, *New England Journal of Medicine* 312 (1985): 1159–1168.

2. N. B. Belloc and L. Breslow, Relationship of physical health status and health practices, *Preventive Medicine* 1 (1972): 409–421.

3. T. Harris and coauthors, Body mass index and mortality among nonsmoking older persons, *Journal of the American Medical Association* 259 (1988): 1520–1524.

4. E. D. Schlenker, Obesity and the life span, in *Nutrition, Physiology, and Obesity,* ed. R. Schemmel (Boca Raton, Fla.: CRC Press, 1980), pp. 151–166; Y. Kagawa, Impact of westernization on the nutrition of Japanese: Changes in physique, cancer, longevity and centenarians, *Preventive Medicine* 7 (1978): 205–217.

5. W. M. Lovenberg, Biochemical regulation of brain function, *Nutrition Reviews* (supplement), May 1986, pp. 6–11.

6. K. Yoshimura and coauthors, Animal experiments on thiamine avitaminosis and cerebral function, *Journal of Nutritional Science and Vitaminology* 22 (1976): 429–437, as cited in A. Cherkin, Effects of nutritional factors on memory function, in *Nutritional Intervention in the Aging Process,* eds. H. J. Armbrecht, J. M. Prendergast, and R. M. Coe (New York: Springer-Verlag, 1984), pp. 229–249; M. K. Horwitt, Niacin, in *Modern Nutrition in Health and Disease,* 6th ed., eds. R. S. Goodhart and M. S. Shils (Philadelphia: Lea & Febiger, 1980), pp. 204–208; C. S. Russ and coauthors, Vitamin B_6 status of depressed and obsessive-compulsive patients, *Nutrition Reports International* 27 (1983): 867–873; J. S.

Goodwin, J. M. Goodwin, and P. J. Garry, Association between nutritional status and cognitive functioning in a healthy elderly population, *Journal of the American Medical Association* 249 (1983): 2917–2921.

7. H. Sandstead, A brief history of the influence of trace elements on brain function, *American Journal of Clinical Nutrition* 43 (1986): 293–298.

8. Goodwin, Goodwin, and Garry, 1983.

9. R. W. Strachan and J. G. Henderson, Psychiatric syndromes due to avitaminosis B_{12} with normal blood and marrow, *Journal of Medicine* 34 (1965): 303–317, as cited in Cherkin, 1984.

10. E. J. Root and J. B. Longenecker, Brain cell alterations suggesting premature aging induced by dietary deficiency of vitamin B_6 and/or copper, *American Journal of Clinical Nutrition* 37 (1983): 540–552.

11. P. J. Garry and coauthors, Nutritional status in a healthy elderly population: Dietary and supplemental intakes, *American Journal of Clinical Nutrition* 36 (1982): 319–331.

12. R. Hullin, Zinc deficiency: Can it cause dementia? *Therapaecia,* September 1983, pp. 26, 27, 30.

13. Garry and coauthors, 1982.

14. E. Pollitt and coauthors, Iron deficiency and behavioral development in infants and preschool children, *American Journal of Clinical Nutrition* 43 (1986): 555–565.

15. D. M. Tucker and coauthors, Iron status and brain function: Serum ferritin levels associated with asymmetries of cortical electrophysiology and cognitive performance, *American Journal of Clinical Nutrition* 39 (1984): 105–113.

16. J. Weinberg, Behavioral and physiological effects of early iron deficiency in the rat, in *Iron Deficiency: Brain Biochemistry and Behavior,* eds. E. Pollitt and R. L. Leibel (New York: Raven, 1982), pp. 93–123.

17. S. Barrett, Claims and cautions: Megavitamin therapy, *Priorities,* Spring 1989, pp. 27–29.

18. H. Smicklas-Wright, Aging, in *Present Knowledge in Nutrition,* ed. M. L. Brown (Washington, D.C.: International Life Sciences Institute – Nutrition Foundation, 1990), pp. 333–340.

19. Position of the American Dietetic Association: Health implications of dietary fiber, *Journal of the American Dietetic Association* 88 (1988): 216.

20. P. J. Garry and coauthors, Vitamin A intake and plasma retinol levels in healthy elderly men and women, *American Journal of Clinical Nutrition* 46 (1987): 989–994.

21. Vitamin D status of the elderly: Contributions of sunlight exposure and diet, *Nutrition Reviews* 43 (1985): 78–80.

22. V. Holt, J. Nordstrom, and M. B. Kohrs, Food preferences of older adults (abstract), *Journal of the American Dietetic Association* 87 (1987): 1597.

23. J. Weinberg, Psychologic implications of the nutritional needs of the elderly, *Journal of the American Dietetic Association* 60 (1972): 293–296.

24. This Spotlight was in part adapted from S. R. Rolfes and L. K. DeBruyne, *Life Span Nutrition: Conception through Life* (St. Paul: West, 1990), pp. 415–456.

CHAPTER 16

Death and Dying

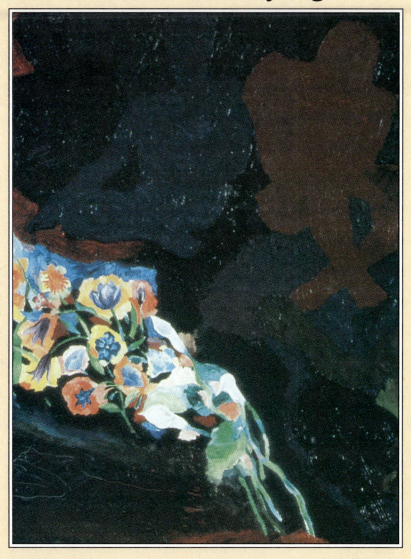

Imagine you were told that you had a limited time to live. What would you do? Would knowing the date of your death change the way you would conduct your life? Do you need to put in order any practical, financial, or legal matters before you die? Do you need to work out any emotional issues with your parents, children, siblings, and friends? Have you postponed talking about anything with anyone? What ideas and traditions do you want to pass on to those who will follow you? Have you arranged for your own funeral?

Now imagine someone close to you has only a few weeks to live. What will you talk about with this person? How will you spend your time together? The value of thinking about questions like this is that it enriches your life. Knowing that your time is limited motivates you to spend it well.

This chapter will help you examine your feelings, beliefs, hopes, and fears about death and to prepare to cope when loved ones die. The purpose is to help you learn to use the gift of life as happily and productively as possible. You can discover life's true meaning if you accept that death is a part of the human experience. If you face the challenge and opportunity of dealing with death, you will grow emotionally and spiritually.

■≡ The Fear of Death

Many people cannot stand to think of death. Our society tries to cope with death mostly by ignoring it: we worship youth and progress.

It is natural to fear death; all creatures strive to live. To express your fear and contemplate your mortality is healthy; to flee and hide from reality is unhealthy. Denying death causes some people to live empty, purposeless lives. People who live as if their days were unlimited find it easy to postpone doing things that are important to them.

To accept that you will die, and to spend time thinking about it, can set your priorities straight. You have a task—to make something of your life within a limited time period. You have a deadline to meet. Whatever you want to accomplish in life, you must do before you die. There is an urgency in this, because you don't know how many days or weeks or months or years you have. This awareness can keep you from frivolously wasting the

FACT OR FICTION: People who think about death are unhealthy and morbid. False. People who contemplate mortality and express their fears about death are healthy.

time you have. Death acts as a reminder not to wait until tomorrow to do what you mean to do today.

This doesn't mean that people have to rush through life, for one great value is to savor every moment. People can live with appreciation and gratitude, especially for the simple things of life that they tend to take for granted. They can learn to focus on the things they have learned to tune out—to notice and take joy in the budding of new flowers in spring, to wonder at the beauty of a sunset. They can take comfort in the smile or touch of another person and watch with amazement the growth of a child. They can share in children's wonderful enthusiasm for living. Acknowledging death helps people to cherish their lives rather than simply pass through them.

To gain the perspective that death gives to life, you first have to deal with your fear of death. Examine the fear—what are you afraid of, exactly? Some people are afraid of the uncertainty of the afterlife—they fear what may await them. Some people fear that everything will end. Others fear the particular process of death; for example, the person with a painful **terminal illness** fears the manner in which death will occur rather than death itself.[1]

To get over the fear of death completely may be impossible, but people fear two things most: uncertainty, and things they are unprepared to face. If you think through the probable events surrounding death and prepare for them as described next, you may fear death less.

≡▶ *It is natural to fear death; most people do. People who are healthy can express their fears about death. Examining the specific fear—whether it be fear of the process of death or doubts about what the afterlife may bring—can help people cope with death.*

terminal illness a progressive, irreversible disease that is expected to end in death in the near future.

■≡ Preparation for Death

Preparation for death has two aspects. One is financial and legal preparation, and the other is emotional and spiritual preparation.

Financial and Legal Preparations

One thing to do in preparing for death is to make a will. Half of the people in the United States die without having done so. When a person dies, the state distributes that person's property according to its laws, and often the family loses much of the property. Typically, much more goes in taxes than is necessary. Without a will, the assets go not to the people the person would have chosen but to the people the state chooses. Usually the end result is not what the person would have preferred.

Even those who don't have any property worth mentioning should not postpone making a will for too long. You may not think of yourself as owning an estate, but you do, even if you own only a bicycle and a backpack. Make a will before the time comes when dying without one would deprive the people you care about of things you would want them to have.

*Reference notes are at the end of the chapter.

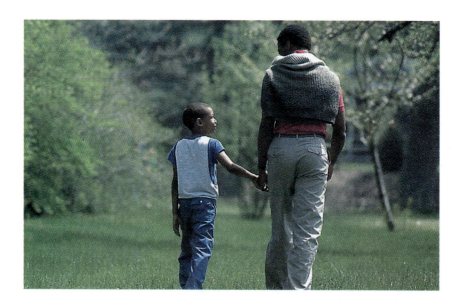

Spending time with a child can help people learn to take joy in the simple things of life.

■ *FACT OR FICTION:* Only wealthy people need to prepare wills. *False.* Everyone should prepare a will, particularly anyone who wants to protect loved ones from avoidable losses.

A good time to make a will is when you first marry or first become a parent. Even if you have little or no property at that time, assume that you will have, and plan accordingly. Then when the thought of your death crosses your mind, that particular fear will be gone. You will have the comfort of knowing you have protected those you love from avoidable losses.

Part of making a will involves appointing a personal representative to pay from the estate all debts, including funeral expenses, costs of the last illness, expenses of administration of the estate, and any other costs. People with a child or children usually name a friend or relative to serve as a guardian in the event that they both die. If people die without naming a guardian, the court will appoint one.

Another thing to do in preparing for death is to obtain adequate health and life insurance. People who develop serious illnesses often find it too late to get insurance. Different kinds of policies are suitable at different times in life and in different situations. It is possible to be underinsured, but it is also possible to squander needed money buying too much insurance. Shop carefully and beware: the salesperson may not have your best interests at heart, because the desire for personal gain can contaminate the salesperson's motives. (Chapter 20 provides details on shopping for health insurance.)

There are other ways to prepare for death. Strictly speaking, these are not health issues, and so they are not covered here. But at some point you might want to learn about the roles of coroners and medical examiners; the reasons for autopsies; the need for, and uses of, morgues; the various options for funerals; the possibilities for donating organs to the living; and the costs and paperwork involved in death.

In the event of sudden death, one thing that can help the bewildered spouse, next of kin, or person with power of attorney is to find in an easily accessible place a page of directions listing all important information and documents and telling where they are kept. Such a list might include:

■ The name and phone number of the attorney who prepared the will (and the attorney should have the original will).

■ A copy of the will.
■ Marriage/divorce documents.
■ Citizenship papers.
■ Military service papers.
■ Health, life, and accident insurance policies.
■ Information about retirement benefits.
■ Safe deposit box information and contents (and where the key is).
■ Real estate papers.
■ Bank accounts, stocks/bonds, savings bonds.

The importance of preparing ahead of time cannot be emphasized enough. One of the most considerate acts parents can perform is to pre-plan, even pre-pay, for the funerals of their choice. Consider the person who is in the position of having to make decisions about the funeral and the disposal of property without knowing the deceased's desires. The family not only has to deal with many financial and legal issues, but also has to face these decisions during a tragic time of grief. This chapter's Critical Thinking section warns against one kind of pressure people need to resist when forced to make decisions during times of emotional crisis.

Another thing to do in preparing for death is to consider signing a **living will**. This protects you in case you lose consciousness and other people have to decide what will happen to you. If you are incompetent to make a decision about your care, your family and health care professionals will make that decision for you unless you have provided a legal document to guide them.[2] These are the questions to think about. If a tragic illness or accident left you with no conscious brain function and no hope for recovery, would you want to be kept alive on an artificial **life-support system**? If you were in the final stages of a terminal illness and unable to express your wishes, would you want to be resuscitated each time your heart stopped? Today, life-support systems can keep hopelessly ill individuals alive even though their minds are gone and their bodies have stopped functioning naturally. Expenses for such treatments can mount to astronomical sums, leaving families penniless, all without enabling the unconscious person to enjoy a single additional day of conscious life. People have the right to refuse such treatments.

Not in all states, but in some, the courts recognize the right of unconscious people to die, provided they have previously made their wishes known regarding their preferences for treatment.[3]

Many states have enacted laws that authorize the use of living wills.[4] In those states, such a will stands as a clear expression of a competent adult's wishes.[5] It gives instructions stating exactly how you want to be treated, should you lose the ability to make decisions for yourself. Some people request that no measures be taken to prolong their lives, to avoid unnecessary grief and expense for their families. They may instruct their families to use no life-support systems after **brain death** has occurred, or they may even instruct their families to "pull the plug" if such measures have been started.

Other people who fear that relatives won't have their best interests at heart may request the opposite—that *every* measure be taken to save their

living will a will a person can make to indicate how he or she would like to be treated on becoming unable to make decisions (for example, in the event of brain death).

life-support system a mechanical and/or artificial means of supporting life, such as machines that force air into the lungs or feedings given into a central vein.

brain death irreversible and total cessation of function of the higher brain centers, reflected in a flat line recorded by the electroencephalograph, in contrast to the irregular wave pattern made by an active brain when awake, asleep, or temporarily unconscious.

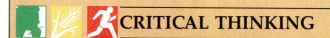

CRITICAL THINKING

The Emotional Crisis Opportunist

Imagine this scenario: A woman's husband dies unexpectedly. Totally unprepared for the tragedy, the woman is trying to face this shocking event. She is at the funeral home, trying to select a casket. The funeral director explains the different selections to her. Her husband passed away without communicating any of his wishes to her in regard to his funeral. The funeral director guides her toward an array of caskets. She begins to select a plain pine box, and the funeral director says, "This one is OK, except, over time, the weight of the dirt will break the top of the box, and the dirt will fall all over your husband." He adds, "I know you want the absolute best for your husband. This is the last thing you can do for him." Then he shows her the more expensive caskets. The woman shells out far more money than she can afford for a coffin her husband will never appreciate.

At weddings, the same sort of thing happens. People get conned into spending far more than they mean to, just to prove their love.

Be aware that during times of emotional crisis, salespeople may try to take advantage of you. They know that people going through emotional times are vulnerable. People like this funeral director know how to use both anguish and joy to their financial advantage. Be on guard—yielding to their tactics may leave you with not only an emotional loss, but a financial one as well.

Don't equate the value of your love for someone with the money you spend on a funeral or a wedding.

■ *FACT OR FICTION:* A living will is a document that bestows some of your property on someone before you die. *False.* A living will is a document that states the degree of medical care that you would desire in the event that you were incompetent and unable to communicate your wishes.

lives, regardless of expense. You need not linger if you do not want to—but you can if you choose. In any case, it is important to take the responsibility for the decision, yourself. It's a heavy burden for someone else to make the choice for you—and in many instances, the law forces heroic life-prolonging measures on people who are brain-dead. An example of a living will is shown in Figure 16–1, together with an address from which forms can be obtained. People can either spell out detailed instructions for conditions under which they would want caretakers to refrain from making efforts to revive them or they can list specific procedures they would want caretakers to withhold.[6]

Some states honor living wills only partially. They may have laws that recognize people's requests with respect to medical procedures, but specifically exclude the right to withhold or withdraw artificial feedings: nourishment or water given through tubes into the vein or stomach.[7] They consider such nourishment to be part of ordinary care and do not allow it to be withheld or withdrawn for any reason. Most living wills fail to deal with the question of artificial feedings, so people who prefer that such feedings be discontinued need to specifically say so in their living wills.[8] The long struggle to win permission for people to exercise their rights to die in this manner is still going on. Its progress to date is detailed in this chapter's Spotlight.

In states that do not authorize living wills, people can and should make their wishes known in writing, nevertheless. In some states, a document

FIGURE 16–1 ■ **A living will.**

To My Family, My Physician, My Lawyer
And All Others Whom It May Concern

Death is as much a reality as birth, growth, and aging—it is the one certainty of life. In anticipation of decisions that may have to be made about my own dying and as an expression of my right to refuse treatment, I,

_____ ,
(print name)

being of sound mind, make this statement of my wishes and instructions concerning treatment.

By means of this document, which I intend to be legally binding, I direct my physician and other care providers, my family, and any surrogate designated by me or appointed by a court, to carry out my wishes. If I become unable, by reason of physical or mental incapacity, to make decisions about my medical care, let this document provide the guidance and authority needed to make any and all such decisions.

If I am permanently unconscious or there is no reasonable expectation of my recovery from a seriously incapacitating or lethal illness or condition, I do not wish to be kept alive by artificial means. I request that I be given all care necessary to keep me comfortable and free of pain, even if pain-relieving medications may hasten my death, and I direct that no life-sustaining treatment be provided except as I or my surrogate specifically authorize. I do (　) I do not (　) desire that nutrition and hydration (food and water) be withheld or withdrawn when the application of such procedures would serve only to prolong artificially the process of dying.

This request may appear to place a heavy responsibility upon you, but by making this decision according to my strong convictions, I intend to ease that burden. I am acting after careful consideration and with understanding of the consequences of your carrying out my wishes. *List optional specific provisions in the space below.*[a]

I sign this document knowingly, voluntarily, and after careful deliberation, this _____ day of _____ , 19 _____ .	Witness _____ Printed Name _____ Address _____ _____
_____ (signature) Address _____ _____	Witness _____ Printed Name _____ Address _____ _____
I do hereby certify that the within document was executed and acknowledged before me by the principal this _____ day of _____ , 19 _____ .	Copies of this document have been given to: _____ _____ _____
_____ Notary Public	_____ _____

[a]The living will should clearly state your preference about life-sustaining treatment. You may wish to add specific statements that concern cardiopulmonary resuscitation, kidney dialysis, mechanical or artificial respiration, blood transfusion, surgery (such as amputation), and antibiotics. You may also wish to indicate any preferences you have about such matters as dying at home.

SOURCE: Reprinted by permission of Society for the Right to Die, 250 W. 57th St., New York, NY 10107. For a copy of "A Living Will" and other information, write or call (212) 246–6962.

durable power of attorney a document that allows a competent adult to designate another competent adult as an agent to make decisions in the event of incapacitation.

known as a **durable power of attorney** offers people the protection of having their wishes carried out (see Figure 16–2).[9] A durable power of attorney allows a competent adult to designate another competent adult as an agent to make decisions in the event of incapacitation.

A living will frees others from the guilt and anxiety of having to make decisions in the case of an irreversible state of unconsciousness. Imagine the anxiety a family member goes through in directing the health care team to stop medical or nutrition support, knowing that it will hasten death. That decision is far easier if a legal document takes the decision out of the family's hands altogether. (Another hard choice is discussed in the accompanying box, Assisting Death.)

FIGURE 16–2 ■ **Durable power of attorney.**

Durable Power of Attorney for Health Care Decisions

To effect my wishes, I designate _____ , residing at _____

_____ (Phone #) _____ ,
(or if he or she shall for any reason fail to act, _____
_____ (Phone #) _____ ,
residing at _____)

as my health care surrogate—that is, my attorney-in-fact regarding any and all health care decisions to be made for me, including the decision to refuse life-sustaining treatment—if I am unable to make such decision myself. This power shall remain effective during and not be affected by my subsequent illness, disability or incapacity. My surrogate shall have authority to interpret my Living Will, and shall make decisions about my health care as specified in my instructions or, when my wishes are not clear, as the surrogate believes to be in my best interests. I release and agree to hold harmless my health care surrogate from any and all claims whatsoever arising from decisions made in good faith in the exercise of this power.

I sign this document knowingly, voluntarily, and after careful deliberation, this _____ day of _____, 19 _____ .

_____
(signature)
Address _____
_____

Witness _____
Printed Name _____
Address _____

_____
Witness _____
Printed Name _____
Address _____

I do hereby certify that the within document was executed and acknowledged before me by the principal this _____ day of _____, 19 _____ .

_____
Notary Public

Copies of this document have been given to:

_____
_____
_____
_____
_____

SOURCE: Reprinted by permission of Society for the Right to Die, 250 W. 57th St., New York, NY 10107. For a copy of a durable power of attorney form and other information, write or call (212) 246–6962.

Assisting Death

Allowing someone to die by doing nothing is different from hastening death by actively doing something. The latter is called **euthanasia**, or mercy killing, and most such acts are illegal, although some physicians quietly perform them. Occasionally, someone other than a physician is forced to confront a similar choice, when a friend who has a terminal illness, but who is fully conscious and alert, asks for assistance in committing suicide.

Until recently such decisions almost invariably involved people who had lived out long lives and were faced with painful terminal illnesses in their later years. Now, however, the young are increasingly facing such choices, because of the AIDS epidemic. AIDS (acquired immune deficiency syndrome) has been striking the young with a ferocity unprecedented among infectious diseases in recent times (as Chapter 17 describes). Because the diagnosis precedes death by months or even years, people with AIDS are faced with inevitable death. While most choose to live as long as possible, some choose to die voluntarily, and sometimes they ask others to assist them in doing so.

Suicide contemplated in a depression, when terminal illness is not involved, is widely opposed, because depression is treatable. Some people argue, however, that suicide in the case of a terminal illness such as AIDS should be viewed differently, and that even assisting such a person should be condoned. "My friend is about to die anyway," a young person says of an AIDS victim. "The quality of his life has been destroyed and he is ready to go. Why shouldn't he choose the time and place, and ask his loved ones to be with him? Why shouldn't I help him?"

People's opinions differ on whether such assistance is ethical. Some feel that it is, and should become legal. They say that a means of dying as surely and painlessly as possible should be made available to those who want it.* People who oppose assisted suicide state that killing is immoral and that one person does not have the right to kill another person. They generally agree, however, that a person facing death should be provided with physical and emotional comfort and that death should be made as painless as possible. They oppose making mercy killing legal, not only based on ethical views, but also because they foresee that promoting this idea may indirectly encourage assisting of killing and suicide in situations that do not involve terminal illness. For example, people without terminal illnesses, facing depression, have already ended their lives by means of using techniques described in a how-to-commit-suicide book written for people with terminal illness.

euthanasia (you-than-AY-zee-uh) mercy killing. Euthanasia differs from simply allowing a person to die, in that an act is performed, such as pulling the plug on life-support equipment (which may be legal in some cases) or injecting a poison (which is illegal).

A person who makes a living will should discuss it with the family and give copies to the people who may need them one day. The person's physician should also know the person's preferences ahead of time and keep a

*An organization that espouses the right to die and to assist someone in dying is The Hemlock Society, P.O. Box 11830, Eugene, OR 97440.

hospice (HOS-pis)   a support system for people with terminal illnesses and their families, which helps the family to let the person die at home with dignity and in comfort.

copy in the medical files, and the physician should note in the person's medical record that the will is there. The person should keep a copy with all other important papers, and carry a card in the wallet stating that a signed living will exists and indicating where it is kept.

In the event of a long-term or terminal illness, an alternative to institutional care may be available. Most people select hospitals and the like for long-term medical care,[10] but given the choice of a place to be ill for a long time and possibly to die, many people prefer to stay at home or in home-like settings.[11] Sometimes it is possible to do this and use a **hospice** for support. A hospice is a support system especially set up by an outside agency for people with terminal illnesses and their families.[12] The intent is to enable the family to care for the person at home, and if appropriate, to let the person die there.[13]

The key phrase of the hospice movement is "death with dignity," and the emphasis is on achieving quality in the dying person's remaining lifetime. People with terminal illnesses who are cared for at home may experience more dignity and comfort than in the hospital, and their families may have less difficulty in adjusting to the impending death.[14]

Hospice services are provided by a team of professionals, each attending to a different aspect of the dying person's care. A team typically includes physicians, nurses, and a psychiatrist or psychologist, and often social workers, clergy, and trained volunteers. The hospice has a twofold purpose: (1) to make the dying person as comfortable as possible by controlling pain and distressing symptoms; and (2) to offer psychological, social, and spiritual support to the client and family. Hospice care for the family continues beyond the person's death into the bereavement period.*

≡▶   *To prepare for death financially and legally, people can make wills, obtain adequate health and life insurance, make living wills, and consider alternative places to die.*

Emotional and Spiritual Preparation

To prepare for death is partly an emotional and spiritual task. Chapter 2 and its Spotlight have already discussed some aspects of emotional and spiritual health; this section describes how an awareness of death can enhance a person's emotional and spiritual life.

To begin with, acknowledging death can enhance the quality of personal relationships. People who are mindful of life's transitory nature can appreciate others while they have them. In contrast, people who do not consider the inevitability of death often feel as though family members or friends are their possessions forever, and they may take them for granted or even begin to value material things over them. Children may undervalue their parents, thinking they will have them forever. Parents may forget how they love their children, yet each day when parents and children are together is a gift, not to be squandered worrying about cookie crumbs in the rug or milk on the couch. The knowledge that a friend can be taken from you in a heartbeat is

*The address for the National Hospice Organization is 1901 N. Fort Myer Dr., Suite 307, Arlington, VA 22209; the telephone number is (703) 243–5900. The National Consumer League publishes a booklet, *A Consumer Guide to Hospice Care,* by B. Coleman, February 1985, available from 600 Maryland Ave. SW, Suite 202-West, Washington, DC 20024.

sobering; people who are aware of this take opportunities now to show their friends that they are cherished.

Live each day as if it were your last. Seize every moment; don't live for the future, waiting for some upcoming event to be happy. Discard this way of thinking: "When I graduate from college, *then* I'll be happy" or "I'll be happy when I get married [have a different job, have children, and so on]." Facing death can help you live in the present, not in the future. The author of the poem "I'd Pick More Daisies" (see box) communicates her desire to learn to live in the present.

People who have considered death in a spiritual and emotional way tend to learn to let go of material values and intensify relationships with those dearest to them. They see the importance of reconciling unmended friendships. They tell their loved ones that they love them. They stop postponing acts of kindness to those who are dear. They find and affirm value in life. All these preparations are things people can do while they're alive—now.

Part of the spiritual preparation for death involves exploring your personal beliefs about life after death. People want to know why they die and what happens to them after they die. Is there a life after death, and if so, what is its nature? People who have strong spiritual beliefs, particularly those who believe in a positive afterlife, may face death serenely, because they find comfort in believing that a better life awaits them. Some examples may help illustrate how believing in a positive afterlife can bring people peace about death.

In some cultures, death is not mourned. Many people from Japan do not fear death. They believe that after people die they go to a pure, beautiful, and peaceful land, a place they call "the other shores."[15] Although the family miss and grieve for the person who has died, they do not feel that the death is tragic. The funeral is a time of celebration, and the funeral carriage is white and festive, not black and somber.

People of the Christian faith believe in life after death, and some are actually eager to experience the afterlife. Heaven is described as paradise,[16] a place of bliss and rest, a place where all tears will be wiped away,[17] where people will be reunited with their loved ones.

≡▶ *Preparing for death is partly an emotional and spiritual task. Learning to appreciate the significant people in one's life and learning to live in the present, giving thanks for each day, is a way facing death can enhance life. A positive view of the afterlife makes death easier to accept.*

Near-Death Experiences

People naturally search for answers about the possibility of life after death. Studies of people who have had narrow escapes from death (other than suicide) have given some insights to the searchers.

Those who have had near-death experiences report that the events dramatically changed their lives. Some say they completely changed their values, switched careers, or altered their lives significantly in other ways. Many people have turned away from competition and making money and focused on helping others and appreciating life and nature.

In a near-death experience, a person seems to leave the body and go to another vivid and inviting realm. People who have had near-death

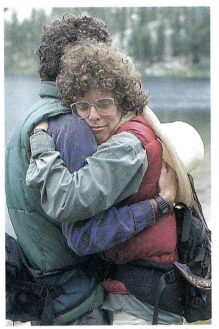

If there are people who should know that you love them, show them.

I'd Pick More Daisies

If I had my life to live over, I'd try to make more mistakes next time.

I would relax.

I would limber up.

I would be sillier than I have been this trip.

I know of very few things I would take seriously.

I would be crazier.

I would be less hygienic.

I would take more chances.

I would take more trips.

I would climb more mountains, swim more rivers, and watch more sunsets.

I would eat more ice cream and less beans.

I would have more actual troubles and fewer imaginary ones.

You see, I am one of those people who lives prophylactically and sensibly and sanely, hour after hour, day after day.

Oh, I've had my moments and, if I had it to do over, I'd have more of them. In fact, I'd try to have nothing else.

Just moments, one after the other, instead of living so many years ahead each day.

I have been one of those people who never goes anywhere without a thermometer, a hot water bottle, a gargle, a raincoat, and a parachute.

If I had it to do over again, I would go places and do things and travel lighter than I have.

If I had my life to live over, I would start bare-footed earlier in the spring and stay that way later in the fall.

I would play hookey more.

I wouldn't make such good grades except by accident.

I would ride on more merry-go-rounds.

I'd pick more daisies.

Nadine Stair, 87
Louisville, Kentucky

experiences claim that they know there is life after death. They say they are no longer afraid to die. The experience leaves them much more alive, not afraid to take risks, not afraid to put themselves out for others. They become more interested in spirituality. People come back with a sense of purpose, with a feeling that their lives have significance.

Reported near-death experiences are amazingly similar. As death nears, there is a brilliant light that seems to be everywhere, or at the end of a tunnel. One feels serenity, clarity of mind, a sense of looking down on one's

■ **FACT OR FICTION:** Most people who have had near-death experiences report that they are no longer afraid to die. *True.*

body as if suspended from above.[18] One experiences a peaceful and calm feeling, being transported out of the body, entering a dark void such as a tunnel and reviewing the past life's events, being reunited with dear relatives, and then being told to return to the physical body. Most near-death experiences have been positive, but some people have been extremely frightened by them and returned from them with a sense of doom and gloom.

Researchers trying to analyze near-death experiences suggest that they may represent a psychological defense to the perceived threat of dying. Some think there may be physiological reasons why people near death experience the sights and sounds they do. However, most conclude that there must be more to it, because the reports are amazingly consistent. One psychologist is convinced that these reports show proof that a spirit leaves the body as death draws near. He says nine traits typify a near-death experience:

1. A sense of being dead. The person's consciousness is still alive, but has left the body.
2. An out-of-body experience. The person is floating above the body and feels confused. The person wonders, "How can I be up here, looking at myself down there?"
3. Peace and painlessness. An illness or accident is frequently accompanied by intense pain, but suddenly during a near-death experience, the pain vanishes.
4. The tunnel experience. This usually occurs after the out-of-body experience. A portal or tunnel opens, and the person is propelled into darkness, heading toward intense light.
5. People of light. After passing through the tunnel, the person meets beings radiating an intense light that permeates everything and fills the person with feelings of love. Often some of the glowing beings are friends and relatives who have died, although they cannot always be identified.
6. The Supreme Being of Light. After meeting several beings of light, there is usually a meeting with a Supreme Being of Light. To some this is God or Allah, to others simply a holy presence. Most want to stay with this presence forever.
7. The life review. The Supreme Being of Light frequently takes the person on a life review during which life is viewed from third-person perspective, almost as though watching a movie. An important difference from cinema, however, is that the person not only sees every action but also its effect on the people in his or her life. The Supreme Being of Light helps put the events of life in perspective.
8. Rising to the heavens. Some people report a "floating experience" in which they rise rapidly into the heavens, seeing the universe from a perspective otherwise reserved for satellites and astronauts.
9. Reluctance to return. Many find their unearthly surroundings so pleasant they don't want to return. Some even express anger at their physicians for bringing them back.[19]

Researchers believe that the near-death experience is a positive experience that transforms personality.[20]

LIFE CHOICE INVENTORY

Are you prepared to die? Imagine you were told that you had a limited time to live. What would you do? How prepared are you to face death? Answer the following questions yes or no.

Financial and Legal Preparations

1. Have you made a will?   Yes   No
2. Is your health insurance policy up to date?   Yes   No
3. Does your life insurance policy read as you want it to and clearly state your beneficiary?   Yes   No
4. Have you made a living will and given copies to your physician and family members?   Yes   No
5. Have you made an easy-to-find list of where these documents are?   Yes   No
6. Do you carry a card in your wallet saying where this list is? and where your living will is?   Yes   No
7. Have you made your funeral arrangements?   Yes   No
8. Have you considered making organ donor arrangements?   Yes   No
9. Have you discussed these issues with your friends and family?   Yes   No

Emotional and Spiritual Preparation

10. Looking back on your life, do you feel you have accomplished most of the goals that are meaningful to you?   Yes   No
11. Have you worked out the important emotional issues or problems with your loved ones?   Yes   No
12. Have you said the most significant things you need to say to the people important in your life?   Yes   No
13. Have you communicated the ideas and traditions you want passed on to those who follow you?   Yes   No
14. Have you faced your fears about death?   Yes   No
15. Are you living a full life in view of death? Yes   No
16. Do you have peace of mind about your after-death destiny?   Yes   No

Scoring: Give yourself 1 point for each yes answer (maximum points = 14).
11–14: You have prepared yourself to face death.
  7–10: You have made a good start, but further preparation would be beneficial to you.
  0–6: You can make your life more meaningful if you give time and thought to the questions to which you answered no.

This chapter began by saying that most people fear death, sometimes so intensely that they don't dare even think about it. Perhaps this discussion has shown that as death becomes more familiar, it becomes less frightening and even contributes value to life. To see how well you have prepared for death, complete this chapter's Life Choice Inventory.

Near-death experiences can give people hope of a positive afterlife. Near-death experiences of different people are amazingly consistent, giving support to the notion of life after death.

■≡ Approaching Death

A person who expects to die within days or weeks typically has a height-ened sense of life and an almost overwhelming need for human contact and communication.[21] At the same time, others may tend to withdraw in the effort to avoid their own pain. One physician admits that when he is with someone in the final stages of a fatal illness, he finds it increasingly hard to communicate with the dying person. A family member noticed that the physician's style of contact with his dying father changed, as his father's condition worsened, from being frequent, warm, and friendly to rare, brief, and detached. People often have a hard time talking with someone who is dying. The dying person loses individuality and becomes a symbol of what every human being fears and knows: that we too must someday face death.[22] People naturally feel pity, anger, and even revulsion at the impending death of someone they love. It is human to want to avoid contact with the dying person. It helps to know that.

Many people find it so hard to face the process of someone's dying that they miss out on many opportunities to give support. But remember, the person who has learned that death is coming is still the same person as before. If the person had lost a fortune, a home, or an opportunity, you would offer sympathy and love. Now that the person is facing the loss of life itself, doesn't it make sense to offer that same sympathy and love? It may be hard to do, but perhaps it's easier if you realize that there is no one right way to go about it. Your personal style is fine, whatever it is. If your habit has been to laugh and joke with the person, then laugh and joke now, too. After all, the person is alive and capable of responding to cheering company. If you tend to show sorrow easily, that's all right, too. Listen well, if the person wants to communicate. Let the person know you care in whatever way feels right to you. The thing not to do is to avoid the person: any kind of contact is better than simply writing your friend off before the end.

The physician mentioned earlier, whose father was dying, naturally had an especially hard time remaining supportive. A physician has to cope not only with the loss a death represents but also with the feeling that, on some level, the impending death is a personal failure. But a physician who overcomes that frustration can still be a healing presence and maintain a continued relationship. The presence of people who care can make the experience of death peaceful and allow people to die with self-respect and without loneliness.

▶ *People approaching death often have a heightened sense of being alive and an intense need for human contact. Conversely, often the people around someone who is dying struggle with how to interact and tend to withdraw because of their own pain. People who can look past their own fear can be a healing presence to those who are approaching death.*

■ Attending the Dying

Birth attendants are professionally trained to assist at the start of life; ideally, people present at death should also be trained.[23] You need to know the signs of impending death and the comforts to offer the dying person. When you can do things, rather than standing helplessly by, it makes it easier to be present.

Everyone knows what it is like to be sick in bed and have to be cared for by others. The experience is the same for a person within a few hours of death. For as long as the person is alive, you are tending a living person, not a dying person. Think of it that way, and you will know better what to do.

A person who is sick, weak, uncomfortable, and possibly in pain has little energy to give to the psychological task you may be facing. The person needs physical comforts: learn what they are and offer them.

The signs of impending death include glazed eyes, open mouth, cold skin, irregular breathing and pulse, and restless arms and hands. The process of dying usually progresses from the lower part of the body upward. Sensation is lost first in the lower extremities. Then control of the digestive system is lost, and it becomes useless to offer food. As long as the person can swallow, though, water helps—just a little at a time so that it won't cause choking. Keep the mouth wet, with a gauze wick if necessary. Be sure the person is not lying flat when facing upward, because water or even the tongue can fall back in the throat and cause choking. In other ways, too, you may perceive that the person is uncomfortable and needs to be helped to change position, to be bathed if sweating, to be helped to breathe, and so forth.

The restlessness of a dying person is often caused by the feeling of being too hot. People often don't realize this, because the skin becomes cold as circulation to the peripheral parts begins to cease. But inside, the person's body is hot, and the circulation is failing to radiate that heat away in the normal fashion. Fresh, moving air helps. Light is comforting; a dying person may ask to be allowed to lie in the sun, and dying people turn toward the light. Soothing music may help, but be sure it's of a kind the person doesn't dislike. And don't whisper nearby; speak audibly or not at all.

According to an authority on dying, it is always easy at the last. There is an interval of perfect peace and often of ecstasy before death, perhaps because pain ceases. The words of people who could speak at the moment of death indicate that they experience no suffering at that point.[24]

≡▶   *People can learn the signs of impending death and how to provide physical and emotional comfort for the dying.*

■≡ Grief

Chapter 3 described the grief process in relation to losses in general, but not in relation to death. The death of a loved one may be a major loss, and the grief surrounding it takes many forms.[25] A person who is dying grieves the loss of life; others who love that person grieve the loss of the person. Grief at death is unavoidable and painful, but education about grief may help people cope when it happens. To review the stages, they are:

■ Denial—"No, it can't be!"
■ Anger—"Why me? It's too soon!"
■ Bargaining—"I'll do anything; just let me live."
■ Depression—withdrawal, loss of hope.
■ Acceptance—"I am ready, now. It's all right."

The stages are experienced both by the dying person and by those nearby, and they are quite universal.[26] It helps to know that you will experience these emotions, sometimes over and over again, in the process of coming to accept death. Not everyone goes through all the stages, however, and not everyone expresses their feelings to the same extent or in the same way.

People can also handle grief better when they realize that they have something to *do* about it: they have "grief work" to do.[27] Our culture has some traditions that, though painful, help people come to terms after a death has occurred. These include arranging for care of the body, writing obituaries, notifying friends and relatives, conducting the funeral ceremony and burial, thanking donors for gifts and letters, and disposing of possessions. At the same time, people need to take care of their own health as well as possible during their grief. Grieving people are advised to continue the same patterns of sleeping, eating, and activity as before the death.[28]

If people avoid doing their grief work, they are likely to suffer more in the long run. They tend to experience delayed grief reactions, or to experience later maladjustment.[29]

When providing support to someone who has lost a loved one, many people make the mistake of being attentive only immediately after the death. The care usually stops when the casseroles stop, a week or so after the funeral. And that, ironically, is just about the time the sense of loss really begins to sink in for most bereaved families. Instead, people can better help the grieving families if they spread the care out so that it doesn't stop after ten days. People can help especially well if they remember the person's loss even years after the death. For example, parents of a child who has passed away will never forget their child's birthday. They'll grieve on that day for the rest of their lives. Being sensitive at times like these can help people cope with grief.

When trying to provide support to a grieving person, it may be helpful to reassure yourself that you can't take away the pain, but you can show how much you care. In speechless situations, the best approach may be a warm touch and the question, "What can I say?" You don't have to learn smart things to say; just be there. The most profoundly anguishing question is "Why?" When one pastor is asked this, he replies, "My theology doesn't tell me why—there's a question mark there."

After someone has died, people often think it's best not to mention the dead person to the survivors. "I don't want to remind them," they think. "Let's stay off the subject. I don't want to stir up their grief." Yet the very opposite is more often advisable. After someone close has died, the memory is still very much alive. People can't suddenly shut off all thoughts of someone they've loved. It actually helps survivors to know you're thinking of the person, too. You should mention the person when the thought crosses your mind. Bring back and share memories: "Sis would have enjoyed this," or "I thought of your mom today," or "Did I ever tell you about the discussion your husband and I had"—remarks like these let the grieving person know that you, too, remember and miss the one who is gone.

For as long as they occur to you, such comments are appropriate. Grief has no time limit. You may have heard that it takes about a year to get over someone's death. The tradition that a widow or widower should grieve for a year has some validity, for that permits every occasion throughout the year to pass, once, without the person with whom it had been shared earlier— religious holidays, birthdays, anniversaries, and all the rest. But grief can spring to the heart years after a loss and be felt as keenly as if the person had died just yesterday. It may never be completely gone, and if you care about

■ *FACT OR FICTION:* To avoid upsetting a bereaved person, it's best not to talk about the person who has died. *False.* Mentioning the person who is gone comforts the grieving person, for it shows that you, too, feel the loss.

■ ■ ■ ■ □ *STRATEGIES:* COPING WITH GRIEF

To help yourself through your grief over the loss of a loved one:

1. Be patient with yourself. Grief lasts far longer than society recognizes.
2. Give yourself permission to cope in your own way, knowing that each person who feels the loss will do it differently.
3. Cry freely as you feel the need. And don't hesitate to laugh; laughing brings the same relief as tears.
4. Anticipate that you will feel anger and guilt, and realize that these are normal reactions, as are thoughts of suicide. Express your feelings as openly as you wish.
5. Tell friends and relatives how they can help. Let them know, for example, that you want to talk about the person who has died.
6. Try to find a balance of time alone and time with others.
7. Be sure to include children in the grieving process. Children may feel to blame for a death; they experience the same grief you do; and they need to feel loved when they grieve.
8. Expect disruptions of your eating, exercise, and sleeping habits. Strive for a balanced diet, moderate exercise, and rest.
9. Expect disruptions of your sexual appetite. Seek affection, and ask for understanding.
10. Use no drugs or alcohol. They delay the grieving process and can lead to addiction.
11. Try not to make major decisions, such as moves and job changes, for at least one year.
12. Don't rush to dispose of the deceased person's possessions, and don't allow other people to take over the task. Deal with belongings bit by bit as you feel ready. It is helpful to talk about the deceased person, look at photographs, and keep the memories alive.
13. Anticipate tough times on holidays, birthdays, and anniversaries. Allow time and space for your emotional needs.
14. Don't be alarmed if you find yourself questioning your basic spiritual beliefs. Talk about it. In the process of examining their faith, many find comfort in accepting the unacceptable.
15. Consider joining a support group to ease the loneliness and promote expression of your grief.

---

the person who is grieving, you will be willing to share in those feelings whenever they arise.

It is considered unhealthy, though, to grieve without relief for an unusually long time. Sometimes people don't seem able to pull out of grief; they get stuck. Such people may need help, and it is not necessarily supportive in such cases to indulge their grief forever. Grief counselors can help people to complete their goodbyes and move on. The accompanying strategies describe the steps involved.

≡▶ *Grief about death occurs in five stages. Understanding these stages can help people cope, at least intellectually, with their pain. People can help those who are grieving by being sensitive and supportive.*

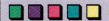

To help a friend grieve:

1. Feel free to hug and cry with your friend if it's appropriate to your relationship. Say that you care and that you're sorry.
2. Accept that you can't make the hurt go away or fully understand the depths of your friend's despair.
3. Don't say "I know how you feel," unless you've truly been in the same situation. Don't compare the death of a child, for example, to the death of a grandparent. Both events are painful, but in different ways.
4. It's better to listen than to offer verbal consolation. Allow your friend to share feelings of anger, frustration, or guilt. Expressing these feelings helps the bereaved person to move beyond them.
5. Be careful about imposing your personal religious beliefs. Your grieving friend may have possessed a strong faith in the past, but now may need to express anger and doubt without being judged. You may want to say that you don't understand the "why" of it, either.
6. Don't look for "positive" things to say. In the case of a child's death, don't tell parents they should be grateful they still have other children, or can replace the missing child. People are not interchangeable.
7. Pay special attention to bereaved children, who usually feel lost in the grieving process.
8. Don't impose a limit on someone else's recovery time. You add hurt to the grief when you imply that the person has the choice to feel no pain.
9. Don't compliment bereaved people by telling them how well they're doing a few months down the road. This implies an expectation of swift recovery and unduly rushes the grief process.
10. Do mention the deceased by name. Don't worry that you'll remind the bereaved of their loss—be assured that they're thinking of it anyway. The fear that nobody will remember is far greater than the pain of remembering.
11. Finally, take care of your own emotional needs. Give what support you can afford and want to give, and don't let guilt push you beyond that.

SOURCE: K. Olsen, Coping with grief: The hurt doesn't leave when the visitors do, *Tallahassee Democrat*, 8 July 1990, pp. 1G, 10G.

The most positive way to prepare for death is to use it as a reminder to live life to its fullest and savor the precious gift of life itself. Are there things that you want to do but keep putting off—because you think there is plenty of time? Whatever things you would do to make your life more personally meaningful before you die, do them *now*, because you *are* going to die—and you may not have the time or energy when you get your final notice.

■≡ For Review

1. Discuss why it is healthy to think about death.

2. Itemize legal ways that people can prepare for death.

3. Describe the value of having a living will.

4. Explain what a hospice is and what services it performs.

5. Discuss how people can prepare for death emotionally and spiritually.

6. Describe how a positive belief about life after death can help people face death.

7. Discuss near-death experiences.

8. Explain how you would go about easing a person's transition into death.

9. Describe the stages of grief.

10. List ways to help yourself grieve and ways to support a grieving friend.

■≡ Notes

1. E. P. Seravalli, The dying patient, the physician, and the fear of death, *New England Journal of Medicine* 319 (1988): 1728−1730.

2. N. G. Smedira and coauthors, Withholding and withdrawal of life support from the critically ill, *New England Journal of Medicine* 322 (1990): 309−315.

3. Avoiding a prolonged death, *Consumer Reports Health Letter* 2 (1990): 57−58.

4. B. Mishkin, Withholding and withdrawing nutritional support: Advance planning for hard choices, *Nutrition in Clinical Practice* 1 (1986): 50−52.

5. J. E. Ruark, T. A. Raffin, and the Stanford University Medical Center Committee on Ethics, Initiating and withdrawing life support−Principles and practice in adult medicine, *New England Journal of Medicine* 318 (1988): 25−30.

6. Living wills: Asserting your right to refuse treatment, *University of Texas Lifetime Health Letter,* March 1990, p. 2.

7. Mishkin, 1986.

8. R. Steinbrook and B. Lo, Artificial feeding−Solid ground, not a slippery slope, *New England Journal of Medicine* 318 (1988): 286−290.

9. Mishkin, 1986.

10. A. Ford, Looking after the old folks, *American Journal of Public Health* 77 (1987): 1499−1500.

11. J. S. Oktay and P. J. Volland, Foster home care for the frail elderly as an alternative to nursing home care: An experimental evaluation, *American Journal of Public Health* 77 (1987): 1505−1510.

12. W. Bulkin and H. Lukashok, Rx for dying: The case for hospice, *New England Journal of Medicine* 318 (1988): 376−378.

13. *Hospice in America* (a brochure available from the National Hospice Organization, 1901 N. Fort Myer Dr., Suite 307, Arlington, VA 22209); S. V. Dobihal, Enabling a patient to die at home, *American Journal of Nursing,* August 1980, pp. 1448−1451.

14. S. T. Putnam and coauthors, Home as a place to die, *American Journal of Nursing,* August 1980, pp. 1451−1453.

15. E. Kubler-Ross, *On Death and Dying* (Hudson River, N.Y.: Macmillan, 1991).

16. Luke 24:4; Revelation 2:7.

17. Revelation 7:17, 21:4.

18. Near-death experiences, *Consumer Reports Health Letter,* February 1991, p. 16.

19. P. Perry, Knowing near death, *Psychology Today,* September 1988, pp. 16−17.

20. Perry, 1988.

21. Seravalli, 1988.

22. Kubler-Ross, 1975.

23. A. Worcester, *The Care of the Aged, the Dying and the Dead,* 2d ed. (Springfield, Ill.: Charles C. Thomas, 1961), pp. 33−61.

24. Worcester, 1961.

25. T. L. Martin, The study of grief: An in-depth look at a response to loss, *American Journal of Hospice Care* 6 (1989): 27.

26. R. Kelly, Teaching a course on death and dying, in *Death and Dying Education,* ed. R. O. Ulin (Washington, D.C.: National Education Association, 1977), pp. 22−23.

27. Kelly, 1977, p. 23.

28. J. Kaprio, Love and death, *Psychology Today,* November 1989, p. 18.

29. Kubler-Ross, 1991.

SPOTLIGHT

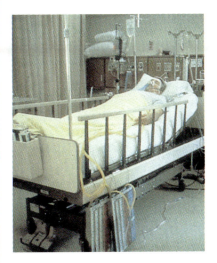

Allowing Death by Withdrawing Artificial Feeding

A person is terminally ill, is unconscious, and has no hope of recovery. The high-tech machines that were supporting the person's life have been shut down. Still the person lingers, seemingly endlessly, in a coma. All the nurses do, now, is keep replenishing the feeding formula that drips through a tube into the person's vein or stomach; changing the bag that collects the person's wastes; and washing and turning the body. Should the tube be withdrawn? Is it time to stop giving even food? The medical and court systems are struggling with the question of whether it is legitimate to withdraw nutrition support in such cases.

Why are they singling out nutrition support to worry about?

Only in recent years has the medical profession become able to provide nourishment to clients unable to eat by mouth. This technical advancement has saved many lives. However, as is true with other medical technologies, the availability of special nutrition support forces health care professionals and society to face ethical issues—specifically, the question of when it is morally and legally appropriate to discontinue use of nutrition support techniques. Health care professionals also ask when such treatments are prolonging life and when they are merely delaying death.

Don't health care professionals normally provide whatever form of nutrition is necessary to support all clients?

Yes, normally they do, if the clients have any chance of recovering and then sustaining an acceptable quality of life. Clearly, health care professionals cannot rightfully withhold nutrition support because of poor judgment or negligence. If a client were to die because nourishment was withheld, the staff and facility would be held responsible, and in all likelihood, a malpractice lawsuit would result.

The decision of whether to feed a client becomes less clear, however, when the client is not expected to recover. How aggressively should the person who is terminally ill or in a persistent vegetative state be supported? How should health care providers respond to elderly or physically disabled clients who refuse nutrition support because they feel the quality of their lives is so poor that they do not wish to be

sustained? Are health care professionals morally and legally obligated to comply with, or to deny, such requests? Furthermore, when clients are incompetent and unable to speak for themselves, who, if anyone, should be allowed to make life-and-death decisions? These questions represent but a few of the unanswered concerns that have evolved along with the technology of nutrition support.

What does the law say on the matter?

The court system has ruled on several cases. Some cases have involved alert adults who were competent to evaluate a treatment and comprehend the risks of refusing or accepting the treatment. Other cases have involved people in a persistent vegetative state. The accompanying box presents a brief review of several landmark decisions. In each case, the court weighs the state's rights against the individual's right to refuse medical treatment. The state is supposed to preserve life, to prevent suicide, and to support the integrity of the medical profession. Table S16–1 lists general conditions under which it is considered appropriate to withhold or provide medical treatment.

With respect to preserving life, the court examines the question of whether a client will return to conscious life or just continue a biological existence. On suicide, the court considers whether withholding treatment would allow the underlying disease to take its course; if so, eventual death is not suicide. Regarding the integrity of the medical profession, the court holds that medical professionals should not be forced against their will to withhold

Landmark Court Cases on Withdrawing Artificial Feedings

1983–1986, Bouvia: A mentally competent 26-year-old quadriplegic woman who required assistance in eating wanted to be allowed to starve to death. Hospital officials believed that to discontinue feeding would make them party to suicide, which is illegal. A lower court rejected Bouvia's request. Two years later, her condition worsened, and she was given a tube feeding against her will. The California Second District Court of Appeals ordered removal of the tube, stating that her right to refuse treatment was absolute, regardless of her motives or whether her illness was terminal.

1985–1986, Requenia: A competent 55-year-old woman refused tube feeding. The hospital objected and arranged for her transfer to another facility. When she refused to transfer, the hospital sued her to leave. The court ordered the hospital staff to honor her request to decline feeding.

1985–1986, Brophy: The wife and family of a 49-year-old man in a persistent vegetative state requested discontinuance of artificial feeding. Brophy had made his wishes known to them prior to his illness, and it was apparent that his active life was over. When his physicians and the hospital opposed the request, the case went to probate court. The judge decided to continue feeding even though he realized that Brophy would decline artificial feeding if competent. The Massachusetts Supreme Judicial Court overruled the lower court and held that Brophy's feeding tube could be removed.

1985–1987, Jobes: The family of a 31-year-old woman in a persistent vegetative state requested discontinuance of her tube feeding. A lower court ruled that the nursing home could continue tube feeding until transfer arrangements could be made. The New Jersey Supreme Court ordered the nursing home to honor the request to discontinue feeding and to continue to provide care until her death.

1986, Corbett: The Florida Second District Court of Appeals allowed the removal of a feeding tube from a 75-year-old woman in a persistent vegetative state. This decision took precedence over Florida's law that specifically forbids clients to decline "provision of sustenance."

1987, Peter: The New Jersey Supreme Court found no distinction between artificial feeding and other forms of life-sustaining treatment and allowed the withdrawal of a feeding tube from a 65-year-old woman in a persistent vegetative state.

1987–1988, Gray: The family of a 49-year-old woman in a persistent vegetative state requested discontinuance of her artificial feeding. When the hospital objected, the Federal District Court of Rhode Island ordered the hospital to honor the request to discontinue feeding.

1988, O'Connor: The daughters of a 78-year-old woman who had severe, irreversible loss of mental function refused to allow a hospital to insert a feeding tube. They believed that their mother would not want any form of life support. The New York Court of Appeals ruled that a feeding tube must be inserted unless there was unequivocal evidence that the client would have chosen to refuse it.

feedings. Arrangements to withhold feedings can, however, be made with physicians who are willing. The emerging consensus seems to support the opinion that individuals do have the right to refuse medical treatment—including artificial feedings (such as by tube or by vein). Authorities seem to agree that people have the right to refuse such treatment even when that treatment is necessary to sustain life.[1]*

Several court cases have argued the distinction between providing medical care and providing nourishment and hydration. They suggest that to "pull the plug" on a life-support machine is acceptable, but that to deny food and water—the basics of life—is inhumane. However, the court system has defined nutrition support as a medical procedure rather than as routine care.[2]

What about the special case when a client is in a coma and cannot refuse or accept medical treatment—when the person's wishes are not known?

Without knowledge of an incompetent person's wishes, the court decides in the client's "best interest." For many families, it becomes their burden to convince the court that discontinuing feeding is in the client's "best interest." Consider the case of Nancy Cruzan, a young woman who suffered permanent and irreversible brain damage after a car crash in January 1983. Since then, she had been in a persistent vegetative state—

*Reference notes are at the end of the Spotlight.

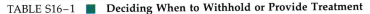

TABLE S16–1 ■ **Deciding When to Withhold or Provide Treatment**

It is considered reasonable to withhold treatment if:
■ The person is clearly going to die, even with treatment.
■ The means necessary to prolong life would be painful or invasive.
■ Those who know the person well are reasonably certain that the person would want such a choice to be made.

It is considered wrong to withhold treatment if:
■ The treatment might conceivably restore the quality of life.
■ The treatment is not painful or invasive.
■ The person would want his or her life prolonged.

As long as they follow these guidelines, medical personnel and the family are generally permitted to make decisions without obtaining court permission. The court is appropriately called in if the decision is urgent and if there is uncertainty about:
■ The client's mental faculties.
■ The probable outcomes with or without treatment.
■ The consent of the client, spouse, or guardian.
■ The good faith or interests of those making the decision.

SOURCE: *Nursing Practice in the Care of the Dying* (Kansas City, Mo.: American Nurses Association, 1982), pp. 7–11.

awake but unaware. Her physicians and parents held no hope for recovery, but given food and water, she might have lived for another 30 years. Her parents' request to discontinue tube feeding was rejected by a lower court, and in 1989 it went to the U.S. Supreme Court as its first "right-to-die" case.

Cruzan's parents tried to convince the Supreme Court that their once independent and vivacious daughter would not want to live in a vegetative state. Their lawyer argued that Cruzan had a right to be free from medical intervention. No one questioned that Cruzan's parents knew their daughter's wishes better than anyone and had the highest and most loving motives. The question for the Court to consider was, Can families (or anyone) make life-and-death decisions on behalf of incompetent persons?

The Supreme Court recognized that competent adults have the right to stop life-sustaining treatments. But, in a 5-to-4 decision, the Court decided that life-sustaining treatment could not be withdrawn without "clear and convincing" evidence that the incompetent person would refuse treatment.[3] The Supreme Court left it to state legislatures to establish laws that would address the issue of whether families (or other third parties) could authorize the withdrawal of life-sustaining treatment on behalf of incompetent persons without such exacting evidence. Then, after another round of court battles, Cruzan's feeding tube was removed on December 14, 1990, and she died from dehydration two weeks later.

Keeping Cruzan alive must have been expensive.

The costs involved in supporting Cruzan were phenomenal. The financial cost of supporting her ran about $130,000 per year (it was paid by the state). The emotional costs were also horrendous. Cruzan's parents first had to face the shock of their daughter's accident. Then, for several years, they held hope that she would regain consciousness. Then, they endured court battles over their child's fate—a fate that held grief whichever way it turned.

Have other such cases occurred?

Yes. The Cruzans were one family. There are, at any given time, 10,000 such families of people who live in a persistent vegetative state. No doubt, the Supreme Court's decision has widespread implications for these people and the health professionals who care for them. In fact, this decision touches all of us, because it influences the extent to which society views life-sustaining treatment as optional for ourselves and our families.[4] It decides how we may be allowed to die.[5]

■≡ Spotlight Notes

1. S. H. Miles, P. A. Singer, and M. Siegler, Conflicts between patients' wishes to forgo treatment and the policies of health care facilities, *New England Journal of Medicine* 321 (1989): 48–50; R. Steinbrook and B. Lo, Artificial feeding—Solid ground, not a slippery slope, *New England Journal of Medicine* 318 (1988): 286–290.

2. R. Dresser, Discontinuing nutrition support: A review of the case law, *Journal of the American Dietetic Association* 85 (1985): 1289–1292.

3. Supreme Court of the United States Syllabus, *Cruzan, by her parents and co-guardians, Cruzan et ux. v. Director, Missouri Department of Health, et al.,* no. 88-1503. Argued December 6, 1989—decided June 25, 1990.

4. M. Angell, Prisoners of technology: The case of Nancy Cruzan, *New England Journal of Medicine* 322 (1990): 1226–1228; B. Lo, F. Rouse, and L. Dornbrand, Family decision making on trial—Who decides for incompetent patients? *New England Journal of Medicine* 322 (1990): 1228–1232.

5. The Court and Nancy Cruzan, *Hastings Center Report,* January/February 1990, pp. 38–50.

CHAPTER 17

Infectious Diseases

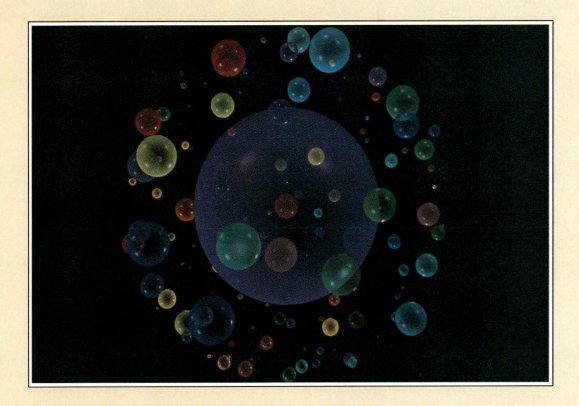

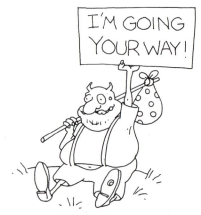

You are surrounded; microbes are all around you.

microbes (microorganisms) minute organisms, too small to be seen with the naked eye, such as bacteria, yeasts, and viruses.

infectious diseases diseases transmitted from person to person caused by microorganisms or their toxins; also called *communicable* or *contagious diseases*. A separate Miniglossary of Infectious Diseases appears on page 462.

endogenous bacteria the normally harmless bacterial residents of the human body, which live on the skin, in the digestive tract, and elsewhere.

pathogens (PATH-oh-jens) disease-causing microbes.

opportunists in general, creatures that take advantage of opportunities that come their way. Of microbes, those that can infect when an altered physiological state of the host provides an opportunity, although they ordinarily cause no harm.

Y ou are surrounded by **microbes**. They are all around you—on the surfaces you touch, in the air you breathe, on the forkfuls of food that you lift to your mouth, and on the surfaces of your body. Most are harmless, but others can cause **infectious diseases**. This chapter describes microbes and their world, along with the risks of infection they present to people. It discusses two kinds of defenses against disease-causing organisms: public health measures and your body's own remarkable defenses. Then it singles out sexually transmitted diseases for special attention and offers strategies for protection.

■≡ Agents of Infection

A microbe is a living thing that is too small for the unaided human eye to see. Early scientists, using crude lenses, could see only the giants of the microbial world—molds, yeasts, algae, the largest bacteria, worms, and other creatures. With more powerful microscopes, smaller and smaller microbes have become visible, some so small that they contain only a few molecules.

Microbes can be beneficial. For example, the normal microbes of the intestines, **endogenous bacteria**, protect against some diseases. If they are reduced in numbers, infections become more likely, because disease-causing microbes, or **pathogens**, encounter less competition and more nutrients when they try to invade. Some normally harmless endogenous bacteria can become pathogenic, given the opportunity. If a person's immune system becomes weakened, or if a wound occurs, these **opportunists** may invade and cause illness.

Table 17–1 lists the general classes of microbes. Within the classes, there are both innocent and pathogenic varieties, but the table gives examples only of a few pathogens within each class. The Miniglossary of Infectious Diseases names and defines a few of the diseases the pathogens produce, and the next three sections describe some of the most common kinds of disease agents.

Bacteria

The **bacteria** are simple, microscopic, single-celled organisms. Though often associated only with disease, bacteria are important in digestion, and in the making of products such as yogurt and cheese. Many bacteria grow and multiply best in an environment like that found in the human body: warm, dark, moist, and nutrient-rich.

Notice that oxygen is not listed as a requirement for bacteria. Some bacteria, the **aerobes**, require it, but others, the **anaerobes**, require environments that are devoid of oxygen. (Some can handle both.) Anaerobes make puncture wounds dangerous, because they can thrive in the interior of the wounds, where medicines applied to the surface cannot reach. Normally, ordinary soap makes it easy to wash pathogens away with water, but a puncture wound requires more. One first aid measure for a puncture wound is to pour the compound hydrogen peroxide into it. Hydrogen peroxide produces bubbles of oxygen that not only wash out the deep bacteria, but also make conditions too oxygen-rich for the anaerobes. Some recommend applying an antibacterial cream on open wounds.

One anaerobe causes the infamous disease tetanus, a disease that, once started, is fatal. Tetanus shots provide immunity against the bacterial toxin that causes the disease. Because of the threat of tetanus, any deep cut or puncture wound demands treatment by a health professional. Remember that Appendix E offers basic first aid techniques. Much more can be learned in a first aid class.

A wound provides an opportunity for bacteria on the inhospitable skin to take up residence in warm, moist, nutrient-rich body fluid, where they can grow and multiply (**infection**). If you fail to treat an infected wound, the bacteria may invade the bloodstream, causing a dangerous, generalized blood infection (**septicemia**). Periodic washing of the skin with soap and water protects against opportunists. Chemicals that prevent growth of bacteria on the skin are **antiseptics**; drugs that prevent their multiplication in the body are **antibiotics**; and chemicals that kill bacteria on surfaces such as tabletops, countertops, and dishes, and in the water, are **disinfectants**.

Bacteria can invade uninjured skin, too. One example is the skin bacteria that aggravate acne when the pores become clogged. Infection sets in when debris collects for the bacteria to feed on and they multiply. (For self-care of acne, see the Spotlight following Chapter 1, "Your Body—An Owner's Manual.") Another example—people who use hot tubs often develop skin rashes and ear infections from the bacteria that thrive in the infrequently changed warm water.[1]* (Hot tubs are harder to keep safe than regular swimming pools, because the heat and rapid water motion promote fast evaporation of the disinfectant chlorine.)

A bacterial infection of the lungs, tuberculosis, is the world's number-one killer disease. Deaths from tuberculosis had declined for years in the United States, but the number of cases is on the rise again.[2] Researchers cite the AIDS epidemic as a contributing factor (more about AIDS in a later section).[3]

≡▶ *Bacteria are one of the potential agents of infection. Pathogenic bacteria can cause disease in the body or on the skin.*

*Reference notes are at the end of the chapter.

bacteria (singular, **bacterium**) microscopic, single-celled organisms of varying shapes and sizes, some capable of causing disease.

aerobes (AIR-robes) microbes that require oxygen to grow. (Some can become anaerobic if the environment changes.)

anaerobes (AN-air-robes) microbes that require an oxygen-free environment to grow. (Some can become aerobic, if need be.)

Appendix E describes types of wounds and first aid for them.

infection growth and multiplication of pathogens within the human body, causing disease.

septicemia (sep-tih-SEE-me-uh) a generalized infection that spreads by way of the blood throughout the body.

antiseptics agents that prevent the growth of microorganisms on body surfaces and on wounds.

antibiotics drugs that prevent growth of bacteria in the body.

disinfectants chemicals that kill microbes on surfaces and in water.

TABLE 17–1   ■   Microbes That Surround Us

	Microbes	Common Pathogens and Diseases	Transmission	Control
 Tuberculosis bacteria.	*Bacteria* Bacteria come in many shapes and sizes. They can be seen through an ordinary light microscope.	*Vibrio cholerae* produces a toxin that causes cholera. *Legionella pneumophila* produces a type of pneumonia (legionellosis). *Mycobacterium tuberculosis* disguises itself by growing inside immune cells; it causes tuberculosis.	Bacteria are everywhere. Some make airborne spores that reproduce when conditions are right. Bacteria can live on surfaces and be transferred when people touch them, breathe in airborne droplets containing them, or ingest water and food containing them.	Antibiotics treat internal infections; antiseptics kill those on the skin. Soap and water remove bacteria, and prolonged pressure, heat, or radiation destroys them. Disinfectants such as bleach can kill them on surfaces.
 AIDS viruses leaving a cell.	*Viruses* Viruses are simpler than cells; each consists of a protein coat that contains a genetic message. They can be observed only through the highest-power electron microscope.	Hepatitis A viruses cause the liver disease hepatitis. T-lymphotropic viruses cause AIDS. Herpes simplex I causes cold sores; herpes simplex II causes genital sores. The common cold is caused by viruses.	Viruses can survive but cannot thrive outside the host body. They are transmitted quickly from host to host by direct contact, by the breath, by excretions, and by shared utensils. They can survive briefly on surfaces.	Viruses are destroyed by high heat and chemical agents. Most are invulnerable to medicines, but vaccines can help people build up immunity to viruses.
 Ringworm fungus.	*Fungi (yeasts and molds)* Fungi come in distinctive shapes and colors; some resemble minute flowers. Fungi are visible under an ordinary light microscope.	Several fungi species of the group dermatophytes cause athlete's foot. *Candida albicans*, a yeast, can infect many body parts, including mouth, fingers, and vagina.	Like bacteria, fungi are everywhere. Many have reproductive spores especially good at air travel because they are light in weight and can survive periods of dehydration.	Chemical agents destroy molds and fungi on surfaces. Drugs can fight the infections fungi cause, although they are not so effective as against bacteria.

TABLE 17–1 ■ continued

Microbes	Common Pathogens and Diseases	Transmission	Control
Parasitic Worms Most parasites live as microscopic organisms for at least part of their life cycles. Typical are worms that damage blood vessels, vital organs, or muscle tissue, before reproducing and being passed on to other hosts.	*Taeniarhynchus saginatus* is a tapeworm found in infected beef. This causes intestinal disorders and weight loss. Roundworms cause inflammation of the rectum, vomiting, rash, and diarrhea. Hookworms cause intestinal bleeding.	Parasites usually are transmitted to human beings when they eat infected meats, seafood, or soil.	Parasites are best controlled by thoroughly cooking all meats and seafood and not ingesting soil.
Rickettsia Rickettsia are viruslike organisms that require a host's living cells for growth and replication.	*Rickettsia prowazekii* causes typhus. *R. rickettsii* causes Rocky Mountain Spotted Fever.	Rickettsia are transmitted to human beings by the bites of arthropods such as insects.	Rickettsia are best controlled by destruction of insects.
Protozoa These are the simplest animal form, one-celled organisms. The group includes ciliates, amebas, flagellates, and sporozoans.	*Naegleria fowleri,* an ameba that reproduces in stagnant water, can cause severe and fatal swelling of the brain and spinal chord. *Plasmodium* species invade blood cells and destroy them, causing malaria. Amebic dysentery and *Giardia lamblia* are caused by protozoa.	Protozoa enter the body through the nose or mouth from an aquatic environment.	Harmful protozoa are best controlled by chlorination of the water supply.

Head of a tapeworm.

Rickettsia.

Giardia lamblia.

■ MINIGLOSSARY
of Infectious Diseases

---

acne a skin disease characterized by chronic inflammation of the sebaceous glands, usually causing pimples of the face, back, and chest.

athlete's foot a fungal infection of the feet, usually transmitted through floors; wearing rubber shower shoes will reduce the likelihood of its transmission.

bubonic plague a bacterial infection causing swollen lymph glands and pneumonia, frequently fatal. Also called *black plague* or *black death,* it caused the near extinction of the human race in the Middle Ages and is still common in India today. It is transmitted to people by bites from fleas, which in turn live on rodents, so extermination of the rodent hosts aids in control of the disease. Immunizations are also effective.

chicken pox a usually mild, easily transmitted disease causing fever, weakness, and itchy blisters that, if scratched, may leave permanent scars on the skin. The herpes virus that causes chicken pox stays in the body for life and may later emerge as the painful skin condition called **shingles**. Once a person has been infected, immunity to chicken pox is lifelong.

cholera (KAH-ler-uh) a dangerous bacterial infection causing violent muscle cramps, severe vomiting and diarrhea, and severe water loss; without treatment, death is likely. People contract cholera by consuming infected water, milk, or foods (especially seafood harvested from contaminated water).

common cold a group of highly contagious, upper respiratory infections that last from two to ten days; many different viruses and a few bacteria cause colds.

diphtheria a bacterial infection of the respiratory system that causes leathery obstructions of the airways; preventable by immunization.

encephalitis inflammation of the brain caused by viral infection. Mosquito control prevents transmission.

flu short for **influenza**, a highly contagious respiratory infection caused by a variety of viruses; symptoms often include coughing, sneezing, fever, chills, and headache that spontaneously abate in two to seven days. Older or ill people need yearly vaccines; the viruses change their identities quickly, and immunity against last year's variety is generally useless against the current type.

hepatitis inflammation of the liver caused by one of several types of viruses that are transmitted mainly by infected hypodermic needles (drug use, tattoos, blood transfusions), by eating raw seafood harvested from contaminated water, and by any contact (including sexual contact) with body secretions from infected people. Sewage treatment and monitoring of commercial fisheries reduce these sources of infections.

infectious mononucleosis a viral infection with early symptoms similar to those of flu; later symptoms may include swollen lymph glands, skin rash, or jaundice (skin yellowing due to liver malfunction). It is not a dangerous disease, but it is long lasting and tends to recur. The mode of transmission is unknown, but kissing is suspected.

influenza see *flu.*

Legionnaires' disease a type of pneumonia caused by aquatic bacteria that can live in air-conditioning systems.

Viruses

viruses organisms that contain only genetic material and protein coats, and that are totally dependent on the cells they invade; they draw upon the cell contents for reproduction.

The **viruses** are a unique life form, in that they depend entirely on the living tissue of other organisms. Outside of living cells, they have no way of reproducing. They do not eat, they do not breathe, they do not grow or mature. Each virus has a body that is the ultimate in simplicity: it is made only of a bit of genetic material that can direct a cell to reproduce the virus, and a protein case in which to carry that material.

■ MINIGLOSSARY
(continued)

malaria a parasite common to the tropics that resides within the red blood cells of the host, destroying the cells and causing high fever, anemia, and other symptoms. Mosquitoes transmit it to people who carry the parasite thereafter.

measles a highly contagious viral disease characterized by rash, high fever, sensitivity to light, and cough and cold symptoms; preventable by immunization.

mono see *infectious mononucleosis*.

multiple sclerosis a slowly developing disease of the central nervous system in which the nerve fiber coverings are destroyed. The cause is unknown, but a slow-acting virus is suspected.

mumps a highly contagious viral disease that causes swelling of the salivary glands and, occasionally, of the testicles; preventable by immunization.

pertussis a respiratory infection characterized by a violent cough with noisy gasping; also called *whooping cough*; preventable by immunization.

pneumonia inflammation of the lungs with high fever, cough, and pain in the chest. A wide variety of bacteria, viruses, and some fungi cause pneumonia.

polio (poliomyelitis) a viral infection that produces mild respiratory or digestive symptoms in most cases but that afflicts some victims with severe, permanent paralysis or death from respiratory failure; preventable by immunization.

rabies a disease of the central nervous system that causes paralysis and death. Mammals transmit it by biting. During the incubation period, treatment with vaccine halts the disease; once it is started, there is no cure.

rheumatic fever a childhood illness that may attack and scar the valves of the heart, leading to heart disease. See also *strep throat*.

rubella a short-duration infectious disease (lasts three to five days) that resembles measles but that does not involve high fever or serious complications for the sufferer; preventable by immunization.

shingles see *chicken pox*.

smallpox a severe viral infection with skin eruptions similar to those of chicken pox but occurring all at once, about three or four days after the onset of the illness. Smallpox, once often fatal and permanently disfiguring to those who survived, is now under control worldwide, thanks to immunizations.

strep throat a severe sore throat, accompanied by fever and other symptoms, caused by *Streptococcus* bacteria. Strep throat or an earache caused by the same bacteria always precedes rheumatic fever, and therefore should be properly diagnosed and treated.

tetanus a disease caused by a toxin produced by bacteria deep within a wound, which causes sustained contractions of body muscles and results in rigidity of the body and death from lack of oxygen or from exhaustion; preventable by immunization. Also called *lockjaw*.

traveler's diarrhea sudden and severe diarrhea with general illness, caused by bacteria or parasites from the water supply; especially likely in countries with unsophisticated public health programs.

tuberculosis a bacterial infection of the lungs.

whooping cough see *pertussis*.

Once inside a living cell, viral genes take over the cell's own genetic machinery and force it to serve their purposes—to reproduce viruses (see Figure 17–1). The cell replicates exact copies of the virus's genetic material and the parts that make up the protein coat, using up the cell's own energy fuels and raw materials in the process. From the pieces, new viruses assemble themselves. Then, typically, the cell bursts open, liberating multitudes of

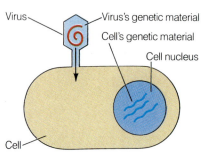

Virus ──── Virus's genetic material
Cell's genetic material
Cell nucleus

Cell ────

(a) Virus attaches to cell and injects its
    genetic material.

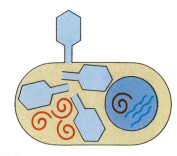

(b) Viral genes take over cell nucleus and
    direct the making of new viral materials.

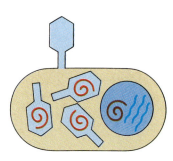

(c) Viral materials self-assemble into viruses.

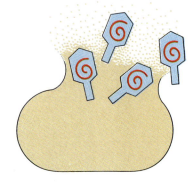

(d) Cell bursts, releasing a multitude of
    new viruses.

FIGURE 17–1 ■ **How viruses multiply
and cause infections.**

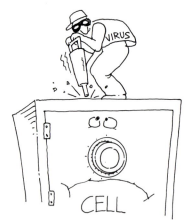

Viruses cause diseases by invading cells.

■ *FACT OR FICTION:* Antibiotics are
among the few medicines effective against
viruses. *False.* Antibiotics are useful against
bacteria but useless against viruses.

viruses that invade neighboring cells and restart the process. The only way
to stop them is to build immune defenses against them within the body, or
to deny them access to the body.

When a person contracts a viral disease, treatment usually consists of
minimizing damage and relieving symptoms while the body responds to the
virus and eventually overcomes the disease. This process is often described
as letting the disease run its course. Antibiotics, effective against bacterial
infections, are useless against viruses and can be dangerous in the long run
(see the accompanying box, How Antibiotics Can Do More Harm Than
Good).

Once the disease symptoms have subsided, the person may be free of the
virus; however, some viruses can take up residence in the body to remain
for life. In later years they can cause disease once again: an example is
shingles, a painful skin condition in adults that is caused by the reemergence of the virus that brought them chicken pox as children. An adult with
shingles can pass the virus to others, who will get chicken pox if they have
not previously had the illness.

≡▶ *Viruses depend entirely on the living tissue of other organisms. They invade
cells and cause disease symptoms until they run their course. Some viruses remain
in the body for life.*

How Antibiotics Can Do More Harm Than Good

Almost everyone has taken an antibiotic for one infection or another. However, these drugs are overused in the United States, and as a result, antibiotic-resistant bacteria are increasingly becoming a threat to health.

Consider a story that begins when a person takes an antibiotic for strep throat. The person starts out with a large population of normal, harmless bacteria in the digestive tract. While the antibiotic is killing the strep bacteria, it also wipes many of these intestinal bacteria—but not all of them. The most sensitive bacteria stop multiplying, but those that are resistant to the drug survive and multiply. Thus a population of drug-resistant bacteria succeeds the original population. These bacteria do no harm at the moment, but their drug resistance sets the stage for a major problem.

Bacteria are sometimes able to give up portions of their genetic material, **plasmids**, to other bacteria. The plasmids jump out of one bacterial body into another nearby. Once a normal inhabitant of the digestive tract has developed drug-resistance, it may transfer this drug resistance by way of plasmids into pathogenic bacteria that happen along later on. Thus it is possible to start a strain of pathogens that will not yield to antibiotic therapy.

The sequence, then, is this. An infection is treated with an antibiotic. The antibiotic elicits drug resistance within the body's normal bacteria. Then along comes another infection; the pathogen picks up this drug resistance; and now the antibiotic cannot cure the infection.

Some people fear that we are rendering one of our most effective weapons, antibiotics, powerless by overusing them. Overuse of antibiotics stems partly from a lack of understanding of what they can and cannot do. For example, most virus-caused diseases, such as the common cold, do not respond to antibiotics, but people take antibiotics for colds anyway. Each such treatment sets the stage for drug-resistant bacteria to develop. People also misuse antibiotics in a way that encourages drug-resistant bacteria to develop: they stop taking the prescription as soon as the symptoms disappear. When enough bacteria have been killed, relief from symptoms occurs, but a few bacteria are left; these must be wiped out by several days more of antibiotic treatment. If they multiply, they will produce billions of new bacterial cells to fill the space formerly occupied by the ones that died. This means they will have billions more opportunities to produce antibiotic-resistant strains, and if such a strain arises it will have an especially good chance of multiplying because the antibiotic has wiped out its competition. Always finish your prescription.

Some people use illegally obtained antibiotics or leftover prescriptions to try to self-treat diseases they would rather not seek help for, such as the sexually transmitted diseases. Not only do they take shots in the dark at their own cures, but they also risk creating and transmitting drug-resistant strains of pathogens. We now have among us antibiotic-resistant gonorrhea, food-poisoning bacteria, and strep throat bacteria.

New, stronger antibiotics, jokingly called "gorillacillins," can still wipe out some resistant strains of bacteria. Whether these, too, will lose their effectiveness after years of overuse remains to be seen.

plasmid a piece of genetic material that can be transmitted from one organism to another and can thus pass on an inheritable trait to the recipient. For example, plasmids can pass drug resistance from strain to strain of bacteria.

Other Agents of Infection

The **fungi** are organisms that absorb and use nutrients manufactured by other organisms, living or dead. Microscopic, one-celled forms of fungi are **yeasts**; the multicellular types are **molds** and mushrooms. The yeasts can be pathogenic, and they cause an enormous variety of illnesses, from athlete's foot to vaginal yeast infections (discussed later).

A **parasitic worm** is an organism that lives at the expense of another (called a **host**); these worms depend on their hosts for the nutrients they need. Common parasitic worms are flatworms, tapeworms, roundworms, pinworms, and hookworms. They make their living by inflicting bites on their hosts to obtain blood. Worldwide, parasitic worms cause many deaths. One of the most prominent is the roundworm that causes trichinosis, which is acquired when a person ingests uncooked infected pork. The worms enter the body and may invade muscle tissue, the stomach, brain, liver, and lungs. Like this roundworm, most parasitic worms cause diarrhea and blood loss—life-threatening to those without access to medical treatment.

The **rickettsia** are viruslike organisms that require a host's living cells for growth and replication. These are transmitted by the bite of an infected insect. Infected ticks transmit Rocky Mountain spotted fever and rickettsial pox.

The **protozoa** are single-celled organisms. They are responsible for many diseases of concern in the United States. The organism *Giardia* causes severe diarrhea. Another disease that has received a great deal of attention recently is a type of pneumonia caused by a protozoan observed in people with AIDS.

With so many pathogens bombarding everyone every day, why aren't people ill from infection most of the time? Actually, it would be so, except that people have defenses. The public health systems provide one, and people's immune systems provide another.

≡▶ *Other agents of infection include fungi, parasitic worms, rickettsia, and protozoa. Some can be life-threatening or cause a variety of mild or severe illnesses.*

■≡ Control of Infectious Diseases

Infectious diseases may occur in single individuals, or may go on the rampage, affecting whole populations. A disease that exists within a population at all times is called **endemic**; an infection that sweeps suddenly through a population is an **epidemic**; and a disease that spreads throughout the world is a **pandemic** disease.

Several factors are required to spread an infection:

1. A pathogen (an infecting organism).
2. A **reservoir** of infection—such as water, air, soil, food, or a host (an animal or a person).
3. A means of escaping from the reservoir (**portal of exit**).
4. A means of reaching the host, such as through the air, water, food, surfaces, sewage, etc. Nonliving transmitters of infection, such as towels or drinking glasses, are called **fomites**; a living thing, such as an insect, that transmits an infection is called a **vector**.

---

fungi organisms that absorb and use nutrients manufactured by other organisms. They include *yeasts* (microscopic and one-celled), and *molds* and mushrooms (visible), some causing diseases.

yeasts microscopic, one-celled fungi, some of which cause diseases.

molds multicellular fungi, some of which cause diseases.

parasitic worm a worm that lives within or upon, and at the expense of, another organism (the *host*).

host the organism at whose expense a parasite lives.

rickettsia viruslike organisms that require a host's living cells for growth and replication.

protozoa single-celled organisms; many are responsible for diseases.

endemic a term used to describe a disease that is always present in at least a few people in a population.

epidemic a disease that appears in many people in the same geographical location at the same time.

pandemic an epidemic that occurs around the globe.

reservoir (of infection) the source of an infectious disease agent, including people, animals, water, air, soil, or food.

portal of exit a site in the body that allows microbes to exit.

fomites nonliving things that transmit infection, such as blankets, dishes, and hypodermic needles.

vector a living thing that carries and transmits a disease-causing organism.

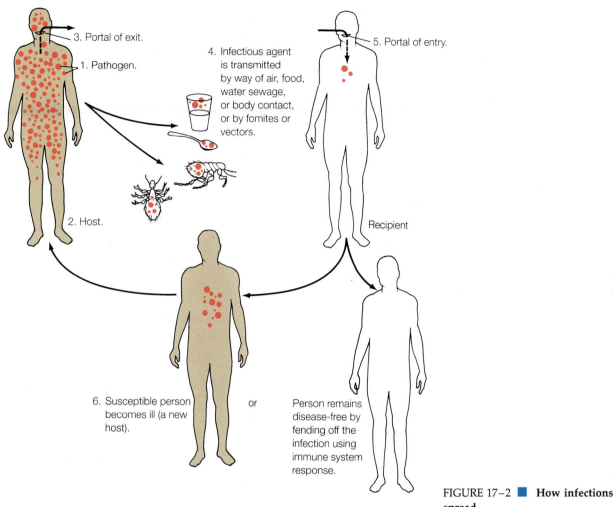

3. Portal of exit.

1. Pathogen.

4. Infectious agent is transmitted by way of air, food, water sewage, or body contact, or by fomites or vectors.

5. Portal of entry.

2. Host.

Recipient

6. Susceptible person becomes ill (a new host).

or

Person remains disease-free by fending off the infection using immune system response.

FIGURE 17–2 ■ **How infections spread.**

5. A means of entering the host's body (**portal of entry**), such as the soft membranes of the mouth, nose, or eyes, or a break in the skin.
6. Susceptibility of the new host to the infection.

Figure 17–2 demonstrates how infections are spread.

To prevent the spread of infection, one of these factors must be eliminated. It may sound easy, but only a sophisticated public health system can succeed.

portal of entry   a site in the body that allows microbes to enter.

Public Health Defenses

The discoveries of the pathogens and of drugs to combat them are two reasons that death rates from infectious diseases have remarkably declined since the early 1900s. The public sanitation measures of developed countries provide chlorination of public water supplies and treatment of sewage that destroy pathogens that could otherwise contaminate drinking water. Where sanitation is poor, sick people pass on diseases such as cholera through untreated water that has become contaminated with sewage. When people travel to developing countries, they must take precautions against water-borne infections, which cause traveler's diarrhea. Two such measures are to avoid raw foods and salads, and to use the local water supply only after boiling it first.

To control fungi, disinfectants are also used. For example, public showers and pool decks are disinfected to prevent transmission of the common fungal infection athlete's foot.

Unlike bacteria and fungi, viruses are transmitted only from one living thing to another and cannot be so easily controlled. Public health programs often control viral diseases by locating the vectors, destroying them, and protecting potential hosts. For example, to prevent people from contracting the viral disease rabies by way of a bite or scratch from an infected animal, health departments require that household pets be immunized and infected animals be destroyed.

Immunizations can prevent some infections in people, too. Immunization involves injecting a **vaccine**—a drug made from the disease agent itself that trains the body's immune system to recognize the active viruses, bacteria, or toxins when they invade. Just as an airplane pilot in training practices on a flight simulator before trying out a real plane, the body practices on the vaccine as a sort of pathogen simulator. If the real invader arrives, the practiced reaction is so fast that the disease never has a chance to develop.

Like the control of viruses, the control of parasites can be achieved by destroying the vectors that transmit them. For example, because the disease malaria is caused by a protozoan transmitted into the blood by way of mosquito bites, spraying insecticide over mosquito breeding grounds helps control malaria.

The status of infectious diseases is constantly changing. Vigilance and effort are needed to keep up with them. At present, the U.S. Public Health Service is working hardest to eliminate these infectious diseases: tuberculosis, hepatitis, pneumonia, polio, measles, rubella, mumps, AIDS (see later section), and hospital infections.[4] In hospitals, the high population density of people with infectious diseases favors the transmission of **nosocomial** (hospital-acquired) **infections**. Clients may be infected by health care personnel, other clients, or visitors. People in hospitals who contract infections unrelated to their original condition greatly extend their hospital stays and expenses.

The examples already given have shown that an understanding of the life cycle and mode of transmission of a pathogen provides keys to its control. Control, however, is all that public health systems usually achieve—they seldom achieve complete elimination. Even the ancient scourge bubonic plague is still endemic in the United States. The "controlled" diseases are simply that—they are under control. Their causes are alive and with us today, waiting in the wings for public health systems to break down, or for drugs to lose their effectiveness. They could still cause disease, should conditions once again permit.

immunizations injections with suspensions of modified infectious agents (vaccine) to induce immune responses and establish long-term resistance to specific infectious diseases.

vaccine a suspension of modified infectious agents used for immunization.

Pneumonia is a group of diseases of the lungs, and is a major threat to the lives of older people.

nosocomial (no-soh-COH-me-ul) **infection** an infection acquired in the hospital.

≡▶ *Public health measures can help control infectious diseases. Chlorination of water, treatment of sewage, immunization of people and animals, and spraying insecticides are all ways the public health authorities help control disease.*

The Body's Defenses

One way the body controls the pathogenic microbes is to keep them out by means of barriers such as skin and membranes. The skin is a well designed protective structure with salty, acidic sweat secretions (most pathogens don't like salt or acid) and one-way pores that let things out but won't let pathogens in. The membranes that line the body chambers have additional defenses, which were described for the lungs in Chapter 11—a layer of mucus that entraps microbes, along with cells and chemicals of the immune system that destroy them. Some membranes also have cilia, tiny beating hairlike structures that sweep the mucus and its contents out of the body. Membranous linings are soft and moist, and somewhat more susceptible to pathogenic attack than the tough outer skin, so most infectious diseases do begin in the digestive, respiratory, reproductive, or urinary tracts. Still, the membranes fend off great numbers of pathogens every day and are part of the body's first line of defense against diseases.

Once an infection penetrates the body's outer membranes, the immune system takes over fully. Usually, the immune system can intercept the invaders in time to prevent disease. Occasionally, though, the pathogens multiply and produce illness. Not all diseases follow an orderly sequence of events, but many do, and five phases of the course of a typical disease have been identified in the Miniglossary: The Course of a Disease.

The prodrome symptoms listed in the Miniglossary are ones you might experience if you contracted one of a number of infections, many of them minor. One warning: if any of the prodrome symptoms listed in Appendix E are present, do not delay seeking help—they can mean the disease is serious.

If you develop an elevated body temperature, think twice before you reach for fever-relief medicine. Fevers have long been feared because they are associated with dangerous diseases, but the fever itself may actually assist the immune system. Fever does stress the body—it raises the heart rate and increases the tissues' demand for oxygen—but low fevers are not bad. When fever is allowed to run its course, it often facilitates the production of immune system cells that fight infection.[5]

≡▶ *The body defends itself against many infectious diseases. Skin and membranes offer the first line of protection in the form of a barrier. The immune system counters infections that make it past this barrier.*

Strategies against Infectious Diseases

Public health and the body's defenses protect the population against many diseases. People can also help protect themselves from infectious diseases. One of the most important steps a person can take to avoid infectious diseases is to keep immunizations up to date. Table 17–2 presents immunizations recommended for children and a proposed schedule of immunizations for adults.

*Do not give children or young adults aspirin. Their illnesses might turn out to be chicken pox or flu which, if treated with aspirin, may result in the life-threatening condition Reye's Syndrome.

■ MINIGLOSSARY
The Course of a Disease

incubation the period after initial invasion when pathogens multiply in the body; the person may be unaware of the infection at this stage and may unwittingly infect others. The immune system may begin to detect the invaders; if the person was earlier vaccinated against the disease, the immune system will launch a full attack and stop the progression of the disease.

prodrome the onset of general symptoms common to many diseases, such as fever, sneezing, and cough. Such symptoms are common to many diseases; in this stage, the disease is easily transmitted. The immune system is beginning to fight.

clinical period the period of symptoms specific to the disease. The immune system is in full battle. (Medical intervention could possibly shorten this and succeeding stages.)

decline the period when the immune system has almost won the fight against the infection, and symptoms are subsiding. Memory cells form.

convalescence the period when the body repairs damage and returns to normal immune operations. The microbe may or may not remain in the body; if it does, the person may remain a carrier of the disease, able to infect others even if no symptoms are evident.

■ *FACT OR FICTION:* Fevers are dangerous, especially when people have infections. *False.* Low fevers are usually not harmful and are part of the body's defense against infection.

Oral temperatures over 104° F: seek medical attention.
Oral temperatures over 100° F: control with acetaminophen, ibuprofen, or in adults, aspirin.*
Oral temperatures 100° F and less: do not treat. (If fever persists, see a health care provider.)

TABLE 17–2 ■ **Suggested Immunization Schedule**

Recipient	Vaccine
Children:	
2-month-olds	DPT (diphtheria, pertussis, tetanus) Oral polio
4-month-olds	DPT Oral polio
6-month-olds	DPT
12-month-olds	Tuberculin test
15-month-olds	Measles, mumps, rubella (MMR) DPT Oral polio
18-month-olds	Hib
4- to 6-year-olds	DPT booster Polio booster
14- to 16-year olds	Tetanus-diphtheria toxoid, adult type; booster every ten years or after a contaminated wound if more than five years have passed since the previous injection
Adults:	
Never-vaccinated young men and women (nonpregnant)	Rubella, to reduce risks to fetuses
Adults born after 1956 never vaccinated for the disease who have never had it	Live measles (people vaccinated between 1963 and 1967 with the killed measles vaccine should be revaccinated with the more effective live vaccine.)
Anyone who has not had the disease or the vaccine	Mumps
Nonimmunized adults over 65 years of age	Pneumococcal vaccine (one-time injection protects against the most common form of pneumonia.)
All adults over 65 years of age and other adults with chronic ailments	Influenza (vaccine changes yearly as the virus changes identity; given in anticipation of the varieties likely to attack.)
People who hold high-risk jobs (health care workers); homosexuals; intravenous drug users	Hepatitis B series
People who travel to high-risk areas, particularly to less developed countries	Any of the above vaccines, plus polio, hepatitis A, plague, rabies, typhoid fever, cholera, and yellow fever

SOURCES: *Parents' Guide to Childhood Immunization,* U.S. Department of Health and Human Services, Public Health Service, Centers for Disease Control, Atlanta, Georgia, 1988; S. Snider, Childhood vaccines, *FDA Consumer* 24 (1990): 19–26; D. Campos-Outcalt, Measles update, *American Family Physician* 42 (1990): 1274–1283; A. Jurgrau, Why aren't we protecting our children? *Registered Nurse* 11 (1990): 30–34; M. E. Pichichero and coauthors, New vaccines and vaccination policies, *Pediatric Annals* 19 (1990): 686–694; A. R. Hinman, Immunizations in the United States, *Pediatrics* 86 (1990): 1064–1066.

What can people do to prevent those diseases for which no vaccine is available? Some illnesses are so widespread and common that you need to be vigilant against them all the time—for example, the common cold. Several hundred different viruses can cause colds, so one vaccine cannot eliminate all colds.[6] Besides, new strains of cold viruses keep arising, to which no vaccines have been developed, so people recovering from one cold can contract another. Although the body may have built up antibodies that protect against the first cold virus, along comes another cold virus for which the body has not yet acquired resistance. The principles of self-protection against colds and other infections are offered in Table 17–3. To see how well you protect yourself against infectious diseases, complete the Life Choice Inventory.

You can often avoid viral and other infections by remembering that for pathogens to cause disease, they must be transmitted from a person or an

---

■ **How to Avoid Infection**

1. Take measures to deter pathogenic growth, both on your body and in your surroundings—maintain a cool, well-lit, dry, clean environment.
2. Use soap and water to remove pathogens from skin; to kill pathogens, use antiseptics on skin and disinfectants on surfaces and elsewhere.
3. Obtain medical treatment for deep wounds.
4. Stay current with immunizations to develop necessary immunity before infection sets in.
5. Avoid unnecessary contact with people who are ill.
6. Do not share objects with people who are ill.
7. Wash your hands often throughout the day, especially before eating and after using the bathroom.
8. Place yourself away from people who are coughing or sneezing.
9. Select foods that support immune system health.
10. Use alcohol in moderation, if at all.
11. Exercise regularly.
12. Do not use tobacco.
13. Control stress.

---

object to you. For example, if your roommate becomes sick with an infection, you may want to provide assistance, but you certainly want to avoid the illness. Caring for someone who is ill does not necessitate becoming ill, yourself. People who work in hospitals learn to avoid illnesses; you can do it, too.

Imagine that the pathogens that have made your friend ill are a quart of red paint that has been sprayed all over the room, and is still wet. The easiest way for them to reach you is for you to touch the surfaces they are on, and then transfer them to your mouth, eyes, nose, or other portal of entry. So avoid unnecessary contact. Comfort the sick person with soothing words from across the room instead of with hugs or kisses.

Objects such as blankets and other bedding, clothing, and dishes can pass pathogens on to others. (Some microbes can live on surfaces for days.) Disinfectants can eliminate some types, but others are unaffected by them. Until the illness is over, pick out some utensils to use, use only those, and wash them separately in detergent and hot water.

People unconsciously wipe their eyes or mouths with their hands many times a day, transmitting pathogens to the body's portals of entry. (Again, picture yourself becoming smeared with red paint.) The best defense is to wash your hands often with soap and water, especially before eating, and especially if those around you show signs of illness.

Millions of pathogens are sprayed into the air by uncovered sneezes and coughs, so provide disposable tissues for someone who is ill. In public places, place yourself a good distance away from someone who is carelessly sneezing or coughing into the air. Wash yourself and even your clothes if you think you've been sprayed.

Despite your best efforts, some pathogens may still reach you. Keep your resistance up by taking care of your immune system; it works best when given a balanced diet. Related to diet is alcohol intake. Alcohol is directly toxic to the immune system, weakening resistance, and it also causes the body to discard its supplies of many vitamins and minerals, weakening it

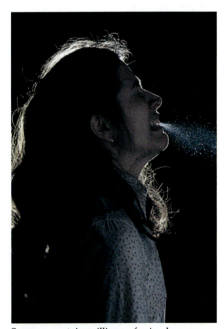

Sneezes contain millions of microbes, some of which may be pathogenic.

LIFE CHOICE INVENTORY

How well do you protect yourself against infectious diseases? If you answer no to any of the following questions, you may be neglecting a way to assist your body's defenses against infection.

1. Do you keep your environment clean, dry, and well lighted?
2. Do you wash your hands several times during the day, before mealtimes and after using the bathroom?
3. Are your immunizations up-to-date?
4. When your local public health department sends out an alert that people should receive special immunizations, do you take the recommended action?
5. Do you avoid sharing food, beverages, utensils, towels, and other objects with people who have symptoms of contagious infections, such as colds, cold sores (fever blisters), flu, or others?
6. Do you, whenever possible, place yourself at a distance from people who have symptoms such as coughing?
7. Is your diet the kind your immune system needs?
8. If you drink alcohol, do you do so only moderately?
9. Are you including exercise in your daily routine?
10. Do you make time for rest and fun?
11. Is stress under control in your life?
12. Do you abstain from using tobacco?
13. If you do get sick, do you follow the full course of treatment to prevent a relapse?

Scoring:
13 yes answers: perfect.
10-12 yes answers: good.
6-9 yes answers: needs improvement.
5 or fewer yes answers: your immune system is crying "Help!" Please improve.

Chapter 4 provides details about stress management techniques.

further. Regular aerobic exercise supports the immune system,[7] while tobacco use impairs immunity. If you don't exercise, start; if you use tobacco, stop.

Stress management is a major part of your strategy against infectious disease. When the immune system is suppressed by sustained stress, illness is likely. Defective resistance to pathogens can permit them to cause cold sores, acne flare-ups, and sore throats. You may have noticed that when you are worried or nervous about something, your throat tends to get sore. This is a warning that before long, unless you manage the stress more effectively, the pathogens already present there will make you ill.

≡▶ *People can take action to minimize their risks of infection. Keeping immunizations up-to-date, maintaining a distance when others are ill, and keeping immune systems strong are all ways to reduce infectious diseases.*

■≡ Sexually Transmitted Diseases (STDs)

sexually transmitted diseases (STDs) formerly called *venereal diseases*, diseases that are transmitted by way of direct sexual contact.

Pathogens that cause **sexually transmitted diseases (STDs)** are passed directly from person to person by way of sexual contact. Most STDs require genital, oral, or anal intercourse for transmission. The delicate, vulnerable membranes of the these orifices make a perfect portal of entry for these various pathogens. Moist, warm, dark environments encourage the growth of sexually transmitted pathogens, and the immune system develops no permanent defense against them. Once in the body, STDs cause numerous symptoms ranging from rashes and lesions to blindness, psychosis, and death. They also cause a host of emotional problems, including relationship problems. Many STDs seriously threaten health; most are treatable, but some are incurable. The reported cases of STDs make up an epidemic of disease in the United States, and the known cases comprise only the tip of the iceberg. By far, most cases are unreported.

The following section focuses on the STDs most common among college students. A short section then covers other infections, those that usually occur without sexual contact. A later section discusses AIDS, and the chapter closes with strategies for how to protect yourself against STDs, including AIDS.

The known cases of STD: the tip of the iceberg.

Common Sexually Transmitted Diseases

Before the discovery of antibiotics, contracting any STD led to severe, progressive, and inevitable consequences. In those days, the medical community had no power to stop the progression of symptoms and experienced the same helplessness as today's medical experts who are trying to help people who have contracted AIDS. This section describes common STDs, roughly in order of their prevalence, and Table 17–4 summarizes some of the most prevalent STDs and those that cause serious illness.

CHLAMYDIA The most prevalent bacterial STD is **chlamydia**.[8] More than 4 million chlamydia infections occur each year in the United States,[9] and college students are especially at risk for contracting this STD.[10]

In men, a chlamydia infection generally begins with inflammation in the urethra and travels to the testes, where it can cause infertility. Infected men who show symptoms typically experience painful urination and a mucous-like white discharge from the penis; some experience testicular pain.[11] But most of the time, men show no outward symptoms.[12]

In women, this pathogen typically begins by invading the cervix, but it may also infect the urethra.[13] If not properly treated, the infection can invade the deeper pelvic structures, spreading to the uterus, fallopian tubes, and ovaries and producing **pelvic inflammatory disease (PID)**. PID can be caused not only by chlamydia, but also by any bacterial infection. The fallopian tubes touch the lining of the abdominal cavity, and in extreme cases the infection can spread throughout this lining or even cause blood poisoning. Chlamydia will sometimes make its presence known in women by causing vaginal or urethral discharges, burning, painful urination, lower abdominal pain, fever, bleeding or pain with sexual intercourse, and irregular menstrual periods. The infection usually progresses with no outward symptoms, however,[14] so women typically seek no treatment for it. As a result, chlamydia often advances to harmful stages. Most do not discover they have contracted it unless they undergo testing.[15]

Several years after a woman unknowingly contracts chlamydia, she may try without success to conceive a child. Her health care provider may then discover that her PID infection has left scar tissue either partially or totally obstructing her already narrow fallopian tubes. When a tube is partly

chlamydia the most prevalent sexually transmitted disease in the United States, caused by the bacterium *Chlamydia*. Its progression is usually silent; it invades the reproductive organs and often causes infertility, especially in women.

Chapter 12 illustrates the organs referred to here.

pelvic inflammatory disease (PID) an acute or chronic sexually transmitted infection of the fallopian tubes initiated by a variety of bacteria that invade the cervix during sexual intercourse. The term PID is widely used to refer to infections of all parts of the pelvic cavity above the vagina. PID increases the risk of ectopic pregnancy and infertility.

■ *FACT OR FICTION:* People who know what symptoms to look for can tell if they have contracted sexually transmitted diseases. *False.* Some sexually transmitted diseases, such as chlamydia, often progress with no outward symptoms.

TABLE 17–4 ■ **Common Sexually Transmitted Diseases**

Name	Symptoms	Treatment	Potential Complications	Prevention
Acquired immune deficiency syndrome (AIDS)	Swollen lymph glands, diarrhea, pneumonia, weight loss, other infections	No cure, symptom relief only	Immune system failure; severe illnesses leading to death in 6 months to 2 years; infants born with immune system failure resulting in death	Abstinence, mutual monogamy with uninfected partner
Chlamydia	Usually no symptoms; burning on urination; vaginal discharge; symptoms of PID; in males, infection of urethra	Specific antibiotics	Ectopic pregnancy, infertility in both men and women, blindness and pneumonia of newborn	Abstinence, mutual monogamy with uninfected partner
Genital warts	Dry, wartlike growths on penis, anus, labia, cervix, vagina.	No cure, control by removal	Recurrence; cervical cancer; penile cancer; possible obstruction of cervix, vagina, anus	Abstinence, mutual monogamy with uninfected partner
Gonorrhea	Possibly no symptoms; vaginal/penile discharge; in males, painful urination, tender lymph nodes, testicular/abdominal pain, fever; in females, painful menstruation or urination, bleeding after intercourse	Antibiotics	Sterility, skin problems, PID, arthritis, infection of heart lining, infection of eyes of newborns	Abstinence, mutual monogamy with uninfected partner

closed, the sperm, which are very small, are often able to make their way through it to fertilize the egg. After fertilization, however, the egg, which is bigger, may lodge in the obstructed tube. In such a case, the fertilized egg implants itself inside the tube rather than in the uterus as it should, resulting in an ectopic pregnancy. As the zygote grows, it gets so large that it ruptures the wall of the tube. This is a life-threatening condition in thousands of women.[16] In the event that the fallopian tubes are totally obstructed, the sperm may be unable to travel to the egg at all. Chlamydia is responsible for most cases of infertility, including those caused by ectopic pregnancies, in the United States.[17]

TABLE 17–4 ■ **continued**

Name	Symptoms	Treatment	Potential Complications	Prevention
Herpes	Painful, blisterlike sores on penis, anus, labia, vagina, cervix, mouth	No cure; prescription medication may lessen severity and frequency of outbreaks	Recurrence, herpes eye infection, infection of newborn during childbirth	Abstinence, mutual monogamy with uninfected partner
Pubic lice*	Itching; lice on pubic hair; eggs, possibly visible, clinging to strands	Prescription or over-the-counter shampoo, lotion, or cream	Skin irritation	Abstinence, mutual monogamy with uninfected partner, not sharing towels or bedclothes with others, good personal hygiene
Syphilis	*Primary* (3 weeks after exposure): chancre on penis, vagina, rectum, anus, cervix *Secondary* (6 weeks after primary): rash on feet and hands; flulike symptoms including anorexia, fever, sore throat, nausea; headaches *Tertiary* (10 to 20 years later): severe nerve damage	Antibiotics	Brain damage; heart disease; spinal cord damage; blindness; infection of fetus, causing death or severe retardation	Abstinence, mutual monogamy with uninfected partner
Trichomoniasis	Possibly no symptoms in men; frothy, thin, greenish discharge; genital itching and pain in women.	Antibiotics	Bladder and urethra infections	Abstinence, mutual monogamy with uninfected partner

*Pubic lice can also be transmitted nonsexually by sharing bedding, towels, or clothing that is infected.

Chlamydia not only is dangerous for adults, but also can damage the fetuses of infected pregnant women. Infants born to mothers with chlamydia are at risk of acquiring the infection themselves during delivery, but it will infect their lungs or eyes, so that they may develop pneumonia or become blind.[18] Health care providers can prevent these tragedies by treating infected pregnant women before delivery.[19]

The silence of chlamydia is detrimental for two reasons. The first has already been mentioned: the disease can progress to a serious state, resulting in ectopic pregnancy, infertility, or infections in newborns, without a person's realizing it. Second, people infected with chlamydia who remain sexually active can pass the infection to others, totally unaware that they have an STD.

Testing for chlamydia is expensive and not routinely done in federally funded and state-funded clinics. In view of the overwhelming evidence that chlamydia is the most common curable STD and a major cause of infertility in women, many health care providers suggest developing funded programs of diagnostic testing for chlamydia.[20] Once detected, the infection is treatable with antibiotics, but only the health care provider should make the choice of which drug to use. Self-prescribed treatments are highly ill-advised (see the Critical Thinking section).

PID can result not only from chlamydia but also from other bacterial STDs. One of these is gonorrhea, discussed in the next section.

gonorrhea a sexually transmitted bacterial disease that, like the chlamydia infection, can cause PID and often advances without symptoms. It can infect the urethra, reproductive organs, rectum, or throat.

GONORRHEA A small, gonococcus bacterium causes the sexually transmitted disease **gonorrhea** (sometimes called "the clap" or "the drip"). Gonorrhea infections occur less frequently than chlamydia infections, but when they do attack, they can infect a man's or woman's urethra, reproductive organs, rectum, or throat.

Gonorrhea often displays itself with a thick, pale yellow penile discharge in men and a burning sensation on urination. Women have a thick, slimy, yellow-green vaginal or urethral discharge and slight pain on urination. As with chlamydia, gonorrhea can advance without giving any symptoms to warn that it is present.

If left untreated, gonorrhea can spread to other parts of the body, leading to arthritis, skin problems, heart problems, and reproductive failure in both men and women. Like chlamydia, gonorrhea can cause PID and can be transmitted to infants at birth. To protect a baby against blindness from a possible gonorrhea infection, health care providers place drops of an antibiotic drug in every infant's eyes within minutes after birth, even if the mother has not tested positive for the pathogen.

The diagnosis of gonorrhea is routine. Just as health care providers can swab infected throats to test for strep infection, so they can swab infected areas to test for gonorrhea. Antibiotic treatment regimens are usually simple and effective, but health care providers must choose the drugs to use, for antibiotic-resistant strains of the gonococcus are spreading.

herpes a common, incurable, easily transmissible sexually transmitted viral disease that produces periodic outbreaks of lesions. The symptoms clear up on their own, but the infection remains and usually recurs.

HERPES Another common STD, **herpes**, is caused by herpes simplex virus-2 (HSV-2). A genital herpes infection usually produces clumps of painful, inflamed, blister-like lesions on the penis, in the vagina, on the vulva and cervix, in the mouth and on the lips, or around or in the anus.[21] The lesions often burn and are tender or itchy. The sores typically break, then crust over and heal in two to four weeks.

The first herpes episode is usually the most severe. In addition to the discomfort of the sores, a person with an initial outbreak often experiences fever, headache, muscle aches, painful urination, and swollen glands. When the initial outbreak subsides, the person is *not* free of the virus. Herpes is incurable, because after the first outbreak, it establishes residence in the nerve fibers, where it is completely safe from the immune system's attempts at wiping it out. After the first outbreak, the virus lies dormant; but it will usually reactivate, causing a person who has acquired the virus to

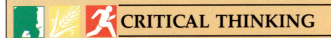

CRITICAL THINKING

Tricks Used to Sell STD Treatments

STDs can be embarrassing. Some people who suspect they may have contracted STDs seek treatment on their own, outside the medical community. There is a black market for antibiotics, and drug pushers make large profits selling them, but the chances of cure from self-treatment are slim to none. More likely, the attempts will delay medical attention, allowing the disease time to disappear from the surface and progress undetected inside the body. Some people take small doses of illegal antibiotics every day in hopes of warding off STDs. This does not work, but it can set the stage for the development of antibiotic-resistant STD microbes as well as other resistant diseases (see box, page 465).

Especially for herpes and AIDS "cures," charlatans abound. The desire for privacy is understandable; reaching for any hope of cure is also natural. But only health care professionals have access to the latest treatments, and people should not let shame or embarrassment deter them from seeking treatment. Health care providers do not waste time pointing accusatory fingers at people who are sick. They are more likely to congratulate them for seeking help.

One person's desire for privacy is another person's opportunity for personal profit. Bypass it; go to a legitimate clinic.

have recurrent outbreaks, often brought on by stress. Most people who have contracted herpes report that with time, the attacks become less frequent and severe. This is because the body has produced some antibodies in response to the initial outbreak, although not enough to keep the virus from reactivating.

The herpes virus is most often transmitted by direct sexual contact with someone who has an active lesion present. Much evidence shows that an outbreak is not necessary, however, for the virus to be transmitted. The absence of sores does not guarantee that herpes will not be transmitted. One study found the virus in semen even when the men studied had no symptoms. This implies that although the risk of herpes transmission may be lower without symptoms, it is still a possibility.[22] Also, a woman may have herpes blisters only on the cervix and no other symptoms, and so may unknowingly pass the virus to her partner.[23]

The virus may also be transmissible *before* lesions appear. Just before an outbreak, some people with herpes experience prodromal symptoms of burning, itching, or tingling at the blister site. This warns that an outbreak is approaching and indicates that the virus is present on the skin and therefore easily transmitted. The virus continues to be easily transmissible until the blisters have completely disappeared and the skin surfaces have healed.[24] To *minimize* risk of infection, people are wise to abstain from sexual activity during the prodromal and acute stages of this infection. (A later section discusses how uninfected people can *eliminate* risk of STDs.)

Another warning is in order about this virus. Herpes simplex virus-2 is closely related to herpes simplex virus-1 (HSV-1), which takes up residence in the nerve fibers of the face and is responsible for fever blisters and cold sores on the lips and mouth. In fact, the two viruses are so closely related that they can take each other's places. A person with HSV-1 on the mouth can transmit this virus to the genitals of a sex partner through oral sex. People with cold sores on the mouth should not kiss or perform oral sex with their partners. People with blisters on their genitals should not have sexual intercourse. Parents are wise to watch that people with fever blisters do not kiss their children.

People experiencing outbreaks must keep the infected areas clean and dry and refrain from touching the blisters. A person can transmit the virus by touching open cold sores and then touching other parts of the body. For example, people with outbreaks who rub their eyes after touching the blisters risk infecting their eyes with the virus.[25]

People who contract herpes suffer in other ways, too. Physical pain and illness may make them lose time from work or school. Additionally, herpes may bring emotional pain. People with the virus experience emotional turmoil, including episodes of depression, loss of self-esteem, and a sense of isolation. A herpes infection may also put a strain on love relationships. An uninfected person whose partner carries the herpes virus may feel anxious during sexual activity, for fear of contracting an incurable STD. Joining a local or national support group offers some people help in coping with the emotional trauma that results from this life-long infection.*

Pregnant women with genital herpes infections put their unborn children at risk of exposure to the virus. The virus can infect the newborn if sores are present when it passes through the birth canal. When babies come in contact with herpes through the birth canal, the virus is not well contained, and it is able to make its way to the brain and bloodstream. Babies who acquire the herpes virus during childbirth face the risks of blindness, severe mental retardation, coma, seizures, brain and nervous system impairments, and even death.[26] Women experiencing a first episode of herpes infection during delivery have a greater chance of transmitting the virus to their babies than women experiencing recurrent infections.[27] A woman who has active herpes lesions when labor begins often requires a surgical delivery to bypass the infected area of the birth canal.

A health care provider can make a diagnosis by physically examining the outbreak. Although herpes is not curable, it is treatable. An antiviral drug, acyclovir (trade name is Zovirax), can be taken by mouth in pill form, or can be spread on the area as an ointment to reduce the frequency, duration, and severity of outbreaks.[28] Acyclovir is available only by prescription, and is not to be confused with ineffective over-the-counter remedies. Unapproved over-the-counter products abound, and may appear on drugstore shelves before the FDA has had the chance to remove them.[29] People searching for treatments are wise to dismiss the wishful thinking that these products might work and see health care providers instead.

GENITAL WARTS Another sexually transmitted disease prevalent among college students is **genital warts** (sometimes called *condyloma*), caused by forms of human papillomavirus (HPV).[30] These viruses sometimes cause

genital warts a viral STD that causes wartlike growths on the infected areas; many strains of the virus that cause genital warts are also correlated with cervical cancer in women.

*An agency of the United Way is *Herpetics Engaged in Living Productively* (HELP), P.O. Box 100, Palo Alto, CA 94302.

growths that resemble the warts people get on their hands or feet, but they are not the same. They may be hard or soft; they may appear isolated or in clusters. Genital warts are sometimes painful, and if not controlled, they can become large enough to obstruct the urethra, cervix, vagina, or anus.[31] This is of special concern when a woman is pregnant; warts may obstruct the cervix or vagina.

More than 50 forms of this virus exist, and many of them may cause cervical cancer.[32] Some researchers claim that human papillomavirus is the leading cause of cervical cancer worldwide.[33] Women who have multiple sex partners place themselves at high risk for cervical cancer.[34]

Many people carry HPV and never experience wart outbreaks; only 10 percent of people who carry HPV ever display warts. Many people unknowingly have wart outbreaks, because warts often go undetected. They are easily hidden underneath the skin of the penis in men and on the cervix or well into the vagina in women. The virus may be present on the genitals, invisible to the naked eye, and can be transmitted by the warts themselves or by semen.[35] For this reason, it is extremely difficult to know who carries the virus. Men with the virus may unknowingly transmit it to their partners, putting them at increased risk for cervical cancer.

A health care provider can make a diagnosis by physically examining the outbreak. If there are no symptoms, a solution can be applied that turns warty growths and any HPV white. In women with barely visible growths or no symptoms, the standard Pap test may identify some strains of HPV. If a woman puts herself at risk by having multiple sex partners, yet has no symptoms, and the standard Pap test responds negative, a health care provider may use more sophisticated tests to detect HPV.*

To treat genital warts, a health care provider must remove them. (Warts seldom clear up on their own.) A surgeon can destroy wart tissue by freezing it, or by using electric heat or laser therapy.[36] A health care provider may topically apply or inject a substance that shrinks or completely clears warts.[37] While removal is painful, it is the only effective treatment. People who try to bypass medical treatment and buy over-the-counter drugstore treatments for regular warts on hands and other body parts are on the wrong track: these remedies are not effective.

Some people have only one episode of genital warts, but most have recurrent outbreaks that repeatedly require removal. Wart infections are similar to herpes in that both are caused by viruses and both remain in the body forever. However, unlike herpes outbreaks, which clear up on their own, warts must most often be removed. Like genital herpes, genital warts also bring a host of emotional problems.

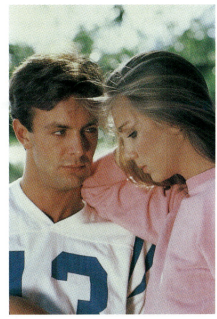

If you care enough to hesitate, you care enough to tell your partner.

SYPHILIS The STD **syphilis** (sometimes called "syph" or "pox") is caused by a spiral-shaped bacterium. Syphilis is not as common among college students as the STDs just discussed, but its incidence is on the rise among minority heterosexuals in the United States.[38]

The consequences of syphilis can be devastating. If untreated, it can cause permanent disability or death in its final stages. It can damage a fetus in the

syphilis a bacterial STD that, if untreated, advances from a sore (chancre) to flulike symptoms to a long symptomless period to a final stage that involves irreversible brain and nerve damage ending in death.

*Other tests are ViraPap, a test to detect the RNA of HPV, and ViraType, a DNA test that can detect three types of HPV. A. Loucks, Human papillomavirus screening in college women, *Journal of American College Health* 39 (1991): 291–293.

Famous and infamous people suspected of suffering from the brain damage and other symptoms of syphilis: Julius Caesar, Cleopatra, Napoléon Bonaparte, Catherine the Great, Peter the Great, Henry VIII, Mary Tudor, John Keats, Franz Schubert, Oscar Wilde, Vincent van Gogh, Friedrich Nietzsche, Ludwig van Beethoven, Thomas Mann, and Adolf Hitler.

chancre (SHANG-ker)   a hard, painless sore that is seen in the first stage of syphilis.

uterus of an infected woman; in fact, unless the mother receives treatment in early pregnancy, her fetus is certain to become infected. Syphilis may kill the fetus or cause birth defects, including severe mental retardation.[39] Many of the most disturbed inmates of mental hospitals, who are 20, 40, 60, and even 80 years old, are there because they were born with syphilis.

The initial symptoms of a syphilis infection usually occur about three weeks after sexual contact with an infected person; thereafter, the disease progresses in stages. (Syphilis can be transmitted during each of these stages.) The primary stage of the infection brings a painless sore (a **chancre**) on the vagina, cervix, vulva, mouth, penis, or anus. The sore is usually obvious in men, but it can easily go undetected in women, because it is painless and often occurs deep in the vagina or on the cervix. It disappears after two to six weeks with *or without* treatment. The secondary stage occurs six to eight weeks after exposure and brings swollen lymph nodes, a skin rash, hair loss, or flulike symptoms. The symptoms of the second stage clear up within two to six weeks with *or without* treatment.

This is why syphilis destroys the lives of so many people even though a cure is available: the symptoms go away on their own. People who pass through the first two stages of this devastating disease can believe they have only contracted minor ailments and have recovered. They seek no medical care, but the syphilis infection goes undetected and untreated, silently advancing until it seriously threatens health.

After the second stage clears up on its own, the disease moves into the latent stage, a long period (maybe as long as 15 to 25 years after contact) during which the infected person feels well. Few clinical signs are detectable, but the infectious agent is silently attacking the internal organs. Eventually, in the late stage, organ damage is both apparent and irreversible. Damage to the cardiovascular system, central nervous system, eyes, and skin is profound. Death is likely.

A health care provider can diagnose a syphilis infection using a specific blood test designed to detect the disease. Antibiotics can kill the pathogen at any stage of infection but cannot reverse the physical damage that occurs in the late stage. To escape the dire consequences of syphilis, then, a person who is infected urgently needs early diagnosis, even if the person feels fine.

trichomoniasis (TRICK-oh-mo-NYE-uh-sis) an STD caused by a protozoan, can cause bladder, urethral, and vaginal infections and PID.

TRICHOMONIASIS The STD **trichomoniasis** ("trich," pronounced TRIK) is caused by a protozoan. These infections are on the rise, increasing by an estimated 120 million new cases each year, worldwide.[40]

Most often, trichomoniasis is transmitted by sexual activity, but on rare occasions it has been transmitted by wet clothes and towels that were contaminated by some vaginal discharge.[41] This may happen occasionally when a woman wears a friend's wet bathing suit. In women, this infection causes a heavy, unpleasant-smelling, foamy, yellow-green or grey discharge; discomfort during sexual intercourse; abdominal pain; painful urination; itching in the genital area; and chronic, painful vaginal infections.[42] In men, symptoms sometimes include a slight tingly feeling inside the penis, painful urination, or a thin, watery discharge. Most men have no symptoms, however, and can unknowingly transmit the disease to their partners.

If left untreated, trichomoniasis can cause infections of the urethra and bladder in both men and women. It can also cause PID in women. An oral antibiotic, taken for two weeks, clears up these infections but often causes unpleasant side effects such as nausea.*

PUBIC LICE The STD **pubic lice** (often called "crabs") is an infestation of tiny parasites that breed in the pubic hair and cause intense itching. The pubic louse attaches itself to the skin around the genitals and lays eggs on the pubic hair shafts. Within three weeks these eggs develop into mature crab lice. If left untreated, they multiply quickly and cause extreme discomfort that intensifies as they spread.

Pubic lice can be transmitted not only through direct sexual activity, but also by any close body contact or by the sharing of contaminated towels, clothes, or bedding. A health care provider or the person with the disease can often make an easy diagnosis based on symptoms and examination.

A health care provider can prescribe creams, lotions, or shampoos to kill the parasites. An infected person can also purchase these treatments over the counter. To prevent reinfection, the person must wash clothes and bedding in hot water and treat furniture.[43] The effort to eliminate pubic lice is a lengthy one. Good personal hygiene can help prevent this disease.

MULTIPLE STDS A person who has one STD may very well have others. This is of special concern because one STD may mask another that poses a more serious health problem. Syphilis is a particularly dangerous second infection—its characteristic early symptom is a painless sore, easily disguised in, say, a cluster of herpes blisters. If the herpes alone is recognized, the syphilis will go untreated and will silently spread through the body. A person who contracts any STD should see a health care provider and request a test for syphilis—and, some health care providers say, for several other STDs.[44] The second-infection threat holds true for all STDs listed in Table 17–4, even pubic lice.

One STD may make it easier for another STD to flourish. AIDS, for example, can be easily transmitted during a herpes outbreak, since the open sores of herpes offer a direct pathway for the AIDS virus to enter the bloodstream. People who engage in sex during a herpes outbreak greatly increase their risks of contracting not only AIDS, but also other bacterial and viral STDs.

Other Infections

The STDs just described are almost invariably transmitted by sexual contact. Other infections of the genital and urinary organs occur that are not STDs, but that, for convenience, are described here. One of the most common of these is the yeast infection of women. This uncomfortable vaginal infection, **candidiasis**, is caused by a yeast (a type of fungus) that normally lives in the vagina. This yeast usually causes no problem but on occasion may multiply out of control and create an infection. Pregnancy, diabetes, use of birth control pills or antibiotics, and douching can cause yeast cells to reproduce quickly.

This infection is always noticed because it causes intense itching, redness, and swelling of the vulva. It is accompanied by a white or cream-colored

pubic lice an STD caused by tiny parasites that breed in pubic hair and cause intense itching.

candidiasis (can-did-EYE-a-sis) an infection caused by a fungus that multiplies out of control in the vagina; commonly called a yeast infection. It causes intense itching and redness of external genitalia and produces a thick, curdled discharge.

*The oral antibiotic is metronidazole (trade name, Flagy).

curdled vaginal discharge. Antifungal creams provide relief and successfully control yeast infections. These are available both by prescription and over the counter. Male sex partners may also be infected, so both partners should be treated. Sexual activity should be avoided during periods of infection. Conscientious self-care, as described in the Spotlight following Chapter 1, helps to minimize vaginal yeast infections. For prevention, women are advised not to use douches; to wear cotton, not nylon, underwear; and to wear pantyhose, if any, with cotton panels.

Many types of bacteria cause **urinary tract infections (UTIs),** or infections of the urethra. Most UTIs are caused by bacteria that commonly inhabit the skin of the anal area. Pathogens or organisms from the digestive tract, which migrate to the genital area, or are transferred there from the rectal area, can cause UTIs.

Most UTIs cause frequent, urgent, and painful urination. Some people notice a dull, aching pain above the pubic bone and blood in the urine.

The health care provider can analyze a urine specimen to determine the specific pathogen causing the infection. UTIs are usually easily treated when the specific organism has been identified. If left untreated, infection of the bladder may progress to infection of the kidneys. A kidney infection is more serious and usually brings additional symptoms of chills, fever, rapid heart rate, and nausea or vomiting. Kidney infections can threaten life.

One out of every four women experiences a UTI at some point in her lifetime. Some women are plagued with recurrent infections. To prevent infections:

1. Drink plenty of fluids. A glass of water every two to three hours is recommended.
2. Urinate frequently and completely. Don't hold your urine. The less time bacteria spend in the bladder, the less likely they are to cause infection.
3. Urinate after sexual intercourse. Then drink more water to force urination several hours after, as well.
4. If you use a diaphragm or cervical cap, don't leave it in place any longer than necessary.
5. Wipe from front to back after urination or bowel movements.
6. Cleanse genitals after sexual intercourse. (Bathe daily, of course.)[45]

This chapter has so far described infectious diseases, emphasizing common STDs and related infections. A major STD is the focus of the rest of this chapter: AIDS.

≡▶ *Infections of the genitals and urinary organs can be caused by sexually transmitted and other pathogens. Some infections are easily prevented and treated, others require more persistent attention.*

■≡ Acquired Immune Deficiency Syndrome (AIDS)

A disease of enormous concern worldwide is **acquired immune deficiency syndrome (AIDS)**. First observed in the human population in the late 1970s,

urinary tract infections (UTIs)   bacterial infections of the urethra that can travel to the bladder and kidneys.

acquired immune deficiency syndrome (AIDS)   an infectious disease transmitted by way of sexual contact or sharing of infected blood. The disease attacks the immune system, rendering the infected person vulnerable to a host of opportunistic diseases.

AIDS has already become a pandemic, emerging in country after country. The reaction of the mass-communication media has bordered on panic—understandably so, for many lives have been lost to this devastating disease that causes so much physical and emotional suffering. Health care authorities are working hard to stop AIDS from becoming a bigger problem.

AIDS is a disease that progresses relentlessly with dire consequences. Our civilization's once steadfast confidence that infectious diseases posed little threat to developed nations has been shattered. AIDS continues to spread, despite intense efforts to obliterate it. So deadly is AIDS that the Centers for Disease Control predict that it will soon be one of the leading causes of death in the United States, surpassing all other causes of death for people between the ages of 25 and 44 years.[46] AIDS is a worldwide health problem, with cases being reported in more than 100 countries and all inhabited continents.[47] Today, the virus that causes AIDS is spreading among college and university students[48] and is even beginning to infect high school students.

New findings about AIDS are reported almost daily. This section provides a basic understanding of the information available so far, so that you can evaluate new information as it becomes available.*

AIDS is unique among infectious diseases because the immune system cannot fight it off. AIDS is caused by the human immunodeficiency virus (HIV), which attacks the immune system itself, disabling its defenses.** It thus makes the body vulnerable to infections that would not otherwise occur or would produce only mild illnesses in people with normal immune responses. AIDS leaves a person vulnerable to certain types of cancers and to a wide variety of serious infections.

Transmission of the AIDS Virus

People infected with HIV can transmit the AIDS virus to others. Although HIV carriers are considered most contagious when the disease is well advanced,[49] they can pass the virus to others before they develop signs of illness,[50] and most HIV carriers are in their symptomless incubation stage.[51] One cannot tell, by looking, who is harboring the virus and who is not.

Sexual activity, including anal sex, is the most common way HIV is transmitted. A person with HIV usually carries the virus in blood, semen, vaginal fluids, or saliva and can pass it to a sex partner by way of the penis, vagina, rectum, or mouth.[52] A person with abrasions, tears, or sores in the mouth, genital area, or rectum (resulting from other STDs or traumatic sexual practices such as anal sex) is most vulnerable, because these irritations are open pathways to the bloodstream. These abrasions are, however, not necessary for transmission to occur; it can occur without them.[53]

Anal sex is a common way in which HIV is sexually transmitted. This accounts for the high prevalence of AIDS among homosexual men.[54] Anal sex is traumatic to the rectal tract; it inflicts tears that make this vulnerable membrane a perfect portal of entry for the AIDS virus. Being part of the

---

*For answers to questions relating to AIDS, call the Public Health Service's toll-free AIDS hotlines: 1–800–342–AIDS (English) or 1–800–344–SIDA (Spanish).

**The virus that causes AIDS is *human T-lymphotropic virus, type III* (*HTLV-III*), or *lymphadenopathy-associated virus* (*LAV*). The name *human immunodeficiency virus* (*HIV-1*) is official. Another related virus (*HIV-2*) is also pathogenic and spreading.

digestive tract, the rectum is an absorptive system anyway, and readily takes up HIV, even without tears.

HIV is also commonly transmitted by way of vaginal intercourse.[55] Heterosexual transmission of HIV is steadily increasing.[56] Contrary to popular belief that heterosexuals are not at risk for HIV,[57] the Centers for Disease Control estimate that as many as 30,000 heterosexuals already have been infected with the AIDS virus through heterosexual activity alone.[58]

HIV can be transmitted during any sexual act in which body fluids are exchanged, including oral sex. Research has shown that some homosexual men, in the attempt to reduce their risks of developing AIDS, have engaged only in oral sex, and still have contracted the virus.[59] Researchers have also shown that people could be infected by having mouth contact with the penises of their HIV-infected sex partners.[60] HIV can directly infect cells in the membranes of the mouth, since tiny lesions in the mouth allow the virus to enter.[61]

Passionate, open-mouthed kissing is also thought to be a potential mode of HIV transmission. This type of kissing can injure the lining of the mouth, making it receptive to viruses such as HIV. In one study of passionate kissing, researchers found traces of blood in the saliva of half of the subjects.[62] Only microscopic traces of blood are needed to convey virus particles from person to person. Authorities warn that although no cases have yet been reported of HIV transmission through passionate kissing, kissing should not be considered a safe activity. (The "no case yet" theory holds no weight; years ago researchers said people could not get AIDS from vaginal sex, because no cases had been reported "yet.") Membranes of the mouths of both partners contain small lesions that come into close contact during kissing, and blood can pass directly from one person to another. The intense rubbing that takes place during kissing favors this passage, and if the blood of one partner contains HIV, the AIDS virus can pass into the bloodstream of the other partner. In addition, people infected with HIV usually carry the virus in their saliva. People infected with HIV usually have lower concentrations of the virus in their saliva than in their blood, semen, or vaginal fluids, so the risk of transmission of HIV through deep kissing is lower than through intercourse.[63] But it is still a risk. Open-mouthed kissing with an HIV carrier is not safe.

Transmission of HIV can occur during a single sexual encounter with an infected person. While steady sex partners of people with AIDS are at the greatest risk of contracting HIV, one-time partners can also contract the virus.[64]

The sharing of needles among **IV drug abusers** is the second most common mode of HIV transmission.[65] IV drug users or athletes who inject steroids or anabolic hormones, and who share needles and syringes with others, can pick up the AIDS virus from one person and transmit it to themselves and others.[66] HIV can be transmitted even if the needle is not directly inserted into a blood vessel.[67] The use of unsterilized needles for any purpose can cause HIV transmission.[68] Uses can include acupuncture, tattooing, ear piercing, and electrolysis (the removal of hair by electricity using a needle).[69]

HIV is transmitted not only by sexual contact and sharing of infected needles, but also by receiving transfusions of blood or blood products that are infected with the virus. Anyone receiving blood transfusions between the late 1970s and March 1985 is at high risk of being infected with the virus,

■ *FACT OR FICTION:* You can get AIDS from passionate, open-mouthed kissing. *True.*

IV drug abusers   people who use hypodermic needles to inject drugs of abuse into their veins (*IV* means "intravenous," or "into a vein").

HIV has been transmitted by anal, vaginal, and oral sex. Passionate open-mouthed kissing is a potential means of HIV transmission. Other means of HIV transmission include sharing of infected needles, ear piercing, acupuncture, tattooing, electrolysis, infected blood transfusions, and infected organ transplants. HIV can be transmitted to infants through pregnancy, childbirth, or breastfeeding.

because blood products were not screened at that time (see ''AIDS Testing and the Blood Supply'').[70] People have also contracted AIDS from organ transplants when the organ donors carried HIV.[71]

HIV can be transmitted to infants. Women who have AIDS or who carry the virus can infect their children during pregnancy, birth, or breastfeeding.[72]

HIV appears *not* to be transmitted by casual contact such as sharing meals, shaking hands, hugging, casual kissing, coughing, or sneezing.[73] The AIDS virus does not seem to be transmitted by mosquitoes or other insects, by saunas, by pools, or by food handled by HIV carriers.[74] HIV is not transmitted *to* people who donate blood using sterilized needles, by vaccines using sterilized needles, or by contact with unbroken, healthy skin.[75] HIV does not appear to be transmitted by touching shared objects, such as toilet seats. Intimate sexual activity, not casual contact, seems to transmit HIV.

≡ ▶ *The deadly disease AIDS is caused by infection by HIV. HIV is readily transmitted by people infected with the virus by way of sexual contact or exchange of blood. HIV does not appear to be transmitted through casual contact.*

The Progression of AIDS

Infection with HIV does not immediately lead to a full-blown case of AIDS. A person who contracts HIV can remain symptom-free for from six months to ten years.[76] Some people who contract the AIDS virus remain in good health for many years (remain asymptomatic); then the disease progresses to an early stage of infections, fever, diarrhea, and fungal infections of the mouth before moving into the stage of full-blown, lethal AIDS.

AIDS begins when the virus selectively uses the immune system cells for replication—specifically, the **T cells**. The virus acts as any other virus does, by invading the cell, taking over the replication machinery, and reproducing, using the cell's resources. The AIDS virus replicates faster than any other known virus—it can make thousands of copies of itself in a very short time. It changes its identity up to a million times more quickly, too, and hides within the immune system's own cells to avoid detection.[77]*

As T cells are destroyed by replicating viruses, their numbers dwindle, disabling their essential function of triggering the other cells to produce antibodies. Those that remain are unable to warn the body of the presence of invaders, including HIV, other microorganisms, and cancer cells.[78] With the immune system thus weakened and unable to fight disease, opportunistic infections thrive unchecked.

HIV infection commonly begins with an initial stage of feeling well or having only mild, vague symptoms such as fatigue. As the disease progresses, it causes persistent swollen lymph nodes and other symptoms, including skin rashes, fever, and diarrhea.[79] It often causes fungal infections of the mouth.

HIV is able to make its way to the brain and nervous system and can cause severe mental deterioration, commonly called **AIDS dementia**, a brain disorder seen only in people with compromised immunity.[80] Other brain and nervous system problems arising from HIV infection, include delirium, mood swings, apathy, withdrawal, agitation, depression, hallucinations,

HIV appears not to be transmitted by casual contact; mosquitoes; food; blood donation; vaccines using sterilized needles; contact with unbroken, healthy skin; or touching shared objects.

T cells cells of the immune system that detect infection and prompt other cells to respond by producing antibodies.

AIDS dementia a severe brain disorder caused by AIDS.

*The way AIDS hides is known as the Trojan horse mechanism. For more about AIDS mechanisms, read S. Broder, *AIDS: Modern Concepts and Therapeutic Challenges* (New York: Marcel Dekker, 1987).

AIDS Testing and the Blood Supply

Shortly after the discovery of the AIDS virus, scientists developed a blood test to detect the antibodies that the body makes in response to HIV.* This test identifies only the antibodies to HIV, not HIV itself, and it can come out falsely positive sometimes. If the test comes out positive, then another test is given to confirm the presence of antibodies and the diagnosis of HIV infection.[a]** The presence of antibodies means that the person will eventually develop AIDS. A negative test result means one of two things: the person may not have the virus or the person may have HIV but has not yet developed antibodies to it.

Most people who contract HIV begin to manufacture antibodies immediately after exposure to the virus, and these antibodies are usually detectable through blood screening within 6 to 12 weeks after contracting HIV.[b] Some people with HIV, however, do not develop enough antibodies to be detected for as long as six months or more after exposure to the virus.[c] It may even take years after exposure to

HIV to develop antibodies. In one study, 27 people known to have the virus itself continued to test negative for HIV antibodies for *seven months to three years*.[d]

The standard blood test for HIV antibodies cannot prove that someone is free of HIV.[e] The accuracy of this testing procedure is important, because this antibody test is used to screen blood products collected for transfusions. Each donor's blood is screened for HIV antibodies, and blood that tests positive is not used. Blood products thus screened are considered safer for use in medical treatments than before this test was developed, but the use of this test has not completely eliminated the risk of contracting HIV through transfusions. A blood donor may have HIV but may not yet have developed antibodies, and so may be able to transmit the virus to a blood recipient.[f]

In response to this problem, some blood products are being treated by methods that deactivate viruses. These processes, designed to destroy any HIV in the plasma, have greatly reduced the risk of transmitting AIDS through transfusion of blood-clotting preparations used to control bleeding.[g] However, this deactivation method may not be 100

*The test that detects antibodies is called the enzyme-linked immunosorbent assay, or ELISA.
**The ELISA test occasionally produces false positives. The test used to confirm the diagnosis of HIV infection is the Western Blot test.

delusions, anxiety, and memory impairment.[81] When HIV invades the nervous system, it affects the muscles, too, causing leg weakness, unsteady gait, and poor coordination.[82]

Finally an HIV infection progresses to a state of severe immune failure resulting in full-blown AIDS. People infected with HIV experience rare types of pneumonia and cancer, as well as many other opportunistic diseases.

The most common opportunistic infection seen in people with AIDS is a severe type of pneumonia caused by a parasite. People with AIDS also contract a variety of infections from other parasites, bacteria, fungi, and

Common progression of HIV infection:

1. Initial stage of infection: no symptoms or mild symptoms.
2. Persistent swollen lymph nodes, fever, diarrhea, and fungal infection of mouth.
3. Brain and nervous system disease.
4. Severe immune failure (full-blown AIDS).
5. Death.

percent effective, for people have developed AIDS from blood transfusions since the screening and treating of blood products began.[h] Health officials estimate that 1 out of every 250,000 units of transfused blood may still be contaminated with HIV due to false-negative test results.[i]

Another problem with the safety of the blood supply is concern about human error. Health care workers in blood banks, plasma centers, and public health clinics are supposed to conduct the antibody test and comply with other safety guidelines.[j] But some blood plasma centers have been closed for violation of health and safety standards.[k] Among the several reasons for closing were shortcuts in donor screening and acceptance of ineligible donors, such as those suspected of being at high risk for AIDS.[l] Persons with signs or symptoms suggestive of AIDS have been asked not to donate blood, but many people at risk for HIV still continue to do so.[m]

People who are planning to have surgery would be wise to donate their own blood to be stored for use, should transfusions be needed. Even this strategy is not foolproof, though. Hospitals usually do not welcome this activity, because it requires additional work on their part to keep track of the blood. Another drawback is that sometimes a person will require more blood than what is donated, necessitating the use of blood from an unknown donor.

a. R. M. Healy and T. Coleman, A primer of AIDS for health professionals, *Health Education* 19 (1988/1989): 4–10.
b. *Casual Contact and the Risk of HIV Infection,* July 1989 (a report of the Special Initiative on AIDS of the American Public Health Association, Washington, D.C.).
c. B. P. Beste and J. Hummer, AIDS: A review and guide for infection control, *Journal of the American Optometric Association* 57 (1986): 675–682, as cited in Healy and Coleman, 1988/1989; *The HIV Antibody Test* (Rockville, Md.: American College Health Association, 1988).
d. R. A. Kaslow and coauthors, The multicenter AIDS cohort study: Rationale, organization, and selected characteristics of the participants, *American Journal of Epidemiology* 126 (1987): 310–318, as cited in W. A. Haseltine, Silent HIV infections, *New England Journal of Medicine* 320 (1989): 1487–1488.
e. Healy and Coleman, 1988/1989.
f. *Answers about AIDS* (Summit, N.J.: American Council on Science and Health, 1988).
g. No risk of AIDS from plasma, *FDA Consumer,* June 1989, p. 4.
h. J. G. Donahue and coauthors, Transmission of HIV by transfusion of screened blood, *New England Journal of Medicine* 323 (1990): 1709; *Answers about AIDS,* 1988.
i. *Answers about AIDS,* 1988.
j. Donahue and coauthors, 1990.
k. S. Snider, Plasma center closed, *FDA Consumer,* October 1990, page 33.
l. Snider, 1990.
m. Donahue and coauthors, 1990.

viruses. They often contract other STDs, which advance with abnormal rapidity. An HIV infection sometimes opens the way for cancers of the lymphatic system and a form of skin cancer (Kaposi's sarcoma) that otherwise is extremely rare. These opportunistic infections in people with AIDS often resist treatment and usually cause death.[83] People with HIV do not die of AIDS itself; they die of other diseases against which they have been rendered defenseless.

AIDS is devastating physically and emotionally. People diagnosed with AIDS soon learn how severely the disease will affect their lives; they learn that it will bring catastrophic losses of health, job, finances, friends, sexual

Common infections seen in people with AIDS:

- ■ Thrush (fungal infection of the mouth).
- ■ Pneumonia; tuberculosis.
- ■ Other STDs, which advance rapidly.
- ■ Lymphatic and other cancers; Kaposi's sarcoma.
- ■ Tuberculosis meningitis (inflammation of the membranes surrounding the spinal cord and/or brain).
- ■ Encephalitis (inflammation of the brain).
- ■ Esophagitis (inflammation of the esophagus).
- ■ Persistent diarrhea.
- ■ Extensive skin inflammation.[85]

relationships and social support. People who test positive for HIV often become psychologically unable to function and emotionally disabled, even to the point of becoming suicidal or homicidal. Many experience intense guilt over the lifestyle behaviors that caused them to contract the disease, and this guilt is compounded by judgmental attitudes from others.[84] Others experience anger when they learn they contracted HIV through an infected blood transfusion or from an infected dentist or other health care provider. People who develop AIDS can expect to lose physical strength, mental acuity, control of life activities, self-esteem, and ultimately, life itself.

No one has recovered from AIDS. Most people infected with HIV die within three years after symptoms develop. With treatments, some people with AIDS are surviving longer than before, but still dying in agonizing ways.[86]

Physicians use drugs, radiation, and surgery to reverse, at least temporarily, some of the various physical manifestations of the disease. Although toxic themselves, the drugs used for AIDS treatment can sometimes forestall the advancement of the disease and prolong life while research seeks new treatments and victims long for a cure in the future.

Researchers have made progress in their search for AIDS therapies. One product of their efforts is the discovery that an anticancer drug, zidovudine,* delays the progression of the disease.[87] However, this drug does not cure AIDS.

More than two dozen other anti-AIDS drugs are being tested.[88] One that shows promise is a drug that suppresses the replication of HIV.[89] Researchers point out, though, that although results sound promising, studies are in the early phases. They advise hopeful health care workers and their HIV-infected clients to suspend judgment until further studies are completed.[90]

A vaccine to prevent AIDS is slow in coming because the AIDS virus alters its identity, effectively hiding from even a healthy immune system. Vaccines and antiviral drugs are presently being tested in efforts to prevent AIDS infection.[91] Because of the extreme lethality of AIDS, testing must be conducted more carefully than for other, less life-threatening diseases. Yet at the same time, researchers are under pressure to rush their research and try possibly hazardous or ineffective treatments on human beings before having tested them adequately on animals. People with AIDS are clamoring for the right to try any drug that offers even the remotest hope of comfort or cure.

Because there is no cure for AIDS, public health authorities agree that massive education is needed to teach individual strategies for prevention.[92] Formal education about AIDS is believed most likely to succeed in extinguishing risky behaviors.[93] Although the incidence of AIDS is highest among homosexual men and drug users, a person does not have to be gay or a drug user to get it.[94] Regardless of whether a person is a member of a high-risk group or not, one can get AIDS if he or she engages in behaviors that transmit the virus, with people who carry HIV. The next section describes strategies for preventing AIDS and other STDs.

≡▶ *The progression of AIDS begins when a person contracts HIV. The person often remains asymptomatic for years before developing AIDS. People with AIDS die from opportunistic diseases that advance when their immune systems severely fail.*

*Zidovudine was formerly called azidothymidine, or AZT.

■≡ Strategies Against STDs

STDs are both life-threatening and life-changing in their consequences. As viral and antibiotic-resistant bacterial STDs have emerged, people are no longer assured of cure.[95] Since there is no cure for some STDs, a person's only protection against them is prevention.

Most prevention strategies propose ways to *reduce* STD risk, and in the past, these guidelines have generally been well received. However, the era of AIDS, which is deadly, has changed the public's acceptance of such recommendations. People are now not satisfied with STD strategies that, at best, merely lower risk. Instead, they want to learn ways to *eliminate* risk. They claim that adopting strategies that hold any degree of uncertainty is gambling with their lives—they feel that there is no acceptable level of risk when death is the consequence.[96]

The first section that follows defines **safe-sex strategies**, those that eliminate STD risk—behaviors that promise, if you adhere to them, that you will not contract STDs through sexual contact. (Remember, though, that sexual contact is not the only way you can contract STDs.) The next section then describes behaviors that will reduce STD risk. The good news is (except in rare cases) that the locus of control is within you—you can decide if you want to completely protect yourself or if you want to somewhat protect yourself (or if you do not want to protect yourself at all). This chapter's Strategy box summarizes these guidelines.

safe-sex strategies behavior guidelines that offer complete protection from contracting STDs.

Safe-Sex Strategies

The following three strategies are the only ones that, if practiced successfully, reduce risk to zero. The first depends on no one but yourself.

SEXUAL ABSTINENCE The most effective way to completely protect yourself from acquiring STDs through sexual contact is to abstain from sexual relations (**celibacy**). Practicing sexual abstinence is a 100-percent-guaranteed safe-sex strategy.[97] Masturbation is included as a safe part of abstinence.

celibacy (SELL-ih-ba-see) complete abstinence from sexual relations.

Abstinence need not be a life-long choice; it can be just "for now." It is a vitally important part of the strategy called "serial monogamy," discussed below: the between-partner part. It is also necessary during relationships from time to time, for example, when distance may separate a couple. Even for people who value sexual involvement highly, abstinence offers rewards. Freedom from sexual relationships for at least part of your life permits you to focus totally on yourself and your goals—to develop your career, work hard for a cause you believe in, or offer all of your energy to a project. In short, abstinence is of greater value than just as a preventive measure against STDs. Some people cherish it as a value in and of itself.

In these days of incurable and fatal STDs, abstinence has never looked better. Some tips on how to practice abstinence include:

■ Reaffirm that it is your personal right to practice abstinence.
■ Decide in advance what sexual activities you will say "yes" to and discuss these with your partner.
■ Tell your partner, very clearly and in advance (not in bed), what activities you will not engage in.
■ Avoid high-pressure sexual situations. (Stay sober, double date, stay out

of the back seat of a car, don't take your date alone back to your apartment, and don't go alone to your date's apartment.)

■ If you suspect you will be sexually pressured, don't go out with the person.

■ Learn to give and receive non-sexual affection.

■ Maintain friendships with other men and women.

■ Learn about available birth control methods should you choose to engage in intercourse. Have a back-up method accessible to you.

■ If you say "no," say it like you mean it. Turn the tables on the date who says "If you loved me you would." Respond by saying "If you loved me, you wouldn't insist."[98]

LIFE-LONG MONOGAMY Another way to completely protect yourself from acquiring STDs is to have sexual relations exclusively with one uninfected partner, who is also monogamous.[99] A prospective partner's infection status is the most important factor in determining if sex can be safe.[100] Having a mutually faithful sexual relationship is a valid ideal, not only for STD prevention, but also because it has the potential to become enhanced by social, intellectual, emotional, and spiritual, as well as sexual, facets. As for the sexual part of the relationship, it need be limited by no restrictions regarding sexual activities. Full freedom is safe, with the exception of anal sex (discussed later). Anal sex is not safe for anyone. Serial monogamy, discussed next, offers this same advantage.

See Chapter 12 for more about psychologically intimate relationships.

SERIAL MONOGAMY Another sure way to protect yourself from contracting STDS is to practice **serial monogamy** (to have a series of mutually exclusive relationships) with uninfected partners. Assuming you are sexually faithful in each relationship, and providing you are *absolutely certain* your partner is both uninfected and faithful, this strategy is 100 percent safe. If you are not completely sure that your partner is uninfected, it is not safe to have sex.[101] Before you can use this strategy, you must determine two things:

serial monogamy a series of mutually exclusive relationships; having one sexually exclusive relationship at a time.

■ Your prospective partner's infection status.
■ Your prospective partner's trustworthiness.

The truly safe-sex strategies of abstinence and monogamy both require periods of abstinence, which makes them unpopular. Being abstinent requires discipline. It is not easy to practice abstinence in opposition to your own sexual desires, and in the context of a society where sex is so freely promoted and expected, even early in relationships. It takes courage to overcome peer pressure and adhere to values that may not be consistent with those of people around you. But be encouraged if you think this is an insurmountable task, for more and more people are choosing celibacy and are learning to change their sexual behaviors and be abstinent.[102] You can learn self-control. People who value themselves, their physical health, and their emotional well-being, and who want to experience the complete fulfillment that an intimate relationship can offer, are learning to practice abstinence. Many people find that practicing abstinence requires a high level of self-esteem.[103] So the first goal when learning to be abstinent is to build self-esteem.

The first goal when learning to be abstinent is to build self-esteem. For more on self-esteem, see Chapter 2.

Next, consider the risks associated with the STDs discussed in this chapter. Changing sexual behavior requires some high incentive and strong motivation. There is no better motivation than the desire to remain alive.

Then, consider the value of having a quality relationship versus casual sex. Casual sex invites deadly diseases, and what it offers is temporary. Consider how long an orgasm lasts: about 12 seconds. Then it's over. There is no lasting satisfaction in that. Most people who contract STDs say that the temporary pleasure of the encounter was not worth the emotional and physical agony that accompanies most STDs.

Next, choose your partner with extreme care. An important part of selecting a partner is to determine the person's infection status. Young people are advised to select potential sexual partners in part by asking about partners' sexual histories. Unfortunately, this advice overlooks the fact that most people do not like to reveal their sexual pasts, and so, quite often, they lie. Many physicians know several clients whom they have treated for STDs who are volunteering no information to their sex partners or are lying to them if they ask. One physician reported that he had asked an AIDS-infected client if he told his sex partner that he had AIDS. The client responded, ''No, Doctor, it would have broken the mood.''

In a survey, 20 percent of men said that in order to get a woman into bed, they would lie about their past sexual experiences and would not reveal that they had an STD if they had one.[104] A study of 400 college students revealed that both men and women used deception when discussing past sexual encounters.[105] Men admitted lying three times more often than women did, but dishonesty was alarmingly frequent among both men and women. If a new partner asked, 47 percent of the men and 42 percent of the women said they'd underestimate their total number of former lovers. In another survey of 665 college students, many people reported telling lies about their histories in order to have sex.[106]

Thus simply asking one's partner about STDs is not enough to eliminate the risk and does not by itself guarantee safe sex. Sexually active people deceive themselves when they rely on the truthfulness of a partner as protection against STDs.

Also, prospective partners may actually be truthful and may not have much of a sexual past, but this doesn't mean they are free from infections. It takes only one encounter to contract an STD, and many infections exhibit no symptoms. Some people erroneously believe that only people of low character get these STDs. But in reality, anyone who has been exposed to STDs can get them, even ''nice'' people. And you cannot tell by looking who is infected and who is not.

The only way to know *for sure* about a prospective partner's infection status is to have the person go for medical tests. Your prospective partner's blood can be screened for HIV antigens, syphilis, herpes, and human papillomavirus antibodies. Your prospective partner can also undergo culture tests for chlamydia, gonorrhea, and trichomoniasis.

Having a prospective partner tested for the common STDs just discussed is costly (it could easily cost more than $500). Many health care authorities recommend, at the minimum, to have a prospective partner tested for AIDS, since this STD is invariably fatal. The reliability of this strategy assumes that the person has maintained a period of abstinence before being tested and maintains sexual abstinence after being tested. For example, if your

■ *FACT OR FICTION:* A reliable strategy for preventing STDs is to ask potential partners about their past sexual experiences. *False.* Simply asking a potential partner about past sexual experiences overlooks the fact that many people lie, and is not an accurate way to assess infection status.

prospective partner is tested one day and the day after the test contracts a disease, this strategy would obviously fail. Also, be prepared to undergo these tests yourself as well.

Once you've determined that a prospective partner is free of infection, you need to assess the person's trustworthiness. You need to know that your partner will be monogamous, as you will be. A committed, long-term relationship is most likely to be monogamous. A prospective partner who has agreed to undergo the medical tests just mentioned must be quite interested in having a long-term, committed, mutually monogamous relationship with you and is probably capable of being, and intends to be, both monogamous and trustworthy.

≡ ▶ *Sexual abstinence and mutual monogamy with an uninfected partner are the only practices that are absolutely safe. These practices offer other rewards beyond those of STD prevention.*

Reduced-Risk Strategies

Abstinence and mutual monogamy with an uninfected partner are the only strategies that are safe.[107] A person who chooses to have unsafe sex can take some action to reduce STD risks. The following guidelines offer only some degree of protection.

If there is any doubt about a partner's infection status, the wise person will assume that the partner is infected. Therefore, the goal is to avoid any exchange of body fluids. This involves two techniques: restricting sexual activities and using barrier methods during sexual activity.

RESTRICT SEXUAL ACTIVITIES This risk-reduction measure must be very stringent, with sexual activity limited to mutual masturbation only, and only when the hands have no cuts or open sores. Body fluids, after all, include saliva, vaginal secretions, semen, urine, blood, and anal secretions, and all of these must be avoided. Therefore, to avoid exchange of body fluids a person must not have mouth contact with the penis, vagina, or rectum, and must abandon deep kissing, oral sex, vaginal intercourse, and anal intercourse.

USE LATEX CONDOMS WITH SPERMICIDE If couples do not restrict their sexual activities, they must use the next-best risk-reduction measure: using latex condoms in absolutely every episode of sexual activity, including oral sex and intercourse.[108] Latex condoms (not natural skin or lambskin) with spermicide may provide an effective barrier, and so may prevent the exchange of body fluids.[109] Natural condoms are sufficiently porous to permit the transmission of pathogens,[110] so this discussion focuses on latex condoms.

Condoms are not perfectly safe, although they are better than nothing. Advertisements that promote condom use as "safe sex" mislead people and give them a false sense of security—implying that as long as they use condoms, they can have sex with infected people safely. Many health officials fear that the campaign to encourage condom use to curb the spread of AIDS and other STDs may be misunderstood, creating a false sense of security in

Abstinence and having a mutually monogamous relationship with an uninfected partner are the only true safe-sex strategies.

■ *FACT OR FICTION:* Condoms are 100% effective at protecting people from AIDS and other sexually transmitted diseases. *False.* Condoms may provide an effective barrier to body fluid, but they are not perfectly safe.

people whose behavior continues to put them in danger.[111] The keys to using condoms to best advantage are to select, store, and use them properly every time (see this chapter's Spotlight).

Chapter 13 and this chapter's Spotlight describe the use of condoms with spermicides.

≡▶ *Avoiding exchange of body fluids by restricting sexual activity and using latex condoms with spermicide may reduce STD risk. These methods are by no means foolproof and are not recommended when failure can result in death.*

Other Suggestions to Reduce STD Risk

The suggestions just given are all the things a person can do to eliminate or reduce risk of STDs. The following are things to avoid.

AVOID ANAL SEX The practice of **anal sex** is common among many homosexual men and is not uncommon among heterosexual partners. Anal sex is associated with health risks for anyone who engages in it. The anus cannot stretch as the vagina does, and is subject to tearing during the sex act. The bleeding that occurs when the anal membrane is ruptured renders the person receptive to sexually transmitted diseases, particularly the AIDS virus. Even without bleeding, the anal passage is like the rest of the digestive tract in that it is an absorptive organ. It picks up pathogens efficiently and transfers them into the bloodstream just as if they were nutrients. Another hazard: the anus may rupture; the resultant excessive bleeding can be life threatening and requires immediate medical attention.

anal sex: inserting the penis into the anus.

Another important point about anal stimulation is that anything that has been inserted into the anus should not be put into the vagina unless it has been thoroughly washed. Bacteria that are naturally present in the anus can cause vaginal infections, so moving from anal intercourse (or finger insertion into the anus) to vaginal intercourse (or finger insertion into the vagina) is risking infection.

AVOID DRUGS Do not use alcohol or other drugs that may impair your judgment. The transmission of STDs is more common among those who abuse alcohol than among those who do not.[112] This may be due to impaired judgment, which leads to sexual relations with a high-risk person or to failure to use a condom.[113]

AVOID SEX WITH HIGH-RISK PEOPLE Do not have a sexual relationship with anyone in a high-risk group: a male homosexual, anyone else who engages in anal sex, an IV drug addict, a prostitute (male or female), or anyone who has multiple partners.[114] Do not have multiple sex partners (male or female). Do not have anonymous sex partners (male or female). Do not have sex with anyone who has rashes or sores. (Remember, though, that the absence of sores does not mean your partner is risk-free.)

SEEK EARLY DIAGNOSIS If you have contracted an STD, treat it early. See a health professional if you have any of these STD symptoms:

■ Unusual discharge from vagina, penis, or rectum.

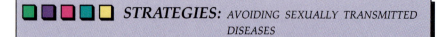

STRATEGIES: *AVOIDING SEXUALLY TRANSMITTED DISEASES*

To completely *protect yourself from contracting STDs:*

1. Practice sexual abstinence.
2. Have a mutually monogamous sexual relationship with an uninfected partner.
3. Have a series of mutually monogamous relationships with uninfected partners.

To reduce *your STD risk:*

4. Avoid contact with partner's body fluids.
5. Restrict sexual activity.
6. Use latex condoms with spermicides in every sexual act whereby body fluids are exchanged (intercourse and oral sex).
7. Do not practice anal sex or any other traumatic sexual activity.
8. Do not use alcohol or other drugs.
9. Do not have sex with high-risk people.

One more strategy against AIDS:

10. If you are addicted to a drug that you administer by injection, seek help for the addiction; meanwhile, use only clean, unused syringes.

■ Pain or burning during urination or intercourse.
■ Pain in the abdomen (women), testes (men), or buttocks and legs.
■ Blisters, open sores, warts, rashes, or swelling in the genital area, sex organs, or mouth.
■ Flulike symptoms: fever, headache, aching muscles, or swollen glands.

Some places to get help include college or university health services, public health departments or community STD clinics, or the offices of private physicians.[115] Follow any prescribed treatment carefully.

PROTECT YOURSELF IN MEDICAL SETTINGS Remember that you can contract AIDS in the following ways, too. Do not receive blood or blood products from unknown donors. Make sure your health care providers wear gloves when doing invasive procedures such as vaginal, rectal, and dental exams. And ask your health care provider the following questions:

■ Are you HIV-positive?
■ Do you use a new set of gloves for each client and disinfect your instruments (including their handles) between clients?
■ Do you follow the universal safety precautions for health care professionals—masks, protective eyewear, and gowns when blood or other body fluids could be dispersed?
■ Do you and the facilities where you practice follow standard universal precautions?

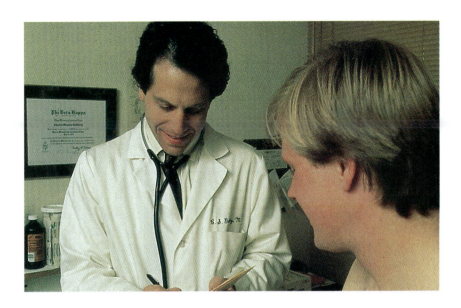

See a health professional.

PROTECT OTHERS If you have HIV or are in a high-risk group, do not donate blood, plasma, organs, tissues, or sperm.[116] If you are sexually active outside of a mutually monogamous relationship with an uninfected partner, get annual checkups and request an STD exam. If you find you have an STD, notify your sex partners, and make sure they've been treated before you resume sexual activity. Otherwise, you and your partner may end up passing the pathogen back and forth several times.

The best way to tell someone you have an STD is simply to do it as directly as possible—in person or on the phone, when you are sure only that person is listening. If telling someone this way is impossible—for example, if you are out of the country when the diagnosis is made—you should send the person a letter. A danger of this method is that letters have a way of getting opened by other people or lost in the mail. If a letter is the only option, include these elements:

■ That you have been diagnosed with an STD and that your partner (or former partner) may therefore have it, too, even if no symptoms have appeared.
■ That the person should see a health care provider or go to a clinic at once.
■ That the person should immediately inform anyone else who might have it.

In many cases the entrance of an STD into a relationship gives partners reason to question the other's trustworthiness. Discovering that a partner has been sexually unfaithful can be devastating and often destroys relationships. The thought of telling a partner of a diagnosis of an STD can be psychologically threatening. But people who are sexually intimate together have rights and responsibilities—the right to be informed if a dangerous disease is a possibility, and the responsibility to inform all sex partners that treatment is needed, if a positive diagnosis has been made. After all, if you value someone enough to worry about losing his or her affection, then a way to prove you care is to warn the person of physical danger. Besides, simultaneous treatment of sex partners is essential to keep them from reinfecting each other.

≡▶ *To reduce STD risk, avoid anal sex, drug use, or sex with high-risk people. Obtain regular STD exams, get early treatment, and inform your partners if you contract an STD.*

Without cures for some STDs, the solution is prevention. Except in rare cases, the locus of control is with you—your behavior dictates your STD risk.

■≡ For Review

1. List the major beneficial roles bacteria play in the body.
2. Compare and contrast bacteria, viruses, fungi, parasitic worms, rickettsia, and protozoa in terms of their requirements for life.
3. Name the factors required for infection to spread.
4. Describe the importance of public health systems in preventing the spread of the most prevalent infectious diseases.

5. Explain how vaccinations work to prevent diseases.
6. Describe the body's lines of defense against microbes and the order in which it uses them when pathogens attack.
7. List several personal strategies that strengthen people's defenses against infectious diseases.
8. Give examples of some sexually transmitted diseases (STDs), and

describe their detrimental effects on the body when they are allowed to progress untreated.
9. Describe some effects of STDs on fetuses and infants.
10. Describe ways in which the transmission of AIDS occurs and how it can be prevented.
11. List some strategies useful to avoid contracting AIDS and other STDs.

■≡ Notes

1. M. S. Insler and B. A. Gore, *Pseudomonas* keratitis and folliculitis from whirlpool exposure, *American Journal of Ophthalmology* 101 (1986): 41–43.
2. WHO warns of TB increase, *The Nation's Health,* January 1991, p. 2.
3. E. Zamula, Tuberculosis still striking after all these years, *FDA Consumer* 25 (1991): 18–23.
4. U.S. Department of Health and Human Services, Public Health Service, *Summary of Healthy People, 2000: National Health Promotion and Disease Prevention Objectives* (Washington, D.C.: Government Printing Office, 1990), pp. 21–22.
5. H. D. Jampel and coauthors, Fever and immunoregulation: 3. Hyperthermia augments the primary in vitro humoral immune response, *Journal of Experimental Medicine* 157 (1983): 1229–1238.

6. J. P. Cohn, Here come the bugs: Cold and flu season's back, *FDA Consumer* 22 (1988): 6–10.
7. J. G. Cannon and M. J. Kluger, Exercise enhances survival rate in mice infected with *Salmonella typhimurium, Proceedings of the Society for Experimental Biology and Medicine* 175 (1984): 518–521.
8. J. Schachter, Why we need a program for the control of *Chlamydia trachomatis, New England Journal of Medicine* 320 (1989): 802–803.
9. *Chlamydia trachomatis* infections: Policy guidelines for prevention and control, *Morbidity and Mortality Weekly Report* 34 (Supplement 3S, 1985): 53S–74S.
10. D. M. White and W. M. Felts, Knowledge and chlamydial infection among university students, *Health Education* 20 (1989): 23–25.
11. *What Are Sexually Transmitted*

Diseases? (Rockville, Md.: American College Health Association, 1988).
12. White and Felts, 1989.
13. White and Felts, 1989.
14. *What Are Sexually Transmitted Diseases?* 1988.
15. H. L. Zimmerman and coauthors, Epidemiologic differences between chlamydia and gonorrhea, *American Journal of Public Health* 80 (1990): 1338–1342.
16. White and Felts, 1989.
17. P. M. Layde, Pelvic inflammatory disease and the Dalkon shield (Editorial), *Journal of the American Medical Association* 250 (1983): 796; D. Ki and coauthors, Prior condom use and the risk of tubal pregnancy, *American Journal of Public Health* 80 (1990): 964–966.
18. Schachter, 1989.
19. J. Schachter and coauthors, Experience with the routine use of

erythromycin for chlamydial infections in pregnancy, *New England Journal of Medicine* 314 (1986): 276–279; *Chlamydia trachomatis* infections, 1985.

20. J. L. Jacobson, *Women's Reproductive Health: The Silent Emergency*, Worldwatch Paper 102 (Washington, D.C.: Worldwatch Institute, June 1991).

21. *What Are Sexually Transmitted Diseases?* 1988.

22. J. F. Rooney and coauthors, Acquisition of genital herpes from an asymptomatic sexual partner, *New England Journal of Medicine* 314 (1986): 1561–1564.

23. *What Are Sexually Transmitted Diseases?* 1988.

24. *What Are Sexually Transmitted Diseases?* 1988.

25. *What Are Sexually Transmitted Diseases?* 1988.

26. R. Whitley and coauthors, Predictors of morbidity and mortality in neonates with herpes simplex virus infections, *New England Journal of Medicine* 324 (1991): 450–454.

27. Z. A. Brown and coauthors, Effects on infants of a first episode of genital herpes during pregnancy, *New England Journal of Medicine* 317 (1987): 1246–1251.

28. G. J. Mertz and coauthors, Long-term acyclovir suppression of frequently recurring genital herpes simplex virus infection, *Journal of the American Medical Association* 260 (1988): 201–206.

29. Unapproved herpes drug confiscated, trail followed, *FDA Consumer* 24 (1990): 34–35.

30. A. Loucks, Human papillomavirus screening in college women, *Journal of American College Health* 39 (1991): 291–293.

31. *What Are Sexually Transmitted Diseases?* 1988.

32. Virus type predicts risky cancer return, *Science News* 136 (1989): 310; HPV viruses linked to cervical cancer,

once again, *The Nation's Health*, August 1989, p. 17.

33. Jacobson, 1991.

34. Barrier contraception blocks cervical cancer, *Modern Medicine* 55 (1987): 25.

35. R. S. Ostrow and coauthors, Detection of papillomavirus DNA in human semen, *Science* 231 (1986): 731–733.

36. *Condyloma* (Daly City, Calif.: Krames Communications, 1988).

37. New treatment for genital warts, *FDA Consumer*, September 1988, pp. 6–7.

38. R. T. Rolfs, M. Goldberg, and R. G. Sharrar, Risk factors for syphilis: Cocaine use and prostitution, *American Journal of Public Health* 80 (1990): 853–857.

39. *What Are Sexually Transmitted Diseases?* 1988.

40. Jacobson, 1991.

41. *What Are Sexually Transmitted Diseases?* 1988.

42. Jacobson, 1991.

43. *What Are Sexually Transmitted Diseases?* 1988.

44. *What Are Sexually Transmitted Diseases?* 1988.

45. What to do about urinary-tract infections, *Consumer Reports Health Letter* 2 (1990): 73–74.

46. J. W. Buehler, O. J. Devine, R. L. Berkelman, and F. M. Chevarley, Impact of the human immunodeficiency virus epidemic on mortality trend in young men, United States, *American Journal of Public Health* 80 (1990): 1080–1086.

47. *Answers about AIDS* (Summit, N.J.: American Council on Science and Health, (1988).

48. H. D. Gayle and coauthors, Prevalence of the human immunodeficiency virus among university students, *New England Journal of Medicine* 323 (1990): 1538–1541.

49. R. A. Kaslow and coauthors, The multicenter AIDS cohort study: Rationale, organization, and selected

characteristics of the participants, *American Journal of Epidemiology* 126 (1987): 310–318, as cited in W. A. Haseltine, Silent HIV infections, *New England Journal of Medicine* 320 (1989): 1487–1488; D. Osmond and coauthors, Time of exposure and risk of HIV infection in homosexual partners of men with AIDS, *American Journal of Public Health* 78 (1988): 944–948.

50. *Answers about AIDS*, 1988.

51. R. M. Healy and T. Coleman, A primer of AIDS for health professionals, *Health Education* 19 (1988/1989): 4–10; Glimpses of AIDS and male prostitution, *Science News* 138 (1990): 380.

52. C. E. Koop, *Understanding AIDS—A Message from the Surgeon General* (Washington, D.C.: Government Printing Office, 1988).

53. *Answers about AIDS*, 1988; Healy and Coleman, 1988/1989.

54. U.S. Department of Health and Human Services, Public Health Service, Centers for Disease Control, Summary of results, data from serosurveillance activities through 1989, in *National HIV Seroprevalence Surveys*, 2d ed., 1990; R. Detels and B. Visscher, HIV and orogenital transmission, *Lancet*, 29 October 1988, p. 1023.

55. Koop, 1988.

56. K. K. Holmes, J. M. Karon, and J. Kreiss, The increasing frequency of heterosexually acquired AIDS in the United States, 1983–88, *American Journal of Public Health* 80 (1990): 858–862.

57. R. Ahia, Compliance with safer-sex guidelines among adolescent males: Application of the health belief model and protection motivation theory, *Health Education* 22 (1991): 49–52.

58. *Answers about AIDS*, 1988.

59. A. R. Lifson and coauthors, HIV seroconversion in two homosexual men after receptive oral intercourse

with ejaculation: Implications for counseling concerning safe sexual practices, *American Journal of Public Health* 80 (1990): 1509–1511.

60. W. Rozenbaum and coauthors, HIV transmission by oral sex, *Lancet* 1 (1988): 1395, and F. D. Konotey-Ahulu, Extensive palatal ecchymosis from fellatio: A note of caution with AIDS at large, *British Journal of Sexual Medicine* 14 (1987): 286–288.

61. Healy and Coleman, 1988/1989.

62. M. Piazza and coauthors, Passionate kissing and microlesions of the oral mucosa: Possible role in AIDS transmission, *Journal of the American Medical Association* 261 (1989): 244–245.

63. H. Jones, N. Ellis, M. Tappe, and G. Lindsay, HIV related beliefs, knowledge and behaviors of ninth and eleventh grade public school students, *Journal of Health Education* 22 (1991): 12–18.

64. *Answers about AIDS,* 1988.

65. Healy and Coleman, 1988/1989; Y. Chu, J. W. Buehler, P. L. Flemming, and R. L. Berkelman, Epidemiology of reported cases of AIDS in lesbians, United States 1980–89, *American Journal of Public Health* 80 (1990): 1380–1381.

66. *Answers about AIDS,* 1988.

67. *Answers about AIDS,* 1988.

68. D. Vittecoq, J. F. Mettetal, C. Rouzious, and J. F. Bach, Acute HIV infection after acupuncture treatments, *New England Journal of Medicine* 320 (1989): 250–251.

69. *Answers about AIDS,* 1988.

70. Healy and Coleman, 1988/1989.

71. *Answers about AIDS,* 1988.

72. S. Logan, M. L. Newell, T. Ades, and C. S. Peckham, Breast feeding and HIV infection, *Lancet* 1 (1988): 1346; S. J. Heymann, Modeling the impact of breast-feeding by HIV-infected women on child survival, *American Journal of Public Health* 80 (1990): 1305–1309.

73. G. H. Friedland, B. R. Saltzman, and M. F. Rogers, Lack of transmission of HTLV-III/LAV infection to household contacts of patients with AIDS or AIDS-related complex with oral candidiasis, *New England Journal of Medicine* 314 (1986): 344–349.

74. Koop, 1988.

75. *Casual Contact and the Risk of HIV Infection,* July 1989 (a report of the Special Initiative on AIDS of the American Public Health Association, Washington, D.C.).

76. *Casual Contact and the Risk of HIV Infection,* 1989; Kaslow and coauthors, 1987.

77. Healy and Coleman, 1988/1989.

78. Healy and Coleman, 1988/1989; *Answers about AIDS,* 1988.

79. Newsfront, *Modern Medicine,* March 1987, p. 16.

80. *Answers about AIDS,* 1988.

81. S. Broder, *AIDS: Modern Concepts and Therapeutic Challenges* (New York: Marcel Dekker, 1987).

82. *Answers about AIDS,* 1988.

83. *Answers about AIDS,* 1988.

84. Broder, 1987.

85. *Answers about AIDS,* 1988.

86. W. E. Lafferty, D. Glidden, and S. G. Hopkins, Survival trends of people with AIDS in Washington State, *American Journal of Public Health* 81 (1991): 215–218.

87. R. D. Gallo and L. Montagnier, AIDS in 1988, *Scientific American,* October 1988, pp. 41–48; K. A. Fackelmann, Early AZT use slows progression to AIDS, *Science News,* 136 (1989): 135.

88. *Answers about AIDS,* 1988.

89. J. S. Lambert and coauthors, 2′, 3′-dideoxyinosine (ddi) in patients with the acquired immunodeficiency syndrome or AIDS-related complex, *New England Journal of Medicine* 332 (1989): 1333–1340.

90. A. S. Fauci, ddi—A good start, but still phase I, *New England Journal of Medicine* 322 (1990): 1386–1387.

91. New AIDS treatment studies, *FDA Consumer,* June 1989, p. 4; R. R. Redfield and coauthors, A phase I evaluation of the safety and immunogenicity and vaccination with recombinant gp160 in patients with early human immunodeficiency virus infection, *New England Journal of Medicine* 324 (1991): 1677–1684.

92. National Academy of Sciences, Institute of Medicine, Committee on a National Strategy for AIDS, *Confronting AIDS: Directions for Public Health, Health Care, and Research* (Washington, D.C.: National Academy Press, 1986).

93. R. Fennell, Evaluating the effectiveness of a credit semester course on AIDS among college students, *Journal of Health Education* 22 (1991): 35–36.

94. *What Are Sexually Transmitted Diseases?* 1988.

95. K. M. Stone, D. A. Grimes, and L. S. Magder, Personal protection against sexually transmitted diseases, *American Journal of Obstetrics and Gynecology* 155 (1986): 180–188.

96. J. J. Goedert, What is safe sex? *New England Journal of Medicine* 316 (1987): 1339–1342.

97. Healy and Coleman, 1988/1989.

98. Adapted with permission from R. A. Hatcher and coauthors, *Contraceptive Technology* (New York: Irvington, 1991), pp. 157–158.

99. N. Hearst and S. B. Hulley, Preventing the heterosexual spread of AIDS: Are we giving our patients the best advice? *Journal of the American Medical Association* 259 (1988): 2428–2432; Healy and Coleman, 1988/1989.

100. Goedert, 1987; Hearst and Hulley, 1988.

101. Koop, 1988.

102. Testimony of Theresa L. Crenshaw, president, American Association of Sex Educators, Counselors and Therapists, *Condom advertising and AIDS,* Hearing before the Subcommittee on Health and the Environment of the Committee on

Energy and Commerce, 100th Congress, 1st session, 10 February, 1987 (Washington, D.C.: Government Printing Office, 1987), pp. 69–78.

103. E. Weinstein, Health educators: Where are you? *Health Education* 19 (1988/1989): 21–22.

104. M. Roberts, Dating, dishonesty and AIDS, *Psychology Today,* December 1988, p. 60.

105. Roberts, 1988.

106. S. D. Cochran and V. M. Mays, Sex, lies, and HIV, *New England Journal of Medicine* 322 (1990): 774.

107. Goedert, 1987.

108. Goedert, 1987.

109. Healy and Coleman, 1988/1989.

110. M. F. Goldsmith, Sex in the age of AIDS calls for common sense and condom sense, *Journal of the American Medical Association* 257 (1987): 2261–2266.

111. L. Gruson, Condoms: Experts fear false sense of security, *New York Times Science Times,* 18 August 1987, pp. C1, C9.

112. L. Penkower and coauthors, Behavior, health and psychosocial factors and risk for HIV infection among sexually active homosexual men: The multicenter AIDS cohort study, *American Journal of Public Health* 81 (1991): 194–196.

113. Alcohol and AIDS connection, *Nutrition Today,* July/August 1988, p. 34.

114. Healy and Coleman, 1988/1989.

115. *Making Sex Safer* (Rockville, Md.: American College Association, 1987).

116. Healy and Coleman, 1988/1989.

SPOTLIGHT

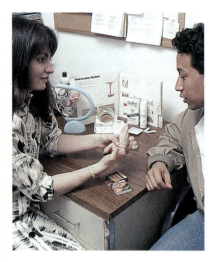

Condoms: Safe Sex Device or a Dangerous Illusion?

Condom use has been promoted by some as a safe-sex strategy. Indeed, next to abstinence or a mutually monogamous relationship with an uninfected partner, condoms are the best protection available, so don't discount them while reading about their drawbacks. But how effective, really, is this second line of defense against transmission of STDs? Condoms offer some protection, but it is nowhere near absolute.[1]* This Spotlight explores the problems with relying on condoms for absolute STD protection.

In the past, people considered STDs as minor inconveniences

*Reference notes are at the end of the Spotlight.

requiring minimal physician attention. Today, however, STDs have shown themselves to be much more threatening. AIDS, of course, is most certainly fatal; genital warts is now known to cause cancer; and chlamydia causes life-threatening pelvic disease. With stakes this high, people must demand higher levels of protection than they would have against the easily curable STDs of the past. For this reason, experts have taken a hard look at the facts concerning the degree of protection against STDs that condoms provide.

If condoms do not offer absolute protection, why are they so widely promoted?

The use of latex condoms with spermicides can minimize the spread of STDs, so experts claim that campaigns that promote the devices are valuable.[2] In large groups, condom use has been shown to reduce STD prevalence.[3] For example, in Sweden, authorities aggressively promoted condom use and demonstrated an 80 percent reduction in the incidence of gonorrhea.[4] For this reason, authorities say encouraging condom use is a valid public health strategy: if most people in a population use condoms correctly and consistently, the number of STD infections drops.

"Most people" doesn't mean "every individual," though. Although fewer people in a *population* get STDs, condom use cannot be guaranteed as a total safe-sex strategy for any *individual*.[5] Promoting condom use, which helps prevent STDs but does not eliminate them, is like promoting vaccinations against the measles. It greatly benefits the population at large, but some vaccinated individuals still get the measles.

How does condom protection against pregnancy compare with condom protection against STDs?

Unplanned pregnancies with the use of condoms are common events. STDs with the use of condoms are probably even more common, because a woman is fertile only a few days a month, whereas she is vulnerable to STD pathogens all the time. Also, bacteria and viruses, being much smaller than sperm, are more able to penetrate through condom membranes.[6] Condom failure rates for STDs are likely to be substantially greater than for pregnancy, even for highly motivated people.

How much protection do condoms offer against STDs?

No one knows exactly. In laboratory experiments, condoms have been shown to effectively block the transmission of sperm, the herpes virus, and HIV.[7] These tests, however, do not accurately duplicate real-life condom use. Laboratory tests use a machine that simulates vaginal intercourse performed by people who are using a condom correctly. To suggest that the results of such research apply to real people is to falsely assume that people always use condoms properly in real life.[8]

Secretions can get around and over a condom even if it does not break. Cases have been reported of women who developed AIDS while depending on condoms for protection.[9]

What are some real-life problems associated with condom use?

In real life, problems with condom use fall into two categories. The first of these is under people's control—

the way they use condoms. People sometimes do not pay close attention when using them: they often put them on or take them off improperly, and they sometimes allow them to slip off or get pulled off. Some people do not or cannot read the directions. People often inadvertently allow condoms to be exposed to heat or light, where they can deteriorate rapidly. Some people use oil-based lubricants with them, such as Vaseline, which cause them to break down.

When people drink alcohol or take other mind-altering drugs before using condoms, their concentration and judgment become impaired. Good intentions to use condoms often disappear in the heat of passion, anyway, and under the influence of alcohol or other drugs, people especially often use condoms improperly or not at all.

Knowing that a great part of condom failure is due to people's using them incorrectly or not at all is, in a way, encouraging. It means people can overcome such failures by using condoms *meticulously every time* they engage in sexual activity. Unfortunately, though, even if people use condoms perfectly and consistently, they are still not guaranteed complete protection, for the condoms themselves may fail.

Condom quality varies, unfortunately, in ways that are out of the user's control. Condoms are known to age, to break, to tear, to leak, or to be damaged in their packages. For example, one study of condom use showed that 5 percent of the people's condoms ruptured even with proper use.[10]

Aren't condoms tested? Don't they have to meet legal standards?

Yes, but some batches are still defective. Condoms have been found to deteriorate dangerously *before* their expiration dates.[11] The FDA recently required three leading manufacturers to recall 100,000 condoms because a spot check had found that an excessive number of them leaked.[12] And the spot check was not conducted until *after* those batches of condoms had already been distributed to the public.

Are there other problems with condoms used for STD prevention?

Condoms have special limitations in regard to preventing transmission of the herpes virus. While they sometimes effectively block the virus in areas they cover, they provide no barrier to viruses from lesions in areas that they do not cover, such as on the vulva, testes, or lower abdomen or legs.

With all the limitations of condoms, are they really worth using?

If you do not practice truly safe sex by abstaining or limiting your sexual activity to one mutually monogamous partner, by all means, use condoms. They will significantly lower your risk, provided you use them *meticulously every time* you have sex.

How can I use condoms properly?

Successful condom use relies upon proper selection, storage, and use.

What should I look for when selecting a condom?

First, do not purchase one from a vending machine that is exposed to extremes of temperatures or to direct sunlight. Extreme temperatures, especially heat, can damage latex condoms.[13] Next, read the label. The condoms should be made of latex

rubber, and the package should say that the condoms are to prevent disease. Do not use novelty condoms; they will not be labeled this way and will not protect against disease. Buy condoms with spermicide; the spermicide nonoxynol-9 kills some organisms that cause STDs. Do not purchase or use condoms past their expiration dates, which are usually listed by the abbreviation "EXP." And store them in a cool, dry, dark, clean place.[14] Closets or drawers are usually good storage places; pockets, wallets, purses, or glove compartments of cars are not.

Describe proper condom use.

When opening a condom, handle the package gently. Don't use teeth, fingernails, scissors, or other sharp instruments, as these may damage the condom. Make sure you have adequate light, and inspect the condom closely after you have opened it. If the material sticks to itself or is gummy, it is damaged—discard it. Check the condom top for other obvious damage, such as brittleness, tears, and holes, but don't unroll the condom to check it, because this could damage it.[15]

Use a new condom for every act of intercourse or oral sex. If the penis is uncircumcised, pull the foreskin back before putting on the condom. Put the condom on after the penis is erect and before any contact is made between the penis and the partner's body. Put a small amount of spermicide inside the condom tip, even if the condom contains spermicide. (Spermicide can kill some pathogens.) If the condom does not have a reservoir top, pinch the tip enough to leave a half-inch space for semen to collect. While pinching the half-inch tip, place the condom against the penis, and unroll it all the way to the base. It must unroll completely to cover the entire penis. Add more spermicide on the outside of the condom.

If you feel the condom slip off or break during intercourse, stop immediately and withdraw. Do not continue until you put on a new condom and apply more spermicide.

Promptly after ejaculation, before the penis gets soft, grip the rim of the condom to hold it on, and carefully withdraw. Then, to remove the condom, gently pull it off the penis, being careful the semen doesn't spill out. Do not reuse it; condoms are not to be recycled. Because condoms may cause problems in sewers, don't flush it down the toilet. Wrap the used condom in a tissue, and dispose of it where others won't handle it. Afterward, wash your hands with soap and water.

Curtail use of alcohol and other drugs that can affect your judgment and ability to use a condom properly.

Never use a lubricant that contains oils, fats, or greases, such as petroleum-based jelly (Vaseline), baby oil, hand or body lotions, cooking shortening, or oily cosmetics such as cold creams. These can seriously weaken latex, causing a condom to tear easily. Use a spermicide as a lubricant, or use a water-based product such as K-Y jelly.

What do I need to know about using condoms for oral sex?

When engaging in oral sex, use a condom without spermicide, or else it may have a bitter taste. One researcher warns that saliva may cause condoms to deteriorate, though, so their use for oral sex may be more risky than commonly realized.[16]

Do condoms provide protection during anal sex?

Condoms fail more often during anal than vaginal intercourse.[17] Because of the friction and stress of anal sex, condoms are likely to slip off and break. Studies have shown condoms to be unreliable for anal sex even in testing conditions, where use is optimal.[18]

Another problem that occurs, even among highly educated and motivated homosexual men, is noncompliance—people don't like to use condoms.[19] Anal sex is a dangerous activity that should not be practiced at all.

Condoms are to be used as only the second-best line of defense for STD protection, next to mutual monogamy with an uninfected partner or sexual abstinence. People who hope condoms will provide full protection against AIDS are in danger. When condoms fail, the consequences can be fatal. People who rely on condoms for complete protection are playing Russian roulette, particularly in regard to AIDS.[20] A lot of people will die in this dangerous game.

■≡ Spotlight Notes

1. Testimony of Theresa L. Crenshaw, president, American Association of Sex Educators, Counselors and Therapists, Condom advertising and AIDS, Hearing before the Subcommittee on Health and the Environment of the Committee on Energy and Commerce, 100th Congress, 1st session, February 10, 1987 (Washington, D.C.: Government Printing Office, 1987), pp. 69–78; J. L. Willis, Latex condoms lessen risks of STDs, *FDA Consumer* 24 (1990): 32–36.

2. L. Gruson, Condoms: Experts fear false sense of security, *Science Times* (*New York Times*), 18 August 1987, pp. C1, C9.

3. J. A. Perlman and coauthors, HIV risk difference between condom users and nonusers among U.S. heterosexual women, *Journal of Acquired Immune Deficiency Syndromes* 3 (1990): 155–165.

4. M. F. Goldsmith, Sex in the age of AIDS calls for common sense and condom sense, *Journal of the*

American Medical Association 257 (1987): 2261–2263.

5. J. J. Goedert, What is safe sex? *New England Journal of Medicine* 316 (1987): 1339–1342.

6. Willis, 1990.

7. M. Conant and coauthors, Condoms prevent transmission of AIDS-associated retrovirus, *Journal of the American Medical Association* 255 (1986): 1706.

8. Willis, 1990.

9. M. A. Fischl and coauthors, Eval-

uation of heterosexual partners, children, and household contacts of adults with AIDS, *Journal of the American Medical Association* 257 (1987): 640–644.

10. P. C. Gotzsche and M. Hording, Condoms to prevent HIV transmission do not imply truly safe sex, *Scandivanian Journal of Infectious Diseases* 20 (1988): 233–234.

11. Gruson, 1987.

12. Gruson, 1987.

13. Willis, 1990.

14. Willis, 1990.

15. Willis, 1990.

16. M. F. Goldsmith, Some advice on using condoms against STDs: What every man (and woman) should know, *Journal of the American Medical Association* 257 (1987): 2266.

17. Gruson, 1987.

18. L. Wigersma and R. Oud, Safety and acceptability of condoms for use by homosexual men as a prophylactic against transmission of HIV during anogenital sexual intercourse, *British Medical Journal* 295 (1987): 94.

19. Goedert, 1987.

20. Testimony of Theresa L. Crenshaw, 1987.

CHAPTER 18

Heart and Artery Disease

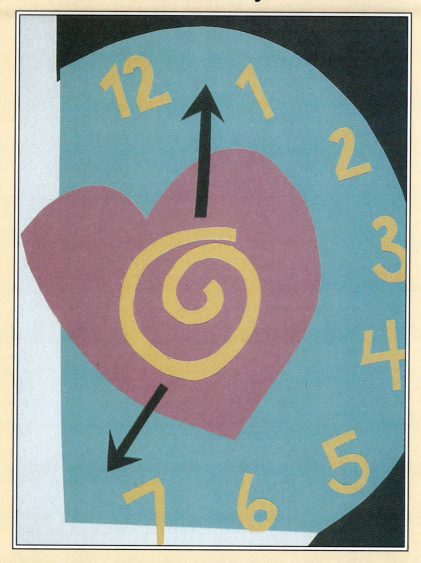

M ost teenagers and people in their 20s feel they have little to fear from heart and artery disease. After all, they reason, people of their grandparents' and parents' ages are the only ones they know with heart disease; young adults need not worry about it. To a point, their feelings are valid, for indeed, few young people do suffer with advanced heart and artery disease. But they are forgetting a critical fact about these diseases: cardiovascular diseases develop slowly over a lifetime. And in developed countries, everyone has some degree of disease, even in early childhood. The hearts of children show early traces of developing heart disease, and these traces steadily worsen through the young adult years; autopsies on soldiers as young as 18 have shown that their arteries were already clogged with accumulated fat. Finally, in middle age or later, the heart and arteries are so damaged that they fail to perform their life-supporting tasks. A fast progression toward disabling disease is not inevitable, though. Experts believe that, many times, the choices people make in young adulthood have everything to do with whether or not their heart and artery disease progresses to the danger point by middle age.

To understand the relationships between lifestyle habits and the health of the heart, you must first become acquainted with the workings of the circulatory system. Then an understanding of how heart and artery disease develops and what the associated risk factors are can give perspective on the risks of anyone's developing it. The last section of this chapter speaks of prevention—actions everyone can take now, to promote the health of the circulatory system before heart and artery diseases take hold.

■■ The Circulatory System

Each of the body's cells is a self-contained, living entity, but not one can live on its own, outside the body. Each cell stays alive about the same way as its single-celled ancestors did living alone in the ocean some 3 billion years ago—by taking up what it needs from the surrounding fluids and releasing its wastes into that fluid. Each cell of the body is bathed in fluid that provides it with a continuous supply of oxygen, energy, water, and building

■ *FACT OR FICTION:* Everyone is developing heart disease, even the young. *True.*

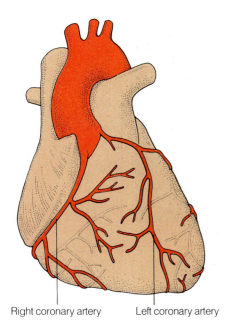

Right coronary artery   Left coronary artery

FIGURE 18–1 ■ **The heart's major arteries.**

materials. This fluid also provides a system of waste disposal, for when cells use up material, they cast off wastes that, if allowed to collect, would damage and ultimately kill the cells.

The system of the body charged with providing cells and tissues with a constant supply of nutrients and oxygen, removal of wastes, and communication between their parts is the **circulatory system**—the heart and its associated blood vessels. Also called the **cardiovascular system**, it pumps around the body the equivalent of 4,000 gallons of blood each day, propelling it by over 85,000 heartbeats.

The heart, at the center of the system, is almost all muscle, with hollow chambers inside that collect blood and then squirt it out again into tough, elastic arteries. The heart has four chambers: two that function as receiving areas and two, as shipping areas. The receiving chambers, the **atria**, pool the blood as it arrives from the body, and the shipping chambers, the **ventricles**, contract powerfully to send the blood on its way again. One atrium and ventricle, on the right side of the heart, collect used blood—blood that has visited the tissues—and send it to the lungs to pick up fresh oxygen supplies and to release its load of carbon dioxide, to be breathed out. The other atrium and ventricle, on the left side of the heart, collect blood that is returning from the lungs freshly oxygenated and force it out to the body tissues again.

The heart derives no direct benefit from the blood within its chambers. It relies for nourishment on its own network of arteries—the **coronary arteries**—and capillaries (see Figure 18–1). This fact becomes important to understanding how the heart is affected by disease.

You have probably listened to your own or someone else's heartbeat and noticed its two-step rhythm, sometimes called *lub-dub*. The first beat (lub) is the sound made when the atria contract to send the blood they have pooled to the ventricles below them; the second beat (dub) is the sound made when the ventricles contract to send the blood on its way to the body (the atria relax and pool more blood during the dub). You may be wondering why the contraction of the heart muscles should make any sound at all, and in reality it does not. The sound comes from the slapping shut of the heart's **valves**, flaps of tissue located at the entrances and exits of the chambers. Normally, the valves allow blood to flow in only one direction on its way through the heart, but if the valves are damaged or unusually shaped, some blood will flow backward, changing the sound (a **heart murmur**). Heart murmurs are usually no cause for alarm, but occasionally they reflect conditions that require medical attention.

The ventricles' jobs are to maintain the correct pressure of the blood in the **arteries** and to keep the blood moving at the rate that best maintains the tissues. The arteries are built to withstand the pressure of the blood pulsing from the ventricles. The arteries branch out, become smaller in diameter and more numerous, and end in networks of **capillaries**—webs of tiny vessels too small to see. No part of the blood can cross the artery walls, but the thin capillary walls allow fluid (lymph) with nutrients, oxygen, and chemical messengers such as hormones to be forced out of the bloodstream into the tissues. The fluid that is drawn back into the blood carries with it wastes from the tissues. The capillaries that carry waste-laden blood then merge with others to form greater vessels, the **veins**, and these transport this used

circulatory system the system of structures that circulates blood and lymph throughout the body. Also called the **cardiovascular system**.

atria (singular, **atrium**) the two upper chambers of the heart.

ventricles the two lower chambers of the heart.

coronary arteries the two arteries that supply blood to the heart muscle.

■ *FACT OR FICTION:* Just listening to the sound of the heartbeat can tell much about the health of the heart. *True.*

valves flaps of tissue that allow the body's fluids to flow in one direction only. The heart's valves are located at the entrances and exits of its chambers.

heart murmur a heart sound that reflects abnormal or damaged heart valves.

arteries: blood vessels that carry blood from the heart to the tissues.

capillaries minute weblike blood vessels that permit transfer of blood and tissue materials.

veins blood vessels that carry used blood from the tissues back to the heart.

blood to the lungs for renewal. Blood in the veins appears to be blue under the skin; the bluish cast appears when blood has been stripped of its oxygen by the tissues. Figure 18–2 diagrams the cardiovascular system.

So, to repeat, as the blood moves through a capillary net, much of its fluid, with its cargo of nutrients and oxygen, is strained out, leaving a high concentration of blood cells and dissolved materials inside the capillaries. This attracts fluids carrying wastes from the tissues, and these fluids seep back into the bloodstream. Thus the tissues are nourished and cleansed (see Figure 18–3). A similar exchange in specialized capillary networks within

FIGURE 18–2   ■   **An overview of the cardiovascular system.**

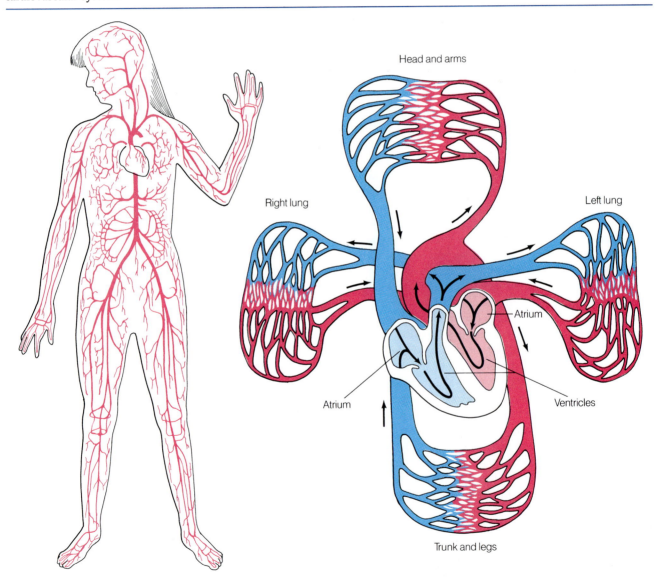

A. Arteries conduct blood away from the heart toward the tissues. Veins are not shown, but they form a similar network conducting blood back to the heart.

B. This is a simplified diagram that depicts the blood flow through the heart, out into arteries, through capillaries, and back to the heart by way of veins.

the kidneys removes certain wastes from the blood and disposes of them into the urine.

A certain blood pressure is vital to the trading of materials between tissues and the bloodstream. The pressure of the blood against capillary walls is what pushes fluids out into the tissues. Blood in the veins is under comparatively little pressure. It must travel uphill against gravity on the return trip from the lower parts of the body, such as the legs, to the heart.

The veins are more delicate than the arteries, and they are equipped with valves at intervals along their length to hold blood up against the downward pull of gravity. These valves can become too weak to hold the heavy blood, which then pools inside the delicate veins, causing them to bulge out visibly under the skin, a condition called **varicose veins**. People who stand on their feet for long periods are especially vulnerable. Elevating the legs for short

varicose veins visible bulging out of the veins, especially in the legs, sometimes accompanied by pain and ulcers.

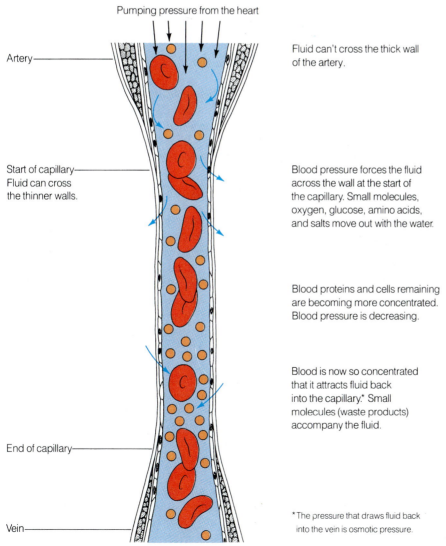

Artery

Start of capillary
Fluid can cross
the thinner walls.

End of capillary

Vein

Pumping pressure from the heart

Fluid can't cross the thick wall of the artery.

Blood pressure forces the fluid across the wall at the start of the capillary. Small molecules, oxygen, glucose, amino acids, and salts move out with the water.

Blood proteins and cells remaining are becoming more concentrated. Blood pressure is decreasing.

Blood is now so concentrated that it attracts fluid back into the capillary.* Small molecules (waste products) accompany the fluid.

*The pressure that draws fluid back into the vein is osmotic pressure.

FIGURE 18–3 ■ **Two kinds of pressure in the capillaries.**

intervals each day may help prevent the condition. Another help is exercise, for the contractions of the muscles that surround the veins help to propel the venous blood upward. Treatment may include elevating the feet each day, wearing supportive stockings, or undergoing surgical removal of the largeset veins. (Tiny, spidery purple marks on the skin are normal and are not related to vericose veins.)

Disease in any part of the circulatory system affects many of the body's tissues. **Heart disease** is any disease that affects the heart muscle or other working parts of the heart. The term **cardiovascular disease (CVD)** covers diseases of all parts of the cardiovascular system, including both the heart and blood vessels. The most prevalent form of CVD is **atherosclerosis**, which can lead to heart attack and stroke (see later sections). Cardiovascular disease is discussed next, with attention to the question of how people can minimize their risks.

≡▶ *The circulatory system consists of the heart and its associated blood vessels. The health of this system is absolutely vital, because it forms the tissues' supply line for nutrients and oxygen.*

■≡ Cardiovascular Disease

Cardiovascular disease is the number-one killer of adults. One in every four people living in the United States suffers from some form of this disease, and many more are developing it.[1]* Many people die of CVD long before they reach retirement age. Everyone is susceptible to heart and artery disease, but fortunately, everyone can take measures to help prevent it.

Atherosclerosis and Blood Clotting

Atherosclerosis, a type of hardening of the arteries, begins with an accumulation of mounds of soft fat along the inner walls of all the arteries of the body. Such mounds gradually enlarge and harden with mineral deposits to form **plaques**, which make the artery walls lose their elasticity and narrow the passage through them (see Figure 18–4). As mentioned, the heart muscle depends on blood flow through its own arteries for nourishment and oxygen—the blood it pumps through its chambers cannot meet its needs. The end result of atherosclerosis, then, may be disease of both the heart and of the arteries that feed other organs and tissues (CVD).

Normally, as blood surges through the arteries, they expand to allow blood to pass, and they contract with each beat of the heart to push it along. Arteries hardened and narrowed by plaques cannot expand or contract, and so the blood must squeeze through them. The pressure inside the arteries increases beyond normal, because the blood backs up at the restricted areas while the heart works ever harder to push it through. This high blood pressure, or **hypertension**, is a major contributor to cardiovascular disease. Hypertension damages the artery walls further and can even cause them to go into spasms, blocking blood flow. The heart, pumping blood against this back pressure, is also under a strain. As pressure builds up in an artery, the

heart disease any disease of heart muscle or other working parts of the heart.

cardiovascular disease (CVD) a general term for all diseases of the heart and blood vessels.

atherosclerosis (ATH-uh-roh-scler-OH-sis) the most common form of CVD, a disease characterized by plaques along the inner walls of the arteries.

plaques (PLACKS) mounds of lipid material, mixed with smooth muscle cells and calcium, that lodge in arterial walls and contribute to atherosclerosis. (The same word is used to describe a different kind of accumulation of material on teeth, which promotes dental caries.)

hypertension high blood pressure. See the section, "Hypertension" later in this chapter.

*Reference notes are at the end of the chapter.

arterial wall may become weakened and balloon out, forming an **aneurysm**. An aneurysm can burst, and when this happens in a major artery such as the aorta, it leads to massive bleeding and death.

The heart is a muscle, and it tries to respond to the extra strain of hypertension by becoming larger and stronger, especially in its left ventricle. Research evidence is mounting that an enlarged left ventricle reflects advancing heart and artery disease.[2] This heart abnormality can be detected by a test that compares the mass of the left ventricle to the other portions of the heart, to produce a score known as the **left ventricular mass index**.

Abnormal blood clotting is another factor that contributes to life-threatening events. Under normal conditions, clots form and dissolve in the blood all the time. Small, cell-like bodies in the blood, known as **platelets**, cause clots to form whenever they encounter injuries—a protective function

aneurysm (AN-your-ism)   the ballooning out of an artery wall at a point where it has been weakened by deterioration.

left ventricular mass index   a comparison between size of the heart's left ventricle and its other portions.

platelets   tiny, disk-shaped bodies in the blood, important in blood clot formation.

FIGURE 18–4 ■ **The formation of plaques in atherosclerosis.**
When plaques have covered 60 percent of the coronary artery walls, the critical phase of heart disease begins.

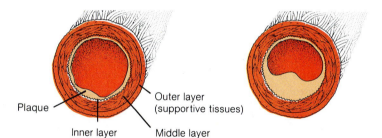

Plaque

Outer layer (supportive tissues)

Inner layer (artery lining)

Middle layer (smooth muscle)

An artery (section) with plaque just beginning to form. Plaques can easily appear in a person as young as 15.

The same artery, years later, half blocked by plaque.

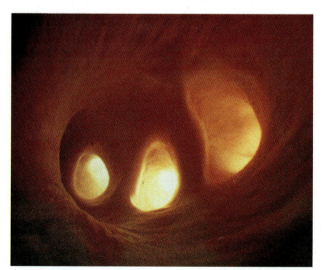

A healthy artery provides an open passage for the flow of blood.

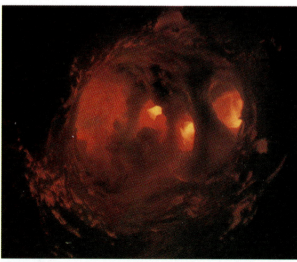

Plaques along an artery narrow its diameter and obstruct blood flow. Clots can form, aggravating the problem.

that prevents blood loss from minor wounds. Clots also form inside the blood vessels when the platelets encounter rough spots such as plaques, but they soon dissolve again unless they are needed to plug a leak. In atherosclerosis, the balance between clot formation and dissolution is disturbed. The platelets are triggered to begin the clotting process more often than normal.

Prostaglandins are hormones that control the action of the platelets, and an imbalance among the prostaglandins may contribute to the formation of clots. Particles released when platelets break down also may worsen atherosclerosis by adding to the growth of plaques. A person who has suffered a minor stroke may feel that the problem is being dismissed lightly when the health care provider orders daily aspirin as preventive therapy. Aspirin, though, modifies the prostaglandins, as described in Chapter 8, and so can suppress the platelet clotting action. In fact, an aspirin a day has been shown to cut by almost half the risk of having a heart attack in healthy men aged 50 and older.[3] Research presently under way is expected to demonstrate the same effect in women.

Atherosclerosis can cause blockage of an artery in any of three ways:

■ The plaques can grow large enough to completely block the blood flow.
■ A blood clot may form on a plaque and gradually grow (a **thrombus**), eventually cutting off the blood supply. In the arteries of the heart, such a blockage is called a **coronary thrombosis** (a type of **heart attack**). A **cerebral thrombosis** is the gradual closing off of a vessel that feeds the brain (a type of **stroke**).
■ A clot can also break loose, becoming a traveling clot (an **embolus**), and circulate until it reaches an artery too small to allow its passage. The sudden blockage of the vessel is an **embolism**.

When an artery is blocked, the tissue normally supplied by the blocked vessel may suddenly die. Tissue death can occur gradually, too, resulting in organ damage. Figure 18–5 shows a thrombus and an embolus.

(Chapter 8 also presents a discussion of prostaglandins.)

thrombus   a stationary clot. When it has grown enough to close off a blood vessel, the event is a *thrombosis* or *occlusion*. A **coronary thrombosis** is the closing off of a vessel that feeds the heart muscle. A **cerebral thrombosis** is the closing off of a vessel that feeds the brain.

heart attack   the event in which vessels that feed the heart muscle become blocked, causing tissue death. Also called **myocardial infarction**.

stroke   the shutting off of the blood flow to the brain by a thrombus or embolus, or by hemorrhage.

embolus (EM-boh-luss)   a clot that breaks loose and travels through the bloodstream. When it causes sudden closure of a blood vessel, the event is an **embolism**.

FIGURE 18–5 ■ **A thrombus and an embolus.**

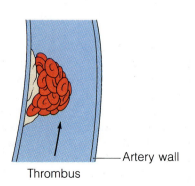

Thrombus

Artery wall

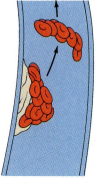

Embolus

As mentioned at the start of this chapter, no one is free of atherosclerosis, and the condition advances with age. The question, then, is not whether you have atherosclerosis, but how far advanced it is. The development of atherosclerosis reaches a **critical phase** at which more than 60 percent of the surfaces of the arteries are covered with plaques. Once in the critical phase, a person faces substantial risks of CVD events, such as heart attacks or strokes.

≡▶ *Atherosclerosis is the formation of plaques in the arteries that worsens hypertension and makes blood clots likely. Atherosclerosis can cause blockage of arteries that feed critical organs, such as the brain or heart.*

Heart Attack

Heart attacks are the most common of the life-threatening events brought on by atherosclerosis. They are especially likely in men in later midlife, but a significant number of heart attacks occurs before age 30. Prior to menopause, women are less susceptible to heart attacks than men are; the onset of CVD is delayed in women perhaps because of the nature of their hormones. Women who take oral contraceptives, however, and especially those who also smoke, are at extra risk for CVD development and for heart attacks.

A heart attack occurs when the arterial blood supply to the heart becomes so restricted that some of the heart's muscle tissue dies. When muscle tissue dies, it is replaced by scar tissue, and the remaining muscle tissue then must work harder to compensate.

Another problem, caused by reduced blood flow and restriction of oxygen to the heart, is pain. When the oxygen supply to the heart is reduced but is still sufficient for sedentary life, a sudden exertion or emotional upset can bring on a pain in the chest, **angina**. Angina is not always a symptom of heart attack, but it can be. A person experiencing angina may deny that a heart attack is occurring and blame the symptoms on "indigestion." Many heart attack victims could have been saved if they had told someone of their symptoms. If you or someone nearby suffers any of the heart attack symptoms listed in Table 18–1, get medical help fast.

Many heart attack victims have no pain and so may not be forewarned of impending heart attacks. Even medical tests designed to predict future heart attacks often fail to diagnose them.[4] Many heart attack deaths are sudden and unexpected.

When heart muscle tissue is threatened by a narrowed artery, the heart begins to compensate by finding alternate vessels through which to deliver the blood. These smaller **collateral blood vessels** act as a detour around the blockages, and many times they can avert much tissue death that would otherwise occur. Some evidence from studies using animals suggests that the heart forms new collateral vessels in response to exercise, especially in the young.[5] In human beings, the development of such vessels may be a factor in the excellent post-heart attack recovery seen in those who exercise.[6]

A person who has suffered a heart attack or infection that has damaged the valves may suffer from **congestive heart failure**. The name does not mean that the heart has stopped pumping altogether, but it certainly is pumping less well. The disabled heart is unable to pump normal quantities

critical phase in atherosclerosis, the stage after plaques have covered more than 60% of the interior surfaces of the arteries, making CVD events likely.

angina (an-JYE-nuh or ANN-juh-nuh) pain in the heart region caused by lack of oxygen. The complete term is *angina pectoris* (peck-TORE-iss or PECK-tore-iss).

collateral blood vessels small, alternate blood vessels in the heart that form a detour around blocked or narrowed larger arteries, permitting the heart to deliver blood and thus preventing tissue death.

congestive heart failure an insufficiency of heart action, causing blood backup in the veins, edema, and breathing difficulties.

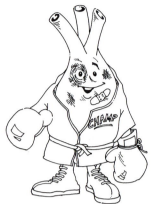

Even if damaged, the heart keeps pumping.

TABLE 18–1 ■ Warning Signs of Heart Attack and Stroke

The symptoms of heart attack:
Even though not every heart attack is announced by clear-cut symptoms, you should get help immediately if you or someone you are with:
1. Feels uncomfortable pressure, fullness, squeezing, or pain in the center of the chest lasting for more than two minutes.
2. Experiences pain that spreads to the shoulders, neck, or arms.
3. Becomes dizzy, faints, sweats for no apparent reason, or has nausea or shortness of breath, especially when other symptoms are present.

The warning signs of stroke:
Report to a physician immediately any of the following:
1. Sudden, temporary weakness or numbness in any part of one side of the body.
2. Temporary loss of speech or understanding of speech.
3. Dizziness, unsteadiness, or unexplained falls.
4. Temporary dimness or loss of vision, particularly in one eye.

---

edema   the accumulation of fluids in parts of the body, resulting from a backup of blood in veins.

digitalis   a drug derived from the foxglove plant that increases the force of the heart's muscle contractions.

pacemaker   a device that delivers electrical impulses to the heart to regulate the heartbeat.

arteriogram   an x-ray procedure used to locate blockages in arteries, such as those that occur in atherosclerosis.

heart transplant   surgical replacement of a diseased heart with a healthy one.

of blood through its chambers, and the blood backs up in the veins that are trying to deliver it to the heart. As blood collects in the veins, fluid is forced out of the capillaries into the tissues, especially into the feet and legs, causing swelling—**edema**. Fluid also can collect around the lungs, making breathing difficult.

Heart attacks do not always end in permanent disability. Many times a person who experiences a minor heart attack can recover fully through treatment and be motivated to adopt habits that could help prevent another. One drug, given within a few hours after the onset of a heart attack, can dissolve clots and thus stop a heart attack in its tracks and prevent much tissue damage.* Other drugs, such as **digitalis,** may be used to strengthen and stabilize the heartbeat. A **pacemaker** is an implanted device that provides electrical stimulation for a failing heartbeat. The latest models even automatically adjust the heartbeat to exercise levels. Sometimes, though, surgery is needed to prevent or forestall further heart attacks. For example, if the exact location of a blockage has been discovered by **arteriogram**, a type of x-ray procedure designed especially for locating such blockages, surgery can remove plaques.

Sometimes the heart is so badly damaged that it no longer pumps sufficient blood to body tissues. In such cases, the person's life can often be saved through a **heart transplant**. Special expert surgical teams perform more than 1,500 heart transplants each year. Of these clients, 85 percent survive their first year with their new hearts, and 80 percent survive for five years. A person who needs a new heart may have to wait years for one to become available, and even after the transplant, rejection of the new organ by the body's immune system is a constant threat. Drugs (immunosuppressants) help to prevent the immune system's attacking the "foreign" organ, but they also leave the person open to more infections. Heart transplant surgery is a last-resort treatment of heart disease.

Since the heart is a pump, and pumps are mechanical devices, scientists are working to develop a mechanical pump to do the work of the living

---

*The drug is plasminogen activator.

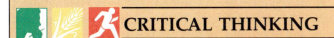

CRITICAL THINKING

Chelation Fraud

People who feel that they are not receiving much help from the medical community are prime targets for a particular kind of quackery, the "medical breakthroughs." One so-called "atherosclerosis cure" is **chelation therapy**. A quack might tell a heart client: "Your doctor never told you about chelation therapy because it works to cure your condition. If all the clients were cured, how would heart surgeons make a living?"

The "therapy" employs a chemical, EDTA, which is known to bind minerals and heavy metals.* The idea is that EDTA will travel through the system to the plaques and pull the calcium out of them, thus breaking them up. Scientific study on this possibility was discontinued in the 1960s when study subjects did not improve. Aside from possible kidney tissue death, bone marrow damage, shock, low blood pressure, convulsions, heart rhythm abnormalities, allergy, and respiratory failure from EDTA, people may suffer from postponement of the legitimate treatments that are available.

In atherosclerosis, legitimate treatments may involve lifestyle changes that take hard work but that carry the benefits of improved heart function, better blood circulation, and improved respiration. EDTA chelation therapy, on the other hand, is an expensive and dangerous placebo.

chelation therapy an unproved therapy for heart disease.

People with medical problems that demand hard work are prime targets for frauds, falsely called "medical breakthroughs."

heart. An **artificial heart** would have the advantage that the recipient's immune system would not recognize it as foreign and so would not reject it.

A common surgical treatment of a failing heart is **coronary artery bypass surgery**, which involves replacing the blocked coronary arteries with sections of the person's own veins or with synthetic tubing. In clients who experience recurring bouts of angina, **angioplasty** may be needed.[7] In angioplasty, a tiny tube is inserted into the artery and expanded to widen the passageway. A laser technique that vaporizes the plaques in the arteries is being perfected, and new drugs that dissolve clots or lower the blood's fat levels are helpful.

Even the most progressive medical techniques are only temporary repairs, though. Nothing has been found that will cure atherosclerosis. Medicine can probably prolong life, but blockages recur, and people may require repeated surgery or treatments. Because medicine isn't perfect, people with heart trouble may be lured into the hands of quacks and receive fraudulent treatments. One such treatment is described in this chapter's Critical Thinking section.

A trend concerning lifestyle factors does seem to be emerging, though. Some evidence indicates that moderate exercise, a low-fat diet, stopping

artificial heart a pump designed to fit into the human chest cavity and perform the heart's functions of moving the body's blood.

coronary artery bypass surgery surgery to provide an alternate route for blood to reach heart tissue, bypassing a blocked coronary artery.

angioplasty a procedure to reduce the size of plaques in arteries by inserting a tube into the artery to put pressure on, and flatten, the plaques.

■ *FACT OR FICTION:* For people who have suffered heart attacks, it is too late for lifestyle changes to be of any help. *False.* Lifestyle factors can be helpful not only in prevention but also in reversal of cardiovascular disease.

*The full name of EDTA is ethylene-diamine-tetraacetic acid. A legitimate medical use of EDTA is to administer it when a person has been poisoned with heavy metals. In such a case, the EDTA binds the metal molecules and carries them out of the body.

Brain damage affects
opposite side of body.

Right brain
damage

Left brain
damage

Paralyzed
right side

Paralyzed
left side

Speech,
language
deficits

Perceptual
deficits

Behavioral
style—slow,
cautious

Behavioral
style—quick,
impulsive

FIGURE 18–6 ■ **The effect of stroke location.**

transient ischemic (iss-KEE-mic) **attack (TIA)**   a small, usually mild, reversible stroke; a warning signal that a major stroke is threatening.

hemorrhage (HEM-or-age)   rapid, uncontrolled bleeding.

FIGURE 18–7 ■ **An aneurysm and a hemorrhage.**

smoking, and stress management are helpful not just in preventing heart and artery disease, but also in reversing its effects once it has set in.[8] Medical advances are exciting, but in the end, health habits may well turn out to be more reliable in preventing, and even permanently reversing, heart disease.

≡▶   *Heart attack is the blockage of blood supply with subsequent damage to the heart muscle. Anyone with signs of a possible heart attack should seek medical help immediately. Treatments of heart attacks and heart disease range from drugs to heart transplants.*

Stroke

Strokes are not as common as heart attacks, but they still claim a substantial number of the lives that are lost to atherosclerosis each year. Sometimes a person will suffer a small stroke, called a **transient ischemic attack (TIA)**— a warning that a blockage is forming. Like a minor heart attack, a TIA may have no lasting effect except to startle a person into taking action to reverse damaging habits.

When a major stroke occurs, a part of the brain is starved for blood and dies. This dead tissue interferes differently with the person's mental and physical functioning, depending on the location of the damage, as shown in Figure 18–6.

Stroke victims are robbed of their former abilities, requiring that they start from scratch to learn such elementary functions as personal hygiene or walking. Most stroke victims can recover basic functioning, but success requires dedication from all participants: the victim, family and friends, and the medical team.

Just as plaques, thrombi, and emboli can lead to heart attacks in the heart, so in the brain they can lead to strokes. Aneurysms are different, though. In the heart region, the bursting of an aneurysm almost invariably leads to instant death, for so much blood is lost so quickly (**hemorrhage**). In the brain, the bursting of an aneurysm can lead to localized hemorrhage, another cause of stroke. Figure 18–7 illustrates an aneurysm and a hemorrhage.

As with heart attacks, strokes require immediate medical attention. The warning signs of stroke were already listed in Table 18–1. If they should

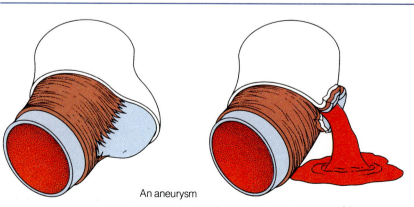

An aneurysm

A hemorrhage

occur, they demand immediate medical treatment. To prevent further strokes, medical treatment, such as anticoagulant medication, is sometimes required.

≡▶ *Strokes are blockages or hemorrhages in the vessels that feed the brain and can impair a person's functioning. Strokes often result from atherosclerosis.*

■≡ Reducing Risks of CVD

Most of the diseases we face today are not those caused by the microbes discussed in Chapter 17, but the diseases of heredity and lifestyle that develop over years. CVD is just such a disease; cancer is another. Even so, when people are diagnosed with CVD, they may be as surprised as if they had just come down with the measles. Yet their inherited susceptibility and many of their own personal choices, made day after day, year after year, may have made the disease practically inevitable.

Risk Factors

The concept of **risk factors** underlies preventive strategies against heart disease. The risk factors for a disease are those factors (hereditary, environmental, and behavioral) that research has found to be associated with the occurrence of the disease—that is, those factors that show a **correlation** with the disease. They are candidates for causes of the disease, not yet pronounced guilty or not guilty. We can say with confidence that the cause of influenza is a virus that attacks a vulnerable system. We cannot, on the other hand, name the cause of heart disease with such confidence, but we can name risk factors, some of which are strongly implicated as causal.

The many risk factors linked to CVD are listed in Table 18–2. Some of the risk factors are powerful predictors of CVD. If you are young and have none of them, the statistical likelihood of your developing cardiovascular disease in the next six years may be less than 1 in 100. If you are older and have all the major ones, the chance may rise to close to 1 in 2. The Life Choice Inventory shows one way of calculating your risk score. The correlation isn't perfect; a few people with many risk factors live long lives without disease, and a few people with only a few or none die young of CVD. On the average, though, the more risk factors in a person's life, the greater that

risk factor a factor that is associated with a disease by correlation but that is not proved to be causal.

correlation an association of two variables, such that when one increases, the other increases (or decreases). A *variable* is anything that varies, such as age, height, or heart attack risk.

TABLE 18–2 ■ **Risk Factors Linked to Cardiovascular Disease**

- ■ Heredity (history of CVD prior to age 55 in family members; gender (being male)
- ■ Smoking
- ■ Hypertension
- ■ High blood cholesterol, high LDL, and/or low HDL (see text)
- ■ Glucose intolerance (diabetes)
- ■ Lack of exercise
- ■ Obesity
- ■ Stress

LIFE CHOICE INVENTORY

How healthy is your heart? Every disease has risk factors; those for heart disease are among the best known. The better you know the nature of the risks you face, the better you can decide what preventive measures may be appropriate. To determine your risk of heart disease, pick the number in each category that most nearly describes you and then score as directed.

1. Gender. If you are:

    Female, 0 points.
    Male, 4 points.

2. Family heart disease history. (Consider just heart attacks and strokes as heart disease here; diabetes comes later.) If you have:

    No relatives with heart disease, 1 point.
    One relative with heart disease over 60 years, 2 points.
    Two relatives with heart disease over 60 years, 3 points.
    One relative with heart disease under 60 years, 4 points.
    Two relatives with heart disease under 60 years, 6 points.

3. Smoking. If you smoke:

    Not at all, 0 points.
    A cigar or pipe, 1 point.
    10 cigarettes or fewer per day, 3 points.

    11 to 30 cigarettes per day, 4 points.
    30 or more cigarettes per day, 6 points.

4. Hypertension. If your diastolic blood pressure (the lower of the two numbers on a blood pressure reading) is:

    Less than 85, 0 points.
    85 to 89, 1 point.
    90 to 104, 2 points.
    105 to 114, 4 points.
    115 or more, 5 points.

    (If you don't know your blood pressure, give yourself 5 points.)

5. High blood cholesterol. (If you don't know your cholesterol level, guess the best you can at the amount of fat in your diet.) If you have:

    Cholesterol below 180 or almost no fat in diet, 0 points.
    Cholesterol 180 to 199 or a low-fat diet, 1 point.
    Cholesterol 200 to 219 or a moderately low-fat diet, 2 points.

person's risk of disease. The following Strategies list ways to reduce CVD risk by controlling those risk factors that you can control. Details about them follow in the next few sections.

Your heredity, of course, is a factor that you cannot control, but you can certainly benefit from learning about it. A health care provider may ask, "Do you have any relatives with heart disease? What did your grandparents die of?" Susceptibility to CVD runs in families.[9] If your parents have it, chances are, you will tend to develop it, too.

Note that to be born with a hereditary *disease* is different from being born with a genetic *tendency* to develop a disease later in life. Hereditary diseases inevitably cause abnormalities in function; they are present at birth; they must be managed throughout life. In contrast, genetic tendencies may or may not result in the disease state itself, depending on lifestyle choices and environmental factors.

Cholesterol 220 to 239 or a typical American diet,
4 points.
Cholesterol 240 to 300 or a high-fat diet, 5 points.
Cholesterol over 300, 6 points.

6. Diabetes. If you have:

No relatives with diabetes, 0 points.
One relative with diabetes, 2 points.
Two relatives with diabetes, 3 points.
Diabetes in yourself beginning after age 40,
4 points.
Diabetes in yourself beginning between 20 and 40,
5 points.
Diabetes in yourself beginning before age 20,
6 points.

7. Lack of exercise. If you engage in:

Strenuous exercise both at work and at leisure,
0 points.
Moderate exercise both at work and at leisure,
1 point.
Sedentary work and intense leisure-time activity,
2 points.
Sedentary work and moderate leisure-time activity,
3 points.
Sedentary work and light leisure-time activity,
4 points.
Little or no activity, 6 points.

8. Body weight. (Use the weight you selected for
yourself in the Life Choice Inventory of Chapter 6; or
use the weight appropriate for you from the chart on
the inside back cover.) If you are:

5 or more pounds below appropriate weight,
0 points.
Up to 5 pounds above appropriate weight, 1 point.
5 to 19 pounds above appropriate weight, 2 points.
20 to 39 pounds above appropriate weight,
3 points.
40 to 60 pounds above appropriate weight, 4 points.
More than 60 pounds above appropriate weight,
6 points.

9. Stress. If you are:

Almost always relaxed and serene, 0 points.
Sometimes tense, 1 point.
Frequently tense, 2 points.
Almost always tense and anxious, 4 points.
Plagued by anxiety and depression, 5 points.

Scoring: Add up the points for each of the nine
answers. Your risk of heart attack is:

0 to 9: Very remote.
10 to 19: Below average
20 to 29: Average. Consider reducing score.
30 to 39: High. Reduce score.
40 to 50: Urgent danger—reduce score!

You cannot change your heredity, but you can be aware of it and pay attention to its significance for you. If several close relatives have CVD, then you should probably adopt additional preventive measures, even if you have no symptoms.

If you have a hereditary tendency toward CVD, or if you want to be screened as a preventive measure, two tests may be worth considering: an **electrocardiograph** (**ECG** or **EKG**) and a **stress test**. The first of these, the ECG, records the heart's own electrical impulses and produces a graph of the heart's beat pattern to check for abnormal heartbeat patterns. A stress test is an ECG taken while the person is exercising on a treadmill or stationary bicycle, and is often used to determine whether a person can safely start exercising after years of sedentary life. Another test, the **echocardiograph**, mentioned earlier, is becoming common as a diagnostic test for CVD. It measures the blood flow through the heart and, using a mathematical

electrocardiograph (ECG or EKG) a record of the electrical activity of the heart that, if abnormal, may indicate heart disease.

stress test an electrocardiograph performed while the person is exercising on a treadmill or stationary bicycle.

echocardiograph a visual image of the heart's blood flow produced by sound waves reflected from the heart and blood.

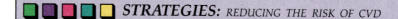

STRATEGIES: *REDUCING THE RISK OF CVD*

To reduce the risk of CVD:

1. Learn about your heredity, and use the information: control the lifestyle factors that may affect you.
2. Don't smoke, or if you do smoke, stop.
3. Keep your blood pressure below 140/90.
4. Keep your blood cholesterol within the normal range (below 200 milligrams per deciliter for people 20 to 29 years of age).
5. If you have diabetes, keep your blood sugar under control.
6. Exercise at least three times weekly (see Chapter 7).
7. Maintain appropriate body weight (see Chapter 6).
8. Control stress—learn to relax.

SOURCE: Adapted from R. E. Olson, How to reduce your risk of coronary heart disease (CHD), *Priorities,* Spring 1990, p. 21.

formula, establishes the likelihood of a serious CVD event such as heart attack.[10] It is also used to determine the left ventricular mass index, mentioned earlier.

If you learn that CVD is developing, then you have the opportunity to begin taking appropriate preventive measures. The four factors that respond best to lifestyle changes and that have emerged as major predictors of risk of CVD are:

■ Smoking.
■ Hypertension.
■ High blood cholesterol.
■ Diabetes.

The chances of having a healthy heart and arteries are much greater if you do not smoke, if your blood pressure and blood cholesterol are normal, if you manage stress skillfully, and if you keep any symptoms of diabetes under control. The first four of these are discussed in the next three sections, and this chapter's Spotlight is devoted to diabetes. As you can see, the other risk factors (lack of exercise and obesity) contribute to the major ones, so they are discussed throughout.

≡▶   *Major risk factors for heart disease are heredity, smoking, hypertension, high blood cholesterol, stress, and diabetes. People whose relatives have CVD should do all they can to reduce other risk factors.*

Smoking

The link between smoking and lung diseases is easy to visualize—hot smoke drawn into the lungs damages the delicate tissues. But the link between smoke in the lungs and disease in the arteries of the heart seems remote until you consider how the damage occurs. The heart and the lungs are both

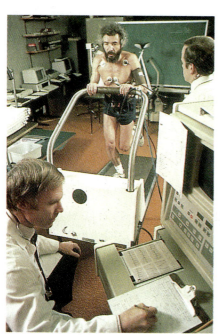

If you have a hereditary tendency toward CVD, consider taking a stress test.

working together on the same unending project: supplying the entire body with ample oxygen so that it can produce energy to do life's work.

When tobacco smoke enters the lungs, it delivers to the blood a load of nicotine, a stimulant that triggers the stress response. This raises the blood pressure and increases the heart rate, and it greatly increases the heart's need for oxygen. At the same time, carbon monoxide from the smoke is mistakenly picked up by the blood, because it closely resembles oxygen—but instead of providing oxygen to the tissues, the carbon monoxide continues to ride in the blood, starving the tissues. Smoking thus increases the demand for heart activity, partly from the stress effect and partly from the oxygen-starved tissues, while starving the heart muscle of the oxygen it needs to support its work. Not only that, but nicotine directly damages platelets, making clot formation more likely.

The action needed to reduce the risk of CVD from smoking is straightforward. Don't smoke, or if you do, make plans to stop. Even people who have smoked for years can reduce their risks by quitting.

≡▶ *Smoking damages the heart by increasing blood pressure and the heart's work load. It also starves the heart for oxygen and damages platelets, making clot formation likely.*

Chapter 11 lists more of the effects of nicotine and smoking on health.

In short, smoking:

- ■ Elevates blood pressure.
- ■ Increases heart rate.
- ■ Increases the heart muscle's oxygen requirement.
- ■ Deprives the heart and other tissues of oxygen.
- ■ Increases the likelihood of clot formation.

Hypertension

The term *hypertension* refers to excess pressure in the arteries. Hypertension has a hereditary component; it runs in families. Learn your own family's characteristics in this respect. People who are middle-aged or elderly, black, obese, heavy drinkers, users of oral contraceptives, or suffering from kidney disease or diabetes are especially prone to hypertension. The most effective single step you can take to protect yourself from CVD is to know your blood pressure, or at least to know whether it is above normal or not. You can see a health care professional to get an accurate blood pressure reading; self-test machines often give inaccurate readings. If your blood pressure is above normal, the reading should be confirmed. Depending on how high it is, and on your age, physical state, and family history, different treatments are appropriate. To understand how the blood pressure can rise too high, consider how the body works to raise it when it falls too low.

Next to lack of air, no condition threatens life so direly as dehydration, which causes the blood pressure to fall too low to deliver fluid to the tissues. In dehydration, the supply of blood is diminished. The kidneys respond immediately; they send out a message to constrict the blood vessels, because the squeezing action will raise blood pressure; and they instruct their own adrenal glands to send out a hormone that will conserve fluid and increase the blood supply. This hormone works by retrieving sodium from the filtered blood constituents. Because water follows sodium, both are conserved, and the blood volume increases. (Most tissues get their water this way—they gather up sodium, and water accompanies it.)

Normally, this response of the kidneys prevents the dire consequences of dehydration (which are described in Chapter 7). In atherosclerosis, though, this same response brings on hypertension.

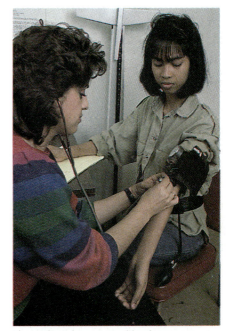

If you don't know your blood pressure, at least know whether it is above normal or not.

When atherosclerosis has narrowed the kidneys' arteries, the kidneys respond as they do to dehydration, because the flow of blood through them is diminished. This time, however, the cause of the problem is different—the reduced blood flow is due to a reduced *delivery* of blood rather than a reduced volume of fluid in the body.

Eventually, the kidneys' response raises the blood pressure high enough to deliver sufficient blood to the kidneys, but now the whole body's blood pressure is too high. Hypertension then burdens the heart—the blood vessels are overfilled, and the heart has to pump harder to push the extra fluid around against constricted arteries. Thus atherosclerosis contributes to hypertension. Hypertension worsens kidney damage; makes strokes and heart attacks more likely; and damages artery walls, increasing the likelihood of plaque formation.

Hypertension produces its harmful effects without a single symptom. You can't rely on your body to warn you; you must actively seek information about your own blood pressure to find out whether you have hypertension.

When blood pressure is measured, two numbers are important: the pressure during contraction of the ventricles of the heart and the pressure during relaxation of the ventricles. The first number is the pressure in the arteries during **systole** (dub); the second number is the pressure during **diastole** (lub). Normal systolic blood pressure is between 100 and 140;* normal diastolic pressure is between 60 and 90. Figure 18–8 shows how to interpret your blood pressure reading.

Hypertension can be controlled, especially if the cause is known, by medication or by means of lifestyle strategies: limiting salty, fatty foods while choosing more nutrient-rich, high-fiber, low-fat foods; losing weight; exercising aerobically; abstaining from alcohol and tobacco use; and reducing stress. You have seen these recommendations before, for besides atherosclerosis and hypertension, many other ills are preventable by the same chosen habits. In severe hypertension, or when other factors increase CVD risk, drugs that lower blood pressure can be a lifesaving treatment.

In some cases, control of hypertension is a matter of reducing body fatness. (A single pound of extra body fat requires miles of extra capillaries to feed it; the heart has to pump the blood around those extra miles.) Distribution of body fat seems important, too. As mentioned in Chapter 6, fat around the abdomen seems to correlate most closely with CVD, especially in men, so a rule of thumb has been developed: if your abdomen protrudes when you lie flat on your back, you may have more body fat than is consistent with good health. (Ideally, if you place a ruler across your hipbones while lying on your back, relaxed, it should touch both bones.)

In some people, restricting dietary salt will produce a drop in blood pressure. Diets high in sodium and chloride are often deficient in other minerals such as potassium and calcium, and these may be needed to regulate blood pressure. But the relationship of salt to blood pressure is not simple; many people can tolerate large amounts of salt without a rise in blood pressure.

It takes time for people's taste buds to adjust to the flavors of food without salt, but eventually the lower levels become the preferred taste. To avoid too much salt, follow these suggestions:

*FACT OR FICTION: You can tell whether your blood pressure is high by the way you feel. *False.* High blood pressure gives no warning signs.*

systole (SIS-toe-lee)   the part of the heartbeat in which the heart ventricles are in contraction, during which the blood is pushed out into the arteries. Systolic blood pressure is the maximum blood pressure in the vascular system and is represented by the first number in a blood pressure reading.

diastole (die-ASS-toh-lee)   the part of the heartbeat in which the heart ventricles relax. Diastolic (die-uh-STAHL-ick) blood pressure is the lowest pressure in the veins and arteries and is represented by the second number in a blood pressure reading.

Foods that are high in salt:

Those prepared in brine, such as pickles, olives, and sauerkraut.

Salty or smoked meat, such as bologna, corned or chipped beef, frankfurters, ham, luncheon meats, salt pork, sausage, and smoked tongue.

Salty or smoked fish, such as anchovies, caviar, salted and dried cod, herring, sardines, and smoked salmon.

Snack items such as potato chips, pretzels, salted popcorn, and salted nuts and crackers.

Bouillon cubes; seasoned salts (including sea salt); soy, Worcestershire, and barbecue sauces.

Cheeses, especially processed types.

Canned and instant soups.

Prepared horseradish, catsup, and mustard.

*Blood pressure is read in millimeters of mercury. The silver column that rises on a blood pressure instrument is a column of mercury; the height to which it is pushed is marked off in millimeters.

When the blood pressure is taken, two measures are recorded: the systole first, the diastole second (example: 120/80). High blood pressure is defined differently for different purposes, but generally, a systolic reading over 140 or a diastolic reading over 90 indicates a too-high blood pressure.

FIGURE 18–8 ■ **How to interpret your blood pressure reading.**

$\dfrac{120}{80}$ { This is the systolic pressure. If this number is above 140, you may have hypertension.

{ This is the diastolic pressure, the most sensitive indicator of hypertension. Interpret this number as follows:

Less than 85:	Normal blood pressure.
85 to 89:	High normal blood pressure.
90 to 104:	Mild hypertension.
105 to 114:	Moderate hypertension.
115 or more:	Severe hypertension.

■ Learn to enjoy the unsalted flavors of foods.
■ Cook with only small amounts of added salt.
■ Add little or no salt to food at the table.
■ Cut down on the foods listed in the margin.
■ Read labels. You may be surprised to learn that some processed foods that are very salty don't taste that way.

In addition to diet, regular aerobic exercise seems to be effective in maintaining normal blood pressure. Although blood pressure rises temporarily at each bout of exercise, the effect in the long run is to significantly lower the blood pressure.[11] Some evidence exists that exercise can lower the blood pressure as effectively as drugs in cases of mild hypertension.[12]

≡▶ *Hypertension is high blood pressure, originated by the actions of the adrenal glands of the kidneys, which conserve water and sodium in the blood and constrict blood vessels. Hypertension damages the kidneys, makes strokes and heart attacks likely, and damages artery walls. Most important is to know your blood pressure, and if it is high, to control it.*

Elevated Blood Cholesterol

Another silent, symptomless risk factor for cardiovascular disease is much talked about but little understood: elevated blood cholesterol levels. Cholesterol is a type of fat, one of the lipids (see Chapter 5); it is found in foods and is also made and destroyed in the body.

Blood cholesterol may be high for any of a number of reasons. Some people inherit tendencies to make too much or to fail to destroy it on schedule. Others have high blood cholesterol for lifestyle reasons: they eat too much fat or too much saturated fat, exercise too little, are obese, or all of these. A blood test to determine high blood cholesterol levels, the **blood lipid profile**, can give you an idea of your standing as to this risk factor. Table 18–3 shows how to interpret your blood cholesterol level.

Note that acceptable cholesterol levels go up as a person ages. Table 18–4 shows how elevated blood cholesterol level combines with other risk factors

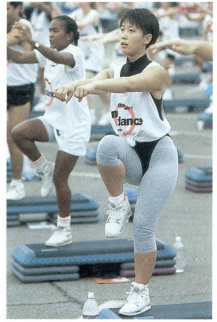

Regular aerobic exercise helps keep blood pressure normal.

blood lipid profile a test that reveals the amounts of various lipids in the blood.

TABLE 18–3 ■ Blood Cholesterol Readings and Risk of CVD		
Age	**Moderate Risk**	**High Risk**
2 to 19	Over 170[a]	Over 185[a]
20 to 29	Over 200	Over 220
30 to 39	Over 220	Over 240
40 and up	Over 240	Over 260

[a]Blood cholesterol is measured in milligrams per deciliter of blood.

SOURCE: Consensus conference statement: Lowering blood cholesterol to prevent heart disease, *Journal of the American Medical Association* 253 (1985): 2080–2090.

lipoproteins   clusters of protein and fat molecules that transport lipids in the blood and lymph.

low-density lipoproteins (LDL)   lipoproteins that carry large amounts of fat and cholesterol from the liver, where the fat and cholesterol are made, to the tissues and also deposit excess cholesterol in arteries, forming plaques.

high-density lipoproteins (HDL): lipoproteins that carry smaller amounts of fat and cholesterol away from the tissues (and from plaques) back to the liver for breakdown and, ultimately, excretion from the body.

■ *FACT OR FICTION:* The most important dietary measure to avoid heart disease is to eat margarine instead of butter. *False.* The primary dietary measure to avoid heart disease is to eat *less total fat;* a secondary measure is to replace some saturated fats, such as butter, with unsaturated fats, such as in soft or liquid margarine or olive oil.

to accelerate atherosclerosis formation. As the table indicates, a person with a cholesterol reading of 300 could delay the onset of the CVD critical phase for 20 years by reducing the reading to 200.[13]

Cholesterol does not travel freely in the blood; it travels in particles called **lipoproteins**.* The reason it must travel this way is that fat and water do not mix; still, within the body, fats must travel from place to place in the watery blood. Proteins mix well with watery substances, so the body uses some of its proteins as vehicles to carry fat around.

The two kinds of lipoproteins that transport cholesterol are **low-density lipoproteins (LDL)** and **high-density lipoproteins (HDL)**. The first type (LDL) carries cholesterol from the liver, where it is made, to the tissues, where it is used for making hormones, building cell membranes, and making vitamin D. LDL also tend to deposit cholesterol along the artery linings when the tissues have all they need. HDL, on the other hand, work to gather up excess cholesterol from the tissues and the arteries and carry it back to the liver to be dismantled.

A high LDL concentration in the blood is a sign of a high risk of CVD.[14] (When the overall cholesterol level in the blood is high, it usually reflects raised LDL.) In contrast, high HDL concentrations are associated with a low risk of CVD. (In this case, the overall cholesterol reading *might* be high, too.) In fact, numerous studies now agree that for men over 50, the most potent single indicator of heart attack risk may be the HDL concentration—the higher the HDL, the lower the risk.

Several factors affect blood cholesterol level. Some of them you can control, and some you can't. First, being female is an asset; women have higher HDL levels than men. Second, nonsmokers have uniformly higher HDL levels than smokers. Maintaining appropriate weight for height is helpful (see Chapter 6). Diet and exercise also affect blood cholesterol. Evidence suggests that regular aerobic exercise lowers LDL and raises HDL in the blood.[15] The role of diet is complex, but the complexities are worth learning.

*Each lipoprotein contains the same three types of lipids, but in different proportions. The three types of lipids are triglycerides, phospholipids, and cholesterol. The four types of lipoproteins are chylomicrons, VLDL (very-low-density lipoproteins), LDL (low-density lipoproteins), and HDL (high-density lipoproteins). Chylomicrons transport all the large lipids a person has eaten from the digestive tract into the body; they are mostly triglycerides. Cells remove triglycerides from chylomicrons as needed, and the liver picks up and disposes of the remnants. VLDL carry mostly triglycerides. LDL and HDL carry mostly cholesterol.

TABLE 18–4 ■ **The Effect of CVD Risk Factors on Life Span**

The age listed is the hypothetical age of onset of the critical phase of CVD risk (60 percent coverage of artery surfaces by atherosclerosis).

Blood Cholesterol	200 mg/dl[a]	250 mg/dl	300 mg/dl
Age of nonsmoker	70	60	50
Age of smoker	60	50	40
Age of smoker with hypertension	50	40	30

The table shows that a nonsmoker with normal blood pressure and cholesterol of 200 would reach the critical phase at age 70. A smoker with high blood pressure and cholesterol of 300 would reach that phase at age 30.

[a]Milligrams cholesterol per deciliter of blood.

SOURCE: Data from S. M. Grundy, Cholesterol and coronary heart disease, *Journal of the American Medical Association* 256 (1986): 2849–2858.

The public has been confused about the relationship of diet to high blood cholesterol, often thinking that cholesterol in foods contributes to high levels of cholesterol in the blood. It does, but regular dietary fat, especially saturated fat, contributes much more. The most important key to lowering blood cholesterol seems to be to eat less total fat. The fat you do eat should be of the unsaturated type, such as is found in soft or liquid margarines based on vegetable oils (polyunsaturated) or in olive oil (monounsaturated).

Of interest in relation to dietary fat are findings on fish oils, which offer a protective effect beyond merely substituting for saturated fat. Fish oils

Saturated fats are:

Solid at room temperature.

Found in and around cuts of red meat.

Found in animal products such as butter, whole milk, cheese, and lard.

Found in a few plant products, such as cocoa butter, coconut oil, and palm oil.

Found in hydrogenated (hardened) vegetable oils, including margarine (the hardened, stick variety), peanut butter, and shortening.

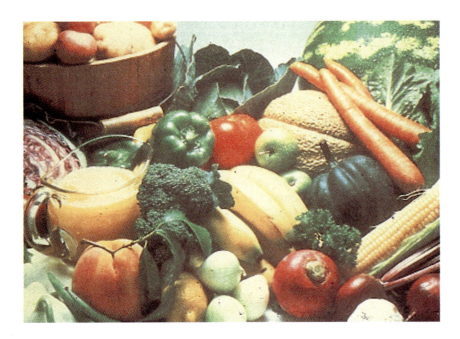

These foods are low in fat, cholesterol, and sodium, and high in fiber and nutrients.

Unsaturated fats are:

Liquid at room temperature.

Found in plant products such as grains, seeds, and nuts.

Found in a few meats, such as fowl and fish.

Found in liquid cooking oils, liquid and soft margarines, and unprocessed peanut butter.

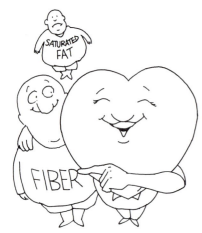

The heart prefers fiber to saturated fat.

contain a type of fatty acid that lowers blood cholesterol.* In addition, the fatty acid alters the prostaglandin balance to favor the dissolving of blood clots over the making of them.[16] One or two fish dishes a week are all it takes to exert a significant effect, and the fattiest cold-water fish are the most effective: mackerel, herring, sardines, bluefish, salmon, tuna, oysters, anchovies, squid, and others.

Dietary fiber may also confer benefits. People on high-fiber diets have been shown to excrete more cholesterol and fat than those on low-fiber diets. One reason is that the high-fiber diet shortens food's transit time through the digestive tract, and so allows less time for cholesterol to be absorbed. When cholesterol from the diet is thus reduced, the body must turn to its own supply to make necessary body compounds. Diets high in fiber are typically low in fat and cholesterol anyway—another advantage to emphasizing fiber. Some people's elevated blood cholesterol does not respond to changes in lifestyle, and such people may be given cholesterol-lowering drugs.

≡▶   *High blood cholesterol is associated with an elevated risk of CVD. The body normally contains and even makes cholesterol, and many factors affect its level in the blood. Exercise and diet also affect it.*

Emotions and the Heart

Up to this point, the risk factors discussed have been powerfully associated with the development of CVD and are considered by some to be proved causes. Emotional health could prove to be equally important in CVD risk, but so far the findings are less clearly correlational, and certainly not proved to be causal. Still, they are intriguing.

An often-cited, but little-proved, link between CVD and emotions involves the theory of type A and type B personalities. According to this theory, the type A person finds it hard to cope with leisure time and likes to be constantly busy accomplishing things. The type B person is able to rest when tired and rarely pushes. Studies that identified people as type A or type B and then followed them over a period of years reported that the type A people had more than twice the rate of CVD as the type B people.[17] Over the years, however, research has yielded little evidence to support this theory. Today, the type A–type B theory has been all but discounted by scientists.[18]

A related theory concerns a link between CVD and job strain. Researchers tested male employees' blood pressures and their left ventricular mass indexes. They concluded that job strain, especially the strain of having much pressure to perform without much power over how things get done, may be a risk factor for both hypertension and for structural changes in the heart that indicate CVD risk. It could be that early research may have detected this link to job strain without recognizing it. Perhaps any personality type would become "type A" under such circumstances and suffer increased risks of CVD.

*The fatty acid is eicosapentaenoic acid (EPA), one of the omega fatty acids.

One personality trait, however, is still strongly suspected as a link to CVD—the tendency to be chronically hostile, angry, and cynical. Several studies have made this connection. It could be that anger-provoking situations trigger unusually strong reactions in chronically angry people, with accompanying shifts in blood lipids and the stress hormones, all elevating risk of CVD.[19]

Research linking personality and CVD continues to be criticized. Its detractors point out that the relationship may be correlational rather than causal. Still, if you identify yourself as hostile and chronically angry (or if school pressures or your job cause you to feel out of control), stress control might help you. The stress hormones are those described earlier that cause water retention, increase the blood volume, and raise the blood pressure. Some people think that the key to prevention lies in control of the stress response.

If this connection holds up, it will help to explain why people with many social ties seem to develop less heart disease than people with few or none. It may explain why married men have less heart disease than single men, and why owners of pets (even pet fish) may have lower blood pressure than other people.

People (at least some people) can learn to lower their blood cholesterol by practicing meditation, prayer, or whatever relaxation techniques work for them. Similarly, plain old affection and love affect the heart and arteries. Clearly, the mystery of CVD, like all the great human mysteries, involves the mind and spirit as well as the body.

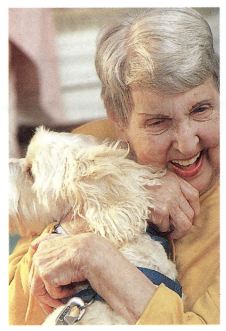

People with pets may have lower blood pressure.

≡▶ *A line of research that links emotions and personality to increased risk of heart disease has yielded inconsistent results. Anger, hostility, and cynicism are strongly suspected as risks for CVD.*

Why is it that making healthful choices is so difficult? Part of the reason is that it sometimes feels like a sacrifice; you have to give up ways of life you like and are accustomed to. And part of it is that society sometimes doesn't support you in doing it. You have to go against the grain of society; pass up the fried, heavily salted (and heavily advertised) fast foods, and instead, search the grocery shelves to pick out the low-fat products. Does this mean that to remain healthy, you must live a Spartan life and bid a final farewell to all pleasures? No, it does not. The effects of life choices are cumulative. If, *most of the time,* you choose low-fat, high-fiber meals, and if, *more days than not,* you exercise, you can indulge in the most outrageous dessert on occasion or loaf for a day without adding to your risks. In fact, "moderation in all things" can be interpreted to mean that you *should* indulge in treats and laziness, but only once in a while. It is the majority that weights the average, so make most of your choices healthful ones, and savor your occasional luxuries.

Throughout this chapter, you learned about CVD and about personal choice making as the number-one strategy against it. The next chapter shows that remarkably similar choices can affect the development of cancer.

■ ≡ For Review

1. Describe the circulatory system, and explain how blood moves from place to place in the body.
2. Explain the role of capillary nets.
3. Describe the development of atherosclerosis.
4. Describe the event called heart attack and its effects on the heart.
5. Define *congestive heart failure*.
6. Name some medical treatments for the post–heart attack victim.
7. Describe the event called stroke and its effects on the brain.

8. Identify the principal risk factors for coronary heart disease and stroke.
9. List some tests used to screen for CVD.
10. Explain ways in which smoking strains the heart, precipitating or worsening heart disease.
11. Explain the relationship of hypertension to CVD.
12. Describe the kidney's role in raising blood pressure.
13. Describe how blood pressure readings are taken and how to

determine whether the reading is normal.
14. Identify methods of controlling high blood pressure.
15. List and describe some ways people can influence their own blood lipid levels.
16. Discuss current thoughts about the relationship of personality, job strain, and stress management to heart and artery disease.

■ ≡ Notes

1. American Heart Association, *1986 Heart Facts* (Dallas: AHA, 1985), p. 1.
2. D. Levy and coauthors, Left ventricular mass and incidence of coronary heart disease in an elderly cohort: The Framingham Heart Study, *Annals of Internal Medicine* 110 (1989): 101–107.
3. Steering Committee of the Physicians' Health Study Group, Final report on the aspirin component of the ongoing physicians' health study, *New England Journal of Medicine* 321 (1989): 129–135.
4. S. E. Epstein, A. A. Quyyumi, and R. O. Bonow, Sudden cardiac death without warning: Possible mechanisms and implications for screening asymptomatic populations, *New England Journal of Medicine* 321 (1989): 320–324.
5. T. B. Jacobs, R. D. Bell, and J. D. Clements, Exercise, age and the development of myocardial vasculature, *Growth* 48 (1984): 148–157.
6. K. Przyklenk and A. C. Groom, Effects of exercise frequency, intensity, and duration on revascularization in the transition zone of infarcted rat hearts, *Canadian Journal of Physiology and Pharmacology* 63

(1985): 273–278.
7. TIMI Study Group, Comparison of invasive and conservative strategies after treatment with intravenous tissue plaminogen activator in acute myocardial infarction, *New England Journal of Medicine* 320 (1989): 618–627.
8. D. Ornish and coauthors, Can lifestyle changes reverse coronary heart disease? *Lancet* 336 (1990): 129–133; C. M. Tipton, Exercise, training and hypertension, *Exercise and Sports Sciences Reviews* 12 (1984): 245–306.
9. P. N. Hopkins and R. R. Williams, Human genetics and coronary heart disease: A public health perspective, *Annual Reviews of Nutrition* (1989): 303–345.
10. R. L. Popp, Echocardiography, *New England Journal of Medicine* 323 (1990): 101–109; P. N. Casale and coauthors, Value of echocardiograph measurement of left ventricular mass in predicting cardiovascular morbid events in hypertensive men, *Annals of Internal Medicine* 105 (1986): 173–178.
11. Tipton, 1984.
12. M.H. Kelemen and coauthors,

Exercise training combined with anti-hypertensive drug therapy: Effects on lipids, blood pressure, and left ventricular mass, *Journal of the American Medical Association* 263 (1990): 2766–2771.
13. S. M. Grundy, Cholesterol and coronary heart disease, *Journal of the American Medical Association* 256 (1986): 2849–2858.
14. M. J. Stampfer, F. M. Sacks, S. Salvini, W. C. Willett, and C. H. Hennekens, A prospective study of cholesterol, apolipoproteins, and the risk of myocardial infarction, *New England Journal of Medicine* 325 (1991): 373-381.
15. S. Rainville and P. Vaccaro, Lipoprotein cholesterol levels, coronary artery disease and regular exercise: A review, *American Corrective Therapy Journal,* November/December 1983, pp. 161–165.
16. A. M. Fehily and coauthors, The effect of fatty fish on plasma lipid and lipoprotein concentrations, *American Journal of Clinical Nutrition* 38 (1983): 349–351; W. S. Harris and coauthors, *Nutrition and Heart Disease* (London: Churchill Livingstone, 1983), as cited in Fish oils, serum lipids and platelet

aggregation, *Nutrition and the MD,* January 1985.

17. R. H. Rosenman and M. A. Chesney, The relationship of type A behavior pattern to coronary heart disease, *Activitas Nervosa Superior* (Prague) 22 (1980): 1–10.

18. D. R. Ragland, Type A behavior and outcome of coronary disease, *New England Journal of Medicine* 321 (1989): 394; D. R. Ragland and R. J. Brand, Coronary heart disease mortality in the Western Collaborative Group Study, *American Journal of Epidemiology* 127 (1988): 462–475; D. R. Ragland and R. J. Brand, Type A behavior and mortality from coronary heart disease, *New England Journal of Medicine* 318 (1988): 65–69.

19. D. C. Helmer, D. R. Ragland, and S. L. Syme, Hostility and coronary artery disease, *American Journal of Epidemiology* 133 (1991): 112–122.

SPOTLIGHT

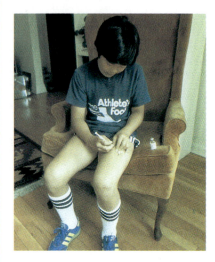

Diabetes

In **diabetes,** the blood sugar (glucose) builds up and is not cleared away normally. One out of every four people in the United States has diabetes in the family, and it is a risk factor for cardiovascular disease. Diabetes ranks among the ten leading causes of death in the United States.[1]* It is a major cause of blindness, kidney failure, leg amputations, and birth defects.[2]

Why doesn't the body handle glucose normally in diabetes?

The answer centers around the hormone insulin, which enables the body tissues to absorb glucose from the blood. Two conditions can interfere with the normal absorption of glucose: either a person's body makes too little insulin, or the tissues lose their sensitivity to the insulin the

*Reference notes are at the end of the Spotlight.

body does make. Without insulin or the sensitivity needed to use it, glucose does not enter the tissues, where it is needed to furnish vital energy. The kidneys normally allow no glucose to escape into the urine. But in diabetes, the concentration of glucose in the blood exceeds the kidneys' capacity to conserve it, and some of the excess is lost in the urine.

Why is that a problem to the body?

The problem lies in the resulting chemical imbalance in the blood. The blood's chemistry is normally tightly controlled, with many centers throughout the body providing checks and balances. In diabetes, the blood contains its normal amount of water, but has too high a concentration of glucose. The body is fooled, and ''sees'' the condition as a lack of water in the blood, so it sends fluid from the tissues into the bloodstream to dilute the glucose to its normal concentration. The tissues then, robbed of needed water, become dehydrated, and thirst results. Then the kidneys detect the excess water in the blood and excrete it, but they can't help excreting with it many other vital blood components as well. Frequent urination causes dehydration. Two of the warning signs of diabetes, excessive urination and thirst, are caused by the movement of water out of the tissues and into the urine. Table S18–1 lists the warning signs of diabetes, and the Miniglossary of Diabetes Terms defines the types.

Without glucose for energy, how do tissues stay alive?

Most cells of the body are equipped to handle long periods of carbohydrate depletion, as would occur

during fasting or starvation. When glucose is not available, the tissues resort to using their other energy fuels—protein and fat—and produce ketone bodies (see Chapter 6). Ketones are the acidic by-products of fat breakdown; they can change the acid-base balance of the blood, and they can disturb brain function if they reach too-high levels. In diabetes, the ketones can overwhelm the brain, producing coma.

I've heard that diabetes affects people's feet, and that they can go blind. Why would sugar in the blood cause trouble for the feet or eyes?

The effects of untreated diabetes on the body seem unlikely, at first glance: disease of the feet and legs, sometimes requiring amputation; kidney disease, sometimes requiring intensive hospital care or kidney transplant; cataracts in the eye, leading to blindness; and nerve damage. The root cause of all these conditions is the same. Diabetes causes destruction and blockage of the small arteries that feed the tissues—with effects like those of atherosclerosis. The tissues of the feet, kidneys, cornea, and other parts

---

TABLE S18–1 ■ **The Warning Signs of Diabetes**

1. Excessive urination and thirst.
2. Weight loss with nausea, easy tiring, weakness, or irritability.
3. Craving for sweets or other food.
4. Frequent infections of the skin, gums, or urinary tract.
5. Vision disturbances.
6. Pain in the legs, feet, or fingers.
7. Slow healing of cuts and bruises.
8. Itching.
9. Drowsiness.

of the body die from lack of nourishment when the arteries that feed them become diseased. That is why uncontrolled diabetes is a powerful risk factor for heart disease or stroke. Hypertension and elevated blood cholesterol are much more common in people with elevated blood glucose than in others.

Is it possible for people with diabetes to avoid developing these conditions?

Yes. Many people with diabetes live long, healthy lives, provided they obtain and follow medical treatment to control their diabetes. In some cases the person with diabetes may attain higher levels of health than a person without the condition, because the person with diabetes is inspired to adopt healthy behaviors. Treatment of diabetes focuses on controlling blood glucose in these ways:

■ Obtaining insulin or oral medication, if required.
■ Monitoring of blood glucose daily.
■ Following a dietary regimen to control blood glucose.
■ Achieving and maintaining appropriate body weight.
■ Exercising regularly.

The person with diabetes is advised to visit the health care provider and to obtain an individualized meal plan from a registered dietitian. Controlling blood glucose increases the chance of avoiding complications.

Can people prevent diabetes from occurring?

Yes, sometimes they can. Diabetes has its own risk factors, some of which can be controlled and others that cannot. One that cannot be controlled is inheritance; people from

families with diabetes stand a greater chance of developing it than do others. Among those risk factors that can be controlled is obesity.[3] Susceptible people who are overweight develop the major form of diabetes as they get older (**type II, or maturity-onset, diabetes**).[4] Type II diabetes accounts for over 90 percent of all diabetes in the United States. Inactivity also can contribute to this type of diabetes, and exercise can be preventive.[5] In addition, women who develop diabetes during their pregnancies (**gestational diabetes**) face a greater risk than normal of developing the disease outright, as well as a higher risk of birth defects in their infants. Gestational diabetes is often preventable by gaining the amount of weight appropriate for pregnancy, without excess.

Is there a type of diabetes that is not preventable?

Yes. About 10 percent of people develop diabetes in childhood (**type I diabetes**). The cause is unknown, but it is suspected that a virus may cause or worsen the condition. In type I diabetes, the immune system attacks and destroys the cells of the pancreas that make insulin, creating an insulin deficiency. A child with the disease usually becomes thin and fails to grow.

Why do some people require insulin shots, whereas others do not?

People with type I diabetes do not make insulin at all. It has to be supplied through injections or other means, such as implanted pumps that deliver the drug automatically. In contrast, people with type II diabetes may produce plenty of insulin but fail to respond to it. Sometimes a person

■ **MINIGLOSSARY**
of Diabetes Terms

diabetes a condition of abnormal carbohydrate metabolism, resulting in too much glucose in the blood and the presence of glucose in the urine. Diabetes is caused by inadequate production of insulin or by the body cells' failure to use the insulin produced. The common form, *diabetes mellitus*, is a major risk factor in the onset of heart disease and stroke and causes many organ diseases.

gestational diabetes a type of diabetes mellitus that develops during pregnancy and is associated with birth defects in offspring; often a forerunner of type II diabetes.

maturity-onset diabetes see *type II diabetes*.

type I diabetes a type of diabetes mellitus that begins in childhood and is characterized by a lack of insulin in the blood, thinness, and failure to grow. Also called *juvenile-onset diabetes*.

type II diabetes a type of diabetes mellitus that sets in during adulthood and is characterized by the presence of adequate insulin in the blood, a lack of tissue response to the insulin, and obesity. Also called *maturity-onset diabetes*.

with type II diabetes benefits from insulin shots or insulin-producing drugs. Some people with type II diabetes can manage the disease by diet and exercise alone.[6]

Is it true that people with diabetes have to avoid eating sweets and ice cream?

In most cases, yes. As mentioned previously, most people with diabetes have type II and are obese. Therefore, a diet that is low in fat and simple sugars can facilitate weight loss and maintain normal blood glucose. This diet contains whole foods that provide starch and fiber and is rich in vitamins and minerals.[7] The recommendations mesh perfectly with those given to prevent CVD and those given to people who need to lose weight.[8]

However, each case of diabetes is as unique as each human being. The goal of the diet is to maintain normal blood glucose concentrations and a healthy body weight. Some people with type II diabetes can incorporate moderate amounts of sugar in their diet and still maintain blood glucose control.[9] Also, in some instances, moderate amounts of ice cream or high-fat foods may be necessary to facilitate weight gain in the underweight individual with diabetes. Since each case is unique, blanket advice regarding diet does not apply to all people with diabetes. For this reason, it's essential to obtain an individual plan developed by three health care providers working together: the physician; the registered dietitian; and most important, the person with diabetes, who must live with the plan every day.[10]

■≡ Spotlight Notes

1. *The Surgeon General's Report on Nutrition and Health: Summary and Recommendations,* DHHS (PHS) publication no. 88–50211 (Washington, D.C.: Government Printing Office, 1988).

2. M. G. Kovar, M. I. Harris, and W. C. Hadden, The scope of diabetes in the United States population, *American Journal of Public Health* 77 (1987): 1549–1550.

3. S. Lillioja and coauthors, Impaired glucose tolerance as a disorder of insulin action, *New England Journal of Medicine* 318 (1988): 1217–1225.

4. G. F. Cahill, Beta-cell deficiency, insulin resistance, or both? *New England Journal of Medicine* 318 (1988): 1268–1270.

5. C. A Beebe, J. G. Pastors, M. A. Powers, and J. Wylie-Rosett, Nutrition management for individuals with noninsulin-dependent diabetes mellitus in the 1990s: A review by the Diabetes Care and Education Dietetic Practice Group, *Journal of the American Dietetic Association* 91 (1991): 196–207.

6. M. L. Wheeler, L. Delahanty, and J. Wylie-Rosett, Diet and exercise in noninsulin-dependent diabetes mellitus: Implications for dietitians from the NIH Consensus Development Conference, *Journal of the American Dietetic Association* 87 (1987): 480–485.

7. J. W. Anderson and coauthors, Dietary fiber and diabetes: A comprehensive review and practical application, *Journal of the American Dietetic Association* 87 (1987): 1189–1197.

8. M. J. Franz, Diabetes and nutrition: State of the science and the art, *Topics in Clinical Nutrition* 3 (1988): 1–16.

9. J. P. Bantle, Clinical aspects of sucrose and fructose metabolism, *Diabetes Care* 12 (1989): 56–61.

10. P. S. Easton, C. S. Harker, C. E. Higgins, and M. C. Mengel, *Nutrition Care of People with Diabetes Mellitus* (Binghamton, N.Y.: Food Products Press, 1991).

CHAPTER 19

Cancer

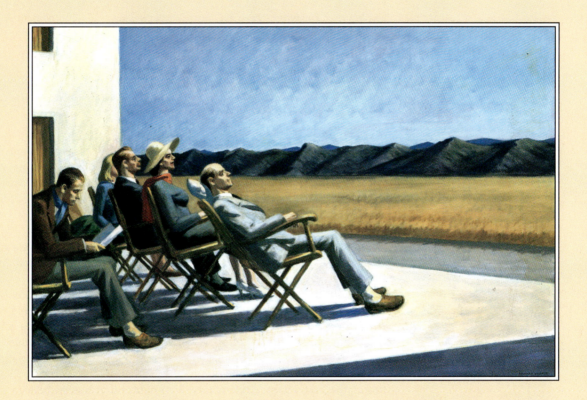

FACT OR FICTION

Just for fun, respond true or false to the following statements. If false, say what is true.

■ You can prevent most cancers by making changes in the way you live. (Page 534)

■ If you must use tobacco, the best choice to minimize your risk of cancer is to use the smokeless types, rather than cigarettes. (Page 538)

■ People who would like to tan without risking skin cancer can do so in tanning booths or with lamps. (Page 540)

■ People with darkly pigmented skin do not need to use sunscreen to prevent skin cancer. (Page 540)

■ Some viruses cause cancer. (Page 543)

■ A person's imagination can help the person deal with the pain of cancer. (Page 556)

cancer a disease in which abnormal cells multiply out of control, spread into surrounding tissues and other body parts, and disrupt normal functioning of one or more organs.

■ *FACT OR FICTION:* You can prevent most cancers by making changes in the way you live. *True.*

tumor an abnormal mass of tissue that has metabolism and replication, but performs no physiological service to the body.

melanoma cancer of the pigmented cells of the skin, related to sun exposure in people with light-colored skin.

myeloma a cancer originating in the cells of the bone marrow.

lymphomas (limf-OH-mahs) cancers that arise in organs of the immune system.

leukemias (loo-KEE-me-ahs) cancers that arise in the blood cell–making tissues, characterized by an abnormally high number of white cells in the blood.

carcinomas (car-sin-OH-mahs) cancers that arise in the skin, body chamber linings, or glands.

sarcomas (sar-KOH-mahs) cancers that arise in the connective tissue cells, including bones, ligaments, and muscles.

Years ago, the forecast for someone diagnosed as having **cancer** was bleak, but today, millions of people are fighting battles against cancer with success and are living normal lives. Although the numbers vary with the type of cancer and how early it is detected, the average rate of complete and permanent recovery from cancers of all types is approaching 50 percent and is predicted to continue improving.

Still, cancer prevention is preferred to treatment, of course.[1]* Researchers estimate that 80 percent of all cancer cases result from the circumstances of people's lives, many of which they can control themselves.[2] For example, the number-one cancer in both men and women is now lung cancer, which is seen only rarely in people who don't smoke. It has been estimated that 30 percent of all cancers could be eliminated if people stopped using tobacco.

Cancer affects one out of every four people in the United States today. Over a hundred diseases are called cancer, and each has its own name and characteristic progression of symptoms, depending on its type and its location in the body. Some cancers are given names that reflect the locations of the tissues from which they arise, with the suffix *-oma*, meaning "**tumor**," added on. For example, cancer of the pigmented cells of the skin, the melanocytes, is called **melanoma**. A tumor of the bone marrow is a **myeloma**— *myelos* means "marrow." The kinds of cancer are so numerous that the terminology can become confusing. For this reason, this chapter will keep naming to a minimum.

Generally, all cancers can be assigned to one of four classes, depending on tissue type:

■ Cancers of the immune system organs are **lymphomas.**
■ Cancers of blood-forming organs are **leukemias.**
■ Cancers of the glands and body linings, such as the skin, lining of the digestive tract or lungs, or other linings, are **carcinomas.**
■ Cancers of connective tissue, including bones, ligaments, and muscles, are **sarcomas.**

*Reference notes are at the end of the chapter.

■≡ How Cancer Develops

Initially, cancer begins with a change in a normal cell. After the change, the cell's metabolism is altered, and it begins reproducing out of control. The steps in the development of at least some cancers are thought to be:

1. Exposure to a type of **carcinogen** called an **initiator.**
2. Entry of the initiator into a cell.
3. Alteration by the initiator of a gene responsible for cell division, creating an **oncogene.** The alteration may be a **mutation,** or may be the liberation of some genetic material from a virus that has been hidden within a cell.
4. Possible acceleration of cancerous alterations by a **promoter.**
5. Out-of-control multiplication of the cells.
6. Tumor or other **malignancy** formation.*

One environmental agent may work alone to initiate cancer, or two or more such factors may work together as **co-carcinogens.**

An example of how initiators and promoters work together is the interaction between alcohol and tobacco in the development of cancers of the mouth, throat, and esophagus (see Figure 19–1). Normally, these cancers are rare. In a person who smokes two packs of cigarettes a day, the risk of developing a cancer is 1½ times greater than for the nonsmoker, but should that person also drink two alcoholic drinks each day, the risk would become 15 times greater. Alcohol alone does not increase the risk for these particular cancers, so it is likely to be acting as a cancer promoter, not as an initiator. The chemicals in cigarette smoke probably act in both ways: they initiate the cancer and promote it, too, to some degree.[3] Figure 11–1 in Chapter 11 showed the composition of mainstream cigarette smoke; many of the chemicals listed there and many others found in the smoke are considered to be either initiators or promoters of cancer.

All of the changes that lead to cancer happen inside an individual's cells, so cancer itself is not contagious. Once it has started, though, it can attack any tissue inside the body, from the solid bone to the fluid blood.

Normally, cells can discriminate when and whether to divide to produce new cells. For example, if some of the tissue of your skin were to become

*Carcinomas and sarcomas result in tumor formation. Leukemias and lymphomas result in uncontrolled multiplication of cells of the body's liquid tissues, the blood and the lymph.

carcinogen (CAR-sin-oh-jen or car-SIN-oh-jen) a substance that causes a growth gene inside a cell to mutate into a cancer-causing oncogene.

initiator a type of carcinogen, an agent required to start the formation of cancer.

oncogene (ON-co-jean) a gene that has been modified and produces irregular cell products that characterize malignant tumors.

mutation (myoo-TAY-shun) a change in a cell's genetic material. Once the genetic material has changed, the change is inherited in the offspring of that cell. A **mutagen** (MYOO-tah-gen) is a substance or event (such as radiation) that causes such changes in genetic material.

promoter a substance that assists in the development of malignant tumors, but does not initiate them on its own.

malignancy a cancerous, harmful, dangerous growth that endangers the victim by shedding cells into body fluids, in which they are carried to new locations to start new cancer colonies. (The general term *malignant* means "growing worse.")

co-carcinogens two or more factors that may be harmless when alone in the body, but that induce cancer when they occur together.

FIGURE 19–1 ■ **Cancer initiators and promoters.**

In cancer research, initiators and promoters are found to work together to produce many more tumors than initiators alone.

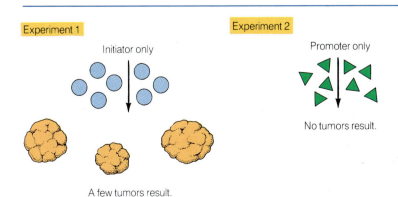

Experiment 1

Initiator only

A few tumors result.

Experiment 2

Promoter only

No tumors result.

Experiment 3

Initiator plus promoter

Many tumors develop.

benign (be-NINE)   noncancerous, not harmful, does not spread from one area to another.

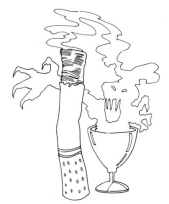

Two factors that work together as carcinogens: tobacco and alcohol.

metastasize (meh-TASS-tuh-size)   to migrate from one part of the body to another, starting new growths with characteristics of the original tumor.

damaged, the remaining healthy cells of the skin would multiply to replace the damaged part and then stop. A cancerous cell, though, appears to have lost responsiveness to the signal that says "stop dividing," and so it divides continuously. In the case of skin, the result is a lump of nonfunctional tissue, a tumor. Sometimes the tumor is harmless or **benign;** it does not spread. It is a well-defined, solid mass that is contained in an external membrane.

The processes that transform normal cells into malignant ones are unknown, but the cells' genetic material is believed to be involved. An oncogene, a portion of a cancer cell's genetic material, is suspected of playing a key role in the transformation process. Oncogenes probably start out as normal genes that undergo mutation—that is, they change. Alternatively, they could originate from the genetic material of a virus left behind from an infection. In either case, an oncogene changes the cell's protein products. These changed products influence the cell's reproduction and metabolism, making it malignant. Because the oncogene is part of the genetic material of the cell, it is passed on to each of the cell's offspring, so that they also are malignant.[4]

As a malignant tumor gains in size, it competes with normal tissues around it for nutrients and space, and eventually interrupts the normal functions of the tissues or organs into which it grows. In cancer of the large intestine, for example, the tumor may block the passage of the intestinal contents; in cancer of the brain, the growing tumor threatens intelligence and body control.

In addition to invading surrounding tissues, cancer cells break loose from the original site and ride the rivers of body fluids to colonize new locations. When the tumor is just beginning, it sheds only a few cells. As it enlarges, however, more and more of these wild cells escape and start new growths in other body parts, and the cancer is said to have **metastasized.** Cancer causes death of the person when it interrupts the functioning of vital organs such as the lungs, digestive system, or brain.

The immune system is on the watch for escaped cancer cells and works to stop these dangerous travelers before they lodge in body tissue. But the immune system is limited in the number of cancer cells it can eliminate at any one time, and when the immune defenses fail, cancer treatment is needed. The success of treatment depends on whether or not it gets under way before the cancer has metastasized.

After the initiating event, some cancers take as long as 20 years to develop. By the time a medical specialist finally detects a cancer, the initiator and promoters that facilitated the long chain of events that led to cancer are long gone. Hence it is hard to know what the original causes of cancer are, but research has uncovered some factors that are known, or strongly suspected, to be causal. Some of them, people can control: lifestyle choices such as smoking, sun and x-ray exposure, and diet. Some, they cannot: genetic susceptibility, gender, age, environmental chemicals, and environmental radiation.

≡▶   *Cancers are invasive diseases, classified according to the type of tissue they affect. Cancers develop in several steps from initiation through promotion to metastasis. A cancer causes death when it interrupts the functioning of vital organs.*

LIFE CHOICE INVENTORY

How well do you protect yourself against cancer? You cannot eliminate all cancer risks from your life, but you can take steps to reduce them. Questions answered no indicate opportunities for improvement.

1. Are you a nonsmoker? Do you avoid using tobacco in any form? Do you request that those around you not smoke?
2. Are you careful not to sunburn? Do you wear sunglasses that block out UV rays when outdoors? Do you obtain regular eye exams?
3. Do you question the necessity of x-ray examinations?
4. Do you read and follow instructions on the labels of chemicals that you use in the home, in the garden, or on the job?
5. Do you choose a variety of foods from a balanced diet that supply adequate fiber, vitamin A, and vitamin C, without too much fat? Do you eat cabbage and related vegetables often?
6. Is your weight within the normal range for your height?
7. Do you limit your intakes of cured and smoked meats?
8. Do you throw away foods that are on the verge of spoilage? (Spoilage suggests the presence of cancer-causing compounds.)
9. Do you limit your alcohol intake?
10. Do you exercise regularly?
11. Do you practice breast or testicular self-examination regularly?
12. Do you select employment with lower occupational hazards?
13. Do you practice safe sex? (The virus that causes genital warts is associated with cervical cancer.)

■≡ Risk Factors That People Can Control

The incidence of many cancers in the United States has not declined over the last 20 years, and researchers are trying to discover which environmental factors might cause them.[5] Environmental factors that can cause cancer include not only agents in air, water, food, and surroundings, but also disease agents (microbes), diet, exercise—in short, every aspect of existence except heredity. This chapter's Life Choice Inventory can help you evaluate the known controllable factors in your life.

Tobacco

Smoking is probably the most familiar of the cancer risk factors, and with good reason—the evidence against it is overwhelming. Hospital studies show consistently that 80 percent of lung cancer victims are smokers; population studies show that an increase in smoking precedes a jump in incidence of lung cancer; and animal studies show that direct application to the skin of condensed chemicals from tobacco smoke causes cancer.

In addition to the connection with lung cancer, smoking is linked to an increased incidence of cancers throughout the body, and to about a third of all cancer deaths. Cancer of the larynx (voice box), mouth, esophagus, urinary bladder, kidney, and pancreas all have been attributed to smoking. (Table 11–1 in Chapter 11 lists cancers whose risks are increased by smoking.)

■ *FACT OR FICTION:* If you must use tobacco, the best choice to minimize your risk of cancer is to use the smokeless types, rather than cigarettes. *False.* Smokeless tobacco products cause more cancers of the mouth and throat than cigarettes do.

People who use smokeless tobacco put themselves at greater risk for cancers of the mouth and throat than cigarette smokers do. Usually painless, white patches (**leukoplakia**) form in the mouths of people who use smokeless tobacco; these serve as a warning sign that changes are occurring that may lead to lethal cancers of the mouth and throat—cancers most frequently seen in tobacco users. Other times, red patches may appear. Both of these warnings should be evaluated by a health care practitioner. If tobacco users also use alcohol, even if not at the same times, they are putting themselves in further danger, for tobacco and alcohol work together to enormously increase cancer odds.

Even living or working with someone who smokes increases the risk of lung cancer. Sidestream smoke from burning cigarettes combines with exhaled smoke to fill the air with carcinogens. Smoke mixes into the air in all parts of the room, and no theoretical boundaries will contain it, although the farther you are from the smoker, the greater the dilution. Make your opinion known, even though it may be unpopular. People who choose to smoke can step outside to do so; they have a right to choose to endanger their own health with tobacco, but not to choose the same for anyone else.

≡▶ *To a great extent, lifestyle choices can contribute to cancer development. Tobacco use is one of the most preventable causes of cancer. Tobacco use causes cancers of the larynx, mouth, esophagus, bladder, kidney, and pancreas, as well as of the lungs. Smokeless tobacco and passive smoking also cause cancer.*

Radiation

People once believed that the sun's rays funneled health into the body. People equated tanning with a healthy way of life. Recently, however, people have learned that these ideas are dangerous, that the look of a tan is actually a mirage or a mask for illness. The modern craving for suntanned skin is becoming less popular as people learn about the proved unwelcome sun effects of wrinkling, skin aging, and cancer. More people are heeding medical warnings that claim that less sun is better and that no sun is best, as they learn the harmful effects of the sun.[6]

The sun's ultraviolet rays are a carcinogenic form of radiation, and too much exposure to them is the leading cause of skin cancer.[7] Skin cancer is a common and preventable form of cancer. Skin color can help predict susceptibility—the darker the skin, the more resistant to cancer, although no one is immune to the sun's harmful rays. Skin cancer risk is greatest among fair-complexioned people who burn easily, especially those with green or blue eyes and red or blond hair.

As the ozone layer is thinning, sun exposure has intensified. Concentrated doses of the sun's radiation, such as the amounts received with sunburns, are most likely to initiate cancerous changes.[8] Melanoma is the most lethal form of skin cancer; formerly one of the less common skin cancers, it is now on the rise.[9] According to one study, a single blistering sunburn in the teen years can double a person's risk of melanoma in later life.[10] People who receive less extreme, daily doses of sunlight tend to develop the more common, easily diagnosed and cured forms of skin cancer: basal cell carcinoma and squamous cell carcinoma. This means that indoor workers on summer vacation in the South and pale-skinned, weekend sunbathers are at the greatest risk for the most serious type of skin cancer, while those who work in the sun stand a greater chance of developing the more common but curable types. Figure 19–2 shows how to recognize the different forms of skin cancer.

Basal cell carcinoma.

Basal cell carcinoma is the most common form of skin cancer. The tumor usually appears as a single, small nodule or bump. It generally appears on the face, ears, head, neck, or hands, and can range in color from flesh tone to reddish brown or black. Occasionally, these tumors may appear on the torso, especially on the back or chest. Its border is often a pearly, translucent color with little evidence of inflammation in the skin surrounding the tumor. These tumors grow slowly, and if left untreated, will begin to bleed, crust over, then repeat the cycle. Although this type of cancer rarely spreads to other parts of the body, it *can* extend below the skin to the bone and do extensive local damage.

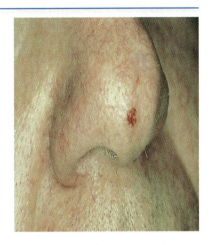

Squamous cell carcinoma.

As the second most common skin cancer, squamous cell carcinoma also favors areas exposed to the sun. The tumors are typically found on the rim of the ears, the face, lips, mouth, or back of the hands. These tumors may be somewhat difficult to discern in their early stages; they sometimes appear as red, scaly patches that may look like basal cell carcinoma. Squamous cell tumors, however, are usually redder or more swollen and tend to grow faster than basal cell tumors.

Squamous cell carcinoma will first appear firm to the touch but eventually form a central crust and, finally, an ulceration with surrounding inflammation of the skin.

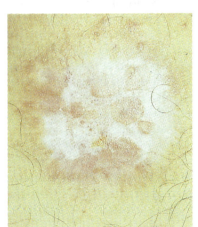

Malignant melanoma.

Melanoma is the deadliest form of skin cancer. When detected early and treated properly, the recovery rate can be very high. However, melanoma can spread throughout the body early in the course of the disease. Melanoma can appear anywhere on the body, not just in sun-exposed areas, enlarging over several months without warning.

Any indication of malignant melanoma is a sign to see your dermatologist immediately. Time is of the essence in treating and curing this form of skin cancer.

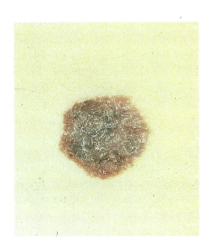

FIGURE 19–2 ■ Forms of skin cancer.

There are three basic forms of skin cancer: basal cell carcinoma, squamous cell carcinoma, and malignant melanoma. Basal cell and squamous cell carcinoma account for more than 90 percent of all cases reported.

SOURCE: Courtesy of The Skin Cancer Foundation, New York, New York.

Skin cancer can be both disfiguring and damaging. It can erode the skin and invade cartilage and bone at the site of the lesion. This can be disfiguring when a tumor occurs near the eyes, nose, or mouth. Skin cancer is a serious health threat, because it can spread through the blood and lymphatic system, ultimately causing death.

All types of sunlamps and tanning booths bombard the skin with radiation and provide no health benefits.[11] According to the FDA, sunlamps can not only cause cancer but also damage blood vessels, cause cataracts,[12] and cause a deadly form of eye cancer.[13]

People can take precautions to avoid dangerous overexposure to the sun. Be aware that ultraviolet rays penetrate clouds, so that even on cool, cloudy days, you can get burned. Use a sunscreen product that will block ultraviolet radiation and prevent burning. The higher a product's sun protection factor (SPF), the more protection it provides. Authorities recommend that all people, even people with dark skin, use waterproof sunscreens of SPF 15 or greater every day during sunny or warm weather.[14] To receive the intended level of protection, a person in a bathing suit should apply a full ounce of product with each application. Plan to enjoy the sun for short times on many occasions rather than on all-day trips, and take along a big hat.

Another warning is in order to those seeking tans by taking tanning pills. These products, which contain canthaxanthin, have not been approved by the FDA and have caused death in one previously healthy young woman.[15]

People are exposed to more radiation than just sunlight. A great deal of background radiation bombards us from the cosmos, from the soil, and from the air and water. Man-made sources of radiation include medical and dental x-ray procedures and above-ground nuclear weapons testing.[16] Researchers believe that throughout life, a person living in the United States normally receives about one-third the minimum radiation required to cause cancer (leukemia can be caused by about three times a person's normal radiation exposure).[17]

Another strategy for avoiding unnecessary radiation exposure is to tell your dentist and health care practitioner that you wish to avoid X rays whenever possible. When they are unavoidable, be sure that the technician takes precautions to protect the parts of your body that are not being x-rayed, especially the abdomen and genitals.

Another potentially risky form of radiation is that from electricity, such as high-voltage power lines and electrical appliances. Most standard home appliances are probably safe, with the exception of electric blankets. Use an electric blanket only to warm the bed, and then unplug it, since a magnetic field lingers as long as the blanket is plugged in. Video display terminals and TVs emit radiation also. People who work at computer terminals should stay 30 inches from the front and 3 feet from the sides and back of the monitor.

■ *FACT OR FICTION:* People who would like to tan without risking skin cancer can do so in tanning booths or with lamps. *False.* Tanning booths or sunlamps are not safer than sunbathing as far as cancer risks are concerned.

The American Cancer Society says, "Fry now, pay later."

■ *FACT OR FICTION:* People with darkly pigmented skin do not need to use sunscreen to prevent skin cancer. *False.* While people with fair complexions who burn easily are at greater risk, everyone needs to use sunscreen to prevent skin cancer from sun exposure.

≡▶ *Sun overexposure causes premature skin aging and skin cancer that can be disfiguring and life-threatening. People who value their health and their long-term personal appearance will shun the sun altogether or use sunscreen. X rays, electronic appliances, and video screens also can initiate cancers, and people should control their exposure to them.*

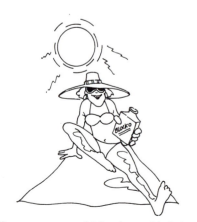

Use sunscreen, and take along a big hat.

Diet and Exercise

People of certain religious groups have remarkably low cancer rates, and scientists have studied them to find out why. One such group, the Seventh-Day Adventists, has rules against smoking, drinking alcohol, and eating spicy foods; the Adventists encourage a vegetarian diet (including eggs and milk). Of course, abstinence from tobacco and alcohol accounts for a large part of the low cancer rate; still, the group's cancer incidence is only half what would be expected in people who do not smoke or drink alcohol.[18]

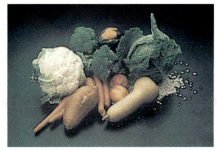

These foods contain nutrients and nonnutrients that are protective against cancer.

These and other studies have led researchers to identify three dietary factors strongly associated with high cancer risk: high meat and fat consumption, low vegetable consumption, and low grain consumption. Vegetarian-type diets are probably protective against certain types of cancers, particularly colon cancer,[19] one of the major health problems in the modern world.[20] The fat, and perhaps the excess protein, in meat may act as cancer promoters. In addition, any meat that has been smoked, charbroiled, burned, or commercially cured may contain carcinogens. Research also suggests that fibers present in vegetables and grains protect against cancer of the large intestine, probably by trapping carcinogens in the digestive tract and hastening their excretion.

Further, evidence suggests that the vitamins that occur in fruits and vegetables may help to prevent the development of certain cancers. For example, the vitamin C of, say, oranges may stop the formation of carcinogens called nitrosamines; and the vitamin A of vegetables and fruits such as sweet potatoes and peaches is important in preventing cancers of the body's external and internal linings, including the skin and lungs.[21] The fibers of plant foods such as whole grains, fruits, and vegetables may play roles as well. Other nutrient candidates for roles in cancer prevention are the vitamins riboflavin and folate, the mineral calcium, and a group of nonvitamins (indoles and others) found in the cabbage family.[22] Taken in whole foods,

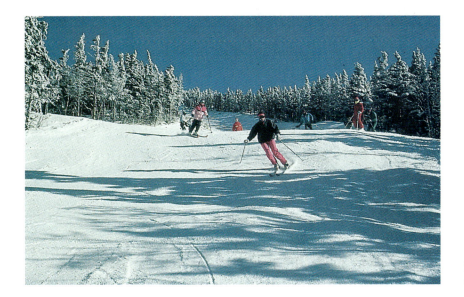

People who exercise regularly may be better defended against cancer.

these arrive in the body together with many other nutrients. A word of caution though: these benefits come from foods, not supplements. Some people promote the sales of useless vitamin and mineral preparations as cancer fighters. Don't waste money on nutrition supplements that provide a false hope of cancer prevention.

Do the recommendations sound familiar? Less fat, more vegetables and grains, and variety are guidelines you have already heard for prevention of obesity, heart disease, high blood pressure, and diabetes, and they are here again for possible protection from at least some types of cancer. Without a doubt, a lifetime of eating nutritious foods and avoiding obesity fortifies the immune system against cancer.

Like diet, exercise may be important in cancer prevention. People who are sedentary may get some types of cancer, especially those of the large intestine, more often than people who exercise regularly.[23]

▶ *People can select a diet that will minimize cancer risk. A diet low in alcohol, fat, and meat and high in grains and vegetables is recommended. Nutrition supplements do not appear to offer the same benefits as whole foods. Exercise may also be important in cancer prevention.*

■ Risk Factors Beyond People's Control

Even if a risk factor cannot be controlled directly, it may still be one you can take steps to minimize. For example, if you learn that light-skinned people are susceptible to skin cancer, and your skin is light colored, you need not feel helpless because you cannot change your race. Instead, you can take seriously suggestions to regulate your exposure to the sun. Generally, wherever there is a risk factor outside of your own control, there are many factors that can work to oppose it, which you can control. Even heredity is one of those, especially in the case of cancer.

Genetics

The genetics of cancer is complex. It is relatively certain that cancer itself, with rare exceptions, is not inherited. Rather, normal genes are thought to change into cancerous ones during a person's lifetime. But whereas cancers usually are not inherited, the tendency to develop certain cancers does run in families. In fact, certain types of cancer correlate more closely with heredity than with environmental factors. One example is cancer of the prostate gland in men. There appears to be no consistent correlation of prostatic cancer with diet, sexually transmitted disease, sexual habits, smoking, or occupational exposure. Cases have been observed in family clusters, however; men who have a brother or father with the disease are at risk.[24] Another example is breast cancer. Women whose mothers or sisters have had breast cancer have two to three times the usual risk for developing breast cancer in their lifetimes.[25]

Because you cannot control your heredity, does this mean you are defenseless against familial cancers? Not at all. As with the inherited risk factors for heart disease, knowing your family history helps you know what preventive steps to take. People with family histories of certain kinds of cancers should, for example, alert their health care providers so that they may obtain tests for them. Early detection gives the most hope of cure.

Blood tests to detect the products that oncogenes produce can help to identify people who are at risk for cancer development. Research into oncogenes and their products is currently very active, for they offer great promise as a screening device. Once an oncogene product is known and detection methods are worked out, families of people with a given form of cancer can be screened for that form of cancer and thus be on the lookout for the disease in the earliest, most curable stages.

Viruses are also being closely scrutinized in cancer research. Like genes, viruses are made of genetic material. The only major difference in composition is that viruses also possess protein coats in which they can travel from one cell to another, as Chapter 17 described. Sometimes, though, viruses don't travel, but insert their genetic material into that of a host cell and remain inactive there for many cellular generations. Each time the cell, with its genes, divides, the viral genes divide, too. But then one day, the viral genes may become active, and when they do, they may produce molecules that cause cancer.

Remember that a virus's genetic material uses the host cell's manufacturing equipment to reproduce copies of the virus. To do this, the virus tricks the cell by imitating compounds that normally give the ''go'' signal for replication of genetic material and certain proteins. That way, the cell works to replace its own parts but produces viral genes and proteins instead.

Scientists think that cancer-causing viruses may also trick the cells into dividing. It may be that the viral oncogenes fool the cells into producing the very molecules that give the go-ahead signal for cell division. Normally, the cells would be triggered to produce this molecule only when cell replacement was required for health, but under the influence of the virus, replication could go on unchecked, forming a tumor. An alternative idea is that people's own genes carry viruslike sections that can be induced by an initiator and start the multiplication.

As an example of a possible cancer-causing virus, the virus that causes genital warts can cause cancer of the cervix in women. The virus appears to cause cancer by altering the genetic material in cervical tissues. The women most likely to get such cancer are those who begin sexual activity at an early age and who have multiple partners, suggesting that in this one case, they may contract, or ''catch,'' the virus as people ''catch'' other diseases. This is an exception to the rule that you can't catch cancer.

Because this sexually transmitted form of cervical cancer is especially likely to attack young women who start having intercourse in their early teen years, women can minimize the risks by practicing the safe-sex strategies described in Chapter 17.

■ *FACT OR FICTION:* Some viruses cause cancer. *True.*

≡▶ *Cancer is not hereditary, but in at least some cases, the susceptibility to it is. Knowing one's family history can therefore aid prevention. Viruses also appear to be related to cancer. A virus known to cause cancer is the one that causes genital warts; it causes cervical cancer in women.*

Gender and Age

Whether you are a man or a woman partially determines your likelihood of developing cancers of all types. Overall, women are slightly more likely to develop cancers than men are, but in men, cancers are more likely to be fatal.

Age plays an important role in a person's chances of developing cancer. Young people rarely contract and die of cancer; older people frequently do. The relationship is linear: the older the person, the more likely he or she is to contract cancer. Like race, age is outside the control of the individual. But a shift in emphasis from prevention alone to prevention and early detection through screening tests can help people to exert maximum control over the disease. The older you are, the more important screening tests become. Screening tests are described in a later section.

≡▶   *Gender and age play a part in a person's chances of developing cancer. Women are more likely to get cancer than men; older people are more likely to get cancer than younger people.*

Environment

Chemical carcinogens, both natural and man-made, surround us, and many of them present cancer risks of varying degrees of severity. City dwellers are exposed to engine exhaust and factory chemicals, while people in the country use pesticides and other agricultural chemicals. Certain occupations also hold greater cancer risks than others.

One job-related chemical carcinogen is asbestos. The asbestos industry discovered, then suppressed, information about the carcinogenicity of asbestos. As a result, millions of workers were exposed to the carcinogen, and hundreds of thousands died.[26] Another example of a potential environmental hazard is cadmium, a metal being used extensively in industry. Public health officials view this metal as a major threat to human health and the environment.[27]

Another example is radon, a radioactive gas, which has recently been recognized as a potential cause of lung cancer. It has probably been responsible for starting many lung cancers in miners of uranium and other underground minerals. Radon has also been found in indoor spaces in unacceptable levels.[28] The presence of radon in homes is an environmental health problem.

As with the other risk factors that you can't control, you are not helpless against environmental agents that cause cancer. Learning what they are is the first step toward prevention. The next steps depend on what you have learned. If an industry is presenting you and your neighbors with an unacceptable risk, you may choose to band together in political action. You may move or seek employment elsewhere. Or you may choose to take all possible precautions against the risks, and hedge your bets by requesting frequent and thorough screening tests as well.

≡▶   *Chemical carcinogens may be harmful not only to the environment but also to human health. Many man-made chemicals create a cancer risk.*

■ ≡ Screening and Early Detection

The treatment of cancer involves sophisticated equipment, powerful drugs, and specialized medical staff, but the detection of common cancers requires mostly routine tests and self-examinations. The sooner a cancer is detected, the better the chances for a complete cure.[29] Table 19–1 lists the cancers that most often cause deaths among young people and the symptoms associated with each. Any of the symptoms listed should be checked by a health care provider immediately.

Often, cancer gives some warning to the person who is developing it. Cancer can develop without symptoms, but it is wise to heed all the messages your body sends you, particularly the following warnings:

■ Change in bowel or bladder habits, such as diarrhea or constipation.
■ A sore that does not heal.
■ Unusual bleeding or discharge.
■ Thickening or lump that suddenly appears anywhere in the body.
■ Indigestion or difficulty swallowing.
■ Obvious change in wart or mole.
■ Nagging cough or hoarseness.
■ Sudden weight loss.

To remember this list, recall that the first letters in the warning signs spell the word *cautions.* Having one of these symptoms does not necessarily mean that you have cancer. A cold or eating too much might bring about some of

TABLE 19–1 ■ Cancers Causing Death in People Ages 15–34

Disease	Early Symptoms	Survival with Early Diagnosis and Prompt Treatment[a]
Brain and nervous system cancer	Personality changes; bizarre behavior; headaches; dizziness, balance and walking disturbances; vision changes; nausea, vomiting or seizures	Poor to good
Breast cancer	Unusual lump; thickening, change in contour, dimple, or discharge from the nipple	Good (about 50%)
Hodgkin's disease	Swelling of lymph nodes in neck, armpits, or groin; susceptibility to infection	Good (54%)
Leukemia	Mimics infection, with fever, lethargy, and other flulike symptoms; may also include bone pain, tendency to bruise or bleed easily, and enlargement of lymph nodes	Poor to good (up to 50%), depending on the type of disease
Skin cancer	Unusual discoloration, swellings, sores, or lumps; change in color or appearance of a wart or mole; tenderness, itching, or bleeding from a lump or mole	Excellent (up to 90%)
Testicular cancer	Small, hard, painless lump; sudden accumulation of fluid in the scrotum; pain or discomfort in the region between the scrotum and anus	Good to excellent (66 to 86%)

[a]The survival rates are estimates based on five years of disease-free survival. For all cancers, survival rates drop dramatically after metastasis.

FIGURE 19–3 ■ **Breast self-examination.**

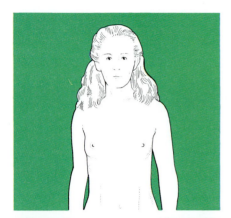

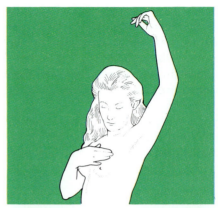

Some women do the next part of the exam in the shower. Fingers glide over soapy skin, making it easy to concentrate on the texture underneath.

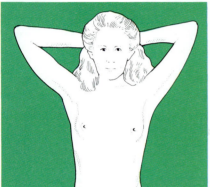

The next two steps are designed to emphasize any changes in the shape or contour of your breasts. As you do them, you should be able to feel your chest muscles tighten.

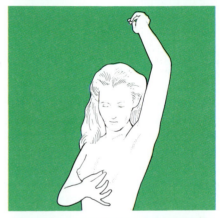

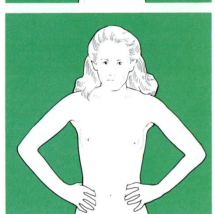

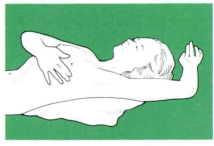

1. Stand before a mirror. Inspect both breasts for anything unusual, such as any discharge from the nipples or puckering, dimpling, or scaling of the skin.

2. Watch closely in the mirror, clasp hands behind your head, and press hands forward.

3. Next, press hands firmly on hips and bow slightly toward the mirror as you pull your shoulders and elbows forward.

4. Raise your left arm. Use three or four fingers of your right hand to explore your left breast firmly, carefully, and thoroughly. Beginning at the outer edge, press the flat part of your fingers in small circles, moving the circles slowly around the breast. Gradually work toward the nipple. Be sure to cover the entire breast. Pay special attention to the area between the breast and armpit, including the armpit itself. Feel for any unusual lump or mass under the skin.

5. Gently squeeze the nipple and look for a discharge. Repeat the exam on your right breast.

6. Repeat steps 4 and 5 lying down. Lie flat on your back with your left arm over your head and a pillow or folded towel under your left shoulder. This position flattens the breast and makes it easier to examine. Use the same circular motion described earlier. Repeat on your right breast.

them, for example. Just remember that when signals last for more than a week, or when they recur, they require the attention of a health care provider.

Self-examinations are particularly useful for early detection of cancer. For example, if you are a woman, you can check your breasts; the test is easy. In young women, lumps in the breasts are most often not cancerous, but they should be checked by a health care provider nonetheless.

Once a month is often enough to check the breasts for cancer. Try to test at the same time each month (women should time the test to follow the menstrual period, because the breasts can be lumpy beforehand). If you start testing now, while you are young, it will be a habit that will serve you well throughout life. The test is especially easy when it is done in the shower, where the skin is slippery (see Figure 19–3). You'll soon easily tell the "normal lumpiness" that occurs before the menstrual period from an unusual lump. Many times, early cancer feels like a little pea buried in the breast. Report anything unusual right away.

If you are a man, you can help protect yourself from cancer of the testes through self-examination (see Figure 19–4). Although it occurs less frequently than breast cancer, testicular cancer is dangerous because it advances rapidly. Once-a-month testing is usually sufficient.

One more test to perform monthly is a once-over visual check of your entire skin. Skin cancer is a real threat, and the more familiar you become with any moles or freckles you may have, the better you will be able to detect changes in them that could mean the start of cancer. Once a month after a bath or shower, stand in front of a full-length or large mirror, and take a look at your skin. Use a hand mirror to help with the back view. If a mole has changed its shape or color or has begun bleeding, have it checked right away. See Figure 19–5 for skin self-examination. Figure 19–6 shows warning signs to watch for.

Self-examinations have proved valuable in early cancer detection. A person who often examines his or her body becomes familiar with it and may be more likely to detect an abnormality than a medical professional who examines the person only once a year or so. (Of course, a professional can

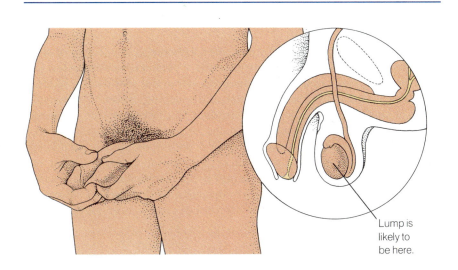

Lump is likely to be here.

FIGURE 19–4 ■ **Testicular self-examination.**

Roll each testicle between the thumb and fingers; the testicles should feel smooth, except for the normal raised organ located on the back of each. Report any hard lump, enlargement, or contour changes to your health care provider.

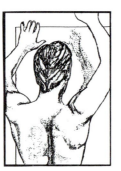

1. Examine your body (front and back) in the mirror, then right and left sides, arms raised.

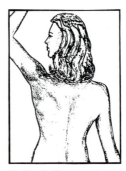

2. Bend elbows and look carefully at forearms and under upper arms and palms. Check between fingers, and take particular note of skin near and under nails.

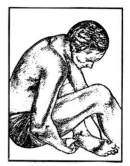

3. Next, look at backs of the legs and feet, including spaces between the toes, and soles of the feet.

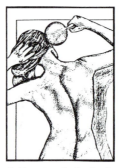

4. Examine the back of the neck and scalp with the help of a hand mirror. Part hair to lift it for a closer look. Be sure to include the area behind and on top of the ears. Also check the top and back of shoulders.

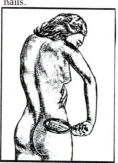

5. Finally, check the back and buttocks area with a hand mirror.

SOURCE: American Academy of Dermatology.

FIGURE 19–5 ■ **Skin self-examination.**

Check all moles, blemishes, and birthmarks from the top of your head down to the soles of your feet. Be sure to note and record anything new, such as changes in size, shape, elevation or color of moles and blemishes, or any sores that do not heal. If you follow these steps on a routine monthly basis, it will be easiest to detect skin cancer in its earliest stage.

detect a lump in places not easily examined at home.) Other forms of self-examination are catching on, too; for example, a person who wants a test for colon abnormalities can buy an inexpensive home test that detects hidden blood in the stools, a primary indicator of developing cancer.* The person collects a small sample at home and sends it to a laboratory for checking. Such tests should not be used as substitutes for periodic screening, however.

Laboratory tests are important, too, and enormous strides have been made in the development of new cancer detection methods. The most accurate detection method for breast cancer is the **mammogram** (x-ray examination), which has helped with early detection of the disease.[30] Because mammograms use X rays, which themselves can cause cancer, they are used

mammogram x-ray examination of the breast, a screening test for cancer.

*The name of one such home test is Hemoccult.

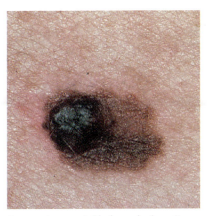

Asymmetry: one-half of a mole doesn't match the other half.

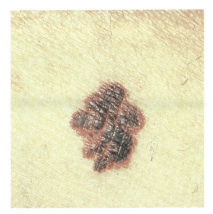

Border irregularity: the edges of a mole are ragged, notched, or blurred.

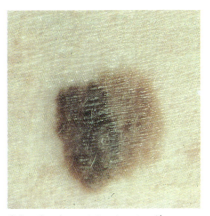

Color: the pigmentation is not uniform. Shades of tan, brown, and black may be present; dashes of red, white, and blue add to the mottled appearance.

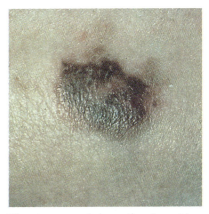

Diameter: any mole larger than 6 mm (size of a pencil eraser) or other growth the size of a mole should be of concern.

SOURCE: Courtesy of The Skin Cancer Foundation, New York, New York. From the brochure "The ABCD's of Moles and Melanomas," © 1985, The Skin Cancer Foundation.

FIGURE 19–6 ■ Warning signs for skin cancer.

The ABCDs of Skin Cancer
Other warning signs of melanoma include changes in the surface of a mole, such as scaliness, oozing, bleeding, or increase in elevation or thickness of a mole. The spread of pigment from the border into the surrounding skin and a change in sensation in the area of the mole, including itchiness, tenderness, or pain, may also be indications of melanoma. See your dermatologist if you suspect *any* change that may indicate skin cancer.

sparingly; many women choose to have one done at age 35 or so to use for a baseline comparison, repeating the test in later life. The National Cancer Institute and the American Cancer Society recommend screening every one to two years for women over age 40.[31] Women with high breast cancer risks indicated by their family histories should be examined by mammography. Table 19–2 lists other medical tests to detect cancer and the appropriate ages at which to seek them.

Women with healthy breasts who are considering breast-implant surgery for enlargement purposes are wise to weigh the associated risks. Silicone breast implants may interfere with the ability to screen for breast cancer; they may obscure malignancies until they've reached a more life-threatening stage.[32]

One standard test for cancer is the **biopsy,** which involves the surgical removal of a small amount of tissue for microscopic and chemical study. In

biopsy surgical removal of a piece of tissue for examination by microscope or other means.

TABLE 19–2 ■ **Medical Tests for the Early Detection of Cancer in Asymptomatic Persons**

Test	Gender	Age 20	35	40	50	60
Pap	F	Every year; then, after two negatives 1 year apart, every 3 years[a]	At least every 3 years	At least every 3 years	At least every 3 years	At least every 3 years
Pelvic examination	F	Every 3 years	Every 3 years	Every year	Every year	Every year
Breast examination (manual)	F	Every 3 years	Every 3 years	Every year	Every year	Every year
Testis and prostate examination	M	Every 3 years	Every 3 years	Every year	Every year	Every year
Thyroid, lymph node, oral region, and skin examination	M, F	Every 3 years	Every 3 years	Every year	Every year	Every year
Mammography	F	—	Once at 35, to establish baseline[b]	—	Every year	Every year
Digital rectal examination	M, F	—	—	Every year	Every year	Every year
Uterine lining tissue sample	F	—	—	—	Once, at menopause	—
Stool slide test	M, F	—	—	—	Every year	Every year
Colon examination	M, F	—	—	—	Every year; then, after two negatives 1 year apart, every 3 to 5 years	At least every 3 years

[a]Start younger if sexually active.
[b]Have additional mammograms on health care provider's recommendation.

SOURCE: Adapted from American Cancer Society recommendations.

CT scan (computerized tomography scan) computer-processed x-ray pictures; the x-ray beam is rotated to cover the body area in question, and the computer organizes the individual images into a whole picture of a thin section of the body tissue, including any tumors that might be present.

the case of small, local tumors such as small skin lesions, a biopsy can be the cure as well as the test. In other cases, it will reveal information vital to the treatment of the disease, such as the tissue in which the cancer originated. Imaging tests are used to discover the size of the mass and the extent of invasion. X-ray examination is often used, including the **CT scan,** a computerized organization of x-ray information into a visual image of the tumor. It is especially useful for areas not easily accessible, such as the brain. Another technique involves **thermography,** the detection of heat produced by a tumor in contrast to the cooler normal tissue around it.

Tests for the most likely cancers—those of the lungs, skin, cervix, prostate, uterine lining, breasts, large intestine, and rectum—are useful. Within these few common locations, the disease can take a great number of forms, and a specific test is needed to detect each one. Specific tests are performed on people with family histories of cancers or with other known risk factors. A health care provider can judge which may be necessary for you. In the future, as mentioned earlier, it may be possible to detect the presence of cancer in the body simply by performing a blood test that detects oncogene products associated with cancer.[33]

Even though the earliest possible detection is crucial to successful treatment, new detection tests may not be the first priority in cancer research. A better use of resources would be to discover how to prevent cancer's occurrence. No disease has ever been cured out of existence. As is now the case with smallpox and polio, widescale success can be claimed only when the disease is prevented from occurring. The rate of cure for cancer, although better than in the past, has been relatively stable for many years, while the number of cases remains high and, for some cancers, is rising higher.

≡▶ *Self-examinations of the breasts, testes, and skin can help to detect cancer early. Other tests can be conducted by health care providers to screen for cancer.*

■≡ Cancer Treatment

Being diagnosed as having cancer can be a frightening experience, and fear can reduce the body's healing response. There are tremendous numbers of treatment success stories, and it is important to know about advances in cancer treatment. For more information about cancer, people can call a cancer hotline number.*

Cancer cells move freely in the body, and surgical removal or destruction of a tumor does not necessarily eliminate all of the cells. Cancer *cure* comes when every cancer cell is either removed from the body or destroyed by treatments.

Surgery is the primary mode of treatment for many cancers. Removal of the tumor stops the cancer growth at the site, especially if the cancer is still small. Figure 19–7 shows cure rates for many types of cancer *by surgery alone;* notice how the cure rate drops off as the tumor invades surrounding tissues and metastasizes. For example, the large intestine may contain precancerous growths called **polyps;** removal of polyps protects against cancer. If the polyp begins to invade just a few millimeters into the tissue, however, its surgical removal no longer guarantees complete freedom from cancer at that site.

A small tumor on the skin or another external membrane sometimes can be destroyed by freezing with liquid nitrogen. Such a procedure is often performed in the physician's office and causes little inconvenience or pain.

thermography a method of detecting tissues of high metabolic rate, such as tumors, by the heat they release.

polyps tumors that grow on stems, similar in appearance to mushrooms. Polyps bleed easily, and some have the tendency to become malignant.

*The National Cancer Institute's information service number is (800) 4CANCER. In Alaska, it is (800) 638-6070; in Washington, D.C., and suburbs, 636-5700 (local number); and in Hawaii, 524-1234 (local number). Spanish-speaking staff are available in some areas. The American Cancer Society is (800) ACS-2345.

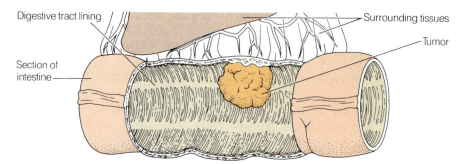

(a) When the tumor is local, surgery alone can cure it 80% of the time.

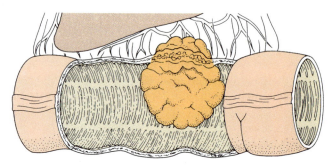

(b) When the tumor has advanced into the surrounding tissues, the cure rate by surgery drops to 40%.

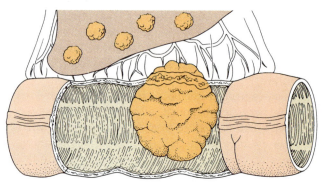

(c) A tumor that has widely invaded the surrounding tissue and has metastasized can be cured by surgery alone only 20% of the time.

FIGURE 19–7 ■ Cancer progression and cure rate by surgery alone.

You have probably heard the name of one type of surgery for breast cancer—the **mastectomy** (removal of the breast). The mastectomy was originally developed only to make clients with advanced cancer comfortable— **palliative therapy**—but even some of these advanced cases were cured by the procedure. Still in use for some cases, the radical mastectomy involves removing muscle, bone, and glands as well as the breast, and it cures the disease about half the time. In more cases, it is possible to remove less tissue, a **lumpectomy,** because the surgery is usually accompanied by other treatments aimed at wiping out cancer cells not removed by surgery.[34] These treatments have been shown, at least by some research, to be as effective as radical mastectomy.[35]

Another treatment for cancer is **radiation therapy.** To kill a tumor with radiation, a beam is focused on the area known to be cancerous. Alternatively, radioactive materials are implanted in the tumor or, in some cases, injected into the bloodstream (when it is known that they will be selectively absorbed by the tumor). Under bombardment from the radioactivity, the fast-growing cells of the cancer become disrupted and die off.

An example of radiation treatment by injection is the treatment of cancer of the thyroid by radioactive iodine. The thyroid normally picks up and concentrates the mineral iodine in its tissues, so it also picks up radioactive iodine, which destroys thyroid tissue. Cancer cells that metastasize from the thyroid to other body locations and the tumors they form exhibit the same iodine-scavenging behavior, so the injected radioactive iodine destroys them, too.

Radiation therapy is similar to surgery in that both are local forms of treatment and both must kill some normal tissue in order to kill cancer tissue. In some cases, as in cancer of the head or neck, radiation is chosen over surgery because surrounding structures may be too delicate to permit surgery.

Radiation is useful only if the tumor proves sensitive to it, as in **Hodgkin's disease,** a cancer of the lymph system that is normally treated with radiation. Sometimes, though, the tumor is not radiosensitive, and the dose of radiation required to kill it would also destroy massive amounts of the surrounding normal tissue. Drugs have been developed that sensitize certain types of cancer so that radiation can be effective. Another problem is that when a beam of radiation is used, some cancer cells may lie outside the beam area and remain unaffected. The problem cannot be solved by irradiating the whole body, because the body cannot tolerate so much radiation.

A well-known disadvantage of radiation treatments is the side effects they cause. People who receive such treatments may suffer from skin irritation, nausea, diarrhea, hair loss, and fatigue. Developments in technology have helped to control these effects by minimizing the damage to healthy tissues.

Chemical treatment of cancer, called **chemotherapy,** has a major advantage—the drugs are taken orally or by injection and are distributed throughout the body to seek out and destroy the escaped cancer cells and any new tumors that may be just starting.[36] More than 40 drugs are now used against cancer in some way, to cure, to inhibit cancer growth, to relieve pain, and to allow the person to lead a more normal life.

A typical anticancer drug works by blocking cell division—for example, by interfering with the action of the vitamin folate. Cancer cells need more folate than other dividing cells, because they are dividing more rapidly, and the anticancer drug is chemically similar enough to folate to fool cancer cells into accepting it instead of the vitamin. When the drug settles into the spot normally occupied by folate, the cancer cells' attempts at division are unsuccessful, and they die. Other drugs work in different ways to accomplish the same thing—blockage of cell division and death of the cancerous tissue. Several of the most effective anticancer drugs are chemicals that occur in nature: an extract of the periwinkle plant and a substance made by ocean

mastectomy surgical removal of the breast and varying amounts of surrounding tissue as the primary treatment for breast cancer. The most extreme form is the *radical mastectomy*, in which the breast, underlying muscle tissue, and lymph glands are removed; a *modified radical mastectomy* involves removal of the breast and lymph glands, but not the underlying muscle; a *simple mastectomy* is removal of the breast only.

palliative therapy measures given to relieve discomfort or alleviate symptoms, without producing a cure.

lumpectomy removal of a tumor with a minimal amount of the surrounding tissue.

radiation therapy the application of cell-destroying radiation to kill cancerous tissues.

Hodgkin's disease a lymphoma that attacks people in early life and is treatable with radiation therapy.

chemotherapy the administration of drugs that have a specific harmful effect on the disease-causing entity but that do not harm the client, or at least usually do not harm the client as much as the disease does.

sponges. Scientists are scanning other wild species for anticancer chemicals, yet unknown.

Anticancer drugs also kill normal tissues, although more slowly than they kill cancerous ones. In the digestive tract, for example, the normal, rapid cell division is disturbed; diarrhea, nausea, and vomiting result. Blood cells are also a rapidly dividing tissue, so their production is impaired in people being treated with anticancer drugs.

New developments in packaging of chemotherapeutic drugs may help prevent such side effects. Microscopic time-release capsules now can be injected directly into the cancer site. That way, the drug stays in the immediate vicinity of the cancer and causes fewer side effects. All anticancer drugs have narrow margins of safety.

A dramatic improvement over any one of these methods alone is attained by the combination of surgery or radiation with chemotherapy, **adjuvant therapy.** Clients are given drug treatments soon after, or sometimes even before, surgery or radiation to prevent the possibility of a tumor's showing up in another location. Radiation and surgery combined are effective for treating breast cancer and produce the fewest possible side effects; surgery for testicular cancer is often combined with chemotherapy for the highest chance of cure.

Researchers in the area of cancer treatment are striding ahead, and some advances sound almost like science fiction. Scientists have been able to magnetize cancer cells lodged in bone and then collect them on a magnet for removal. Bone marrow transplants are looking promising, too: during cancer therapy, a person's bone marrow, both the diseased and the healthy, is destroyed. The person is then injected with marrow cells from a donor that repopulate the bones with healthy marrow. Another method under development: cancer cells are sensitized to red light that passes harmlessly through healthy tissue to the cancer cells and destroys them. Another approach involves the bleaching of cancerous skin pigment cells to reverse the cancer. Researchers also have discovered that cells called mast cells are responsible for creating the new blood vessels that nourish growing tumors. Soon it may be possible to interfere with the mast cells and cut off the cancer's blood supply.

A new treatment with great promise, although still experimental, is **immunotherapy.** Immunotherapy consists of activating a person's own powerful immune system against the cancer.[37] Currently, researchers at the National Cancer Institute are testing a drug (interleukin 2) that works to activate the immune system's killer cells against cancer. So far, the results look promising—even advanced cases of inoperable cancer have been improved by the therapy. Another approach is to use the person's own cancer cells to make a vaccine to activate the immune system against the cancer.[38]

Described here are only a few of the new avenues of approach in the treatment of cancer. A person who gets cancer has reason to be hopeful about possibilities for a cure, but should be on guard against cancer frauds, described in this chapter's critical thinking section.

adjuvant therapy   cancer treatment through a combination of surgery or radiation with chemotherapy.

immunotherapy   cancer treatment that involves activating a person's immune system to fight the cancer, also called cell-transfer therapy.

≡▶ *Cancer treatment is most successful when it is started promptly after early detection. The most common treatments include surgery, radiation therapy, chemotherapy, and adjuvant therapy (a combination of treatments). Many avenues are being explored with great promise.*

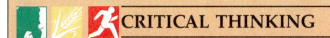

CRITICAL THINKING

Deception of the Desperate

Not all cancer treatments called "cures" are effective. Frauds in health are always cruel, but those aimed at cancer victims are especially so—they prey on people who are already suffering. Laetrile (also called amygdalin or vitamin B_{17}) is a cancer-cure hoax, not a vitamin by any stretch of the imagination. Another such hoax is called immuno-augmentative therapy, or IAT; this one involves traveling to foreign countries for dangerous blood transfusions that not only do not fight cancer, but spread AIDS and hepatitis to the already sick victims. There also are countless other vitamin, mineral, and drug "therapies."

Sometimes people will report that a phony cancer cure worked. A famous quack-buster, Victor Herbert, has identified five possible scenarios to account for this: the person never had cancer; the cancer was cured by conventional therapy, but the quack took the credit; the cancer is silently progressing, and the person only *thinks* that cure has taken place; the person has died of cancer, but is represented as cured; or the person's cancer went away by itself, and the quack took the credit.

The proponents of bogus treatments capitalize on people's fear of cancer and scare them into believing that the medical establishment frowns on their methods for dishonest reasons. "The doctors don't care if you die," they say, "so long as you pay huge sums for their services." Loving life, wanting to trust someone, and wanting to hope that a cure is possible, victims of cancer easily fall prey to this sort of deception, as do relatives and friends who are willing to try anything to help their loved ones get well.

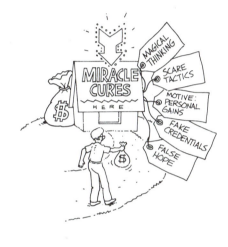

People who are scared and desperate are easy prey for quacks.

■ ≡ Living with Cancer

With respect to cancer treatments, the focus is necessarily on machines, drugs, and techniques that battle a seemingly inhuman tissue. That the tissue is within a living, feeling human being and that the treatments often invade the person's life in intimate ways often go unappreciated. People diagnosed with cancer have to struggle to maintain those areas of wellness that remain open, while dealing with the disease. They have fears to cope with, and their emotions may need to move through the stages of grief before they can take part in their own treatments and recovery. Psychological counseling can be helpful at such times, as can contact with self-help groups such as Cancer Care.*

Some people, of course, face the crisis with courage; they take an active part in treatment and recovery. They are spurred into action, not despair; they cultivate a sense of humor in the midst of fear. Such people maintain strong family bonds and bonds of friendship throughout the illness, and they have that indefinable asset to recovery—the will to live.

*Write to Cancer Care at 1180 6th Ave., New York, NY 10036 or call (212) 302-2400.

> ■ ■ ■ ■ ■ **STRATEGIES:** HELPING A LOVED ONE WITH CANCER
>
> *To help a loved one with cancer:*
>
> 1. Be there. Don't avoid your friend, who needs your presence now more than ever before.
> 2. Touch him. A hug or other physical gesture oftentimes can say more than words.
> 3. Let her talk. Don't avoid the word *cancer.* Ask your friend if she wants to talk about her illness. She may not, but if she does, let her vent her emotions freely.
> 4. Make specific offers of help. Ask if you can mow the grass, clean the house, do the shopping, fix dinner, take care of the children, or do any other task that needs to be done—and then follow through.
> 5. Help the client's family. Your friend's family is suffering, too. Ask family members if you can care for him while they run errands or simply get away for a few hours.
> 6. Recognize her limitations. Involve your friend in as many of your normal activities as possible, but remember that she may tire easily. Don't be offended if she has to cancel an outing or cut a visit short because of pain or fatigue.
> 7. Be positive. No matter what the prognosis, every cancer client needs laughter, hope, and talk of the future.
>
> SOURCE: Adapted from When someone you know has cancer, *University of Texas Lifetime Health Letter,* January 1990, p. 2.

positive imaging a technique used to help achieve the relaxation response; the person imagines achieving positive outcomes to present experiences; also called **guided imaging.**

■ *FACT OR FICTION:* A person's imagination can help the person deal with the pain of cancer. *True.*

A form of positive self-talk, known as **positive imaging,** or **guided imaging,** is useful for people struggling with the pain of cancer. A therapist who teaches positive imaging may tell the person to relax with eyes closed and picture the pain as a mad dog. Then the therapist tells the person to approach the dog, reach out to it tentatively, try to coax it into stopping its snarling and growling, and gradually tame it to the point where it begins to wag its tail and respond in a friendly fashion. Because the dog represents the pain, the client begins to relax when confronted with it, soon befriends it, and learns that it is possible to deal with it. The pain then becomes less of an enemy. Cancer clients who used positive imaging have been shown in some experiments to survive longer than those who did not.[39] The healing effect of the mind on the body is explored further in this chapter's Spotlight.

Family and friends of a person with cancer are also affected by the illness and need to receive, as well as give, support and love. Family and friends can help by taking over chores, filling out insurance forms, and the like. But even more important, they can acknowledge that the person with cancer is the same as before—loved as before, accepted with the diagnosis as much as without. Friends who listen, talk about fears, and continue their friendships can assist the person who must work through many feelings. The disease should be discussed freely, but other topics should be brought in, too; everyday conversation can help lessen the focus on the disease. See this chapter's Strategies for ways you can help a friend or loved one with cancer.

Sometimes cancer is not curable. In that case, the person must accept that death will occur from the disease and, meanwhile, live the remainder of life with cancer. Chapter 16 focused on coming to terms with death.

People who have been cured of cancer may live in fear of its recurrence. The stress of this fear can be enormous. Self-help groups can help people adjust to the fear of cancer's return and provide emotional support.[40] The American Cancer Society can direct you to groups in your area.

≡▶ *People with cancer face extraordinary struggles when coping with the illness. People can maintain strong bonds with others and face the crisis with courage. Family and friends are crucial in providing support and love.*

■≡ The Things That Matter

A young book salesman approached an old farmer who was out plowing in his field to show him a marvelous new book about modern technology in farming. After inspecting the book, the farmer handed it back to the young man and said, "Son, this is a fine book, but I already don't farm half as well as I know how." The point is this: we do not need more new technologies to enjoy better health; we simply must do what we already know how to do.

People may be led by sensationalism to worry about, and try to control, such generally harmless factors as food additives. Those same people may choose to ignore real dangers such as tobacco use, alcohol abuse, overeating, and lack of exercise. When you ask the question "How many deaths each year are related to food additives?" the answer would be "almost none." Compare that with the effects of using tobacco and abusing alcohol, which present the risk factors and causes of the great majority of deaths each year. Choose carefully where you spend your health care energy and money. Some things truly matter—concentrate on them.

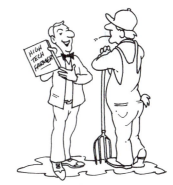

Keep things in perspective.

≡▶ *People are wise to keep the facts about cancer prevention in perspective and concentrate on the things that really matter.*

Chapters 18 and 19 have dealt with the nation's number-one and number-two killers of adults, heart disease and cancer, and have provided a sampling of the many options available for both prevention and cure. Chapter 20 offers perspective on the whole health care system, and shows how consumers can use it to protect their health in many other ways.

■≡ For Review

1. Describe the characteristic course of cancer development and the factors that affect it.

2. Explain the terms *carcinogen* and *promoter*, and name one of each.

3. Delineate the differences between malignant tumors and benign tumors.

4. Describe how cancer spreads.

5. Identify and describe the major risk factors for cancer.

6. List some steps to take to reduce cancer risks.

7. Describe how cancer and genetics are related.

8. Describe the possible role of viruses in cancer development.

9. List cancer's warning signals.

10. Identify and state the usefulness of several home screening tests for cancer.

11. Describe medical or laboratory screening strategies used for early detection of cancer.

12. Name and describe several types of cancer treatments.

■ ≡ Notes

1. F. L. Megskens, Coming of age—The chemoprevention of cancer, *New England Journal of Medicine* 323 (1990): 825–826.

2. U.S. Department of Health and Human Services, National Institutes of Health, *Cancer Prevention,* NIH publication no. 84-2671, 1984.

3. E. Whelan and F. Stare, Alcohol: How does it affect your body? *ACSH Media and Activity Update,* Spring 1981, pp. 8–9.

4. B. J. Druker, H. J. Mamon, and T. M. Roberts, Oncogenes, growth factors, and signal transduction, *New England Journal of Medicine* 321 (1989): 1383–1391.

5. J. C. Bailar and E. M. Smith, Progress against cancer? *New England Journal of Medicine* 314 (1986): 1226–1232.

6. A. Greeleg, No safe tan, *FDA Consumer,* May 1991, pp. 17–21.

7. J. Fuchs and coauthors, Acute effects of near ultraviolet and visible light on the cutaneous antioxidant defense system, *Photochemistry and Photobiology* 50 (1989): 739–744; M. Elesha-Adams and D. M. White, Sun smart: A peer-led lesson on the effects of tanning and sunning on the skin, *Health Education* 21 (1990): 54–55.

8. J. Fuchs and coauthors, Impairment of enzymic and nonenzymic antioxidants in skin by UVB irradiation, *Journal of Investigative Dermatology* 93 (1989): 769–773.

9. NIH panel recommends daily sunscreen use, *FDA Consumer,* October 1989, p. 3.

10. R. A. Lew and coauthors, Sun exposure habits in patients with cutaneous melanoma: A case control study, *Journal of Dermatologic Surgery and Oncology* 9 (1983): 981–986.

11. Indoor tanning, *For Consumers,* September 1988 (a leaflet available from the Federal Trade Commission, Bureau of Consumer Protection, Office of Consumer/Business Education).

12. High-intensity tanning lamps, *FDA Consumer,* June 1985, p. 5.

13. J. M. Seddon and coauthors, Host factors, UV radiation and risk of uveal melanoma, *Archives of Ophthalmology* 108 (1990): 1274–1280; M. K. Memmer, Preventing eye damage from the sun's ultraviolet light: What health educators should teach, *Health Education* 20 (1989): 42–47.

14. NIH panel recommends daily sunscreen use, 1989.

15. R. Bluhm and coauthors, Aplastic anemia associated with canthaxanthin ingested for "tanning" purposes, *Journal of the American Medical Association* 264 (1990): 1141–1142.

16. A. E. Reif, The causes of cancer, *American Scientist,* July/August 1981, pp. 437–447.

17. N. A. Dreyer and E. Friedlander, Identifying the health risks from very low-dose sparsely ionizing radiation, *American Journal of Public Health* 72 (1982): 16–29; N. A. Dreyer and coauthors, *The Feasibility of Epidemiologic Investigations of the Health Effects of Low-Level Ionizing Radiation, Final Report,* U.S. Nuclear Regulatory Commission publication no. NUREG/CR-1728, 1980, p. 33.

18. *Health Quackery: Consumer Union's Report on False Health Claims, Worthless Remedies, and Unproved Therapies* (Mount Vernon, N.Y.: Consumer's Union, 1980), pp. 194–196.

19. U. G. Allinger and coauthors, Shift from a mixed to a lactovegetarian diet: Influence on acidic lipids in fecal water—A potential risk factor for colon cancer, *American Journal of Clinical Nutrition* 50 (1989): 992–996.

20. C. A. Molgaard and coauthors, A public health evaluation of a population-based colorectal cancer education and screening program, *Health Education* 21 (1990): 49–52.

21. R. L. Phillips, Role of life-style and dietary habits in risk of cancer among Seventh Day Adventists, *Cancer Research* 35 (1975): 3513–3522.

22. B. S. Reddy and coauthors, Nutrition and its relationship to cancer, *Advances in Cancer Research* 32 (1980): 238–345; J. L. Werther, Food and cancer, *New York State Journal of Medicine,* August 1980, pp. 1401–1408.

23. Inactivity may increase risk of colon cancer (Newsfront), *Modern Medicine,* February 1985, p. 33.

24. R. F. Gittes, Carcinoma of the prostate, *New England Journal of Medicine* 324 (1991): 236–245.

25. P. S. Houts and coauthors, Using a state cancer registry to increase screening behaviors of sisters and daughters of breast cancer patients, *American Journal of Public Health* 81 (1991): 386–388.

26. D. E. Lilienfeld, The silence: The asbestos industry and early occupational cancer research—A case study, *American Journal of Public Health* 81 (1991): 791–800.

27. M. P. Waalkes, Cadmium and human health, *Health and Environment Digest,* May 1991, pp. 1–3.

28. J. M. Samet and A. V. Nero, Indoor radon and lung cancer, *New England Journal of Medicine* 320 (1989): 591–593.

29. S. J. Ackerman, Modern diagnostics help detect cancers early, *FDA Consumer,* December 1990, pp. 12–15.

30. J. M. Liff and coauthors, Does increased detection account for the rising incidence of breast cancer? *American Journal of Public Health* 81 (1991): 462–465.

31. E. S. King and coauthors, How

valid are mammography self-reports? *American Journal of Public Health* 80 (1990): 1386–1388.

32. M. J. Silverstein and coauthors, Breast cancer diagnosis and prognosis in women augmented with silicone gel-filled implants, *Cancer* 66 (1990): 97–101.

33. E. T. Fossel, J. M. Carr, and J. McDonagh, Detection of malignant tumors: Water-suppressed proton nuclear magnetic resonance spectroscopy of plasma, *New England Journal of Medicine* 315 (1986): 1369–1376.

34. B. A. Mann and coauthors, Changing treatment of breast cancer in New Mexico from 1969 through 1985, *Journal of the American Medical Association* 259 (1988): 3413–3417.

35. B. Fisher, C. Redmond, and E. R. Fisher, Ten-year results of a randomized clinical trial comparing radical mastectomy and total mastectomy with or without radiation, *New England Journal of Medicine* 312 (1985): 674–681.

36. G. T. Wolf and coauthors, Induction chemotherapy plus radiation compared with surgery plus radiation in patients with advanced laryngeal cancer, *New England Journal of Medicine* 324 (1991): 1685–1690.

37. S. A. Rosenberg, Adoptive immunotherapy for cancer, *Scientific American,* May 1990, pp. 62–68.

38. S. A. Rosenberg, Observations on the systemic administration of autologous lymphokine-activated killer cells and recombinant interleukin-2 to patients with metastatic cancer, *New England Journal of Medicine* 313 (1985): 1485–1492.

39. O. C. Simonton, S. Matthews-Simonton, and T. F. Sparks, Psychological intervention in the treatment of cancer, *Psychosomatics* 21 (1980): 226–233.

40. Group therapy aids cancer survival, *Science News* 136 (1989): 302; D. Spiegel and coauthors, Effect of psychosocial treatment on survival of patients with metastatic breast cancer, *Lancet,* 14 October 1989, pp. 888–891.

SPOTLIGHT

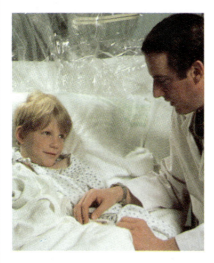

Faith and Healing

A classic story about the mind's power to bring about healing is that of Norman Cousins's bout during the 1970s with a debilitating illness. Cousins, the editor of the famous *Saturday Review* magazine, took a stressful trip overseas and returned home exhausted. A week later, he found himself hardly able to stand up, and he had to go to the hospital.

Didn't he have some sort of miracle recovery?

Yes. At first, he was told that the diagnosis was a degenerative disease of the connective tissue of the spine, almost invariably fatal. His physicians predicted that he would remain an invalid for the rest of his life and that his spine would deteriorate until he was paralyzed. Stress and exhaustion had led to disease, the disease was expected to be totally disabling, the expectation caused further stress, and the end was to be tragic.

Lying in his hospital bed, Cousins considered what he already knew about stress, diseases, and cures. It occurred to him that if negative emotional experiences could harm the body, then positive emotional experiences might restore health. To his way of thinking, the most positive emotional experiences would be "hope, faith, laughter, confidence, and the will to live." Finding the hospital an unpleasant environment, Cousins checked out and moved, with his physician's approval, into a hotel room, where he could be equally well taken care of without so much medicine and illness around. There, he watched comedy films and had funny stories read to him. Having spent weeks with hardly any sleep and being now in acute pain, he made the wonderful discovery that after a hearty laugh, he could relax and sleep soundly for an hour or two at a time. (He also believed in the curative power of vitamin C for diseases of connective tissue and so employed large doses as part of his cure regimen.) The laughter, relaxation, and sleep (and, according to Cousins, the vitamin C) brought about a healing that no amount of medical attention could have achieved. The long of the story is in Cousins's article "Anatomy of an Illness," which was published in the *Saturday Review* and the *New England Journal of Medicine* as a landmark in medical history.[1]* The short of it is that Cousins recovered completely, and was able after some weeks to walk on the beach, to use all of his limbs, to return to work, and to lead a normal life.

*Reference notes are at the end of the Spotlight.

Well, how do you suppose he did it? What accounts for his recovery?

There has been much speculation about that, but most people (including Cousins himself) agree that there was certainly an element of placebo effect. A placebo is an inert, or dummy, substance labeled "medicine," used for its psychological effect. The placebo effect is the healing that occurs in people given such medication. In this case, the vitamin C was the placebo.

How common is the placebo effect?

It is not unusual for experiments using placebos to record benefits in 30 to 60 percent of subjects. That is, people given only distilled water or sugar pills will recover, about half the time, as completely as if they had received a curative medication.

Placebos, given with persuasive encouragement ("This will make you better"), are sometimes so effective that physicians have on occasion prescribed them when they didn't know what else to prescribe. The curious thing is that people will recover, given placebos, when they would not recover without them. In other words, the placebo effect is

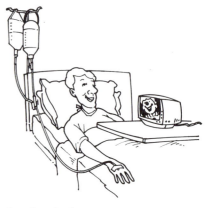

Laughter heals.

valuable; it is an important weapon against illness.

Are you telling me that my physician may give me fake medicine?

No, that would be unethical. But the point is that your response, even to the real drug, may be aided by your faith in the treatment, whether you or your physician know it or not.

We want to warn you, though: quacks will sell you placebos every chance they get. Since 30 to 60 percent of people given anything will recover, there will be plenty of testimonials extolling the virtues of the quack's miracle cures.

How does the placebo effect work?

Recall how the nervous system works. The person is anxious, wonders what might be wrong, feels helpless, and worries so much that symptoms become aggravated. Then the person goes to a famous healer. The healer names the disease, and the person feels reassured: the expert has the answer. The healer then prescribes a treatment, and the person relaxes. Help has replaced helplessness. The stress response diminishes, and symptoms begin to disappear. The placebo actually brings about a measurable physiological response: blood pressure falls, pulse rate slows, and so forth.[2] With resistance restored, the client proceeds to get well, whatever treatment has been prescribed.

So you think the placebo effect works through the relaxation response?

That certainly must be part of it. Research has often illustrated the effect. For example, it had been thought, at various times, that ulcers

were caused by poor circulation to the stomach or intestine, by hot foods, by cold foods, by coarse foods, by spices such as pepper, by alcohol, and by caffeine. People with ulcers were cautioned against all these things. One physician, however, attempted to treat ulcers simply by giving shots of distilled water with the guarantee that they would heal the ulcers. His clients recovered.[3] We now know that the common thread in all such ulcers is anxiety. In such cases, the placebo effect reliably works its magic. Faith heals.

"I have seen a paper with some writing on it, strung round the neck, heal such illness of the whole body, and in a single night. I have seen a fever banished by pronouncing a few ceremonial words."

Plato, 500 B.C.

I see what you mean. I suppose witch doctors, shamans, and all healers work their cures the same way.

Probably so. Don't forget, too, that the body will often heal itself, given time. Frequently, all that healers have to do is to wait out the duration of

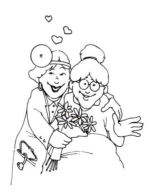

Love heals.

the malady. If they can offer reassurance and confidence, they will be providing support as important as any chemical or physical procedure might be. In fact, health care providers in training are taught not only to manage their clients' medical care, but also to dole out liberal doses of TLC, tender loving care. Children given TLC recover far faster than those deprived of it. They even grow better.[4]

Does the placebo effect work for pain?

Yes. A physician describes a study in which people in pain had to go through some medical procedures. Some people were fully informed in advance; others were deprived of the comfort of knowing what to expect. The informed people needed only half as many pain-killing drugs and were discharged from the hospital an average of two and a half days earlier.[5] This suggests an effect specifically in those nerves that register pain.

Research on exactly how brain and body chemistry interact is only beginning, but some clues have already been collected. They point to natural brain chemicals (endorphins) that relieve stress and pain. People in pain, given placebos, often experience relief of their pain; those given placebos with naloxone, a chemical agent that blocks the brain's production of these natural pain-killers, experience no such relief. This shows that placebos relieve pain by triggering endorphin production.

How powerful can the placebo effect be?

The endorphins are more powerful painkillers than morphine, which has been used for centuries to relieve extreme distress, such as that caused by wounds in war. The endorphins don't necessarily produce a cure; you still need a surgeon to operate on the wound, but mobilizing the body's natural resources speeds healing.

In this connection, some fascinating stories are told about healing in the hospital. Just physically touching people has been documented as hastening healing. Not only do researchers now know it works; they are beginning to find out how and why.[6]

So faith really heals. But I'm skeptical—to say the least—about those faith-healing scenes we sometimes see on television.

Rightly so. Anything as dramatic as faith healing is bound to attract quacks in multitudes. Fraud is most successful when it mimics amazing true events. A viewer should always watch such scenes skeptically and judge each one on its own merits. Just remember, though: the fact that a shyster can try to rip off the public, faking "miracle cures," does not negate the value of the effect of confidence. Faith does heal—or at least it helps enormously—in any situation where stress has contributed to illness.

I see what you mean. I think you've partially explained the healing effect of love, too.

You may be right. Anything that makes people feel cared for helps them to produce their own internal tranquilizers and strengthens their immune systems. As Dr. Francis Weld Peabody, of Harvard University, put it, "The secret of the care of the patient is in caring for the patient."

■ Spotlight Notes

1. N. Cousins, Anatomy of an illness (as perceived by the patient), *New England Journal of Medicine* 295 (1976): 1458–1463. The sequel, which explores further the attitudes of physicians and clients and the importance of the clients' involvement in their own cure, is also stimulating reading: N. Cousins, What I learned from 3,000 doctors, *Saturday Review,* 18 February 1978, pp. 12–16.

2. O. Fennema, The placebo effect of foods, *Food Technology,* December 1984, pp. 37–67.

3. A. M. Gill, Pain and healing of peptic ulcer, *Lancet,* 8 March 1947, p. 291.

4. E. M. Widdowson, Mental contentment and physical growth, *Lancet* 1 (1951): 1316–1318.

5. Dr. Herbert Benson of Beth Israel Hospital and Harvard Medical School, as quoted by B. Sullivan, Placebo effect: Medicine losing a valuable tool, *Miami Herald,* 8 April 1981, p. E1.

6. N. Chesanow, Is it time to take psychic healing seriously? *Family Health,* January 1979, pp. 22, 24, 26, 28.

CHAPTER 20

The Consumer, Health Information, and the Health Care System

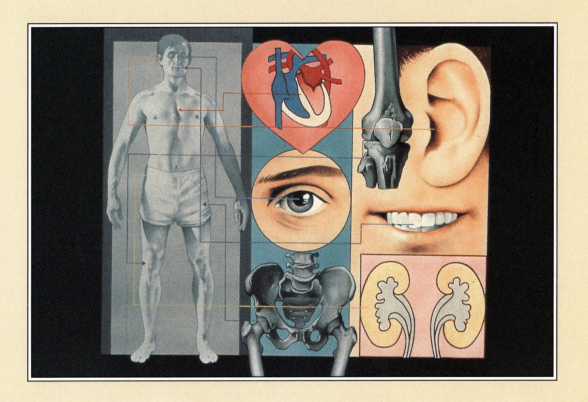

The previous chapters have emphasized personal responsibility for health. They have shown how you can take charge of your lifestyle habits and make choices that will support your well-being. Only a few areas remain to be examined, and they have to do not with your own actions but with your relationship to your environment. This chapter helps develop your skill in evaluating and applying health information, and in using the health care system to serve your needs.

■≡ The Sources of Health Information

First of all, where do you get health information? Not all sources, of course, are equally valid, although they may all claim that their statements are facts. Take, for example, advertisements in which actors, dressed as scientists or physicians, appear on the television screen or on the magazine page and make solemn statements about "research." When you look closely, you find no evidence to back their claims. As a consumer of health information, you need to develop skill in distinguishing between valid and invalid health information.

How to Evaluate Health Claims

When you encounter a claim for a product or service, first ask and find answers to the following questions: Who is making the claim? What are the person's qualifications for making such a claim? What type of education, training, skill, reputation, and credentials does the person have? What is the context of the claim: is it on a billboard, or in a valid scientific publication? How strong is the scientific evidence that backs the claim? (Also ask what language and logic the claim is stated in, as discussed in the Spotlight following this chapter.)

A simple rule governs the evaluation of claims on the basis of who is making them. If the person or organization making the claim stands to profit by selling you something you would not otherwise buy, discount the claim.

It is as simple as that. To get honest, unbiased information on any product or service, find an outside expert who can make an assessment. An example familiar to most people is buying a used car. The salesperson's word alone isn't sufficient, nor is the word of someone who wants to sell you a different car; you need an independent garage mechanic to assess the car. The mechanic has nothing to gain by lying to you, and in fact stands to gain most by telling the truth. As a satisfied customer, you will recommend the mechanic's work to other customers.

If the person making the claim does not appear to be motivated by personal gain, you should still be skeptical. Inspect the person's qualifications for making the claim. A noted poet's words on physical fitness may sound beautiful, but the trainer of Olympic athletes possesses more accurate information. A famed heart surgeon knows hearts, but not sex therapy. The governor of a state is not an authority on nutrition—and so forth.

When an authority makes pronouncements on a topic, ask yourself whether the person is qualified to speak on that particular topic. To do this, focus on five characteristics in sizing up a person's qualifications as an expert. Education is first, and is indispensable; there is no substitute for the hundreds of hours of book learning that provide the foundation for a person to become an authority. Training is another, for book learning must be applied in real-life situations. Skill is a third; it normally develops as the result of practice and time—experience. Fourth comes reputation: a person earns that by developing the first three assets. Finally come the person's credentials—such as membership in professional societies and a license to practice in the profession. This last deserves a moment's attention.

Be careful when evaluating memberships in professional societies, for not all are of high quality. People who belong to legitimate professional societies such as the American Medical Association must meet strict standards for education, training, and skill. Other organizations may have similar names—a society might name itself the National Medical Federation, for example—but may require only payment of membership fees to belong. You can tell which is which by looking them up in the *Encyclopedia of Associations* (ask the librarian).

Besides membership, professional societies impose other controls on quality of practitioners: **certification** and **registration** are examples. Each professional society screens its candidates after completion of their course work and some work experience, by administering an examination. Those candidates who pass are then listed on the society's register of approved practitioners. Many societies require periodic updating of registration, for example, by taking approved course work. When you see the terms *certified nurse practitioner (C.N.P.)*, *certified health education specialist* (CHES), or *registered dietitian (R.D.)*, for example, it means the practitioner has passed the screening test and fulfilled the maintenance requirements of the registering society.

States also impose controls on quality in the form of the **license to practice**. Each state has a health licensing agency, which regulates the practice of health occupations within its borders. Do not visit a health professional who has no license to practice. Of course, in every health care profession you may find fake certifications, registrations, and licenses, so the buyer must still beware—see the Critical Thinking section, Genuine and Fake Credentials. Still, the legitimate titles are workable controls on quality.

certification approval granted by an organization, signifying that an individual is qualified to perform a service according to a certain standard.

registration with respect to health professionals, a listing signifying that the professional has met requirements such as course work, experience, and the passing of an examination, and so may use the title and practice the profession.

license to practice permission under state or federal law to use a certain title (such as medical doctor, osteopath, attorney, etc.) and to offer certain services, obtained by passing a state-administered examination.

bogus fake. There are bogus doctors, bogus professional organizations, bogus accrediting agencies, bogus licenses to practice, bogus certifications, bogus registrations—you name it; it can be bogus.

accreditation approval; in the case of college or university departments, approval by a professional organization qualified to judge the quality of the educational program offered. Professional societies will accept for membership only people who have received their education in accredited programs.

For every valid symbol of legitimacy, there is a counterfeit that copies it.

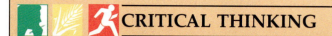

CRITICAL THINKING

Genuine and Fake Credentials

Most degrees listed next to health care practitioners' names are valid degrees that equip people to practice their specialties competently. However, **bogus** degrees complicate the picture. Not everyone who posts a doctor's diploma on the office wall has spent all those years studying and has passed all those examinations. Some organizations, calling themselves colleges or universities, simply sell official-looking diplomas for $50 or $75 by mail. One highly respected health authority exposed a pair of such scams by filling out applications for membership in two "professional societies" using the names of his cat, Charlie, and his dog, Sassafras. His pets were given the memberships without question.

To find out whether a college or university is a genuine educational institution, do some research. It should have an address, some buildings, and a faculty consisting of people with valid degrees and credentials of their own. If you ask to speak to the dean of graduate studies, such a person should exist. A post office box number without a street address is practically a guarantee that the degree-granting institution is a fraud. Also, the university should have **accreditation** from a professional accrediting association—for example, the American Medical Association (AMA) for physicians and the American Psychological Association (APA) for psychologists. But watch out. There are also bogus accrediting agencies and bogus licenses to practice. The rule seems to be that for every valid symbol of legitimacy, there is a counterfeit that copies it. If you can apply to an institution for a degree, a diploma, or a license to practice in the name of your pet poodle—and get it—then you have uncovered a fraud.

Another thing to notice about a health claim is the context. Did you see or hear it in a newspaper or magazine? On the radio, on television, or on a billboard? In a shopping mall? A storefront? Manufacturers make health claims through advertisements and commercials in order to sell products, of course, so you know they provide biased views; you cannot use them to compare competing products or services. Health statements also appear as news, in newspapers and magazines, but these seldom present balanced pictures of whole research areas; they are more likely to present single, new findings, often chosen because they are sensational. Exciting stories help to sell newspapers and magazines, of course, but you cannot use these stories to guide you—they may well be discredited by tomorrow's research.

Some newspapers and popular magazines do make an effort, at times, to review whole research areas accurately and in depth, and when they do this well, they perform a real service for the public. Among those noted for the excellence of their stories are *Time, Newsweek, U.S. News and World Report,* and the *New York Times.* But to be certain you are reading accurate science information, you have to probe further. This book cites newspapers and magazines only when reporting news events, not when reporting scientific facts.

Health statements also appear in books, and these come in several varieties. Some are written to entertain; some to inform; and some, unfortunately, to sell questionable products and services or even to perpetrate outright fraud.

Some time ago, a certain Doctor R, who ran a famous health clinic, published a book that claimed to finally reveal the answers to questions everyone always asks: how to stay young, avoid cancer, recover from heart attacks, become sexually attractive, and become physically fit. The book launched Doctor R on a successful career of radio and television interviews and lectures, and it attracted many people to Doctor R's clinic, where these health wonders were offered. In short, it brought in huge profits to the author.

From these facts alone, you cannot tell whether the book and the health treatment offered at the clinic were based on truth or lies or a mixture of the two. But every consumer should know that the authors of books like this are under no legal obligation to publish true information or safe advice.

The **First Amendment,** which guarantees freedom of the press, makes it possible for people like Doctor R to express whatever views they like, whether sound or unsound or even dangerous. This freedom is a cornerstone of the U.S. Constitution, and it puts the burden on consumers to read books critically and to use their own judgment when evaluating them. The writers of books are ethically obligated to purvey accurate information, but they are not legally obligated to do so; as a result, seeing a statement in the pages of a book is no guarantee that it is a fact.

Books on health written for the public are so unreliable that most professional organizations maintain committees to combat misinformation. A list of organizations that provide reliable scientific information appears in Appendix A; contact them to check out the authenticity of scientific information in a health area. If your question is about a medical book, product, or service, write to the American Medical Association; if it's about an anticancer book, product, or service, write to the American Cancer Society; and so forth. Many of the professional organizations have also banded together to form the National Council Against Health Fraud (NCAHF), which has branches in many states. The NCAHF monitors radio, television, and other advertising; investigates complaints; and maintains a bimonthly newsletter to warn consumers of the latest health scams.*

If books written for the public are so unreliable, what about textbooks? They, too, can contain misinformation, but textbook buyers are likely to reject textbooks that do. This motivates writers and publishers of textbooks to check carefully the validity of the information in them.

Consider, finally, another source of scientific information: the scientific journal (see Figure 20–1 and the accompanying Miniglossary of Research Terms). Scientific findings backed by strong evidence are first published in journals—and not just any journals, either, but *refereed* journals of professional organizations. Such journals accept articles for publication only after experts in the field, called *referees*, have critiqued the work and approved it (a process called *peer review*). Because of this, researchers who believe they

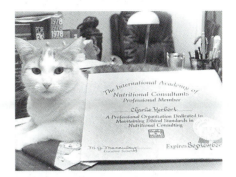

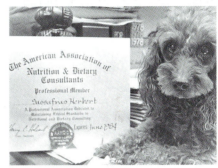

Victor Herbert, M.D., paid money to prove that his pets, Charlie and Sassafras, could obtain fake degrees—he uncovered a fraud.

First Amendment the first amendment to the Constitution of the United States, which guarantees freedom of the press, even the freedom to publish misinformation.

■ *FACT OR FICTION:* An author who makes a statement about health in a published book has a legal obligation to tell the truth. *False.* Authors who write health information for publications are ethically, but not legally, obligated to tell the truth. The First Amendment to the U.S. Constitution protects the right of people to publish health misinformation.

*You can write to the NCAHF at P.O. Box 1276, Loma Linda, CA 92354.

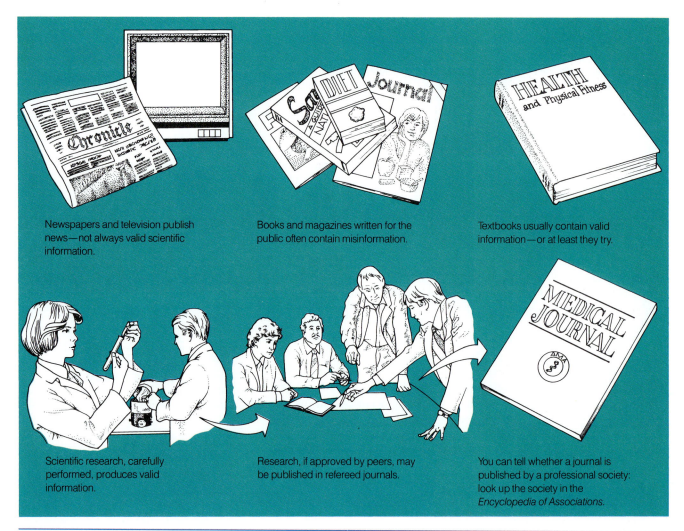

Newspapers and television publish news—not always valid scientific information.

Books and magazines written for the public often contain misinformation.

Textbooks usually contain valid information—or at least they try.

Scientific research, carefully performed, produces valid information.

Research, if approved by peers, may be published in refereed journals.

You can tell whether a journal is published by a professional society: look up the society in the *Encyclopedia of Associations*.

FIGURE 20–1   ■   **Sources of health information.**

have discovered new, important information attempt to publish it in refereed journals; this will promote acceptance of their work by the scientific community and will enhance the authors' reputations.

Why should the consumer (you, for example) even be bothered to know that scientific journals exist and are managed this way? Not because you should feel compelled to read them; a single glance at the shelves upon shelves of volumes in a single research area is enough to intimidate even the most information-hungry soul. But you do need to know that they exist, as a standard of comparison against which to measure reports of scientific findings or claims made by people attempting to sell health products and services. A portion of the table of contents of an issue of the *New England Journal of Medicine* is shown in Figure 20–2, to give you some idea of its seriousness.

Even experiments reported in peer-reviewed journals do not tell "the whole truth" about a health claim. Scientists who report their findings from scientific experiments are simply telling what they did, how they did it, and

The New England Journal of Medicine

Established in 1812 as The NEW ENGLAND JOURNAL OF MEDICINE AND SURGERY

Abstracts in the advertising sections

VOLUME 325   OCTOBER 10, 1991   NUMBER 15

THE NEW ENGLAND JOURNAL OF MEDICINE (ISSN 0028-4793) is published weekly from editorial offices at 10 Shattuck Street, Boston, MA 02115-6094. Subscription price: $89.00 per year. Second-class postage paid at Boston and at additional mailing offices. POSTMASTER: Send address changes to P.O. Box 803, Waltham, MA 02254-0803.

FIGURE 20–2 ■ **A portion of the table of contents of a scientific journal.**

This is a reliable source of health information.

what they found, but this adds only one piece to many others. To get the total picture, you must look at many experiments on the same topic.

A shortcut for those who wish to look at the total picture is reviews of the scientific literature (see the Miniglossary again). Reviews compile the critical points from many single reports and present an overview of what is known on a subject. For an even broader picture, you can gather all such sources on a given topic by turning to indexes in the library, where the names of many such reviews are listed together.

blind (experiment) an experiment in which the subjects do not know whether they are members of the experimental or the control group. (A *double-blind* experiment is one in which the investigators also do not know which subjects are which, until after the experiment is over. It is a good idea to perform such experiments using a *crossover* design; that is, to switch the groups and show that the effect shifts with the treatment.)

control group a group of individuals similar in all possible respects to the group being treated in an experiment.

correlation the simultaneous occurrence of two things. Correlational evidence in science is similar to circumstantial evidence in court; it proves that two things are associated, but not that one is the cause of the other.

index with reference to scientific information, a volume in the library that lists all the research in a given area, by topic, so that readers can locate the original experiments.

peer review review of a proposed publication by two or more of the author's peers, a process used by scientific journals to guarantee the accuracy of what they publish.

randomization a process of assigning members to experimental and control groups in a random fashion.

refereed journal the journal of a reputable scientific society, which publishes reports of scientific findings only after peer review and approval.

review with respect to scientific information, a publication that reviews and critiques the scientific work done on a subject.

scientific journal a publication that contains reports of scientific experiments.

A review article lists its references so that you can look them up and verify that they say what the reviewer says they say. You cannot assume, though, that all reports that list their references are accurate. Many a popular book contains long lists of scientific-looking references, and their names may be familiar. Yet the particular articles listed may not be accurately quoted or interpreted, or may not be in the references at all. And of course, if an article does not cite its sources, you cannot even check them; the article may contain correct information, but it may not. This book's references are cited at the ends of its chapters, and the original sources are obtainable through libraries.

The ways of sizing up health authorities and their claims are summed up in Table 20–1. The next section describes how to recognize the research from which valid health claims come.

≡▶   *To evaluate a health claim, look critically and skeptically at the person making it. Check the person's motives and qualifications, and examine the publication in which the claim is made.*

How to Recognize Scientific Health Research

Sometimes a claim made in the news or in a book is backed by descriptions of the experiments that led to it. Just what does the evidence from an experiment show? If, in a country where it snows, most people die of heart disease, does that prove that snow causes heart disease? This is a silly question, of course, but when the claim being made sounds plausible, it's harder to see through. The general rule is that a correlation is not a cause. When a correlation between two events has been shown, even many times, it suggests, but does not prove, that the two are causally related.

Another kind of evidence gleaned from scientific studies is that available from experiments using animals as subjects. Animals are useful experimental subjects: large groups can be tested under controlled environmental conditions; they can all start with the same hereditary endowment; and one test substance or routine can be tried at a time. If a scientist exposes one of two identical groups of animals to a treatment and demonstrates a difference in outcome between the two groups, that scientist has gathered persuasive

---

TABLE 20–1   ■   **Evaluating Health Claims**

To evaluate health claims:
1. Ask who is making the claim. Does that person stand to gain from your believing it?
2. Ask about the person's education, training, skill, and reputation.
3. Ask about the person's credentials: membership in legitimate professional societies, registration or certification, and license to practice.
4. Ask where the claim is published: newspaper, magazine, book written for the public, textbook, journal?
5. Consult the professional society concerned with the subject matter in question.
6. Write to the National Council Against Health Fraud.
7. The ultimate test: ask whether the claim is derived from research published in the refereed journals of reputable scientific organizations.
8. Look at and verify the list of references.

evidence that the treatment caused the outcome. If removal of the treatment reverses the outcome, that is still more persuasive. In addition, if the two groups can be switched (in a so-called *crossover* experiment) and the outcome follows the treatment across groups, that is often taken as virtual proof.

Before you can be confident that a conclusion is valid, you have to know much more. An experiment is not valid if the *experimental* group of subjects is not matched by a correctly chosen *control* group. The choice of which members to assign to which group must be made randomly. If one group is given pills of an experimental medicine, the other must receive identical, but inert, pills (placebos) on the same schedule, and both groups must be kept in ignorance of which they are getting (blind). Those who score the results must also not know which subjects are which, so as to avoid introducing bias into the judgments made. These and other factors relating to research on health questions are explained in the Miniglossary of Research Terms.

An inspection of the basic characteristics of a sound research experiment will show how great a contrast there is between findings generated with such care and the rumors people trade informally about health products: "I just took those pills and I felt better immediately." "She went to Madame R's salon and came back 10 pounds thinner; it must be the cream they rubbed on her skin." Such is the stuff of popular health fads, and it bears no resemblance to research. A person who tries the pills or the cream based on such "evidence" does so at considerable risk.

In contrast to claims backed by published scientific evidence gathered by experiment is another class of claims—those backed not by evidence but by logic. These can be remarkably persuasive, and it is hard to resist them. They begin with a statement or two that are true and then draw a perfectly plausible conclusion. For example, everyone knows that car parts wear out the more they are used. Logic might apply the same generalization to the parts of the human body: to save them, use them as little as possible. The flaw in this logic, of course, is that most body parts respond to use by becoming stronger and better able to do their jobs, not worn out. The way to determine what is good for people's health is not just to reason it out, but to do experiments and find out for sure. Logic and reasoning can suggest experiments to do—and the more scientific knowledge they are based on, the better—but logic and reasoning alone can never produce new scientific facts.

To identify scientifically derived information accurately, it helps to be able to recognize its opposite—health fraud or quackery. This chapter's Spotlight offers many examples of such misinformation and deceit. Now, how do you put health facts to work in your own life?

≡▶ *To recognize scientific health research, don't be fooled by correlational evidence; it isn't proof of cause. Distinguish research from rumors, and distinguish between logic and evidence.*

■≡ The Health Care System

The health care system is a big system, consisting of big businesses and big suppliers. It is designed to help people, but sometimes it harms them, for

LIFE CHOICE INVENTORY

How well do you know and use the health care system? For each yes answer, give yourself 1 point:

1. Do you take responsibility for your own health insurance? (Someone else may pay for it, but did you obtain your own policies, and are you acquainted with their contents?)
2. Are you familiar with the five types of health insurance you may need? (Can you name them?)
3. Do you know what breaks you can obtain on health/medical insurance, based on your lifestyle choices?
4. Have you ever compared a health maintenance organization (HMO) with the traditional medical care system? (Could you explain to someone else what an HMO is?)
5. Given the choice, when you need prompt medical treatment, do you work out a way to go to a clinic or health care practitioner's office, rather than to the hospital emergency room?
6. Before paying a bill for medical care, do you (or would you) check it to make sure that you received all the services it lists?
7. Should you move to a new location, would you know how to go about selecting a health care practitioner (personal physician or other)? (Can you name several steps you would take to find the appropriate one?)
8. Do you know what is reasonable to expect during a general physical checkup? (Can you identify the steps the health practitioner should take in examining you?)
9. If you meet a "doctor," do you keep in mind that the person may not be an M.D.? (Can you name several other possibilities?)
10. Can you spot a quack? (Extra credit: give yourself an extra point if you have ever reported quackery to a regulating agency.)

Scoring: 9 or more: You are a skilled consumer of health care services.

7 or 8: You know the system fairly well, but have a little more to learn.

5 or 6: Your skill at using the health care system needs improvement.

4 or less: You don't use the health care system well; in fact, you may be losing out in significant ways.

---

many of its transactions are governed by the motives of profit, power, and prestige. This section offers the information you need to use the health care system to best support your health. The Life Choice Inventory can help you discover how much you already know about the system and how skilled you are in using it.

Let us suppose you are going to have three problems this year, all currently unknown to you. For one thing, you are going to get a severe sore throat, which, unless promptly treated, will develop into a major, whole-body infection. Second, you are going to break your arm. And third, you are developing a heart condition (even though you may be as young as 18), although you will not have any noticeable symptoms for 15 years.

Now consider three different scenarios. The first is the simplest: you have no insurance, no personal health care provider, and no health care plan. When the sore throat strikes, you try to live with it until you are so ill that you have to go to the hospital emergency room. There, you have to pay $100 in advance to be seen; you are given a lab test and some medicine for another $100; and you are dismissed. You are still so sick that you lose a week of classes or work. When you break your arm, you again rush to the hospital only to find that they will not even set your broken arm in a cast until you have again paid in advance—this time, $1,000. Total cost of treatment for the year: $1,200, a week of missed classes or work, and failure to detect your advancing heart condition.

In the second scenario you have insurance, so your experience is slightly different. You might pay, say, $100 a month for coverage as an individual. When you went to the hospital on your two trips, you might be admitted without question, and afterward, you might find that the insurance company paid the bills. (If you had to pay the bills at first, you would soon receive reimbursement.) Total cost to you: still $1,200 for the year, but in 12 equal installments of $100 rather than in two surprise lump sums; still a week of missed classes or work; and still, no detection of your heart condition.

Now suppose you have your own personal health care provider, who not only treats but also tries to prevent illness. When your sore throat develops, you telephone this person's office and are seen immediately; prompt treatment spares you the loss of a week's classes or work days. When you break your arm, you still go to the hospital emergency room, and you pay $1,000, as before. Your health care provider gives you a routine physical examination this year, detects the threat of heart trouble, and instructs you to alter your diet and physical activity, so as to postpone the onset and reduce the severity of your heart condition, years later. Your insurance does not cover your general physical examination, so you are out $100 for that—but with health benefits to come in the distant future that outweigh the price paid now. Insurance does pay for the sore throat treatment and for the arm, so your costs are $1,200 for insurance, $100 for the general physical exam, and no loss of a productive week.

As a student, you may have an option similar to this but less expensive: the student health center. For nonstudents, another less-expensive option, at least for the sore throat, is the community public health center. To decide what combination of options will work best for you, you will have to work out answers to the following questions:

1. What kind(s) of insurance do I need, if any?
2. What hospitals are available near me? Which will be best for me?
3. Should I consider joining a health maintenance organization (HMO)? Are other alternatives available?
4. Should I have a personal health care provider? Should this person be a physician (M.D.)? What are the alternatives?

The sections that follow contain information to help you assess your own needs.

Insurance

"I'm sorry, but your insurance policy doesn't cover this. Pay in advance, please." You can avoid the pain of being confronted with this situation, but only if you use considerable know-how in shopping for your health insurance. The suggestions in the margin sum up what is involved.

When buying insurance, think of all the health care costs you will want to cover: accidents, hospitalization, surgery, physician services, medicines, and disabilities. Different kinds of health insurance cover each of these—see the Miniglossary of Health Insurance Types. Accident treatment, hospital costs, and costs of surgery may be combined into single policies, but when

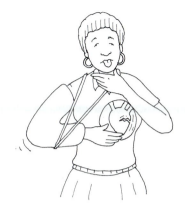

Suppose you are going to have three things happen to you this year.

When purchasing insurance:

1. Be sure to cover these five areas:
   Hospitalization.
   Surgical.
   Medical.
   Major medical.
   Disability.
2. Read each policy to be sure it meets your needs. What is the deductible? (How much must I pay before the company will begin to assist payment?) Does it cover:
   In-hospital and outpatient costs?
   Diagnostic tests?
   Second opinions?
   Medicines?
   Prevention?
   Education?
   Ambulance service?
   Psychological counseling?
3. Use your healthful lifestyle habits to obtain reduced insurance rates.

accident insurance insurance for expenses incurred due to accidents; often duplicates other policies and need not be purchased separately.

disability insurance insurance to replace lost income if a person should suffer a long illness.

hospitalization insurance insurance to pay the cost of a hospital stay. See also *Medicare, Medicaid.*

major medical insurance insurance to pay extraordinarily high bills not covered by other insurance.

medical insurance insurance to pay physicians' fees, lab fees, and fees for prescription medications.

Medicaid hospitalization and medical insurance available for people who qualify as needy, funded by federal and state tax dollars.

Medicare hospitalization and medical insurance for people who are entitled to Social Security, funded by federal tax dollars.

surgical insurance insurance to pay the surgeon's fees. See also *Medicaid.*

■ *FACT OR FICTION:* If you have medical and surgical insurance, you are probably covered for most medical expenses you might incur. *False.* You may need as many as five different kinds of insurance to be adequately covered against medical expenses; even then, long-term care might well not be covered.

malpractice insurance a type of insurance that can be carried by any person offering a service or selling a product. If the person is sued by someone claiming to have been harmed by the service or product, it pays all or part of the fines awarded by the court.

you shop for insurance, be sure your policies cover them all, or that you have *intentionally* left out one or more. In each area, policies differ; read them with attention to your particular needs. For example, if you are planning to start a family soon, be sure your insurance covers the cost of prenatal care, delivery, and newborn care—and be aware that if you are already pregnant when you buy the policy, the costs of your current pregnancy will not be covered.

If your lifestyle compares favorably with that of other buyers, you may be able to obtain reduced insurance rates. Some policies offer reduced rates for nonsmokers (or people who can prove they have quit), some favor people of normal weight, some consider nonuse of alcohol to be worth a reduction in rates, and some even offer discounts to people who exercise regularly. In the future, the reverse may also be true; insurance companies may charge extra on premiums for people who are obese, who smoke, who fail to exercise, who use alcohol, who don't wear safety belts, and whose blood cholesterol and blood pressure are high.[1]*

Other types of health insurance that apply to special groups are Medicare and Medicaid. Medicare provides coverage for senior citizens who are entitled to Social Security benefits. Medicaid provides coverage for those who receive public assistance (welfare) and for others who are identified as financially needy. This type of health insurance is funded by federal and state tax dollars.

Insurance has saved the financial skins of millions of individuals who have faced unexpected medical costs, but no matter how much insurance you have, you cannot be sure of covering every eventuality, particularly in the later years, when long-term care may be needed. Increasing numbers of families today are finding themselves in a nightmare of limited options when they discover that extended care facilities are not covered by Medicare or conventional health insurance policies. Many people think Medicare includes nursing home care, but it does not. Nursing homes can cost tens of thousands of dollars a year, up to $60,000 and higher. Medicare pays less than half, and it may not pay at all, unless the person is receiving specific types of medical care. Clients and their families pay most of the costs, so insurance is not a substitute for careful financial planning.[2]

Insurance is imperfect in another way: it can be abused. The chief insurance abuse contributing to the high cost of medical care today is the abuse of **malpractice insurance.** Malpractice insurance is not for you; it is for physicians or other health care providers. If you sue a provider for negligence, ignorance, or error, and you win, the insurance will pay you. Unfortunately, unscrupulous people and their attorneys exploit malpractice insurance, sometimes winning awards from the courts undeservedly. Each time a client wins a suit, the client's lawyer draws a third to half of the award as the fee—so attorneys are powerfully motivated to encourage clients to sue.[3] Although only a few physicians are unethical or incompetent, all feel compelled to protect themselves with insurance against such lawsuits. And because malpractice awards can be extraordinarily high, some exceeding a million dollars, the premiums are high, too: they can amount to as much as a third of a physician's annual income. This forces physicians and hospitals to raise their fees, and the person who ends up paying is you, the consumer.

*Reference notes are at the end of the chapter.

Not all nations' health care systems operate as the U.S. system does, with a massive, complex, and competitive insurance industry as its main financial provider. For example, Canada has a national program of hospital and medical care insurance that is standardized and covers more than 99 percent of its citizens.[4] Germany has controlled medical care cost increases much more successfully than has the United States.[5] Improvements have been proposed for the United States as well, which has been accused of having no national health program or policy.[6] But the medical, insurance, and attorneys' lobbies have successfully opposed changes that would reduce their power and profits.

■▶ *Insurance is available to cover accidents, hospitalization, surgery, health care provider services, medicines, and disabilities, but it does not cover everything, and it is no substitute for careful financial planning.*

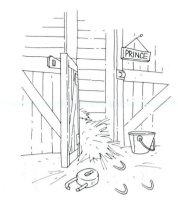

This is not the time to discover that you do not have insurance.

How to Use Hospitals and Other Facilities

Each hospital has its own strengths and weaknesses, including specialties in emergency treatment. The Miniglossary of Hospitals and Related Facilities defines the major types. The better you know what is available to you ahead of time, the better you can choose which one to go to in time of need (see Table 20–2).

Several strategies can help you save money and needless struggles. If at all possible, make appointments to see health care practitioners during office hours—do not go to a hospital emergency room. If you need special tests or surgery, ask to schedule them in the health care practitioner's office. Before submitting to extensive tests or surgery, though, get a second opinion. Some operations, especially **tonsillectomies** and **hysterectomies,** are overperformed—that is, often recommended when they are not necessary. (So are cesarean sections, as described in the Spotlight following Chapter 14.) Insurance covers the price of obtaining second opinions for some operations; if the two opinions differ, consider getting a third, even if you have to pay for it yourself.

tonsillectomy removal of the tonsils (in the throat), an operation sometimes performed unnecessarily.

hysterectomy removal of the uterus, an operation performed more often than necessary.

TABLE 20–2 ■ **Selecting and Using Medical Care Facilities**

When selecting and using medical care facilities:
1. Know what facilities are available and what their specialties are.
2. Avoid emergency room visits.
3. Get a second opinion.
4. Consider alternatives to hospital tests and surgery.
5. Use the hospital on weekdays in preference to weekends.
6. Discover each facility's policy on payment.
7. Find out the physician's and hospital's ways of handling insurance claims. Get help filing for insurance, if available.
8. Protest if the bill is in error.
9. When choosing a place to live, consider the availability of hospital care.
10. Be sure the hospital you choose will take you as a client.
11. Be willing to go out of state, if necessary, for specialized medical care.

■ MINIGLOSSARY
of Hospitals and Related Facilities

birthing center   a center where people can give birth in a homelike atmosphere with the family in attendance.

convalescent home   a center where people can recover from illness or surgery, similar to a hospital but without intensive care, surgical, and emergency treatment facilities.

extended care center   a center for the care of the chronically ill, similar to a convalescent home, but with more medical and nursing services.

government hospital   a hospital run by the federal or local government, for example, a Veterans Administration—that is, VA—hospital.

health center   a center to serve the routine health care needs of a special group.

nursing home   a center for the care of the elderly who can no longer live independently. Essentially a residential, not a medical, facility. See also *extended care center*.

private (also called proprietary) hospital   a hospital run by individuals for profit.

teaching hospital   a hospital that serves a medical and/or nursing school as a place where students can learn their professions.

trauma center   a center for the care of complicated and extreme emergency cases.

voluntary hospital   a nonprofit hospital run by a community for the benefit of its own citizens.

walk-in emergency center   a center for emergency care, similar to the emergency room of a hospital, but operated as a separate institution. Some emergency centers may also be trauma centers.

walk-in surgery center (also called one-day surgery center)   a facility that performs surgery that doesn't require overnight care.

women's health center   a health center that focuses on the routine health care of women and, sometimes, their infants and children.

If you have to go to the emergency room, here are a few hints to make your visit easier:

■ Have only one person go with you, not the whole family.
■ Have identification and your insurance card with you.
■ Tell the person at the admissions desk if you have been there before; if you have, they can use your file and ask you fewer questions.
■ Always wear your ID bracelet or carry a card to alert health professionals to any chronic condition you may have, such as diabetes.
■ Know your own medical history and what medicines you are taking. Carry a short record with you, if your memory is not reliable.

If you need special tests or surgery, you still have choices to make. For simple surgery, you can use a walk-in center rather than the large, general hospital; that way, you will not have to pay for an overnight stay. For surgery requiring hospitalization, schedule your tests before you go in. Check into the hospital on a weekday and check out before the weekend, if possible: the weekdays are when the work gets done. If you need a vacation, you can go to a fine hotel for less than the cost of a hospital room.

Many hospitals must give some care to people who cannot afford to pay. Look for the sign "Notice—Medical Care for Those Who Cannot Afford to Pay" in the admissions area.* Hospitals that serve as teaching facilities where medical and nursing school students can learn their professions often are required to take all clients in return for the federal money that supports their programs.

As a hospital client, you have certain rights. You are entitled to considerate care, privacy, confidentiality, accurate information about your diagnosis and treatment, and continuity of care; furthermore, you have the right to refuse treatment. You are also entitled to an explanation of your bill.

About payment: the time when you receive your bill is not the time to discover that you do not have adequate insurance coverage. *Before* the need arises, check your insurance policies—today, for example. When you are scheduling an operation or other treatment, ask in the physician's office whether your insurance will cover it and what help will be available in filing your claim. Many hospitals and physicians' offices expect you to pay the bill immediately, then file a claim to get your insurance company to reimburse you. Some will help you file the claim; some will do it for you. Other hospitals and physicians' offices will *not* require you to pay, but will collect directly from your insurance company and then bill you (sometimes weeks or months later) for the portion not covered.

Up to 90 percent of hospital bills contain errors.[7] Read through your bills to verify that you did receive all the services for which you are being asked to pay. If you question the accuracy of a bill, ask for an itemized list of services rendered, and send it to your insurance company with an *unsigned* claim form. If the insurance company agrees that the charges are too high, it may be possible to get them reduced. As a last resort, appeal to the peer review committee or grievance committee of the local medical society.

---

*Ask for an application and for a copy of the "Individual Notice." After you have turned in the application, the hospital must inform you, within two working days, if you are eligible for free care. If you can't get a copy of your determination of eligibility, complain to your Department of Health and Human Services (DHHS) regional office. U.S. Department of Health and Human Services, Public Health Service, *Free Hospital Care* (leaflet), HHS publication no. (HRA) 80-14520, August 1980.

The hospital system can be highly successful in treating illness. No drama surpasses the swift sequence of events of a medical emergency beginning with rushed transit in an ambulance and ending with cure and dismissal. Such dramas are played out daily in the world's great medical centers, but they don't always end so happily. At every step are obstacles to the client's receiving the needed care.

The problems are many. One is supply: there are not enough care facilities or health professionals to serve the population. Another is distribution: especially in rural areas, people may find themselves far from needed services. Sometimes it is hard to find the exact services needed, and it is possible to be turned away for lack of funds, even in an emergency (people have died after being turned away from a hospital emergency room because they could not pay for their care). Still another problem is quality control: although the medical profession attempts to police itself, mistakes, incompetence, and even dishonesty occur.

Another problem is cost—which is high and rapidly growing higher, not only because of inflation. Besides malpractice insurance, already mentioned, factors that contribute to the spiraling cost of health care include the high cost of hospital technology; the self-serving decisions of some medical providers; and the **fee-for-service system,** which rewards health care practitioners for each service they perform, tempting them to perform unneeded services.

The problems of supply and distribution of health care practitioners and health services may respond best to alternative approaches: institutions other than hospitals, personnel other than physicians. An example is the community clinic, staffed by people trained in particular aspects of health care—such as nurse practitioners trained to deliver women's health care and well-baby care, or nurse midwives trained to supervise normal births. Another example is the **health maintenance organization (HMO),** which charges a flat monthly fee to its members, regardless of what services they require (a **prepayment system,** in contrast to the fee-for-service system.)

The HMO consists of a group of health care providers (physicians and associated staff) who are still associated with a hospital, but with a difference. The HMO offers comprehensive health care, including out-of-hospital and in-hospital services. It also offers preventive health services, which it emphasizes more strongly than traditional hospitals do. The HMO's prepayment system enables people to budget in advance for their medical costs and reduces the need for some kinds of insurance, although major medical coverage is sometimes still necessary. It also encourages people to come in for preventive health services—such as checkups and advice—because they don't have to pay extra for them. Table 20–3 compares the HMO system with the traditional medical system.

HMOs are one form of response to consumer needs that have not been satisfactorily met by the traditional hospital system. Many variations on the types described here exist; others will doubtless evolve in the future.

As for quality control, some elements of the health care system are intended to deal with that, and they do so with some success. The American Hospital Association has an accreditation board that approves hospitals that qualify. Accreditation is a seal of approval that indicates to you, the consumer, that a hospital has met certain standards for health care. Think twice before choosing one that has not.

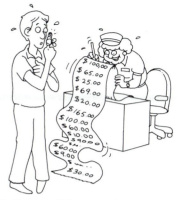

Verify that you did receive all the services listed on your bill.

■ *FACT OR FICTION:* If a person arrives at the hospital bleeding to death, the hospital has to provide emergency treatment. *False.* Hospitals can turn away people who can't afford to pay, even if they need emergency treatment.

fee-for-service system   the system of payments for medical care that charges a fee for each service.

health maintenance organization (HMO)   a group practice organization based on a prepayment system.

prepayment system   the system of payments for medical care that charges a fixed monthly fee regardless of the services provided in a given month.

■ *FACT OR FICTION:* HMO stands for home medical operation—minor surgery that people can perform for themselves. *False.* HMO stands for health maintenance organization. People should not perform surgery on themselves!

TABLE 20–3 ■ Comparison of HMO and Traditional Medical Care

Characteristic	HMO Care	Traditional Care
Philosophic emphasis	Preventive care	Sickness care
Mode of payment	Partial or complete prepayment by group insurance; occasional small fees per visit[a]	Fee for service (can be reimbursed by individual's insurance if applicable)
Provision for out-of-town care	Visit to an out-of-town physician or facility as approved by HMO; reimbursement by HMO	Visit to an out-of-town physician or facility at consumer's discretion; reimbursement by insurance
Needs covered	"One stop": emergency, out-of-hospital care, preventive services,[b] home visits,[c] lab, pharmacy	Many stops: each service provided by a different supplier or facility
Client referral	Initial visit between client and intake specialist; referral to appropriate physician; alternatively, same as in traditional care system	Management of client care by one personal physician; referral to others only for special treatment as needed

[a]Alternatively, in some instances, services are paid by members' insurance companies.

[b]Preventive services include regular checkups; screening and immunization programs; counseling and classes to help people control their blood pressure and weight, develop personalized exercise and diet regimens, plan their families, stop smoking, and learn first aid and safety; and others.

[c]Some HMOs also offer a limited number of mental health visits; service in intermediate and long-term care facilities; service in vision, dental, and more extensive mental health facilities; fertility and family planning services; and rehabilitation therapy.

SOURCE: *HMO—Is It for You?* a booklet available from Metropolitan Life Insurance Company.

≡▶   *To use health care facilities to your advantage, compare those available, choose the ones that will serve you best, and assert your rights to appropriate treatments and reasonable costs. Problems in the health care system include high costs, limited supply, poor distribution, and uneven quality.*

■≡ Health Care Providers: Physicians and Others

Among professional health care providers, important distinctions exist. A person who gets sick usually will think in terms of "going to the doctor"— but what is a doctor? Anyone can adopt the title doctor, but not all are trained the same way, and not all offer beneficial services. The next two sections are devoted to medical professionals—first, the legitimate ones; then, some who may not be legitimate.

The Health Care Provider

The health care provider most people think of when they think of medical care is the medical doctor, or M.D. (this book refers to such a person as the *physician*, except in anecdotes). This is as it should be, for medical school training equips the M.D. to handle many kinds of medical problems.

A physician pursues a long course of education to obtain the M.D. degree and the license to practice medicine. Another type of health care provider, the osteopath (D.O.), takes the same course of training as an M.D., but in a school of osteopathy, which specializes in disorders of the musculoskeletal system. People with D.O. degrees can take the same examination given to

■ MINIGLOSSARY
of Autonomous Health Professionals

autonomous health professional a person authorized to offer a health service without supervision.

dietitian a person trained in diet planning. A *registered dietitian (R.D.)* is a dietitian who has graduated from a state-approved program of dietetics, has passed the professional American Dietetic Association registration examination, and has served in an internship program to practice the necessary skills. Some states require licensing for dietitians; others do not.

medical doctor (M.D.) a *physician*; a person trained to provide medical care and licensed by the state to practice.

nurse a general term for any person who provides health care. A *registered nurse (R.N.)* is a nurse who has graduated from a state-approved school of nursing, has passed the professional nursing state board examination, and has been granted a license to practice within a given state.

nurse practitioner (N.P.) a registered nurse (R.N.) who has received additional medical training to assess the physical and psychosocial status of individuals and families and can manage some of the common illnesses of people in a colleague relationship with a physician. Look for the credential of a *registered nurse practitioner* (R.N.P.), meaning someone who has passed the required state examinations in this specialty area.

osteopath (D.O.) a health care provider who takes the same course of training as a physician, but in a school of osteopathy, which specializes in disorders of the musculoskeletal system.

physician see *medical doctor (M.D.)*; *osteopath (D.O.)*.

physician's assistant (P.A.) a person with medical training, authorized to perform medical services under the supervision of a physician (and therefore, strictly speaking, a semiautonomous health professional). Training includes two to four years of college and two years of specialized training. In some states, physician supervision can be by telephone, and in some, P.A.'s can prescribe certain drugs.

registered dietitian see *dietitian*.

registered nurse see *nurse*.

medical doctors and, on passing it, receive a license to practice medicine and surgery in all states. They may be granted staff privileges, internships, and residencies in accredited hospitals, and so in many ways they are equivalent to physicians.

Following four years of college, the person seeking to become a physician attends medical school, a three-year program. This is followed by a two-year internship and a one-year residency. Then the person is required to pass a state examination to receive a license to practice. Even more schooling is necessary to become a specialist.

A physician is an autonomous health professional—that is, a person who is licensed to provide medical care under his or her own authority. Other such professionals are the nurse practitioner (N.P. or R.N.P.) and the physician's assistant (P.A.). These people have received considerable medical school training and are equipped to handle all routine medical problems—but they consult physicians when necessary. The Miniglossary of Autonomous Health Professionals lists these and other legitimate health care providers, describes their qualifications, and offers details of what they are empowered to do.

How do you go about choosing a health care provider? For many ordinary health concerns, of course, you can provide your own care, but for some, you should at least see the staff at a health center. (The Spotlight following Chapter 1 itemizes the elements of care you might want to learn to provide for yourself.) And for continuity of care, you may want to have a personal health care provider. This person will learn your medical history and will be able to refer you to others whom you may need to see—for example, a gynecologist for women's special problems, an obstetrician for care through pregnancy and childbirth, a pediatrician for the medical care of your children. For some periods in your life, you may visit only the one person periodically; for other periods, you may be in frequent contact with several specialists.

A reasonable first step in selecting a health care provider is to call the county medical society—or simply to ask friends whom they recommend. Then, check the recommended providers' credentials: look for the degrees mentioned in this chapter's Miniglossaries, and find out what you can about the reputations of the institutions where they obtained their degrees.* For physicians, look in the *AMA Directory* or *Directory of Medical Specialists* in the local public library.

Once you have found a qualified health care provider, call the person's office, and ask the questions listed in Strategies: Choosing a Health Care Provider, which follow. On your first appointment, you can gather your own impressions of the person and staff. Most people want a health care provider who listens. If the health care provider and staff willingly furnish all of the information you are requesting, the match may be a good one. It is a good idea, especially if you are easily intimidated or hurried, to write things down before and during your appointment. Beforehand, write out your questions for your own reference, and your observations and thoughts on your condition. Give your notes and questions to the person at examination time, and then write down the answers you receive as the interview takes place.

Expect a thorough **history**—that is, a question-and-answer session about your past medical experiences. How well you communicate with the person in this session is of great importance. The history provides about 70 percent of the information needed for an accurate diagnosis; time spent communicating will likely save money on medical costs later.[8] A truly well-informed health care provider will ask you about your exposure to occupational and environmental threats to health, use of safety belts, eating and exercise habits, sexual history, and stress management and coping skills, as well as many other questions.

Also expect a thorough **physical examination,** head to toe. The person who gives you a once-over-lightly is not starting by getting to know your physical condition well enough to be able, later, to detect symptoms that point to abnormal conditions. Expect certain tests as aids to diagnosis—for example, a blood and urine analysis, a chest x-ray procedure if you have been having trouble breathing; or an electrocardiogram (EKG) if any heart trouble is indicated.

history (medical)   an interview in which a health care professional obtains information from a client relating to past medical experience.

physical examination   an examination performed as part of a general checkup or to achieve a diagnosis.

*If you are especially concerned with finding a physician who has strong credentials and experience, then after you have some names, make sure the person is a member of the American College of Physicians (or American College of Surgeons, if a surgeon). Also, ask the hospital to provide you with a list of staff physicians and their ranks and privileges; this will give you some sense of the extent to which the person has earned the respect of fellow physicians.

> ■■■■■ **STRATEGIES:** CHOOSING A HEALTH CARE PROVIDER
>
> *When choosing a health care provider:*
>
> 1. Ask for recommendations.
> 2. Check the provider's credentials.
> 3. Ask these questions:
>   What are the fees for office visits? Other visits?
>   Will you accept my insurance as complete payment for the care you provide?
>   What are the office hours?
>   Can I obtain advice by phone? At what times?
>   Do you recommend that I have periodic checkups? How often?
>   If I am sick, will you visit me at home? What is the fee for this service?
>   Who handles the calls when you are not available?
> 4. Try a first appointment, and notice how it goes.
> 5. Expect to be listened to.
> 6. Expect a thorough history.
> 7. Expect a thorough physical examination.

Expect to be told the diagnosis and to have it explained. When a treatment is prescribed:

■ Write down the directions you are given. Follow them.
■ If in doubt, ask about alternative treatments.

By the time you leave the office, you should feel satisfied that you have been well received, understood, and instructed. The person has spent adequate time with you, has listened well, has learned everything important about your previous medical history, has examined you carefully, has made an expert diagnosis (or taken the first necessary steps in that direction), and has answered all your questions. If this description does not apply to your interaction, you may want to find another health care provider.

Once your choice is made, periodic contact over the years should help to establish a mutually respecting and trusting relationship. Your health care provider can become an increasingly valuable resource. On occasion, you can obtain advice efficiently just by telephoning. (Do not abuse this privilege, though. If you have more than a simple, routine question, go to the office and pay the fee.) At other times, your health care provider can provide preventive care. (Remember that heart problem we threatened you with, earlier in this chapter? Preventive medicine could help forestall that.)

You needn't have a complete physical examination every year, though. Research has shown that complete physical examinations every year are no more efficient in catching developing health problems than less-frequent examinations. The most effective strategy seems to be for everybody to adopt some broad preventive measures, and then for individuals with specific risk factors to adopt some additional measures tailored especially for them. Periodic checkups—not too often, not too infrequent—give you the best chance of arresting any disease in its early stages.

≡▶ *The match between you and your primary health care provider should be a satisfying one. Select this person with care, and don't accept second best.*

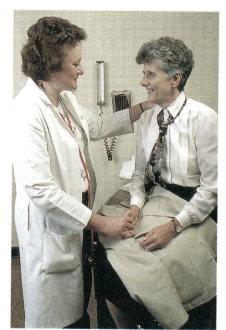

When visiting a health care provider, expect to be listened to and to have your questions answered.

■ MINIGLOSSARY
of Other Health Practitioners

acupuncturist a health practitioner who punctures the body with needles to relieve pain and achieve other physiological effects. Needles inserted at nerve synapses can alter the transmission of pain sensations. Acupuncture is an ancient art in China; depending on the practitioner, it has been found to be of some usefulness in the United States for pain management.

allopath see *naturopath*.

chiropractor a person who is trained to treat people with pain said to be caused by misalignment of the skeleton. Chiropractic treatments use "adjustments"— that is, manipulations of the joints that can, at best, relieve pressure on nerves, and at worst, cause permanent disability.

clinical ecologist a practitioner who claims to be able to cure people's illnesses by diagnosing and treating allergies to substances and materials in the environment.

homeopath the practitioner of a scientifically unproved practice of using small doses of poisons to prevent or relieve harm caused by those poisons.

> *homeo* = same

iridologist a person who claims to be able to diagnose illnesses by studying the patterns of color in the iris of the eye. "Training" consists of payment of $400 to purchase a chart of the iris and a list of diseases indicated by various color patterns.

lay midwife a birth attendant who may or may not be an R.N. and may be educated in any number of ways, from informal observation of births to three-year lay midwifery programs. There are no licensing boards for lay midwives.

naprapath a person who treats connective tissue and ligament disorders by manipulation and massage.

> *napra* = connective (tissue)

naturopath a person who uses "natural" products such as foods and herbs to treat people's illnesses. Naturopaths distinguish themselves from traditional medical practitioners, whom they call *allopaths*—people who use medicine, surgery, x-ray examinations, and other "unnatural" tools to treat illnesses.

> *allo* = other (than natural)

nutritionist a person who specializes in the study of nutrition. Some nutritionists are registered dietitians, some have considerable course work in nutrition, and some are self-described experts whose training may be minimal or nonexistent.

orthomolecular psychiatrist a psychiatrist who uses "natural" treatments, especially vitamins and minerals, to rectify mental illnesses, assuming they are caused by wrong amounts of nutrient molecules in the system.

Other Professionals—Including Some Not So Professional

An assortment of health practitioners of varying quality is listed in the Miniglossary of Other Health Practitioners. Some of these people may be well qualified to help you with what ails you or even to help you improve and prolong your already good health. Some have skills within limited realms that are useful. Some may be out-and-out frauds waiting to ambush anyone with full pockets and an unsuspecting nature. In other words, the quality of these people is more uneven that that of the health care providers described in the previous section, so the consumer has to be more discriminating in selecting among them.

New "specialties" spring up all the time to deceive unwary victims. Anyone can claim the title doctor; there are penalties only for falsely claiming to have an M.D. degree from a particular medical school. Thus where credentialing and licensing are not standardized, the guarantee that a health care provider will give you useful service is not secure. Medical doctors are of different stripes, too; not all are the fine, upstanding, ethical persons we wish them to be. Some are dishonest, incompetent, or impaired—but the chance that this is so is less than it used to be, because the safeguards are greater.

One thing to remember when consulting any health care provider: each health care specialist is qualified to provide care within the specific area of expertise. If you visit a psychologist and begin to receive nutrition advice, this should alert you that this person is speaking beyond his or her area of education and experience. In the same way, a registered dietitian is not professionally qualified to speak about psychological problems. Ethical health care providers will provide information only in their particular fields of training.

■ *FACT OR FICTION:* Anyone can adopt the title "doctor," but there are penalties for falsely claiming to be a medical doctor (M.D.). *True.*

≡▶ *Health care providers other than physicians, physician's assistants, and nurse practitioners are many and varied. None are as well trained as those specialists, and many are untrustworthy.*

The wise consumer uses all the strategies, resources, and services mentioned in this chapter, and more. The person who can evaluate health claims, knows how to avoid health fraud, and knows how the health care system works is way ahead of the game when it comes to self-care. One other area of health remains to be examined: the larger environment, both local and global. Chapter 21 explores that environment.

■≡ For Review

1. List elements a person should consider when evaluating health claims, and explain why they are important.

2. List sources through which to check the authenticity of health products or services and health associations.

3. Explain why scientific journals represent a standard against which to measure other sources of health information, such as the popular press or the mass communication media.

4. List and describe sources of reliable health information.

5. Describe some of the elements of a well-designed scientific experiment.

6. Describe some characteristics of false health claims.

7. Describe various kinds of health insurance.

8. List strategies for purchasing an appropriate health insurance package.

9. Describe insurance abuses and their effects on health care providers, medical care facilities, and consumers.

10. List strategies for selecting and using medical care facilities.

11. Compare a traditional fee-for-service medical care with a health maintenance organization.

12. List elements important in choosing a health care provider.

13. Describe what to look for during an initial visit to a health care provider.

14. List and describe various health care providers, both professional and unprofessional.

▣≡ Notes

1. F. E. James, Study lays groundwork for tying health costs to workers' behavior, *Wall Street Journal,* 14 April 1989.

2. Long-term care: Who pays? *NCL Bulletin,* May/June 1986, pp. 1, 6.

3. G. J. Church and coauthors, Sorry, your policy is canceled, *Time,* 24 March 1986, pp. 16–20, 23–26.

4. V. R. Fuchs and J. S. Hahn, How does Canada do it? A comparison of expenditures for physicians; services in the United States and Canada, *New England Journal of Medicine* 323 (1990): 884–890.

5. J. K. Iglehart, Health policy report: Germany's health care system, *New England Journal of Medicine* 324 (1991): 503–508.

6. M. Allukion, Presidential address: Something is wrong with our non-system, *The Nation's Health,* November 1990, p. 9.

7. Equifax, an insurance benefit consulting firm, as cited by G. Akers, Containing the high cost of health care: New play-or-pay rules for health insurance, *Radcliffe Quarterly,* June 1985, pp. 31–32.

8. J. Creamer, The talking cure (Medical News), *American Health,* June 1985, p. 14.

SPOTLIGHT

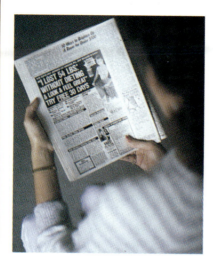

The Consumer and Health Quackery

A theme throughout this book is consumerism. Consumers face many problems in a free-enterprise market where competitors eager to capture their dollars push their wares aggressively and not always honestly. Many advertisements twist the truth to create problems for us, exaggerate the problems, or scare us with them, and then they twist the truth again to persuade us that they have the solutions we need. To give just one example, suppose you have a freckle or two (or ten thousand). A television commercial might start there, and take these steps:

■ You have freckles (that's true).
■ They make you look younger than you are (that might be true, but it's OK).

■ That's a problem (the commercial wants you to think freckles are not OK, so that it can go on to say. . . .)
■ You need Product X to hide those freckles.

Consumers buy many "Product Xs" they don't need because they have been led to follow such untruths and twisted reasoning.

A common case of created problems is premenstrual syndrome (PMS), which has been said to "disable" women before their menstrual periods each month. PMS is not a fiction; it does seriously afflict some women. However, advertisers and news reporters make it out to be more common than it is, and claim that it needs treatment when it does not. Women who have no unusual discomfort are led to think they do, and then to purchase remedies for it. This is a classic trick of quacks, and the informed consumer sees through it. But everyone, no matter how sophisticated, has some difficulty recognizing the difference between real needs and created needs, for some ads are phrased in highly persuasive terms.

When a woman has cosmetic surgery to improve her appearance, is she meeting a real or a created need?

The need is often a created one. Women in our society are under especially heavy pressure to be thin, wrinkle-free, and shapely. By forcing this image on them, profiteers make millions yearly sucking out their fat, giving face lifts, and taking nips and tucks, often with painful and disfiguring results. But cosmetic surgery has a legitimate side, too. After an accident, for example, a skillful

cosmetic surgeon can help restore a person's normal facial appearance or hand function, and with it, the person's self-esteem and employability.

Before you go further into health quackery, remind me of what health products people do need.

Remember the first Spotlight in Chapter 1? You need soap, to wash your body and your hair. You need clean water, too. Baking soda makes an effective toothpaste, toothbrushes and dental floss both help clean the teeth, and talcum powder helps keep the skin dry (an antibacterial measure) and prevent chafing (which can lead to infection).

In addition to these health care products, people are wise to keep items on hand with which to meet common medical needs. Appendix E makes suggestions for stocking a medicine chest.

What common products do people buy unnecessarily?

People buy a multitude of products unnecessarily for supposed health or medical reasons. If you wish to restrict yourself to what you truly need, you will be astonished at the number of items and the amount of expense you can eliminate from your life. Health quackery provides the motivation to make some of these purchases. An example is medical devices. The Food and Drug Administration (FDA) has grouped quack medical devices into nine categories:

■ Figure enhancers (examples: bust developers, penis enlargers, muscle developers).
■ Arthritis and pain-relieving gadgets.

- Sleep aids.
- Hair and scalp devices (example: most baldness cures).
- Youth prolongers (example: wrinkle removers, royal jelly).
- Sex aids (example: cures for impotence).
- Air purifiers.
- Disease diagnosers.
- Cure-alls (example: anemia preparations).[1]*

We would add a list of unnecessary medical products:

- Mouthwashes (they don't eliminate the germs that cause bad breath; they only wash a few away for a very short time).
- Cold medicines; arthritis medicines; sleeping pills and potions; headache remedies (see Chapter 8).
- Cancer preventives and "cures" (see Chapter 19).
- Health foods and nutrient supplements (see Chapter 5).
- Fad diets and diet aids (see Chapter 6).
- Colon treatments (example: enemas for irritated colon, hemorrhoid ointments); laxatives (they create a dependency that can make the situation worse).
- Vaginal deodorant sprays and douches (the natural odor is not offensive; a bad odor indicates a hygiene problem or a medical problem).
- PMS medications.

How do promoters succeed in selling so many unnecessary things?

Most advertising of such products involves the basic scheme already presented: promoters induce alarm, then offer reassurance or promise a

*Reference notes are at the end of the Spotlight.

benefit in the form of bottles, jars, tubes, or devices. Promotional advertisements use testimonials, opinions, exaggerations, and vague generalizations, stating no specific facts. Other techniques are the many kinds of claims familiar to every television watcher today:

- Our product is better than theirs (appeal to brand loyalty).
- Everyone uses our product (bandwagon appeal).
- Rich people use our product (snob appeal).
- Famous people use our product (fame appeal).
- We will give you bonuses and free merchandise if you buy our product (bribery).
- Our product is new and improved. You can tell, because the packaging has changed (newness appeal).
- Ordinary people use our product (just-plain-folks appeal).
- Funny, happy people use our product (smile appeal).
- Beautiful people use our product (vanity appeal).
- Scientific people approve our product (science appeal).

Consumers who use their heads instead of the product wonder where the science is in all of this. Where are the statistics, surveys, professional health organization endorsements, or laboratory test results? Sometimes ads use these, too, but seldom with the serious expectation that the consumer will make a rational analysis of the results. The promotions may be sophisticated and hard to see through.

Quacks also offer special machines (technology appeal), secret formulas (chemistry appeal), and medical breakthroughs (miracle appeal). These

appeals work; but the products do not.

Sometimes advertisers seem to try to confuse consumers in order to sell their products.

Yes, they twist logic and reasoning. Consider the following example: "Tiredness is a sign that you need iron pills." While it is true that an iron deficiency produces tiredness, the reverse is not true, for tiredness is also a symptom of other conditions. Tiredness is a sign that you need a diagnosis. Don't be seduced into action by a symptom without a diagnosis.

Symptoms commonly used to draw in the unsuspecting consumer are those everybody has—tiredness, aches and pains, occasional insomnia, colds. Another class of such symptoms includes those everyone can see because they involve external parts of the body: the skin, hands, face, hair, scalp, eyes, fingernails. Do you have pimples? Use Product A. Dry hands? Product B. Dandruff? Product C—and so on. In all these cases, the thinking is confused, for many causes can produce these symptoms. Cures must be cause-specific, not symptom-specific.

Can't you spot false claims by their language, too?

Yes. Many buzzwords and phrases can alert you to false or misleading information—among them, the following:

- *Organic, health, herbal, natural.* These terms have no legal meaning as used on labels, and although intended to imply unusual power to promote health, they do not.

■ *Contains no X.* Often, the ingredient whose absence is being boasted was never there in the first place—for example, "contains no cholesterol" in a vegetable oil, or "contains no caffeine" on a can of ginger ale. Often, too, the fear of X is an irrational fear not based on a real threat.

■ *Contains X.* Often X is not beneficial or is present in such a small amount as to be insignificant.

■ *Scientific breakthrough, medical miracle.* Seldom do popular reports prove true when they make statements in defiance of current scientific fact —a new cure for cancer, a way to lose weight without cutting calories, a tiny pill with enormous power. In advertisements, claims that a product is "new," "quick," "secret," or "amazing" almost never prove true.[2]

■ *Doctors agree, authorities agree.* When the identity of the doctors is not revealed, or when no reference to an authoritative publication is provided, these statements are meaningless. They may mean only that the advertiser persuaded three doctor friends to agree.

What other tricks do quacks use?

Some claims are outright tricks that work because we consumers can be children who frighten easily and delight in magic. The tricks are simple, but they are still attractive. Who hasn't been tempted to buy a product or try a service because it sounds so easy ("no effort"), because it costs so little and produces such a big reward ("something for nothing"), because it will protect people from terrible things (scare tactics), because it will restore vitality or youth or beauty or all of these (magical thinking), or because it will relieve people of some natural characteristic they are being taught to despise? Learn what you can control and what you can't control, what is truly desirable (your health) and what is not (someone else's success in selling you a product). Promote your wellness in the ways that truly work—they involve your lifestyle choices. None of them is magic.

I know those tricks do work, though. I'm afraid I've had several experiences in which they were successful with me. With so many grasping fingers reaching for my wallet, how can I protect myself? Can I get any help from the government?

Yes, you can. Four major federal agencies are charged with aspects of consumer protection: the FDA (Food and Drug Administration), the FTC (Federal Trade Commission), the Consumer Product Safety Commission, and the U.S. Postal Service.

The FDA has jurisdiction over the ingredients of foods, drugs, medical devices, cosmetics, and labeling. Foods and cosmetics must by law be safe, and the FDA is empowered to test or order testing to see that they are. Drugs and medical devices must be both safe and effective, and the FDA can require proof and order them seized or withdrawn from the market if such proof is not presented. The FDA's efforts against quackery have been weakening, though. Originally founded in 1906 to fight unsafe and fraudulent foods and drugs, the FDA now spends only $1 of every $200 to do so. Since 1960, the FDA has spent much of its effort regulating the labeling of foods and drugs.[3]

The FDA is ineffective against health fraud perpetrators for several reasons. For one thing, the FDA is slow, and while it takes the time to fulfill federal regulations in pursuing a fraud, the fraud can easily make a quick move and go free. A former FDA commissioner confesses, "There are too many quacks, too skillful at the quick change of address and product name."[4] For another, the penalties are not stiff enough, and are not levied soon enough, to deter frauds who get away with millions before they are caught. A case in point is Dreamaway, a fraudulent product that was supposed to make people lose weight while they slept. By the time the district attorney in the California county where Dreamaway originated had instituted a suit against the company, it had already raked in a profit of over $1 million. It agreed not to market the product any more in California, and had to pay over $150,000 in court costs, but it walked away several hundred thousand dollars richer and free to defraud the public again in 49 other states.

Another reason why health fraud is flourishing is because lawsuits are time-consuming, labor-intensive efforts. The FDA cannot begin to prosecute all perpetrators; it has to go after the most medically dangerous. Those that are merely economic frauds go free.

What about the other agencies you mentioned?

The FTC's province is to fight the concentration of economic power and to investigate unfair or deceptive business practices, including deceptive advertising. The FTC has also been weakening, as its powers

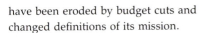

have been eroded by budget cuts and changed definitions of its mission.

The Consumer Product Safety Commission is charged specifically with safeguarding the public against products that injure or poison people, and so it gets involved with extreme cases of health quackery. The U.S. Postal Service deals with mail fraud cases, which amount to $500 million a year or more. Inspectors are available to investigate reports of such fraud, and when a case is uncovered, the Postal Service can take several actions. For example, it can refuse to deliver mail to the perpetrator of a fraud, thus shutting down the operation. It can sue and demand a $1,000 fine for each individual mailing made in perpetration of a fraud, or impose`

a five-year imprisonment penalty per mailing.

Besides these federal agencies, don't some private agencies also deal with consumer issues?

Yes. The *Better Business Bureau* investigates consumer complaints and uses its influence to prevent unethical business practices in communities. Consumers Union systematically studies new products and services from the point of view of the consumer. *Consumer Reports,* a magazine it publishes, informs individuals about products and services judged to be safe, effective, and economical.

Also, the National Council Against Health Fraud (NCAHF) deserves a mention.* Its members, vigilant

against fraud wherever it occurs, keep the central headquarters informed; and the newsletter passes the word on to consumers. However, agencies cannot predict or prevent fraud; they can pursue quacks only after they have *injured* many people. Frequently, you will face the choice of whether to get involved in a health scam before you have heard anything from the authorities about its safety or effectiveness. It is up to you to beware. This book has provided pointers to help you on the way, but keep your eyes and ears open. There are a lot of snakes in the grass.

*Report cases of health fraud to the NCAHF at P.O. Box 1276, Loma Linda, CA 92354. Provide clear copies and include complete references of materials cited; graphics can be sent by FAX to (714) 824-4838.

■≡ Spotlight Notes

1. U.S. Food and Drug Administration, *The Big Quack Attack: Medical Devices,* HHS publication no. (FDA) 80-4022, 1980.
2. J. F. McKenzie, A checklist for evaluating health information, *Journal of School Health* 57 (1987): 31–32.
3. D. Colburn, Quackery: Medical fraud is proliferating and the FDA can't seem to stop it, *Washington Post* (national weekly edition) 8 July 1985, pp. 6–7.
4. A. H. Hayes, Jr., as cited in Colburn, 1985.

CHAPTER 21

The Environment and Personal Health

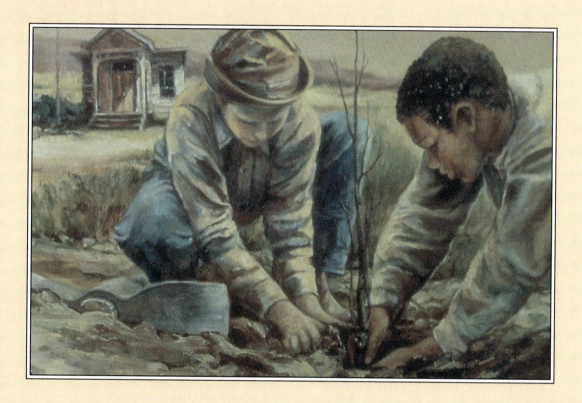

The Air, the Sun, and Green Plants
The Water Supply
The Land: Solid and Toxic Waste
Natural Environments

The Population Problem
A Way to the Future
■ **SPOTLIGHT** Personal
   Strategy—Voluntary Simplicity

Just for fun, respond to the following true or false statements. If false, say what is true.

■ The greenhouse effect is beneficial to the earth, because it promotes the growth of plants. (Page 597)
■ A lake that is clear is a healthy lake. (Page 600)
■ Pure water can pollute the environment if it is of the wrong temperature. (Page 601)

■ To minimize environmental impact, human sewage should be returned to the earth after treatment, not to the water. (Page 603)
■ When birds can't survive in an environment, that is a sign that people's health is likely to suffer there, too. (Page 614)

environment everything "outside" the living organism—air, water, soil, other organisms, forms of radiation.

Technically, an **environment** might be defined as all things that exist or originate outside of an individual. Several environments might be described that way—the home environment, the cultural environment, the biological environment, and so forth. But to define an environment as *outside* implies a separateness that is not real. When you are breathing, is the air outside of you, or inside? When you are conversing with a teacher, where do the thoughts you are sharing come from—inside or outside of you or the teacher? Materials, energy, and information constantly flow into and out of us. We and our environments are not only interdependent but also continuous, part of the same whole. Our biological environment, for example, supplies the materials our bodies are made of and the forms of energy (light, heat, and sound) that make our lives possible. Conversely, we alter and interfere with the environment in many ways.

Healthy environments support personal health; damaged environments detract from it. Consider your needs. Ideally, wherever you lived and worked—inner city, farm, or wilderness—the air would be clean, the water pure, the food nourishing and safe, the surrounding scenery and sounds enjoyable, the space sufficient for play, the people nearby stimulating and loving, the events interesting, and all other elements, both seen and unseen, in harmony together. It is unrealistic, of course, to think that everyone in today's world can enjoy such a life, and it is also untrue that such perfect conditions are indispensable to health. It is true, however, that we will survive or thrive only so long as we maintain our environments sufficiently so that they can sustain us. This chapter focuses on our biological environment—the planet earth.

You may wonder why a book about individual health should have a chapter on such a large subject as the global environment. The book's philosophy, stated in Chapter 1, is that to a great extent you control your health; the book's mission is to help you do a good job of it. The emphasis throughout is on your choices. But in what sense do you make choices that affect your "environmental health"?

You make such choices all the time. The declining health of the planet today is the result of human activities, yours included. You do not leave the earth the same from one day to the next. Each day of your life, you breathe its air, eat its food, leave your wastes on it—and you either restore more of its resources than you consume, or you do not. To make your choices consciously, you have to be informed about the impact you are having on the earth as you interact with it. This chapter is intended to expand your consciousness, partly so that you can make many little choices every day with that awareness.

It is in your interest to learn to do this, for the environment also has an impact on you. If its air is clean, your lungs can be healthy. If its water is pure, you can drink it without fear. If its soil is free of toxins, it will bring forth food that will sustain your life. Because you are a biological creature, you depend on the environment for the physical necessities of your life—air, water, soil, climate, and living plants and animals. You may be unaware of the vast changes taking place in your environment today, but once your eyes are open you can see these changes all around you and recognize their effects. Your awareness is important, because it can lead to action.

Once you have become conscious of your own impacts on the environment, you will be conscious of the impacts of others—and not only of individuals but of groups, including industry, agriculture, and government. To remedy the problems that we human beings are creating on the earth, we must not only act responsibly as individuals, but must, by the millions, demand that industry, agriculture, and governments do the same. After all, these systems are not above the law, and we human beings make the law.

You have the right to a healthy environment. You have the right to demand of your fellow human beings that they maintain it so as to support you and your children and grandchildren. You have the right to clean air, pure water, uncontaminated food. So this chapter has a second mission—to increase your awareness of the ways other people's choices impinge on you. Together with your neighbors, you can demand that other people respect your rights. As large as the world's environmental problems may be, they are all caused by people's choices. They can also only be solved by people's choices, and you can influence those choices. Every time you drop a word of awareness into someone else's consciousness, you start a ripple that may grow into a wave.

Some of the choices are small—for example, that of the motorist who keeps the car running while it sits for ten minutes in a traffic jam: turned off, it would pollute the air a little less. (The mere sharing of that thought might be all it would take to solve that problem.) Some choices are big—for example, that of the hospital administrator who chooses, for profit's sake, to have disease-carrying refuse dumped into the nearest river rather than disposing of it properly. (Effective legislation backed by vigilant police work and stringent punishments for violations might be needed here.) In any case, all such choices begin with consciousness of what the problems and their causes are, so that is where this chapter begins.

The chapter is divided, somewhat artificially, into realms: the air and green plants first, then the water, then the land—but of course, these realms are interconnected, and anything that affects one of them affects them all (see Figure 21–1). The Life Choice Inventory allows you to assess your sense of responsibility toward the earth, and the Spotlight ends the chapter with an emphasis on personal choices you can make, based on that sense of responsibility. The following Critical Thinking section warns you against being taken in by "green" labels on products that do not merit the name.

FIGURE 21–1 ■ **All things are connected.**

The Earth *before* Human Impact

THE AIR

Animals and people take up oxygen (●) and release carbon dioxide (●).

The sun's rays, passing through clear air, provide energy for plants and algae to free oxygen (●) from carbon dioxide (●).

Green plants on land and algae in the ocean take up carbon dioxide (●) and return oxygen (●) to the atmosphere.

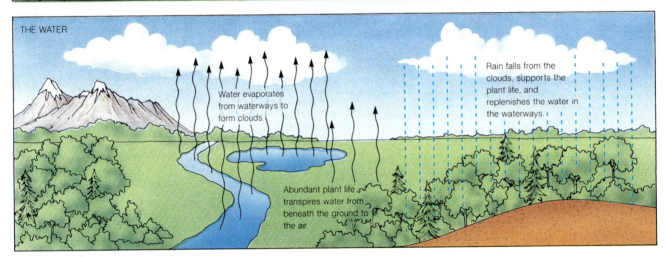

THE WATER

Water evaporates from waterways to form clouds.

Rain falls from the clouds, supports the plant life, and replenishes the water in the waterways.

Abundant plant life transpires water from beneath the ground to the air.

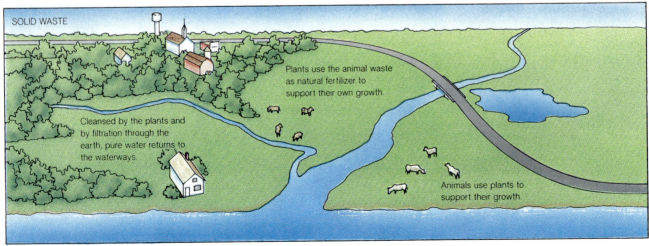

SOLID WASTE

Plants use the animal waste as natural fertilizer to support their own growth.

Cleansed by the plants and by filtration through the earth, pure water returns to the waterways.

Animals use plants to support their growth.

FIGURE 21–1 ■ continued

The Earth *with* Human Impact

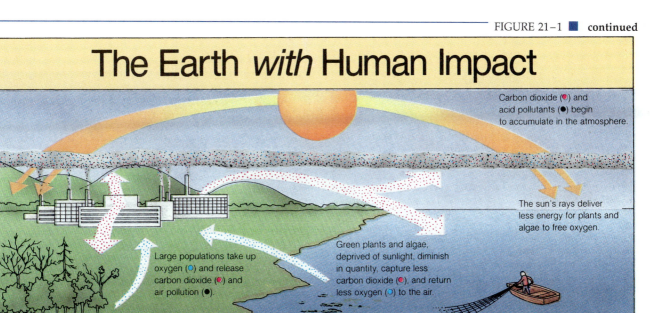

Carbon dioxide (●) and acid pollutants (●) begin to accumulate in the atmosphere.

The sun's rays deliver less energy for plants and algae to free oxygen.

Large populations take up oxygen (○) and release carbon dioxide (●) and air pollution (●).

Green plants and algae, deprived of sunlight, diminish in quantity, capture less carbon dioxide (●), and return less oxygen (○) to the air.

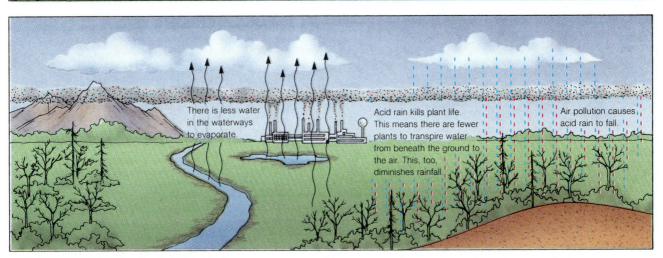

There is less water in the waterways to evaporate.

Acid rain kills plant life. This means there are fewer plants to transpire water from beneath the ground to the air. This, too, diminishes rainfall.

Air pollution causes acid rain to fall.

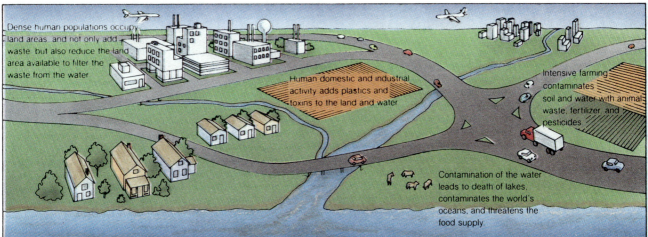

Dense human populations occupy land areas, and not only add waste but also reduce the land area available to filter the waste from the water.

Human domestic and industrial activity adds plastics and toxins to the land and water.

Intensive farming contaminates soil and water with animal waste, fertilizer, and pesticides.

Contamination of the water leads to death of lakes, contaminates the world's oceans, and threatens the food supply.

LIFE CHOICE INVENTORY

How well do you care for the environment? The following questions are from a checklist entitled "65 Things You Can Do to Help Save Tropical Forests and Other Natural Resources."

In your home, do you:

1. Recycle everything you can: newspapers, cans, glass bottles and jars, scrap metal, used oil, etc.?
2. Use cold water in the washer whenever possible?
3. Avoid using appliances to do things you can do by hand (such as electric can openers)?
4. Reuse brown paper bags to line your trash instead of plastic liners? Reuse bread bags, butter tubs, etc.?
5. Store food in reusable containers rather than plastic wrap or aluminum foil?

In your yard, do you:

6. Compost your yard waste?
7. Pull weeds instead of using herbicides?
8. Fertilize with manure and compost, rather than with chemical fertilizers?
9. Compost your leaves and yard debris, rather than burning them?
10. Take extra plastic and rubber pots back to the nursery?

On vacation, do you:

11. Turn down the heat and turn off the water heater before you leave home?

12. Carry reusable cups, dishes, and flatware (and use them)?
13. Dispose of trash in trash containers (never litter)?
14. Buy no souvenirs made from wild or endangered animals?
15. Stay on roads and trails rather than trampling dunes and fragile undergrowth?

About your car, do you:

16. Keep your car tuned up for maximum fuel efficiency?
17. Use public transit, whenever possible?
18. Ride your bike or walk, whenever possible?
19. Plan to replace your car with a more fuel-efficient model when you can?
20. Recycle your engine oil?

At school or work, do you:

21. Recycle paper whenever possible?
22. Use scrap paper for notes to yourself and others?
23. Print or copy on both sides of the paper?
24. Reuse manila envelopes and file folders?
25. Use the stairs instead of the elevator whenever you can?

A warning: this chapter describes some monumental environmental problems. Do not be disheartened. Work your way through them to the end, where solutions are proposed to which you can contribute. We all owe it to ourselves and to one another to face and overcome these problems together.

■≡ The Air, the Sun, and Green Plants

The air supports life in such obvious ways that we tend to take it for granted. To animals, including humans, it offers oxygen and receives carbon dioxide. To green plants, it conveys the energy of sunlight, and they use that energy to consume the carbon dioxide and restore the air's oxygen as they grow. In brief, the air, the sun, and green things are indispensable to life. To support life, the air must be reasonably fresh (oxygen-rich), clear (so that sunlight can penetrate it), and pure (carrying few harmful gases or particles). And to receive the energy of sunlight and return oxygen to the

When you're shopping, do you:

26. Buy as little plastic and foam packaging as possible?
27. Buy permanent, rather than disposable, products?
28. Buy paper rather than plastic, if you must buy disposable products?
29. Buy fresh produce grown locally?
30. Buy in bulk to avoid unnecessary packaging?

In other areas, do you:

31. Volunteer your time to conservation projects?
32. Encourage your family, friends, and neighbors to save resources, too?
33. Write letters to support conservation issues?

Scoring:

First, give yourself 1 point for answering this quiz.

Then, give yourself 1 point for each habit you *know* you should adopt, but haven't yet (total possible points = 33): _____

Then, give yourself 2 more points for each habit you *have* adopted (or would if you could—total possible points = 66): _____

Total score:

1 to 25: You are a beginner in stewardship of the earth. Try to improve.

26 to 50: You are well on your way. Few consumers do even as well as this, yet.

51 to 75: Excellent. Pat yourself on the back, and keep on improving.

76 to 100: Outstanding. You are a shining example for others to follow.

Keep a copy of these suggestions in the drawer where you put your monthly bills. Review them every month, and try to adopt another conservation habit every time you read the list. If everyone does these things, it will significantly help our planet's health.

SOURCE: Conservation Action Checklist, adapted from material produced by the Washington Park Zoo, Portland, Oregon, and available from Conservation International, 1015 18th St. NW, Suite 1000, Washington, DC 20036; (202) 429–5660. Call or write for copies of the original or for more information.

---

air, there must be green plants. The more carbon dioxide in the air, the more green plants there must be to convert it back to oxygen.

Next to the earth's surface, normal clean air consists of about one-fifth oxygen and four-fifths nitrogen, with trace amounts of inert gases mixed in. Natural processes add variable amounts of water vapor (from evaporation), carbon dioxide (from forest fires, volcanoes, and the life processes of living plants and animals), and small quantities of a few other gases contributed by the decomposition of protein matter. Any components other than these that get into air are **contaminants**—forms of **pollution**.

The air has never been perfectly fresh, clear, and pure. The natural processes just described have always released temporary bursts of contamination into the air, but these have always dispersed, leaving the atmosphere as before. However, polluted air surrounds the earth today. The reason is that the earth now sustains a vast population of human beings that uses **fossil fuels** intensively for both domestic living and industrial processes. Natural

contaminants chemicals that ordinarily do not occur (and therefore do not "belong") in a given environment, especially toxic chemicals.

pollution contamination of the environment with any substance or influence that impairs its ability to support life.

fossil fuels fuels, mainly oil, coal, and natural gas, that have been formed over millions of years by the decomposition and compression of plant materials that have lived in past geological ages.

Products to buy, to benefit the earth:

Compact fluorescent light bulbs (because they replace many incandescents and use much less energy).

Shopping bags (because they eliminate the need for both paper and plastic bags at the grocery store and other stores).

Cloth diapers, dishcloths, napkins, and towels to replace the throwaway types.

Dishes, cups, glasses, and tableware to replace the disposable versions. (Yes, it costs fuel and hot water to wash them, but not as much as the fuel and water it costs to keep manufacturing and shipping disposables to you.)

Low-flow shower heads and other devices that help you save water and the fuel to heat it with (remember, electricity is usually made by burning fossil fuel).

Energy-efficient appliances (if you must have them at all).

Haircuts, rather than permanent waves and blow-dries (since the haircut is a service, while perms and blow-dries involve chemicals, containers, and fuel).

A bicycle (if you will use it in place of a car).

Secondhand items (garage-sale items, used clothing, and the like).

It is seldom better for the earth to buy a product than to refrain from buying one.

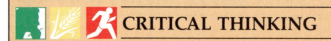

CRITICAL THINKING

Environmental Hype in Marketing

With today's widespread concern about the environment, many consumers are earnestly trying to do their best to shop carefully. "Refuse, reuse, recycle," are the bywords among such consumers. They mean, first, don't buy anything you don't need. Second, avoid disposables (including unnecessary throwaway packaging), and keep using what you do buy. And third, if you must buy disposables, make sure you recycle them. Many corporations are assisting consumers in making these choices, by providing reusable, minimally packaged, recyclable goods for them.

Unfortunately, though, some companies mislead consumers by labeling products "green" (good for the environment) that don't merit the label. A prime example is goods labeled "recyclable" that, realistically, are not. Many plastic items fall in this category. Plastic containers now are imprinted with recycle symbols numbered 1 to 6. In many communities, however, only the 1s and 2s are recycled, and often only the beverage containers among those. The other plastics, even if they bear the symbol, are as useless as ever.

Another scam is the label "recycled" on paper products that actually contain no paper that has been through human hands. Paper makers have always picked up the trimmings off their own mill floors and returned them to the paper-making process; now they call this recycling, when it is nothing of the kind. Real recycled paper is *postconsumer* paper, meaning paper that has been used as such, printed on, and read; then retrieved, de-inked, re-pulped, and re-made into paper. Ideally, consumers will use only recycled paper with a high postconsumer waste content.

Other misleading labels claim that polystyrene foam cups "help preserve our trees and forests." True, they are not made of wood, but the making of foam, a petroleum product processed with ozone-destroying gases, is highly destructive to the environment on which plants depend.

As in every other area of health, consumers seeking to support the health of the environment must sharpen their skills at distinguishing truth from falsehood. Don't buy a product just because it's labeled "green," and remember, it is seldom better for the earth to buy a product than to refrain from buying one. The only exception is when the product is one you need, and also one that eliminates the necessity of buying many others.

air pollution contamination of the air with quantities or types of gases or particles not normally found there.

air pollution is, in general, intermittent and diffuse, whereas people-generated pollution is continuous, concentrated, and in many cases, growing more intense from year to year.

People-generated air pollutants come from four main sources: oil and gasoline burned to run cars and other forms of transportation; oil, coal, and natural gas burned to generate electricity for homes, businesses, and industry; waste products from manufacturing; and cities' solid wastes being burned for disposal. The effects of these pollutants on the earth's climate, plants, animals, and people are often harmful, and potentially catastrophic.

≡ ▶ *Human-generated air pollution, largely from the use of fossil fuels, can harm life on earth.*

Warming of the Climate

A prime example of a human-generated air pollutant is carbon dioxide. Carbon dioxide is a natural substance, but the quantities now accumulating are abnormal. In its normal quantity, which until recently had remained about the same for billions of years, carbon dioxide blocks the escape of heat into the outer atmosphere, and helps to keep the earth warm. Without it, the earth would have been some 50 degrees colder for all those years, and life as we know it would have been impossible. In the past 300 years, however, agricultural and industrial development has increased the concentration of atmospheric carbon dioxide by 25 percent, mostly as the result of increased burning of coal and oil. The result is that the earth is warming up—the so-called **greenhouse effect.**[1]*

The greenhouse effect is expected to raise the earth's average temperature by 3 to 8 degrees in the next half-century (before 2050)—an amount that may not sound like much, but that is expected to have major effects. Most scientists believe that these effects are already occurring. Worldwide, summer heat is setting new high temperature records. Rainfall is declining across the corn and wheat belts in the United States, Europe, the Soviet Union, and Asia, resulting in drought and loss of crops. The water level below the ground is falling. Inland, the rivers are shrinking, creating hardship for areas that depend on their water. Along the coastlines, salt water is invading underground areas where fresh water formerly kept it out; both vegetation and people suffer. In the oceans, the water is expanding as it warms while the polar ice caps are melting, so the sea level is rising. Governments are faced with the choice of seeing coastal cities and shores going under water or building dikes and levees to hold the water back. Forests and agricultural crops, adapted for thousands of years to a certain climate, are stressed by rising temperatures and are becoming weakened to disease. Whole species of animals and plants, including agricultural crops that human beings depend on, may become extinct as the earth's climate changes by only a few degrees. In thinking that the earth would never change, and that its self-correcting processes would continue into the future as they have for billions of years, we forgot that we ourselves could upset the balance. Now that we are seeing that happen, many nations are beginning to take action to curb their use of fossil fuels.

≡ ▶ *In the last 300 years, human agricultural and industrial activities have intensified to the point where they have raised the atmosphere's carbon dioxide concentration. As a result, the planet is growing warmer.*

Thinning of the Ozone Layer

Another atmospheric effect of air pollution is taking place far out, in the outer atmosphere. Normally where intense sunlight strikes the outer atmo-

greenhouse effect the heating effect of trapping carbon dioxide in a closed space that is warmed by the sun. In a greenhouse, the glass and the trapped carbon dioxide keep heat from escaping and facilitate plant growth. The same effect in the air surrounding the earth keeps the earth warm, but now is occurring to excess and warming the earth too much.

■ *FACT OR FICTION:* The greenhouse effect is beneficial to the earth, because it promotes the growth of plants. *False.* The greenhouse effect will produce more damage than benefit to the planet, because most of its effects are harmful to life.

*Reference notes are at the end of the chapter.

ozone layer a layer of ozone in the outer atmosphere that protects living things on earth from harmful ultraviolet radiation from the sun.

ozone holes holes in the ozone layer at the North and South Poles, caused by air pollution.

chlorofluorocarbons (CLOR-oh-FLOR-oh-car-bons), also known as **CFCs** chemical compounds containing chlorine, fluorine, and carbon. They are produced by industrial processes and, when released, react with ozone to destroy it.

sphere, a layer of gas known as the **ozone layer** continuously forms and breaks down from oxygen. The ozone layer has for billions of years screened out 99 percent of the ultraviolet rays of the sun, allowing just enough radiation through to support plant growth. Life probably did not begin until after the earth's protective ozone layer was formed.[2]

Now, air pollution from all over the earth is thinning that layer, especially at the North and South Poles—creating the so-called **ozone holes**. Diffusion of the remaining ozone from the rest of the earth's atmosphere re-covers the poles after each season, but at the cost of thinning the layer over the rest of the earth. As a result, ultraviolet radiation of higher and higher intensities is reaching the earth's surface each year. This radiation causes cancers and mutations in animals and people, and damages plants and crops.

Chief among the pollutants that destroy ozone are compounds known as **chlorofluorocarbons** (trade name, **Freon**). The chlorofluorocarbons that destroy ozone are used to cool refrigerators, freezers, and air-conditioning systems; to create foams (including some styrofoams); and to expel liquids under pressure from aerosol cans.

People and nations have been taking action to reduce chlorofluorocarbon output. Since 1978, aerosol deodorant sprays, window-cleaning sprays, and other sprays used by individual consumers have been largely replaced by roll-ons and pump devices. Industrial use of chlorofluorocarbons is still rising, however, and because these molecules rise slowly to the outer ozone layers, the destruction of ozone may continue for several decades after their production has ceased.[3] At the current rate of increase, according to several independent predictions, the ozone layer will be seriously depleted within 100 years. Skin cancer rates, already on the increase, are expected to rise proportionately—to 1 in 90 by the year 2000 and 1 in 3 by the year 2075; melanomas may already be doubling every ten years.[4] But individual cases of cancer do not constitute the biggest threat. Ultraviolet rays in excess of the norm disrupt the genetic material in all living tissues, damaging all future generations of forests, agricultural crops, grasslands, gardens, and animal life on land and in the seas as well.

The threat of ozone destruction is so serious that it was the first global trend in history to lead to international *preventive* action. At a conference in Montreal in 1986, 30 nations agreed to reduce their output of chlorofluorocarbons by 50 percent within the following decade. (The United States, unfortunately, agreed only to reduce the rate of *increase* of its chlorofluorocarbon production.) This historic event reflects a new and hopeful trend in history—the world is now united as never before by instantaneous mass-media communications, and governments can respond more quickly than ever before to global problems.

≡▶ *Ozone-destroying chemicals produced by human activities are destroying the protective ozone layer in the earth's outer atmosphere, and as a result, threatening life processes on earth. International efforts to cease releasing these chemicals are beginning.*

Health Effects of Local Air

Although global warming and ozone destruction threaten the future of life on earth, most people are blissfully unaware of these processes. They cannot see or smell carbon dioxide accumulating, and they cannot feel the increasing intensity of ultraviolet radiation, so they are not alarmed. Even closer to home, where air pollution threatens individual health, people may not be fully aware of it, for the processes that pollute the air have intensified gradually, and people have grown accustomed to their effects. Take **smog**, for example. Wherever traffic and industrial processes are intense, this type of air pollution arises, as sunlight strikes certain pollutants in the air. One of its components is **ozone**—the very compound that, in the outer atmosphere, provides protection from the intense rays of the sun. Ozone nearby is *not* protective: it can damage people's lungs and reduce their ability to perform work or exercise. And it breaks down before it reaches the outer atmosphere, so it cannot help to replenish the ozone layer. People so commonly take smog as a fact of life, though, that in many cities it has become part of the *weather* report.

Another air pollutant always surrounds automobile traffic: carbon monoxide, from tailpipe exhaust. Electrocardiograms of people with heart disease reveal changes after time spent in heavy freeway traffic, where the concentration of carbon monoxide is high. People with heart disease, lung disease, or anemia (reduced oxygen-carrying capacity of the blood) can be severely disabled or even killed by carbon monoxide levels that merely impair function in healthy people. Even at relatively low concentrations, carbon monoxide impairs mental and visual function and alertness.[5]

Another form of air pollution is **thermal pollution**, which occurs locally, particularly in cities and on cleared land where trees are absent and reflecting surfaces concentrate the heat. Thermal pollution adds significantly to the stress people in such environments face, and it contributes to global climate warming.

≡▶ *Air and thermal pollution near the earth's surface threaten health and the environment and contribute to global warming.*

Acid in the Air

Air pollution cannot help but affect the water and soil, as well as the air. Each time it rains, the air is scrubbed of its pollutants; they fall to the earth. Many of them, when combined with water, form acids, which affect living things profoundly. It doesn't matter what compound forms the acid—it can be a compound of carbon, sulfur, nitrogen, or any other element. The effects are similar, because the acid part is always the same: a tiny, charged particle of hydrogen. This chemical busybody disrupts cell membranes, distorts the proteins that do the work of living cells, and changes the characteristics of fluids so that they cannot support normal life processes.

Just as there has always been air pollution, so too there has always been **acid rain**. But in the last 100 years, the world has become increasingly industrialized, and the air's acid burden has grown greater, primarily because of the burning of coal and petroleum.

Rainfall is normally slightly acidic, but today in some places it is strongly acidic. Of particular concern to North Americans is the rain in the Northeast, made acid by pollution from the burning of coal and oil that drifts northeastward from the industrial Ohio Valley. Thousands of lakes in New England and Canada, once filled with fish and waterfowl, now stand clear and lifeless. You might think that a lake that is clear is a healthy lake, but

smog a form of air pollution that arises when sunlight strikes certain compounds in the air.

ozone a photochemical oxidant, toxic when in direct contact with lung tissue; an air pollutant.

thermal pollution accumulation of abnormal amounts of heat in the environment (air, water, or earth).

acid rain rain that has picked up chemicals from the air that convert to acid when combined with water; a form of pollution.

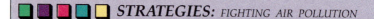

STRATEGIES: *FIGHTING AIR POLLUTION*

To fight air pollution:

1. Learn the sources and causes of air pollution affecting your area
2. Learn and apply energy conservation methods to cut down on fossil fuel use.
3. Learn about alternative energy sources such as solar energy, and use those you can.
4. Bring pressure to bear where it will be effective in improving the pollution problem.

such is not always the case. The clarity of the water may be a sign that all life in the lake has been destroyed.

When acid rain falls on the earth, compounds (bases) in the soil neutralize it at first, but ultimately, these compounds are used up. Then the soil itself turns acid, and the plants and trees growing on it become unable to grow well or to resist diseases and insect pests. Millions of acres of agricultural crops and forests in many areas of the world, including U.S. mountain ranges, the Black Forest in Germany, many parts of China, and elsewhere, have been defoliated and deforested by acid rain. Air-borne acid also eats into public buildings and monuments—the sphinxes in Egypt are now deteriorating after standing unchanged for thousands of years, even though they stand in the dry desert. And acid particles in the air are also directly harmful to human lungs, second only to cigarette smoking as a cause of lung disease.[6]

Air pollution tends to grow worse as people's numbers increase. The more people there are in an area, the more cars and other traffic, the more industry, and the more burning of fossil fuels and production of waste materials there will be. When sufficiently concentrated, air pollution destroys green plants, including trees, nature's air-cleansing machines, creating a vicious cycle.

No individual can, alone, solve problems such as those posed by air pollution. But to run away from them is a mistake we cannot afford to make. Learn to conserve energy so as to cut your fossil fuel use. Your car (now or in the future) and your home appliances are especially significant fuel consumers; use the most efficient ones you can, and use them as little as possible. Learn alternatives—solar energy is becoming a cost-effective alternative to fossil fuels in many applications. And support efforts to clean up the air in your region, as suggested in the accompanying Strategy box.

≡ ▶ *Air pollutants captured into rain produce acid rain, which acidifies lakes and soil, disrupts living systems, and eats away at public buildings. The main contributor is the use of fossil fuels; these can be used less and can be replaced by alternative energy sources.*

■≡ The Water Supply

When you draw water from the tap into a glass and drink it, it is not only water that you are drinking. It may contain chlorine (added intentionally as a disinfectant); nutrients (such as fluoride and calcium); harmful minerals (such as lead); live microorganisms; and a variety of other compounds, some of which are toxic.

The microorganisms in water are mostly from human and animal wastes (sewage, dung dropped by dairy and beef cattle on pastureland, and manure used as fertilizer on agricultural fields). Many of these microorganisms are harmless, but some are pathogens. Sewage treatment plants remove the solid materials from waste water that passes through them, and then chlorinate the water to reduce the microbial count, but they leave many microbes in the water. When the treated water is released into the water supply, the resulting dilution makes the water safe for human use. (The treatment of sewage, because it yields sludge that is deposited on the land, is described further in the next section, ''The Land: Solid and Toxic Waste.'')

High standards for sewage treatment in the developed countries ensure that most people have drinking water that does not carry disease-causing microbes, but for the rest of the world, microbial contamination remains the primary cause of human diseases and epidemics. Two of the most basic public health needs of the world's people are the needs for safe drinking water and safe waste disposal. Even in developed countries such as the United States and Canada, a major epidemic of disease would occur should we allow the public health system to go unsupported.

Among the harmful compounds in water are many contributed by agricultural fertilizers and pesticides, as well as by industry. In the wilderness, water-borne contamination either falls on the ground and then is filtered by the soil before arriving in underground waterways, or if it falls in a river, its contaminants quickly disappear back into the earth as the river flows along its course, leaving the water pure again. But neither the earth nor its rivers can purify completely the water polluted by today's intensive agricultural and industrial processes. Water leaving a factory may contain concentrations of contaminants so high that some are still present in the water after it has been treated and released. The water soaks back into the earth, still contaminated, and when water is drawn from the earth for re-use, the contaminants are still there. When the factory uses some of this water again, the concentrations of pollutants grow higher. The law requires polluting industries and water-processing plants to adhere to set standards, but enforcement often fails. Both government and consumer groups must be vigilant in detecting, reporting, and preventing dangerous levels of contamination, because our water is a vital resource.

Some forms of water pollution first affect living things other than ourselves. When chemicals such as nitrates and phosphates (usually from sewage or fertilizer) are released into lakes and ponds, microorganisms in the water use them as nutrients to grow on. Life in lakes and ponds declines by a process known as **eutrophication**. First, the nutrients support the growth of large quantities of algae—so large that some are shaded out, die, and sink, filling the lake or pond with dead plant material. Bacteria thrive on this dead matter, and as they break it down, they use up the water's oxygen. The ultimate result is death of all life forms in the lake, including fish.

Thermal pollution of lakes and streams also takes its toll on living things. Consider a factory that discharges hot water into a trout stream. The discharge may be pure H_2O, but it still kills the fish, because it is of the wrong temperature.

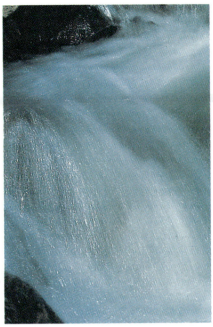

An abundant supply of fresh water is vital to all life forms on earth.

eutrophication (YOU-tro-fih-CAY-shun) death of waterways caused initially by nutrients, then algae and bacteria, and finally oxygen depletion.

■ eu = well
■ troph = to grow

■ *FACT OR FICTION:* Pure water can pollute the environment if it is of the wrong temperature. *True.*

The discussion of water to this point has focused on water *quality*. Water *quantity* is also of concern, as already mentioned. Not only droughts and encroachment of salt water but also the agricultural and industrial use of water strain the supply. Used by agriculture for irrigating and by industry for transporting, dissolving, washing, rinsing, cooling, flushing away waste, and many other purposes, water in huge quantities is diverted from its original, natural uses. Rain repeatedly returns fresh water to the earth, but with global warming, rainfall quantities are becoming erratic, and with air pollution, the purity of rain is no longer assured. In the future, it may be the water supply that first limits the size the human population can achieve.

As with the air, your responsibilities with respect to the water require first that you be aware of the problems. Then, for your personal health's sake, keep an eye on the purity of your local water supply. Watch for news about it, and probe for its significance. Learn about threats to the water supply; learn where they come from; and as a citizen take strong stands, when necessary, to protect yourself and your water.

≡▶ *Contamination of the earth's water is an environmental problem of concern. Depletion of water is another. Consumer vigilance is necessary to protect water supplies.*

■≡ The Land: Solid and Toxic Waste

Like the air and the water, the land has a job to do in supporting human life, and all life, on earth. Today, when large masses of land lie under highways, parking lots, and city sidewalks, we no longer ask that *all* the soil be uncontaminated. But it remains essential that *some* of it be so, because it is in the soil that our food supply grows, and it is the soil that filters and purifies water after human, agricultural, or industrial use.

Two classes of contaminants are deposited directly in the ground as the result of human life and activity. One is **solid wastes** (nontoxic wastes such as ordinary sewage, garbage, and trash); the other is **toxic wastes** (including some household wastes, as well as agricultural pesticides and industrial waste products).

Solid Waste

People and animals have always excreted solid wastes onto the earth. Bacteria break the waste material down and return its constituents to the soil. Plants then use those compounds as fertilizers—that is, building materials. Later, the plants either die or are eaten and are themselves similarly recycled. Everyone knows that manure makes excellent fertilizer. Human manure is no exception—provided that it is not contaminated with toxic minerals, and that it is treated to remove pathogens. However, today's large populations generate more sewage than can practically be used on the land areas that they occupy, and much of it is dumped into the water instead.

In nature, one ten-member wolf pack occupies a 25-acre territory; they and the other animals on that territory excrete a burden of waste that the land can easily handle. The waste is within the land's **carrying capacity**. By contrast, human beings live in densities of up to hundreds per acre in some

solid wastes   a term used primarily to refer to sewage and animal waste and secondarily to nonpoisonous artificial materials such as paper, glass, plastic, and metal.

toxic wastes   waste materials, primarily from industrial processes, that are toxic to plants, animals, and people.

carrying capacity   the total number of living organisms that a given environment can support without deteriorating in quality.

cities, the cities are paved with tar and concrete, and the land is not able to recycle the waste. Cities burden the land far beyond its carrying capacity. The people in a single city the size of Philadelphia excrete fecal matter amounting to millions of gallons of sewage a day; after its water is removed, 100 tons of solid waste have to be disposed of each day. The mass of a typical city's **sludge** would, within a year, cover the whole city to a depth of 17 feet.

Where does it all go? Most people flush their toilets and think it disappears. Ideally, it undergoes three steps of treatment—(1) removal of the sludge; (2) treatment of the remaining water to kill pathogenic microorganisms; and (3) release of the treated water onto land (not into waterways) to deposit its dissolved nutrient fertilizers where plants can use them, rather than where aquatic weeds will grow and strangle waterways. After this treatment, the water returns to the waterways free of contamination. The solid matter can be treated to purge toxic contaminants and kill microorganisms and then can also be returned to the land as fertilizer.

Few cities treat even part of their sewage this way, and of course it doesn't really disappear. It often flows into the nearest river or bay untreated; it often ends up in the ocean. Along the coasts, pollution of the ocean with sewage threatens human health; in the deeper ocean it is causing diseases among numerous species of sea plants and animals, including fish, sea turtles, seals, dolphins, and whales.

Another form of solid waste is what people throw away—their garbage and trash. In so-called advanced civilizations, many people enjoy immediate removal of their throwaways and never have to wonder what becomes of them. Of course, garbage and trash do not just disappear; they must be burned (polluting the air), buried (polluting the soil and groundwater), released into waterways (polluting rivers and the ocean), or stockpiled in landfills (using up space). Nothing ever really goes away.

It is hard to comprehend how massive the problem of solid waste is, but you can get some idea of it by simply becoming conscious of the amount of trash you throw away in a day—the average per American is over 3 pounds a day. Multiply that by 200 million people (the population of the United States alone), try visualizing all that trash piling up *each day* just from personal consumption in one nation—and ask where it all *does* go.

At best, items discarded by people undergo **recycling**; that is, they are transformed into materials that can be used again. Food garbage, for example, once rotted in the soil, makes excellent fertilizer (**compost**) for the next crop of plants; but if put down the sink, it fertilizes water weeds to choke waterways instead. Materials that don't occur naturally, such as glass, paper, and metal, can be reused if communities organize themselves to recycle them.

In the simplest case, everything that is **biodegradable** would be allowed to recycle naturally, while everything that is **persistent** would be recycled commercially or banished from use. The case is oversimplified, however; human communities are overwhelmed with excess items and materials that cannot be treated either way.

A case in point is plastics, most of which are nonbiodegradable. Hundreds of tons of plastic debris litter landscapes all over the world, and vast quantities have found their way into the ocean. Each year, thousands of seabirds and sea mammals get caught in plastic debris or swallow it and die. Another case is toxic waste (next section).

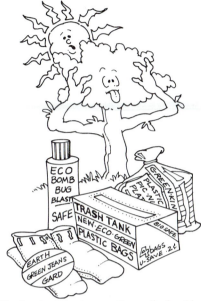

The burden we place on the earth should not exceed its carrying capacity.

sludge the solid material that remains after fluid has been drawn off (as from sewage or industrial waste).

■ *FACT OR FICTION:* To minimize environmental impact, human sewage should be returned to the earth after treatment, not to the water. *True.*

recycling using materials over again in the same process as before.

compost rotted vegetable and animal matter, used as fertilizer.

biodegradable of chemical compounds, those that can be decomposed by living organisms to harmless waste products so that they do not persist in the environment.

persistent a term that refers to chemicals that cannot be broken down to harmless waste products and that therefore accumulate in the food chain (see Figure 21–2).

In summary, human waste materials can cycle through the natural world in ways that benefit life on earth or at least do no harm—but when there are too many of them, and when they are dumped in the wrong places, they can spread disease among people, pollute the water, and threaten all life forms. Know how the sewage in your area is treated, and support responsible sewage treatment. Know what becomes of the litter and trash in your area, and support source reduction and recycling.

≡▶ *Solid wastes, in the form of both biodegradable solids from sewage and persistent solids such as plastics, are accumulating in the environment. Efforts to dispose of them must improve.*

Toxic Waste

Another form of waste that people throw away is toxic wastes—poisons and other chemicals used in homes, pesticides used in agriculture, and wastes from industrial processes. Toxic wastes, if they are biodegradable, may disappear in time. If they are persistent, though, they accumulate in the organs of living things and become concentrated at the top of the **food chain**, in big fish, birds, carnivorous animals, and human beings, as shown in Figure 21–2.

food chain the sequence in which living things serve as foods for one another—actually, a pyramid (see Figure 21–2).

FIGURE 21–2 ■ **Accumulation of toxic compounds at the top of the food chain.** A person whose principal animal protein source is fish may consume about 100 pounds of fish in a year. These fish will, in turn, have consumed a few tons of plant-eating fish in the course of their lifetimes. The plant eaters, in their lifetimes, will have consumed several tons of photosynthetic producer organisms. If the producer organisms have become contaminated with toxic chemicals, these chemicals become more concentrated in the bodies of the fish that consume them. If none of the chemicals are lost along the way, *one person* ultimately eats the same amount of the contaminant as was present in the original *several tons* of producer organisms.

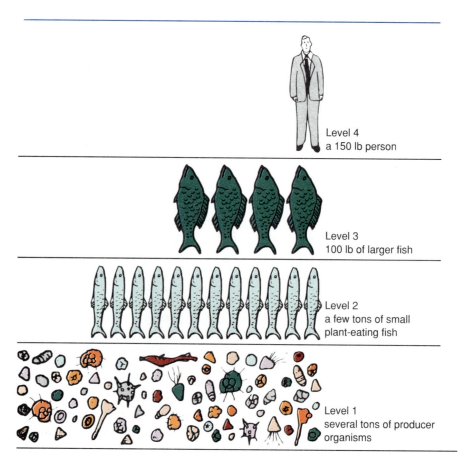

Level 4
a 150 lb person

Level 3
100 lb of larger fish

Level 2
a few tons of small plant-eating fish

Level 1
several tons of producer organisms

What can be done with toxic waste? The earth, large as it is, is a limited place, and wherever we dump our wastes, they have a way of coming back to haunt us. Unfortunately, they often don't come back quite in time to haunt those who dumped them; rather, they affect innocent bystanders who happen to settle unknowingly on the land near the dump site, where waste-containing drums leak poisons into the environment.

Of great concern because of their toxicity are agricultural pesticides that find their way into foods. Pesticide use worldwide is increasing; the hazards may be considerable; and many of them are unknown. The largest contributor of pesticides to the environment is commercial agriculture, and the consumer's chief defense against pesticides is to wash all fresh fruits and vegetables before eating or cooking them. This strategy does not, however, deal with the pesticides that may contaminate the water supply or, through it, the plant and animal tissues that people eat.

On occasion, too, mishaps occur with pesticides, such as spills, mixing of the poisons into animal feed or food destined for human consumption, or illegal overuse. Then these chemicals, no longer a gradually growing threat to life, become deadly contaminants of air, water, and food. For example, a manufacturer may use grain, treated with a deadly poison, in a distillation process and then sell the grain residue, illegally, to farmers. Unaware of the hazard, they may then feed it to their cattle, whence it may find its way into milk, ice cream, and meat products over a wide area. Or a truck or train carrying poisons may overturn, spilling them into a river, killing the fish and poisoning people's wells. Such episodes are rare, but when they occur, they are devastating.

In the crush of other environmental emergencies, the toxics problem may seem to be just one more, but it is one of the most pressing problems. Scientists are alarmed by the growing use of toxic chemicals: tens of thousands of chemicals are in commercial use in the United States, and only a few have been tested for their health effects. Screening, regulation, and monitoring of their use and disposal are urgently needed.

More subtle, but no less lethal, are gradual releases of poisons into the soil and water supply. These threaten everyone's ability to produce safe food or to obtain pure drinking water.

An example of a pollutant in our domestic environment today is the heavy metal, lead. Symptoms of mild lead poisoning include reduced ability of the blood to carry oxygen, intestinal cramps, fatigue, and kidney abnormalities; these symptoms may be reversible if exposure stops soon enough. More severe lead poisoning, however, causes irreversible nerve damage, paralysis, mental retardation in children, spontaneous abortions, and death.[7]

Lead is readily transferred across the placenta, and its most severe effects on the fetus are on the developing nervous system. Absorption of lead is five to eight times greater in children than it is in adults, and it tends to stay in their bodies.[8] Only one year of exposure can irreversibly damage the brain, nervous system, and psychological functioning.[9] Furthermore, recent experiments have shown that the effects occur with lower doses than had been thought in the past. Even children who have only moderately elevated blood lead levels and who have never had high exposures show deficits in school performance—in speed, dexterity, verbal memory, language functions, concentration, and reasoning. Based on these experiments, 1 million children in the United States may now be showing permanent damage caused by lead.[10] Three trends are occurring simultaneously. Scientists are discovering that lead poisoning has more *subtle* effects than had heretofore been appreciated; these effects are more *permanent* than had been known earlier, and they are being found at *lower levels of exposure* than before. At least 1 out of every 50 children in rural areas and more than 1 out of every 10 inner-city children are afflicted with lead poisoning—an average of about 4 percent of all children.[11]

Lead appears in all foods, and is also the nation's most significant contaminant in drinking water. Whether some of it is naturally present is not known, but much of it is known to come from industrial pollution. People use lead in gasoline, paint, batteries, pesticides, and industrial processes that release it into the air and water. Exposures are higher in urban and industrial areas, near highways, and in slums, where children may accidentally ingest leaded paint by teething on old furniture, toys, and the railings of old buildings. Old plumbing is made of lead, and it dissolves into water—especially soft water. A major source of lead is canned food, including evaporated milk, because many cans are sealed with lead solder. Food is also contaminated in the fields by the air pollution from leaded gasoline, by way of rainfall and soil. No monitoring system keeps track of the amounts to which people are exposed.

A strategy known as **source reduction** is advocated to deal with persistent pollutants, and especially toxic wastes such as lead. The idea is that, if cleaning up a toxic material after it has been produced is unsuccessful or impossible, then its production should be stopped. (Cleaning up after release is known as **end-of-pipe technology**.)

In the case of lead, source reduction is proving largely successful. The reduction of the use of leaded gasoline for automobiles and the application of new technology and materials in the canning process are helping to limit the amounts of lead in the environment and in food, and children's blood levels of lead have declined. Preschool children's lead levels are still of concern in 4 to 6 percent of cases, however, and more leaded gas is still being sold than anticipated, so considerable lead is appearing newly in the soil. Consumers would be wise to take ultraconservative measures to protect themselves, and especially their small and unborn children, from lead poisoning.*

Lead is only one of many pollutants in the environment. Another is dioxins, which are formed when chlorine combines with certain nitrogen compounds. Dioxin formation occurs wherever chlorine disinfectants and bleaches are in use. Massive dioxin contamination occurs around all pulp and paper mills, for example, because they use tons of chlorine bleach. These mills always locate on waterways, so dioxins and related compounds generated by the bleaching process have destroyed the life in whole rivers, bays, and large areas of the ocean along the Pacific Northwest, Gulf, and Atlantic coasts. If source reduction were applied in this instance, no paper bleached with chlorine would be produced; all mills would have to shift to a nontoxic bleach such as hydrogen peroxide, or produce unbleached, slightly gray paper.

source reduction limiting the production of a substance or product, a strategy for dealing with persistent, and especially, toxic, substances and materials.

end-of-pipe technology technology applied to dispose of a persistent or toxic substance after it has been produced, such as efforts to collect and degrade the substance.

---

*Obtain the booklet *Lead and Your Drinking Water*, EPA publication no. 87–006, from the U.S. Environmental Protection Agency, Office of Water, or call your local public health department.

These examples serve to illustrate the severity of individual toxic waste cases, but not the magnitude of the problem as a whole. Multiply the worst cases by 10,000, spread them all across the United States, and you will have some idea of the problem's extent and seriousness (see Figure 21–3).

Disposal of toxic wastes is profoundly difficult and expensive. Often it fails. Once millions of gallons of toxic liquid or hundreds of tons of poisoned earth have been removed from a site, after all, what can be done with them? Should they be stored in drums, which will become old and start to leak? Should they be buried somewhere? Where? In whose backyard should they be placed to contaminate the earth again?

Ideally, toxic waste should be converted chemically to harmless, inert, or useful compounds. Sometimes, that is possible. But for the most part, the only way to deal satisfactorily with the toxins produced by agricultural and industrial processes is to outlaw them—to stop them at the source, before they even enter the air, soil, or water.

Some citizens' groups think that present laws are insufficient to protect our rights to pure air, water, and food. They believe that the laws should have more "teeth" in them—that is, the laws should punish polluters more severely than they do now. "Someone else" will not control runaway technologies, these groups say, nor will the polluters voluntarily control

FIGURE 21–3 ■ Hazardous wastes in the United States.

The sites shown are those listed at the top of the Environmental Protection Agency's Superfund list. The Superfund is a multi-million dollar fund intended to pay for the cleanup of those sites, but it is inadequate to cover the costs, and only a few sites are receiving attention. Alaska has no sites; sites in U.S. territories are not included.

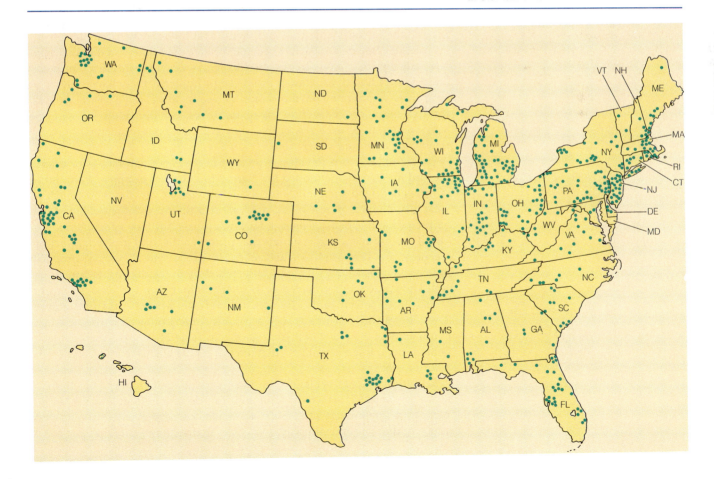

themselves. Indeed, according to one consumer group, much of the chemical industry is actively fighting *against* government curbs on toxic exposures.[12] Citizens must band together to make their demands heard—marshalling the scientific evidence, lobbying Congress, litigating in court, alerting the press—to force industry, our government, and our neighbors to curb the hazards. Producers of toxic wastes need to know in advance that their actions have consequences, and that they cannot get away with crimes against the environment.

≡▶ *Toxic wastes accumulate in the environment from many sources. End-of-pipe technologies are seldom successful in cleaning them up; source reduction, when used, is effective. Consumer vigilance and activism can help stop the production of toxic wastes at their sources.*

Radioactive Waste

Outranking the other toxic wastes in the hazard it presents is radioactive waste, so it deserves a section of its own. The term **radioactivity** refers to the property some elements have, of giving off radiation. Like the ultraviolet radiation from the sun, this radiation chemically alters molecules, including the genetic material in living cells. This harms at least the organisms it strikes, because it causes burns, cancers, and birth defects; it can also damage all future generations of those organisms by causing mutations in their gametes—ova and sperm cells. If a person's genetic material is mutated, then all the person's children, and theirs, and theirs, may carry the defect.

Materials that are radioactive become inactive over time, but the time may be of any duration: days, weeks, months, years, or even centuries. The most hazardous radioactive materials produced by human activity have extremely long lives, numbering in thousands of years. Since radioactivity passes through most barriers as if they were not there, it is difficult to store radioactive materials in such a way that they will not damage nearby life unalterably for all future generations.

Some radioactive materials are present in the earth naturally—for example, radon, already mentioned in Chapter 19. Another example is uranium, which is collected from mines for use in nuclear power plants and nuclear weapons. Nuclear power plants are intended to improve the quality of life by providing inexpensive energy for human use, but they generate quantities of radioactive waste materials that present a disposal problem. Nuclear weapons are supposed to stabilize world peace, but they, too, produce radioactive wastes, and they are threatened by accidents and terrorism. A well-known accident occurred in 1986 at Chernobyl in the western Soviet Union and spewed radioactive waste over the whole world (see Figure 21–4), but it was only one of such accidents—many others have occurred. A chronology of the worst of them is shown in Table 21–1. With such a record behind them, it seems unlikely that nuclear plants will have an accident-free record ahead.

Radioactive waste spills are the most serious spills known. No human sense can detect radioactivity, and so it can do immeasurable harm before people are even aware of it. Such accidents can be prevented in only two ways—either by eliminating the sources so that accidents can't happen or by

radioactivity   the release of radiation from the nuclei of atoms.

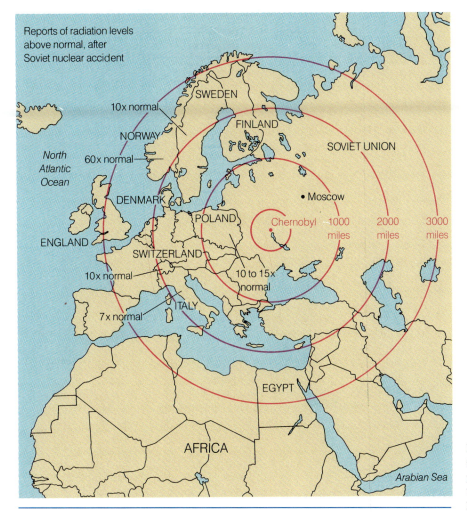

FIGURE 21–4 ■ Radiation levels after the Chernobyl nuclear accident, 1986.
Radiation levels rose briefly worldwide; in the United States, they were highest in Boise, Idaho.

making the nuclear power plants and arsenals totally safe from accidents or vandalism. Many believe that only the first alternative will work.

≡▶ *Radioactive materials are a special category of toxic wastes because all of them can alter genetic material, producing cancers, birth defects, and inheritable abnormalities. Radon gas is a naturally occurring source. Nuclear power plants and arsenals are human-operated sources, and the spills and wastes they produce represent an unsolved disposal problem.*

■≡ Natural Environments

The earth's natural environments produce the resources we need to sustain our lives. Natural environments renew themselves naturally; recycling is a way of life for them. Plant life captures carbon dioxide and returns oxygen to the air. Forests and wetlands cleanse water, restore soil, and serve as

TABLE 21–1   ■   **A Chronology of the World's Worst Nuclear Accidents**

When and Where	What Happened
December 2, 1952, Chalk River, Canada	Employee error leads to 1 million gallons of radioactive water leaking inside an experimental nuclear reactor, forcing a six-month cleanup.
October 7–10, 1957, Windscale Pile, Liverpool, England	A fire in a plutonium-production reactor leads to the largest then known accidental release of radioactive material. Government later attributes 39 cancer deaths to it.
1957, Ural Mountains, Soviet Union	A nuclear accident occurs, probably at a weapons facility. From available information, it is believed that hundreds of square miles had to be evacuated.
May 23, 1958, Chalk River, Canada	A second accident, sparked by an overheated fuel rod, leads to another long cleanup.
January 3, 1961, Idaho Falls, Idaho	A steam explosion at a military experimental reactor kills three servicemen.
October 5, 1966, Enrico Fermi plant, Detroit, Michigan	In an experimental breeder reactor, part of the fuel core melts, producing high radiation levels within the plant.
October 17, 1969, Saint-Laurent, France	A fuel-loading error leads to partial meltdown.
November 19, 1971, Monticello, Minnesota	A power company reactor's waste storage space overflows, releasing 50,000 gallons of radioactive water into the Mississippi River.
March 22, 1975, Browns Ferry reactor, Decatur, Illinois	A worker using a candle to check for air leaks starts a $150 million fire that lowers cooling water to dangerous levels.
March 28, 1979, Three Mile Island, Middletown, Pennsylvania	A partial meltdown occurs, and some radioactivity is released into the atmosphere in what some consider the worst U.S. commercial nuclear mishap. The plant was still being decontaminated years later.
August 7, 1979, Top secret fuel plant, Erwin, Tennessee	Accidental release of enriched uranium exposes 1,000 people to above-normal doses of radiation.
February 11, 1981, Sequoyah 1, Tennessee Valley	More than 100,000 gallons of radioactive coolant leak into the containment building; eight workers are exposed to radiation.
April 19, 1984, Sequoyah 1, Tennessee Valley	A second accident occurs when superheated radioactive water erupts during a maintenance procedure.
April 26, 1986, Chernobyl, Soviet Union	A fire starts, meltdown occurs, and a cloud of radioactive fallout spreads worldwide. 2,000 people near the plant are affected; 11 die; many receive bone marrow transplants; many more are expected to contract cancer and other illnesses and to pass on genetic defects to their unborn children.

SOURCE: Adapted from A chronology of notable nuclear accidents worldwide, *Tallahassee Democrat*, 30 April 1986.

breeding grounds for each season's new generations of animal life. Air, water, and soil support the plants and animals that provide our food. Today, however, the world's rapidly growing human population is displacing the natural environments on which life depends.

People and Land

Even without industrialization, a large enough mass of human beings upsets the life-sustaining balance in an area. The migration of human beings down the western coast of North America caused the extinction, by hunting, of all the species of large animals that used to live in that area. The mountains of China are now bare over thousands of square miles because people of earlier times, living in primitive conditions, burned all the trees for firewood. Now, erosion has worn the mountains to bare rock, and the land has become an uninhabitable moonscape. The cedars of Lebanon were wiped out in the same way, beginning in biblical times, and even the Sahara

Desert is a desert partly because of human misuse of once-fertile land.[13] All over the world, deserts are growing. Dust blown from the ever-growing Sahara Desert now darkens the air all the way to Florida. Irrigation of wheatlands to feed beef cattle, and trampling of rangelands by those cattle, are making deserts out of much of Texas and other western states. (Irrigation produces deserts because, as water evaporates it leaves salts behind, as well as less water with which to continue irrigating.)

The vast wastelands of China, Lebanon, and the Sahara were created by people living *primitively*—cutting trees for homes, for firewood, and to clear the land for agriculture. People living in modern industrialized societies use many times the fuel and generate many times the waste, and faster, so they use up the land faster. Witness the fact that the United States produces 3,000 pounds of toxic wastes for every man, woman, and child, every year.[14] The two factors together are especially destructive: the sheer numbers of people we add up to, combined with our use of polluting processes and products, makes each of us a tremendous polluter.

Where there is human habitation, there is also light and noise—and **light and noise pollution**. Pure darkness is needed for the renewal of many kinds of wildlife. (Baby turtles hatch on the beach on moonless nights and instinctively crawl toward the reflections of stars on the water; but when a highway is built too near the beach, they crawl instead toward the highway lights and are killed by passing cars.) Silence also is needed. (When the noise of cars and radios is audible within half a mile of the nests of water birds, they become unable to raise their young and abandon the nesting site.) Periods of darkness and silence are also human needs, and excessive light and sound are forms of stress.

light pollution abnormal amounts of light in the environment, which disrupt life processes.

noise pollution abnormal amounts of noise in the environment, which disrupt life processes.

≡▶ *Human populations tend to wipe out forests and fertile lands, produce deserts, and disrupt natural environments with light and noise pollution. Wild lands and wildlife diminish as human populations spread.*

The Rainforests: A Case in Point

The disappearance of wild lands through human intervention today is nearing its final stages. A case in point is the rapid loss of the world's tropical rainforests. These forests are fast disappearing all over the globe; in the Amazon River valley alone they are being destroyed at the rate of an area the size of Massachusetts every month. Because the tropical rainforests contain more than half of all the species that remain on earth, the loss of those forests is now bringing about the greatest destruction of life forms that has ever occurred on earth.

The rainforests have existed for millions of years. They are vast—three-dimensional—miles wide, miles long, and over a hundred feet deep. Millions on millions of species of animals and plants not yet known to science thrive in their honeycomb of multitudinous spaces. Within 1 acre of these forests dwell 800,000 pounds of living things.[15]

The forests are destroyed for many purposes people call "development." One such purpose is to grow beef cattle. If an acre of rainforest is cleared to plant grass and grow beef, its soil fertility lasts for only about eight years. Within that eight years, the acre will produce 50 pounds of cattle per year—

400 pounds in all. Of that, 200 pounds is usable meat, enough to yield 800 4-ounce hamburgers. The trade-off: 55 square feet of forest, representing half a ton of forest life, lost permanently for each hamburger.[16]

At the end of eight years of such use of the land, large applications of fertilizer, pesticides, and irrigation are needed to prolong the land's usefulness. These inputs both poison and deplete the water supply and the soil. When the whole region's forest is gone, the land becomes uninhabitable, not only for cattle but also for all other life, including human beings. The last of the soil washes away, leaving bare clay, and ultimately, rain ceases to fall. This is one of many ways in which natural environments are turning to deserts all over the world.

Loss of soil, worldwide, is one of the greatest threats facing the human race. It is increasing every year. At present, it amounts to 25 billion tons a year, enough to fill Yankee Stadium 175,000 times.[17] Nature (where there are trees) creates new soil at the rate of a centimeter every 80 to 280 years, but soil loss due to human misuse of the land today is taking place at a much greater rate.

The reasons why deforestation and soil loss are occurring are complex, but they often have to do with land ownership and greed. The poor own little land, and as they multiply, they are forced onto "undeveloped" government land (wild land) to attempt to support their families. They make roads into the rainforest and start the process by which "development" can take place. They can make money by clearing the land, but they can live on it only for a short while; without the protective cover of trees and the annual allotment of nutritive litter the trees drop on the land, it quickly loses its soil, moisture, and fertility. So the poor move on and clear more land, and speculators follow behind them on the roads that they have made. Having reaped what profits they can, they, too, move on, leaving the land barren behind them. By way of this process, about half of the world's rainforests have been cleared or severely degraded within the last half century. Within 20 more years, the process will be over, for no more forest will be left. In many countries, the end has come already.

Even though we consumers may not personally be clearing rainforest land, our demands for products are driving the process. U.S. companies annually purchase more than 330 million pounds of beef a year from Central American countries alone—an amount that represents 90 percent of that region's beef exports.[18] The demand comes largely from our innumerable fast-food hamburger establishments. Consumers buy the beef, and the trees continue to fall.

Clearly, development as traditionally practiced—by devouring natural resources and destroying natural environments—cannot permanently achieve solutions to any of the world's problems. It cannot even bring prosperity to people in the regions where it is taking place, for what they may gain in temporary income, they lose in the loss of the resources that produced that income. If development produces dollars at the cost of natural resources, no profit is really taking place, except on paper. What is rainfall worth? Soil? Forest vegetation? Animal life? The clean air and water that they generate? A true accounting of their worth would provide a guideline for development worth following.

The traditional concept of development by exploitation must be replaced by that of **sustainable development**. This kind of development supports the

sustainable development   development that betters people's economic well-being, not only in the short term, but also in the long term.

resources it depends on, replacing what it uses. It borrows water, but it returns it pure. It cuts trees, but it plants an equal number of them. It may work within natural ecosystems, but it disrupts them minimally.

≡▶ *Deforestation and soil loss are causing loss of the world's rainforests. Sustainable use of these resources could halt these processes.*

The Value of Species Diversity

The preservation of natural environments matters, not only in terms of air, water, and land for people, but also for wild species that otherwise will become extinct. So far, scientists have studied, for medicinal use, only about 2 percent of all the likely plants and animals on earth, yet every single day several plant and wildlife species become extinct because people destroy their habitats. By the end of this century, if extinction continues at the present rate, we will have lost 1 million of the 5 to 10 million species we now still possess. This may mean hundreds of thousands of lifesaving drugs, for more than 50 percent of such drugs prescribed today trace their origins to such species. A dramatic example is penicillin, a lifesaving drug from a wild mold. Also, drugs prepared from a tropical forest plant, the rosy periwinkle, are used to treat young people with leukemia, and have improved their chances for remission from 1 in 5 to 4 in 5. Commercial sales of drugs from this one plant alone now total around $100 million per year. The total spent on all drugs of plant origin is around $20 billion a year.

More examples are these: some types of birth control pills from the Mexican yam; digitalis (a heartbeat strengthener) from the purple foxglove; reserpine (a tranquilizer) from the root of a small Asian shrub; and quinine (an antimalaria drug) from the bark of the cinchona tree. The octopus yields an extract that relieves hypertension; a sea snake produces an anticoagulant; and a Caribbean sponge manufactures a compound that acts against viruses, much as penicillin does against bacteria. Experts might look forward

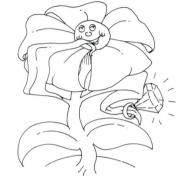

Wild species possess many still-undiscovered treasures.

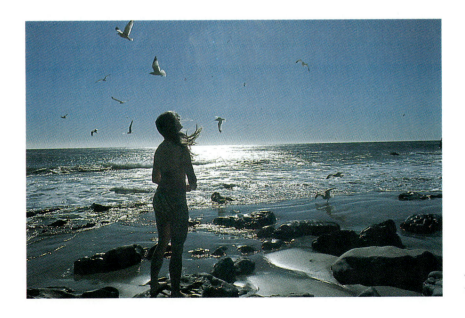

To support healthy fisheries, oceans must be unpolluted.

to many more discoveries as important to health as penicillin, if only the species still exist to be studied.

Another reason we should attempt to preserve the quality of our environment is that the needs of all living things are similar. If the trees, grasses, birds, and flowers in our surroundings are not flourishing, then whether we perceive it or not, the conditions that we need to survive are deteriorating. Biologists know that "birds are indicators of the environment, a sort of litmus paper. Because of their furious pace of living and high rate of metabolism, they reflect subtle changes in the environment rather quickly; they warn us of things out of balance."[19] In fact, the biological quality of a region can be measured by the abundance and variety of its bird life. Miners know this, too; the practice of taking a canary into the mine is the miner's way of self-protection. If the canary sickens and dies, it's time for the miner to hurry out of the mine, for the air is becoming too foul to support human life.

To some people, the extinction of species matters simply for its own sake, as well. We affiliate with other organisms; we need them deeply.[20] The preservation of other species is a moral and ethical responsibility; it concerns us in a deep, spiritual way. Our Native American predecessors, the Indians, have always known:

> This we know. The Earth does not belong to man; man belongs to the Earth. This we know. All things are connected like the blood which unites one family. All things are connected. Whatever befalls the Earth befalls the sons of the Earth. Man did not weave the web of life, he is merely a strand in it. Whatever he does to the web, he does to himself. —Chief Seattle, 1854

≡▶ *Loss of species accompanies the loss of natural environments, a loss with both economic and ethical significance.*

■≡ The Population Problem

The beginning of this chapter promised that if you would work your way through the huge problems described in these sections, some solutions would await you at the end. There is hope—because the world's nations are able to act as a unit, and to act quickly, for the first time in history. Two current trends make this possible: the explosion of scientific knowledge about environmental problems and the world's increasing use of fast communications to make that knowledge available to all governments simultaneously. Information is a form of stored energy, and energy can do work. Information and awareness shared among people can bring about rapid decision making and action. The new global awareness of our shared problems is the source of our hope.

Every expert agrees that all the other problems described up to this point are tied to the greatest problem of all—the world's exploding population. This second-last section therefore focuses on that problem. If we are aware of it and face it, as a single species working together, we can solve it. The chapter ends with "global strategies" to which you can contribute with your own personal awareness and sense of urgency.

These three trends are occurring simultaneously, threatening life on this earth:

1. The spread of industrialization.
2. The destruction of natural environments.
3. The multiplication of people.

The effects of each trend compound those of the others, because, as already emphasized, every person in an industrialized society devours the earth's resources and pollutes the environment much more heavily than a person in a primitive society.

Our present dilemma has been developing throughout human history. It took us a million years to arrive at a population size of a billion in the mid-1800s. A mere 80 years later, we numbered 2 billion; in the 50 years following, we more than doubled again. As this book goes to press, we number over 5 billion, and each year, the number of people added to the population is greater than the number added the year before. If the growth rate remains steady, in less than 50 years, the number of people on earth will reach the maximum that the earth can support—close to 10 billion people.[21] At that level, life for most people will barely be possible, and conditions will be much worse than they are today. Already millions are starving; agricultural and grazing lands are eroding and being paved over; soils are becoming more salty; water shortages are worsening; rainfall is dwindling as the world's forests shrink; ocean pollution and overfishing are leading to smaller catches and less variety; and widespread extinctions of plants and animals are taking place. As shortages develop, people and nations become needy and irrational, and the threat of global destruction through nuclear war looms ever greater.

Even the richest and most protected people on earth are now feeling the effects of the population's growth. People in growing cities are noticing greater crowding, more noise, more cars, more toxins, more crime, more illness, and simultaneously less peace, less quiet, less greenery, less oxygen, less clean air and water. They also experience the effects of population growth indirectly, in the scarcity of resources that once were common. The more people crowd into cities, the more land outside the cities is needed to produce food for those people, but as the suburbs advance, less land is available—hence the shortages and rising costs of food, water, fuel, and other resources.

People in industrial societies often fear that to stop population growth would be to stop progress. This view assumes that growth and progress are the same thing, but they are not. Growth means only greater numbers; progress is intentional movement toward a goal. Further increases in population will drain the economy, not foster its growth, because rising numbers of people mean more people living in poverty. Progress toward meeting the basic needs of our present population could take place better without growth. People who must scramble for food and water have no energy to strive for higher purposes. In fact, growth must stop for real progress to continue; people must limit their numbers.

Two factors hinder success in population control. One is that people who want to use birth control methods often can't get them; the other is that many people resist using them. They want too many children. Of the two problems, the first is easier to solve, but it is no small task. It requires materials, experts, transport, planning, money—and political support. Not only are the resources hard to obtain, but also the political support is unpredictable.

It is even harder to change people's traditional attitudes, such as the desire for large families, but political decisions can override them. The leaders of China, for example, have tried to limit the offspring of each family to one child by offering tax incentives and other motivators. The first hints of such initiatives in the United States are now appearing as well.

In the name of public health, precedents already exist for regulations that limit individual rights. Mandatory vaccinations and safety belt laws are two familiar cases in this country. With an issue as urgent as population control, each society must look at needs both within and beyond its borders and meet those needs with programs that are socially and politically right for them—and for the earth.

≡▶   *The world's population has reached 5 billion and is growing at an unprecedented rate. This growth combined with increasing industrialization constitutes the greatest environmental problem the planet faces. Initiatives to control population growth offer hope.*

■≡ A Way to the Future

An encouraging development in work toward the world's future is that some of the best minds are bringing their powers to bear on these problems. For example, much powerful, positive thinking is coming from the Worldwatch Institute—an independent, nonprofit research institution created to analyze and focus attention on global problems.* Worldwatch is funded by private foundations and by the United Nations, and its papers are written for a worldwide audience of decision makers, scholars, and students. Its *State of the World* report, which comes out annually, not only keeps track of trends in all areas, such as deforestation and fuel use, but also goes beyond stating problems to analyze and compare possible solutions. *State of the World* is used as a text in more and more college courses, and is helping to make tomorrow's leaders aware of the areas on which they need to focus their attention.

The Worldwatch Institute has made an ingenious suggestion: rather than everyone's trying to tackle all the world's problems simultaneously, the nations that have the greatest power to affect each problem should focus on that problem. For example, of the 83 million people added to the world's population last year, China and India accounted for a third of the total. Those two countries should emphasize population control the most heavily, and be encouraged to do so by the others. Similarly, of all the world's increases in carbon dioxide and global warming, caused by the burning of fossil fuels, half appears to be caused by only three nations—the United States, the Soviet Union, and China. Similarly, three nations contain more than half of the remaining tropical rainforests—Brazil, Indonesia, and Zaire—so efforts at conservation should focus on them. Substantial changes can be brought about if the right efforts are made by the right groups.

*Worldwatch Institute, 1776 Massachusetts Ave. NW, Washington, D.C. 20036.

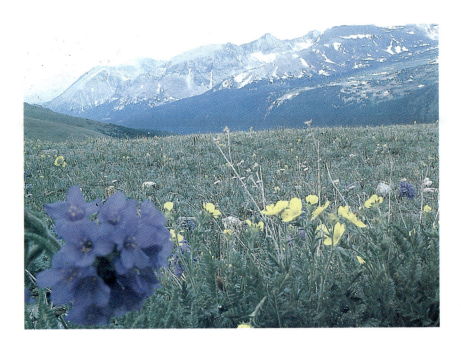

The earth is better off where there are fewer people on it.

One of those groups is American consumers. Major categories of pollutants generated by individuals include fuel burned to run cars and other forms of transportation, and fuel burned to heat and cool homes and run home appliances. These reflect personal, individual choices—our own lifestyle choices. The days when we could blame major industrial polluters for most of our problems are over—they still do their share, but small consumers are now the major contributors to the pollution of our environment. When asked at a major conference on the rainforest what we as individuals could do to help reverse the growing deforestation tragedy, several world experts said, "Convince U.S. consumers to change their own lifestyles." Many avenues are open to us—we can demand that our cars be designed to get 200 miles to the gallon—already a feasible possibility. Or we can demand that they be fueled in the future with hydrogen, whose waste product is pure, nonpolluting water. We can also eat less beef.

≡▶ *Unprecedented public and private efforts are under way to halt the world's environmental decline. Individual initiatives toward conservation can also help.*

To make choices consistent with environmental sustainability will require that citizens learn to live by a less materialistic value system than in the past. To do so will help considerably to reduce the burden we human beings place on the earth's carrying capacity. It can also bring each of us great personal satisfaction, as this chapter's Spotlight reveals.

■≡ For Review

1. Define the term *environment,* and describe the relationship that exists between human beings and their external environment.

2. Describe how air, water, and soil support human life and how human beings can in turn support them.

3. Explain what the greenhouse effect is, why it is occurring, and what its effects are expected to be.

4. Explain why ozone depletion is occurring in the earth's outer atmosphere, and why this is of concern to human health.

5. List the effects of human-generated air pollutants on human health and on the physical environment.

6. Describe harmful compounds found in water and their impacts on human health.

7. Explain why water quantity is as important as water quality.

8. Discuss two classes of contaminants deposited directly on the soil as the result of human life and activity, and describe measures to manage them.

9. Define the term *carrying capacity.*

10. Explain why toxic waste is a pressing environmental problem.

11. List examples of toxic waste that pose particular problems, and explain why they offer cause for special concern.

12. Distinguish between source reduction and end-of-pipe technology as ways of dealing with toxic waste.

13. List personal strategies to deal with environmental hazards.

14. Explain why human beings are likely to suffer detrimental effects from the continuing extinction of plant and animal species.

15. Discuss the relationship between population size and industrialization, as well as the impact of both on human beings and on the environment.

16. Describe current trends in population growth, along with outcomes that are likely if those trends continue.

17. Describe measures designed to cope with the population problem.

18. List long-range objectives for worldwide environmental protection.

■≡ Notes

1. W. C. Clark, Managing planet earth, *Scientific American,* September 1989, pp. 47–54.

2. J. D. Bernal, *The Origin of Life* (Cleveland: World Publishing, 1967), pp. 100–109.

3. R. Crum, More on less ozone, *Harvard Magazine,* May/June 1987, pp. 4, 6.

4. Skin cancer increases, *Health Gazette,* March 1989, p. 4.

5. R. W. Shaw, Air pollution by particles, *Scientific American,* August 1987, pp. 96–103.

6. Three of the nation's leading doctors, testifying before a U.S. Senate subcommittee on environmental pollution, according to P. Shabecoff, Acid rain seen as posing risks for U.S. health, *New York Times,* 4 February 1987, p. A12.

7. E. N. Whitney, C. B. Cataldo, and S. R. Rolfes, *Understanding Normal and Clinical Nutrition,* 3d ed. (St. Paul, Minn.: West, 1991), pp. 344–347.

8. Whitney, Cataldo, and Rolfes, 1991.

9. Whitney, Cataldo, and Rolfes, 1991.

10. Whitney, Cataldo, and Rolfes, 1991.

11. Whitney, Cataldo, and Rolfes, 1991.

12. Undated letter, 1986, from Public Citizen, a consumer group founded by Ralph Nader in 1971.

13. M. W. Mikewell, The deforestation of Mount Lebanon, *Geographical Review,* January 1969, pp. 1–28; J. J. Cloudsley-Thompson, Recent expansion of the Sahara, in *Key Environments: Sahara Desert,* ed. J. J. Cloudsley-Thompson (Oxford, England: Pergamon, 1984), pp. 8–14.

14. Did you know? *Inform,* 1986 (a newsletter available from 381 Park Ave. S, New York, NY 10016).

15. C. Uhl and G. Parker, Viewpoint: Our steak in the jungle, *BioScience* 36 (1986): 642.

16. Uhl and Parker, 1986.

17. T. Peterson, Hunger and the environment, *Seeds,* October 1987, pp. 6–13.

18. J. D. Nations and D. I. Komer, Rainforests and the hamburger society, *Environment,* April 1983, pp. 12–20.

19. R. T. Peterson, as cited by B. Yokel, president, Florida Audubon Society, in a letter to the members, 25 June 1986.

20. E. O. Wilson, *Biophilia: The Human Bond with Other Species* (Cambridge, Mass.: Harvard University Press, 1984), pp. 119–140.

21. B. Bull, Voodoo demography: What population problem? *Amicus Journal,* Fall 1984, pp. 36–40.

SPOTLIGHT

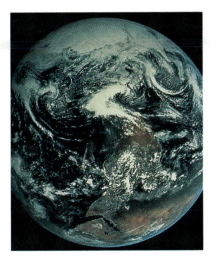

Personal Strategy— Voluntary Simplicity

The problems of the environment and the world's multiplying population may appear so great that they seem approachable only by way of worldwide political decisions. But consider this: you can change the world. To describe some ways in which an individual can accomplish this is, perhaps, the most fitting way to conclude a book about personal choices. After all, a society is the sum of its individuals; as we go, so goes our world.

I feel much too insignificant to have any effect on the way the world goes. In fact, when I think about what's happening around me, I feel overwhelmed, depressed, and pessimistic.

Every thoughtful person feels that way at times and is tempted to give up. Optimism can be cultivated, though, and many people are intentionally doing just that.[1]* They know that optimism gives them energy and makes their efforts to shape the world's future more effective.

How do I go about cultivating optimism?

By living your own life. Don't try to solve all the world's problems. Mentally draw a small circle around yourself, and work as energetically as you can to better yourself through education, spiritual growth, and physical health. Work, too, to better the small world within the circle around yourself.

That sounds simple enough, but I don't see how it will help anything. In fact, it almost sounds selfish.

It will help, though. Every move you make leaves the world a better or worse place. Your actions have a ripple effect, often far beyond what you may think. Tending compassionately to the lives nearest you, including your own, is your first responsibility. Many great religious teachings express that value.

Your second responsibility is to make sure you can answer yes to the question, If everyone lived as I do, would the children of today grow up in a better world? Those who study the future are convinced that the hope of the world lies in everyone's adopting a simple lifestyle. As one such person put it, "The widespread simplification of life is vital to the well-being of the entire human family."[2]

*Reference notes are at the end of the Spotlight.

Are you implying that everybody needs to adopt a life of poverty? I can't envision how my being poor would help anyone. Besides, wealthy people would never agree.

No, the suggestion is not that everyone become poor. It is said that "poverty is repressive, simplicity is liberating. Poverty generates a sense of helplessness . . . simplicity fosters creativity. Poverty is mean and degrading . . . simplicity is enabling."[3] In other words, to become poor would solve nothing—poverty obstructs personal growth; simplicity opens the way to it. You are also right that few people would willingly give up their wealth, even if it did help. What *is* advocated has nothing to do with wealth. It is a lifestyle, a commitment to live more simply in view of the world's limited resources.[4]

Think in terms of *elegance*, not poverty. Streamlined things, things that have no unnecessary frills, are elegant. Life is, too. Don't carry extra baggage around; it only burdens you.

What does living a life of voluntary simplicity involve?

A thousand small decisions—of which we will offer a hundred. Before reading them, be sure to understand that they are not "the" rules, but only a sampling deemed appropriate by one school of thought. *Voluntary* is a key word, just as *simplicity* is. Each individual must look within to discover a personal sense of what is appropriate. "Crucial to acting in a voluntary manner is being aware of ourselves as we move through life. This requires that we not only pay attention to the actions we take . . . but also that we pay attention to the person [ourselves]."[5]

TABLE S21–1 ■ Ninety-nine Ways to a Simple Lifestyle

Heating and Cooling	Other Home Conserving	Food	Gardening	Solid Waste
Save heat and insulate	Light house efficiently	Consume less meat	Garden on available land	Avoid disposable paper products
Keep furnace operating properly	Save water	Select unprocessed foods	Grow vegetables	Refrain from purchasing plastic-wrapped items
Regulate humidity in heated homes	Avoid aerosol sprays	Avoid non-nutritious food	Plant fruit trees	
Conserve cooking energy	Use few cleaning products	Reduce intake of refined sugar	Fertilize wisely	Ban nonreturnables
Refrigerate wisely	Budget resources	Eat wild foods	Use natural pesticides	Sort trash
Design buildings with ecology in mind	Build a yurt	Learn to preserve food	Compost and mulch	Use flush-less toilets
Cut hot-water costs	Make home repairs	Conserve nutritional value of food	Keep bees	
Economize with modular heating	Paint the home	Be aware of agribusiness		
Cool conservatively and ventilate	Make, repair, and reuse furniture	Organize a food co-op		
Dehumidify in summer	Eliminate unnecessary appliances	Bake bread		
Air-condition minimally		Prepare various food products		
Convert to renewable fuel sources (organic, solar, wind)[a]		Drink homemade beverages		
		Advocate breastfeeding		
		Question pets and pet food		

Clothing	Fulfillment	Health	Transportation	Community
Choose fabrics wisely	Have a hobby	Use simple personal products	Know bicycle benefits and servicing	Live communally
Pick quality clothing	Become artistic	Select safe cosmetics	Bike safely	Refurbish old homes
Make clothing	Decorate the home simply	Beware of hair dyes	Encourage mass transit	Provide pure drinking water
Mend and reuse garments	Create toys and games	Do not abuse drugs	Share the car	Join a craft cooperative
Do not wear fur from endangered species	Preserve a place for quiet	Stop smoking cigarettes	Avoid unnecessary auto travel	Care for the elderly and ill
Protect the feet	Camp and backpack	Curb alcohol abuse	Buy cars thriftily	Have simple funerals
	Enjoy recreational sports	Prepare for environmental extremes	Choose proper gas	Influence legislation
	Exercise without equipment	Guard against home hazards	Drive conservatively	Consumers beware
		Recognize signs of chronic disease	Seek proper maintenance and service	Battle utilities
		Care for teeth		Demand corporate responsibility
		Watch weight		Start recycling projects
		Learn to rest and relax		Fight environmental pollution
				Improve land use
				Create work and study opportunities

[a]The book from which this list was adapted devotes a chapter each to organic, solar, and wind fuel sources. These therefore count as three of the 99 topics in the book.

SOURCE: Center for Science in the Public Interest, Simple Lifestyle Team, *99 Ways to a Simple Lifestyle* (Garden City, N.Y.: Anchor Books, 1977).

Each person needs to find a balance—a path, suitable for that individual, that leads between the extremes of poverty and self-indulgence.

That makes sense. Now tell me: what are the 100 ways?

Here are 99 of them, in Table S21–1. They were developed by a team of researchers who had been given the assignment of describing the elements of a simple lifestyle. They wrote 99 short chapters under ten headings: heating and cooling, other methods of home conservation, food, gardening, solid waste, clothing, fulfillment, health, transportation, and community. The book from which the list was taken offers many more pointers under each heading, of course, but you can get a sense of what a simple lifestyle comprises just by reading the chapter titles listed in the table.*

But you said there were 100 ways. What's the last one?

To better yourself. Improving yourself is the first step toward improving the world—remember the ripple effect.

*Another book of excellent suggestions for meeting personal responsibilities to the world is one produced under the auspices of the American Friends Service Committee: J. Bodner, ed., *Taking Charge of Our Lives: Living Responsibly in a Troubled World* (San Francisco: Harper and Row, 1984).

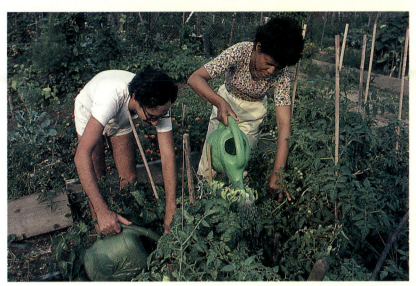

A spot of shared earth enables city dwellers to grow their own vegetables, promoting both mental and physical health.

Learn all you can; work on your emotional and spiritual growth. You will then be better equipped to participate fully and responsibly in the world community.

Do you really think that if everyone made choices like these, it would help the state of the world?

Yes. Every agency that has studied the future has reached the same conclusion: voluntary simplicity can work. It does not mean living primitively; most people prefer beauty and ease to ugliness and discomfort. It does mean seeking a life free of distractions, clutter, and pretense—a life that includes self-discipline. The words of an old poem speak to this idea, and they are a fitting close to this discussion:

Beyond a wholesome discipline, be gentle with yourself. You are a child of the universe, no less than the trees and the stars; you have a right to be here. And whether or not it is clear to you, no doubt the universe is unfolding as it should. Therefore be at peace with God, whatever you conceive him to be, and whatever your labors and aspirations . . . keep peace with your soul.

Desiderata, author unknown; found in Old St. Paul's Church, Baltimore, dated 1692

▪≡ Spotlight Notes

1. E. Cornish and the World Future Society, *The Study of the Future: An Introduction to the Art and Science of Understanding and Shaping Tomorrow's World* (Washington, D.C.: World Future Society, 1977), pp. 34–37.

2. D. Elgin, *Voluntary Simplicity: Toward a Way of Life That Is Outwardly Simple, Inwardly Rich* (New York: Morrow, 1981), p. 25.
3. Elgin, 1981, pp. 32–34.
4. R. E. Pestle, T. A. Cornille, and K.

Solomon, Lifestyle alternatives: Development and evaluation of an attitude scale, *Home Economics Research Journal*, December 1982, pp. 175–182.

5. Elgin, 1981, pp. 32–34.

■≡ Abuse

Abuse Hotline
1-800-342-9152

Domestic Violence Hotline
1-800-333-SAFE
(Hearing impaired)
1-800-873-6363

■≡ Accident Prevention

American National Red Cross
National Headquarters
Washington, D.C. 20006

New York City Poison Control Project
Bellevue Hospital Center
27th Street and First Avenue
New York, NY 10016

National Safety Council
1-800-621-7619

■≡ AIDS

National Hotline
1-800-342-2437

AIDS Action Council
729 8th Street, SE #200
Washington, DC 20030
(202) 293-2886

American Foundation for AIDS Research
40 West 57th Street
New York, NY 10019
(212) 719-0033

Fund for Human Dignity
666 Broadway
New York, NY 10012
(212) 529-1600

National Association of People with AIDS
2025 Eye Street, NW, Suite 415
Washington, DC 20006
(202) 429-2856

National Council of La Raza
AIDS Project
20 F Street, NW, 2nd Floor
Washington, DC 20001
(202) 628-9600

National Minority AIDS Council
714 G Street SE
Washington, DC 20003
(202) 544-1076

■≡ Alcohol and Alcohol Abuse

National Clearinghouse for Alcohol Information
Box 2345
Rockville, MD 20850

Alcohol and Drug Abuse
1-800-252-6465

National Council on Alcoholism
733 Third Ave
New York, NY 10017
1-800-NCA-CALL

Alcoholics Anonymous
P.O. Box 459, Grand Central Station
New York, NY 10163
(212) 686-1100

AL-Non/Alateen Family Group Headquarters, Inc.
P.O. Box 182
Madison Square Station
New York, NY 10159
1-800-356-9996

National Association for Children of Alcoholics
31582 Coast Highway, Suite B
South Laguna, CA 92677
(714) 499-3889

Toughlove
P.O. Box 70
Sellersville, PA 18960

■≡ Blind Services

Blind American Council
1-800-424-8666

Blind Services
1-800-342-1828

Blind and Physically Handicapped Library
1-800-342-5627

Recording for the Blind
1-800-221-4792

American Foundation for the Blind
1-800-232-5463

■≡ Cancer

Cancer Information Service
1-800-4-CANCER

Cancer Response System
1-800-ACS-2345

American Cancer Society
1-800-ACS-2345

Cancer Information (Spanish)
1-800-432-5955

Breast Cancer
1-800-626-2273

■≡ Child Health

National Center for Education in Material and Child Health
P.O. Box 28612
Washington, DC 20005
(202) 842-7617

National Commission to Prevent Infant Mortality
330 C Street, SW, Room 2006
Washington, DC 20201

Incest Survivors Anonymous
P.O. Box 35623
Los Angeles, CA 90035
(213) 464-4423

Child Abuse Hotline
1-800-422-4453

Childbirth Education
1-800-624-4934

Child Find of America
1-800-426-5678

Sudden Infant Death Syndrome
1-800-638-7437

Healthy Baby Hotline
1-800-451-2229

Infant Nutrition Hotline
1-800-523-6633

■≡ Consumer Information

Consumer Information Center
Dept. 609K
Pueblo, CO 81009

Consumer Product Safety
1-800-638-2772

Food Safety and Inspection Service
1-800-535-4555

National Council Against Health Fraud
P.O. Box 1276
Loma Linda, CA 92354

Center of the Science in Public Interest
1755 S. Street, NW
Washington, DC 20009

Office of the Secretary
Federal Trade Commission
Washington, DC 20580
(202) 523-3598

Senior Citizen Hotline
1-800-262-2243

Student Financial Assistant Service
1-800-241-4710

Parents Anonymous
1-800-421-0353

The National Assoc. for Home Care
Dept. P
519 C St., NE
Washington, DC 20002

The National Council on the Aging
Dept. P
600 Maryland Ave, SW
West Wing 100
Washington, DC 20024

Continuing-Care Accreditation Commission
Dept. P
1129 20th St., NW, Suite 412
Washington, DC 20036

Runaway Hotline
1-800-231-6946

Runaway Switchboard
1-800-621-4000

■≡ Cosmetics

Food and Drug Administration
5600 Fishers Lane
Rockville, MD 20852

■≡ Diseases

Alzheimer's Disease Hotline
1-800-272-3900

American Diabetes Association
1-800-ADA-DISC

Arthritis Clinical Center Communications
Building 10, Room 1-C 255
Bethesda, MD 20892

Arthritis Hotline
1-800-282-9487

American Parkinson Disease Assoc.
1-800-223-2732

American Diabetes Assoc.
1-800-232-3472

Epilepsy Foundation of America
1-800-EFA-1000

Diabetes/Juvenile Diabetes Foundation
1-800-223-1138

Disease Prevention Hotline
1-800-336-4797

Kidney Disease/Financial Aid
1-800-638-8399

Lung Disease
1-800-222-5864

Reye's Syndrome Access
1-800-222-4767

Sexually Transmitted Disease Hotline
1-800-227-8922

National Multiple Sclerosis Society
1-800-624-8236

Lupus Foundation of America
1-800-558-0121

Medic Alert Foundation
1-800-ID-ALERT

National Foundation for Ileitis and Colitis
1-800-343-3637

American Liver Foundation
1-800-223-0179

Dental Association
1-800-621-8099

Cystic Fibrosis Foundation
1-800-344-4823

Arthritis Information Clearinghouse
P.O. Box 9752
Arlington, VA 22209

American Dental Assoc.
211 E Chicago Ave
Chicago, IL 60611

American Diabetes Assoc.
2 Park Ave
New York, NY 10016

American Heart Association
7320 Greenville Ave
Dallas, TX 75231

American Medical Association
535 N Dearborn Street
Chicago, IL 60610

High Blood Pressure Information Center
120/80, National Institutes of Health
Bethesda, MD 20205
(703) 558-4880

■≡ Drugs and Drug Abuse

Chemical Referral Hotline
1-800-262-2463

Cocaine Hotline
1-800-262-8200

Cocaine and other Substance
1-800-662-4357

Drug Abuse
1-800-662-4357

Food and Drug Administration
5600 Fishers Lane
Rockville, MD 20852

National Clearinghouse for Drug Abuse Information
5600 Fishers Lane, Room 10A-56
Rockville, MD 20857

Narcotics Anonymous, World Service Office
16155 Wyandotte St.
Van Nuys, CA 91406
(602) 944-0141

■≡ Environmental Safety

Public Information Center (PM-215)
Environmental Protection Agency
Washington, DC 24060
(202) 755-0707

Safe Drinking Water Hotline
1-800-426-4791

■≡ Food and Food Safety

Food and Drug Administration
5600 Fishers Lane
Rockville, MD 20852

Food Safety and Inspection Service
Washington, DC 20250
(202) 472-4485

■≡ Handicapped People

Clearinghouse on the Handicapped
330 C Street, SW
Washington, DC 20202
(202) 245-0080

National Information Center for Handicapped Children and Youth
1555 Wilson Blvd.
Suite 600
Rosslyn, VA 22209
(703) 522-0870

Disabled Persons Advocacy
1-800-342-0823

■≡ Health

Office of Health Maintenance Organizations
Department of Health and Human Services
12420 Parklawn Drive
Rockville, MD 20857
1-800-638-6686

Burn Shrine Hospital
1-800-282-9161

Dyslexia Society
1-800-222-3123

Eye Care Free
1-800-222-3937

Hearing and Speech
1-800-638-8255

Hearing Hotline
1-800-424-8576

Paralysis Association
1-800-526-3456

Poison Control
1-800-282-3171

Toxic Substance Hotline
1-800-367-4378

National Headache Foundation
1-800-843-2256

Overeaters Anonymous, World Service Office
2190 190th St.
Torrance, CA 90504
(213) 542-8363

Overcomers Outreach
2290 W. Whittier Blvd., Suite D
La Habra, CA 90631
(213) 697-3994

■≡ Infertility

RESOLVE, Inc.
National Office
P.O. Box 474
Belmount, MA 02178

National Committee for Adoption
Suite 326
1346 Connecticut Ave, NW
Washington, DC 20036

■≡ Mental Health

National Mental Health Association
1021 Prince St.
Alexandria, VA 22314
(703) 684-7722

The National Alliance for the Mentally Ill
1901 North Fort Myer Drive, Suite 500
Arlington, VA 22209
(703) 524-7600

National Clearinghouse for Mental Health Information
5600 Fishers Lane, Room 11A-33
Rockville, MD 20857
(301) 443-4513

■≡ Nutrition

Human Nutrition Information Service
Federal Center Building
Hyattsville, MD 20752

American Dietetic Association
430 N Michigan Ave.
Chicago, IL 60611

American College of Sports Medicine
(317) 637-9200

Women's Sports Foundation
1-800-227-3988

Aerobics and Fitness Foundation of America
1-800-BE-FIT-86
or (818) 905-0040

Academy for Sports Dentistry
University of Iowa Hospitals
Iowa City, IA 52242
(319) 356-2294

American Academy of Orthopedic Surgeons
222 S. Prospect Ave.
Park Ridge, IL 60068
(708) 823-7186

American Academy of Podiatric Sports Medicine
1729 Glastonberry Rd.
Potomac, MD 20854
(301) 424-7440

■≡ Occupational Safety

Office of Information on Consumer Affairs
Room N3637
200 Constitution Ave. NW
Washington, DC 20210
(202) 523-8151

■≡ Pregnancy

National Center for Education in Maternal and Child Health
P.O. Box 28612
Washington, DC 20005
(202) 842-6717

Birth Control/Abortion
1-800-772-9100

Lamaze Hotline
1-800-368-4404

■≡ Self-Help Groups

Self Help Center
1600 Dodge Ave.
Evanston, IL 60201

The National Self-Help Clearinghouse
33 West 42nd Street
Room 1227
New York, NY 10036

Bulimia/Anorexia Self Help
1-800-762-2273

Eating Disorders
1-800-332-2832

Debtors Anonymous
314 W. 53rd St.
New York, NY 10019
(212) 969-0710

Emotions Anonymous
P.O. Box 4245
St. Paul, MN 55104
(612) 647-9712

Gamblers Anonymous
P.O. Box 17173
Los Angeles, CA 90017
(213) 386-8789

■≡ Smoking

Technical Information Center
Office on Smoking and Health
5600 Fishers Lane, Room 1–16
Rockville, MD 20857

Smokenders
1-800-243-5614 (east of Mississippi)
1-800-828-4357 (west of Mississippi)

American Institute for Preventive Medicine
1911 West Ten Mile Road
Suite 101
Southfield, MI 48075

Many countries have developed nutrient standards. Those of the United States (the Recommended Dietary Allowances, or RDA) are presented here. The main RDA table is presented in Table B–1. The energy RDA are presented in Table B–2. The estimated safe and adequate daily dietary intakes of selected vitamins and minerals appear in Table B–3, and Table B–4 presents the estimated minimum requirements of electrolytes.

TABLE B–1 ■ Recommended Dietary Allowances (RDA), 1989[a]

Age (years)	Weight (kg)	Weight (lb)	Height (cm)	Height (inches)	Protein (g)	Vitamin A (μg RE)	Vitamin D (μg)	Vitamin E (mg α-TE)	Vitamin K (μg)	Vitamin C (mg)	Thiamin (mg)	Riboflavin (mg)	Niacin (mg NE)	Vitamin B_6 (mg)	Folate (μg)	Vitamin B_{12} (μg)	Calcium (mg)	Phosphorus (mg)	Magnesium (mg)	Iron (mg)	Zinc (mg)	Iodine (μg)	Selenium (μg)
Infants																							
0.0–0.5	6	13	60	24	13	375	7.5	3	5	30	0.3	0.4	5	0.3	25	0.3	400	300	40	6	5	40	10
0.5–1.0	9	20	71	28	14	375	10	4	10	35	0.4	0.5	6	0.6	35	0.5	600	500	60	10	5	50	15
Children																							
1–3	13	29	90	35	16	400	10	6	15	40	0.7	0.8	9	1.0	50	0.7	800	800	80	10	10	70	20
4–6	20	44	112	44	24	500	10	7	20	45	0.9	1.1	12	1.1	75	1.0	800	800	120	10	10	90	20
7–10	28	62	132	52	28	700	10	7	30	45	1.0	1.2	13	1.4	100	1.4	800	800	170	10	10	120	30
Males																							
11–14	45	99	157	62	45	1,000	10	10	45	50	1.3	1.5	17	1.7	150	2.0	1,200	1,200	270	12	15	150	40
15–18	66	145	176	69	59	1,000	10	10	65	60	1.5	1.8	20	2.0	200	2.0	1,200	1,200	400	12	15	150	50
19–24	72	160	177	70	58	1,000	10	10	70	60	1.5	1.7	19	2.0	200	2.0	1,200	1,200	350	10	15	150	70
25–50	79	174	176	70	63	1,000	5	10	80	60	1.5	1.7	19	2.0	200	2.0	800	800	350	10	15	150	70
51+	77	170	173	68	63	1,000	5	10	80	60	1.2	1.4	15	2.0	200	2.0	800	800	350	10	15	150	70
Females																							
11–14	46	101	157	62	46	800	10	8	45	50	1.1	1.3	15	1.4	150	2.0	1,200	1,200	280	15	12	150	45
15–18	55	120	163	64	44	800	10	8	55	60	1.1	1.3	15	1.5	180	2.0	1,200	1,200	300	15	12	150	50
19–24	58	128	164	65	46	800	10	8	60	60	1.1	1.3	15	1.6	180	2.0	1,200	1,200	280	15	12	150	55
25–50	63	138	163	64	50	800	5	8	65	60	1.1	1.3	15	1.6	180	2.0	800	800	280	15	12	150	55
51+	65	143	160	63	50	800	5	8	65	60	1.0	1.2	13	1.6	180	2.0	800	800	280	10	12	150	55
Pregnant					60	800	10	10	65	70	1.5	1.6	17	2.2	400	2.2	1,200	1,200	300	30	15	175	65
Lactating																							
1st 6 mo					65	1,300	10	12	65	95	1.6	1.8	20	2.1	280	2.6	1,200	1,200	355	15	19	200	75
2nd 6 mo					62	1,200	10	11	65	90	1.6	1.7	20	2.1	260	2.6	1,200	1,200	340	15	16	200	75

[a]The allowances are intended to provide for individual variations among most normal, healthy people in the United States under usual environmental stresses. They were designed for the maintenance of good nutrition. Diets should be based on a variety of common foods in order to provide other nutrients for which human requirements have been less well defined.

SOURCE: Reproduced from Food and Nutrition Board, *Recommended Dietary Allowances*, 10th ed. (Washington, D.C.: National Academy of Sciences, 1989), with permission.

TABLE B–2 ■ **Median Heights and Weights and Recommended Energy Intakes (United States)**

Age	Weight		Height		Average Energy Allowance			
(years)	(kg)	(lb)	(cm)	(inches)	REE[a] (kcal/day)	Multiples of REE[b]	kcal per kg	kcal per day[c]
Infants								
0.0–0.5	6	13	60	24	320		108	650
0.5–1.0	9	20	71	28	500		98	850
Children								
1–3	13	29	90	35	740		102	1,300
4–6	20	44	112	44	950		90	1,800
7–10	28	62	132	52	1,130		70	2,000
Males								
11–14	45	99	157	62	1,440	1.70	55	2,500
15–18	66	145	176	69	1,760	1.67	45	3,000
19–24	72	160	177	70	1,780	1.67	40	2,900
25–50	79	174	176	70	1,800	1.60	37	2,900
51+	77	170	173	68	1,530	1.50	30	2,300
Females								
11–14	46	101	157	62	1,310	1.67	47	2,200
15–18	55	120	163	64	1,370	1.60	40	2,200
19–24	58	128	164	65	1,350	1.60	38	2,200
25–50	63	138	163	64	1,380	1.55	36	2,200
51+	65	143	160	63	1,280	1.50	30	1,900
Pregnant (2nd and 3rd trimesters)								+300
Lactating								+500

[a]REE (resting energy expenditure) represents the energy expended by a person at rest under normal conditions.
[b]Recommended energy allowances assume light to moderate activity and were calculated by multiplying the REE by an activity factor.
[c]Average energy allowances have been rounded.

SOURCE: *Recommended Dietary Allowances*, © 1989 by the National Academy of Sciences, National Academy Press, Washington, D.C.

TABLE B–3 ■ Estimated Safe and Adequate Daily Dietary Intakes of Selected Vitamins and Minerals[a]

Age (years)	Vitamins	
	Biotin (µg)	Pantothenic Acid (mg)
Infants		
0–0.5	10	2
0.5–1	15	3
Children		
1–3	20	3
4–6	25	3–4
7–10	30	4–5
11+	30–100	4–7
Adults	30–100	4–7

Age (years)	Trace Elements[b]				
	Chromium (µg)	Molybdenum (µg)	Copper (mg)	Manganese (mg)	Fluoride (mg)
Infants					
0–0.5	10–40	15–30	0.4–0.6	0.3–0.6	0.1–0.5
0.5–1	20–60	20–40	0.6–0.7	0.6–1.0	0.2–1.0
Children					
1–3	20–80	25–50	0.7–1.0	1.0–1.5	0.5–1.5
4–6	30–120	30–75	1.0–1.5	1.5–2.0	1.0–2.5
7–10	50–200	50–150	1.0–2.0	2.0–3.0	1.5–2.5
11+	50–200	75–250	1.5–2.5	2.0–5.0	1.5–2.5
Adults	50–200	75–250	1.5–3.0	2.0–5.0	1.5–4.0

[a]Because there is less information on which to base allowances, these figures are not given in the main table of the RDA and are provided here in the form of ranges of recommended intakes.

[b]Because the toxic levels for many trace elements may be only several times usual intakes, the upper levels for the trace elements given in this table should not be habitually exceeded.

SOURCE: *Recommended Dietary Allowances*, 10th ed., © 1989 by the National Academy of Sciences, National Academy Press, Washington, D.C.

TABLE B–4 ■ **Estimated Sodium, Chloride, and Potassium Minimum Requirements of Healthy Persons**

Age (years)	Sodium[a] (mg)	Chloride (mg)	Potassium[b] (mg)
Infants			
0.0–0.5	120	180	500
0.5–1.0	200	300	700
Children			
1	225	350	1,000
2–5	300	500	1,400
6–9	400	600	1,600
Adolescents	500	750	2,000
Adults	500	750	2,000

[a]Sodium requirements are based on estimates of needs for growth and for replacement of obligatory losses. They cover a wide variation of physical activity patterns and climatic exposure but do not provide for large, prolonged losses from the skin through sweat.
[b]Dietary potassium may benefit the prevention and treatment of hypertension and recommendations to include many servings of fruits and vegetables would raise potassium intakes to about 3,500 mg/day.

SOURCE: *Recommended Dietary Allowances*, 10th ed., © 1989 by the National Academy of Sciences, National Academy Press, Washington, D.C.

Terms used to describe common emotional problems are defined in Chapter 3. The following glossaries define terms describing major emotional problems, therapies used to treat them, and therapists who do so. A section on family violence follows the glossaries.

■ GLOSSARY of
Terms Describing Major Emotional Problems

adjustment disorders maladaptive reactions to life changes. They set in within three months of the change and significantly impair the person's functioning socially or on the job or cause symptoms in excess of the expected reactions to such stresses.

bipolar disorder a mental disorder in which a person alternates between contrasting moods. The most common such disorder is manic depression.

catatonia (CAT-ah-TONE-ee-uh) a state characteristic of severe mental disorders; the catatonic person is in a stupor and may be mute or rigid or exhibit purposeless, excited activity or bizarre postures.

delusions false beliefs, held despite obvious proof to the contrary; a sign of mental illness.

hallucinations disturbances in the form of imagined sights, sounds, and events that often occur in emotional disorders such as schizophrenia.

hypochondria (hy-poh-KON-dree-uh) a disorder in which a person experiences physical symptoms that are of little significance but interprets them as signals of serious disease, often refusing to believe firm evidence that nothing is physically wrong.

insane a legal term; persons who are declared insane are not legally responsible for their actions, and they can be involuntarily committed to a mental institution.

mania elation characterized by hyperactivity; a decreased need for sleep; inflated self-esteem; and loud, disconnected speech.

manic depression the most common bipolar disorder, in which a person's mood alternates between mania and depression.

neurosis (noor-OH-sis) a mental disturbance characterized by symptoms that the individual recognizes as unacceptable and finds distressing. The person is in touch with reality, and the behavior does not violate social norms in major ways, even though functioning may be markedly impaired.

organic psychosis psychosis based on brain pathology related to disease, gunshot wound, accident, or other physical causes.

paranoia an unfounded belief characteristic of severe mental illnesses. The belief may be that one is being persecuted; that one is an unrecognized king, genius, or the like; or that one's spouse or loved one is being unfaithful.

para = beyond
nous = mind

phobia (FOH-bee-uh) extreme, irrational fear of an object or situation.
phobos = fear

psychogenic pain pain with no physical basis, inconsistent with the state of the nervous system.
psych = mind
gen = arising

psychosis (sigh-KOH-sis) an emotional disorder that involves behavior and perceptions that are out of touch with reality; the popular term is *insanity*, referring to the person's extreme irrationality and insensitivity to social and behavioral norms.

psychosomatic illness an illness of the body that originates in the mind.

schizophrenia (SKITZ-oh-FREN-ee-uh) a mental disorder characterized by adeterioration in level of functioning in work, social relationships, and self-care. The symptoms are many and varied, and no single one is always present.
schiz = split
phren = mind

syndrome a cluster of symptoms that, taken together, indicate a particular disease or abnormal condition.

■ GLOSSARY of Therapies

aversive conditioning   a mode of therapy related to behavior modification that associates unpleasant consequences with undesirable behaviors. Later, memories of the unpleasant experiences are linked to the behavior and so extinguish it.

behavior modification   a mode of therapy directed at behavior change; may encourage or eradicate a behavior by offering or denying reinforcement (reward). Chapter 1 gave details of the principles involved.

gestalt (geh-SHTALT) therapy   a kind of therapy that takes place in groups that typically focus on one person at a time. The group gives the person its attention while the therapist guides him or her in role-playing exercises that are often intensely emotional and can lead to new understandings and resolution.

hypnosis or hypnotherapy   a therapy aimed at behavior, in which suggestions are given to a willing and profoundly relaxed subject to implant ideas that will later elicit desired behavior. Contrary to popular belief, it is not possible, with simple hypnosis, to persuade people to do things they do not consciously want to do.

psychoanalysis   a specialty within psychiatry, developed by the founders of modern psychotherapy—Sigmund Freud, Carl Jung, and Alfred Adler. It involves a historical approach: deep exploration into the person's unconscious mind and personality structure in the attempt to discover why the person is experiencing problems in the present. Analysis of the person's dreams may be an important part of therapy.

rational-emotive psychotherapy   a form of psychotherapy developed by the psychiatrist Albert Ellis. Ellis trains people to assess their experiences rationally, as inconvenient or unpleasant rather than awful, and to say they *hope* or *want* certain things to happen rather than that those things *must* happen. The reassessment leads to changed emotions as described in Chapter 3.

reality therapy   a type of psychotherapy developed by the therapist William Glasser. Glasser believes that people can adjust to virtually any reality—and must do so if they are to be emotionally healthy. Rather than allowing them to get caught up in wishing, hoping, fearing, and avoiding reality, he encourages them to confront and deal with reality, whatever the temporary pain this process may entail.

systematic desensitization   a kind of psychotherapy directed specifically at phobias and anxieties in which the therapist instructs clients to visualize the situations that frighten them and teaches them to relax at the same time; this approach is used in progressive stages.

■ GLOSSARY of Therapists

counselor   a term for a helping person, not particularly definitive; people with a number of different qualifications can practice under this description. A graduate degree in counseling (M.S. or Ph.D.) from an accredited university is the degree to look for. Many states require licensing for counselors to practice.

psychiatrist   a physician (M.D.) who, after completing medical school, received additional special training to treat emotional problems and is licensed to prescribe drugs.

psych = mind, soul
iatros = doctor

psychoanalyst   a psychiatrist who specializes in analysis, seeking the root psychological causes of emotional problems.

psychologist   a person with a graduate degree (M.S. or Ph.D.) in psychology from a university. This person, although called "Doctor," is not licensed to write prescriptions; a desirable credential for a psychologist is certification by the American Psychology Association (APA).

Many states require licensing for psychologists to practice.

social worker   a person with a graduate degree in social work (M.S.W.), a respected degree that includes training in counseling.

Other practitioners may call themselves by many titles. Some may be truly helpful individuals, but unless they have the appropriate credentials, you can't be sure of their qualifications to practice therapy.

Family Violence

Recently the issue of family violence has become recognized as a serious problem. It is estimated that each year more than a million children in the United States are abused by their parents, guardians, or others. Two to five thousand of these children die as a result of the injuries caused by the abuse. Abused children suffer from a deprivation of necessities, physical major and minor injuries, emotional maltreatment, and sexual abuse.

The single most common cause of injury to women is battery. Over 4,000 women are killed by battery each year. A 1976 survey reports that 18 million wives are severely assaulted by their husbands each year. A prominent sociologist believes that 20 percent of all wives in the United States are assaulted at some time in their marriages by their husbands. According to other sociologists, over one million abused women seek medical help for injuries caused by battering from their spouses each year. Men commit 95 percent of all assaults against spouses. FBI data indicate that 30 percent of the women who are murdered in the U.S. die at the hands of their husbands or partners.

Incest is estimated to occur in 14 percent of all families. The incidence of sexual abuse of children has increased sharply during the 1980s.

Two-thirds of the people who commit violent crimes have been drinking alcohol. Alcohol consumption is associated with violent crimes of all types, including family abuse and incest.

The Center for Women Policy Studies says that an estimate of 500,000 to 1,000,000 cases of elder abuse occur annually.

Violence by children is also on the rise, says a University of Pennsylvania study. It found that in 1982, 500,000 children attacked their parents with a knife or gun.

States now require reporting of child abuse cases by most any observer. The AMA issued a diagnostic guideline so that physicians can comply with the laws. Six states (Delaware, Maine, Minnesota, North Carolina, Oregon, and Utah) have laws mandating the arrest of the abuser. Twenty-seven other states give police more arrest power; they can arrest without warrants. More than half of the states have funds for services for families suffering violence. Twenty-one states have laws mandating the reporting of elder abuse. Children's Trust Funds were created in 1985 in 30 states. They are federal funds used for protecting abused children. Monies for the state Children's Trust Fund comes from surcharges on fees for birth certificates, marriage licenses, divorce decrees, or by donations.

Over 130 YWCAs have programs for battered women and their children. Close to 800 shelters exist for battered women, abused children, and services for the elderly. The National Child Abuse Hotline is 1-800-4-A-CHILD.

SOURCES: J. Saltman, The many faces of family violence, *Public Affairs Pamphlets* - Soc HN-5-p8 no. 634-650, *Domestic Violence: Terrorism in the Home,* Hearing before the Subcommittee on Children, Family, Drugs and Alcoholism of the Committee on Labor and Human Resources, United States Senate - One Hundred First Congress Second Session, April 19, 1990, Doc Y4.L11/4: S.hrg. 101-897.

Food-processing techniques have brought to the marketplace many products different from farm-fresh foods. The processed products may save time and trouble, may last longer, may appear more desirable, or may be new foods or have improved flavors. They may also bring with them unfamiliar ingredients, and their nutrient contents may be altered. This appendix is for people who want to know what those ingredients are doing in their food, and how to choose foods intelligently based on the information given on a label. The following few paragraphs are devoted to the most important terms that describe our staple grain food, bread, and the Glossary that follows defines many other terms.

Wheat is North America's most widely used staple, used in the majority of all breads and cereals. The more wheat products consumers use, the more important it is to understand the terms commonly used to describe them: **refined, enriched,** and **whole grain**. Grain has to be treated before it is used for food, because it has an inedible external coat (the chaff) that has to be removed. Except for the chaff, however, the whole grain is edible, and it includes some especially nutritious portions—the bran and the germ—which, for nutrition's sake, should be retained in the milling process. In some milling processes, however, especially the more modern ones, *all* the rough parts are removed, including the bran and the germ, so that all that is left is the starchy endosperm. White flour can be made from the endosperm, and this refined flour is popular for baking, but it is so lacking in nutrients as to cause nutrient deficits when used as a staple; it displaces other, more nutritious foods from the diet.

During the 1930s in the United States, a survey revealed that people were actually suffering from nutrient deficiencies due to the replacement of whole-grain products with refined products. The nutrients known at the time to be affected were the mineral iron and the B vitamins thiamin, riboflavin, and niacin. The Enrichment Act of 1942 required that these lost nutrients be returned to flour. Thus in *enriched* bread, these few nutrients have been restored to levels similar to those found in whole wheat. This doesn't make a single slice of bread "rich" in these nutrients, but people who eat several or many slices of bread a day obtain significantly more of them than they would from plain, refined white bread.

But this is not the whole story. When the grain is refined, many nutrients not known in 1942 to be important are also lost. As more and more foods other than bread are refined and processed, other nutrients may begin to be lost from the diet. For example, fiber needs are not being met as fiber is refined out of many foods, not just from bread and cereal. Whole grains are preferred over enriched products, also, because they contain more magnesium, zinc, folacin, and vitamin B_6. If breads, cereals, and other grain products are staple foods in your diet—that is, if you eat them every day—you would be well advised to learn to like the hearty flavor of whole-grain products.

Two other terms related to these, which appear on labels of foods, are **fortified** and **supplement**. These terms indicate that nutrients have been added in amounts greater than those occurring naturally in the original, unrefined products. *Fortified* means the nutrients are added to some unspecified amount above the natural level; *supplement* means they are added to levels at least 50 percent above the U.S. RDA.

This Glossary lists these and many other terms found on food labels. Some of these terms are also explained further, elsewhere in this book. To locate any other information about a term, look in the index.

■ GLOSSARY of
Food and Vitamin Label Terms

Accent see *monosodium glutamate (MSG)*.

acetic acid see *antimicrobial agents*.

agar see *stabilizers (thickeners)*.

alanine see *amino acid*.

aloe a tropical plant of widely acclaimed, but unproved, medicinal value. The gel of the plant is often added to lotions and creams, and sometimes is included in preparations for internal use.

alpha tocopherol see *tocopherol*.

aluminum phosphate see *anticaking agents*.

amino (a-MEEN-oh) acid a building block of protein. On a label, you might see any of the following: glycine, alanine, valine, leucine, isoleucine, serine, threonine, aspartic acid, glutamic acid, lysine, arginine, cystine, cysteine, methionine, tyrosine, phenylalanine, tryptophan, proline, histidine, glutamine, asparagine.

anticaking agents substances added to keep products such as salts and powders free flowing. Examples are magnesium carbonate, calcium silicate, aluminum phosphate, or similar compounds.

antimicrobial agents compounds added to products to prevent spoilage by bacteria or molds. Familiar among them are acetic acid (vinegar) and sodium chloride (salt). Others are benzoic, propionic, and sorbic acids; nitrites and nitrates; and sulfur dioxide. See also *irradiated food*.

antioxidant a compound that protects others from oxidation by being oxidized itself. Oxidation is a chemical reaction in which oxygen or a similar substance changes the nature of other chemicals, usually to the detriment of the product or the nutrients it contains. Examples of antioxidants are BHA, BHT, and propyl gallate.

arabic see *stabilizers (thickeners)*.

arginine see *amino acid*.

ascorbic acid one of the two active forms of vitamin C (the other is dehydroascorbic acid). Many people consistently and incorrectly refer to all vitamin C by this name.
   a = without
   scorbic = having scurvy

aspartame the generic name for an artificial sweetener that is ten times sweeter than sugar, derived from two amino acids (aspartic acid and phenylalanine). Aspartame breaks down at high temperatures, and therefore cannot be used in cooking; in the body, it is broken down to its component amino acids and methane, a common waste product that is excreted. People with phenylalanine intolerance (PKU) must limit use of the sweetener. See also *Nutrasweet* and *Equal*.

aspartic acid, asparagine see *amino acid*.

BHA, BHT see *antioxidant*.

bee pollen a product sold with the claim that it boosts athletic performance, but that in reality has no such effect.

benzoic acid see *antimicrobial agents*.

beta-carotene an orange pigment found in plants. The food industry uses it to color foods; the body converts it to active vitamin A, so it is both a food additive and a nutrient. See *coloring agents*.

bicarbonate see *leavening agents*.

bioflavonoids substances found in foods, that supply no nutritional need. Some are called ''vitamin P'' (erroneously) by faddists.

biotin a B vitamin, supplied abundantly in foods and required in supplement form only by people with a rare metabolic disorder. A varied diet supplies all the biotin needed, but biotin pills are often recommended by quacks.

bleaching agents substances used to whiten foods, such as flour and cheese, and to speed up the maturing of cheese. *Peroxides* are examples.

bone meal powdered bone, intended to supply calcium to the diet. Calcium from bone is not well absorbed and often contains toxic minerals such as lead and cadmium.

brewer's yeast see *nutritional yeast*.

brown sugar sugar crystals contained in molasses syrup with natural flavor and color, 91 to 96 percent pure sucrose. (Some refiners add syrup to refined white sugar to make brown sugar.)

buffer a substance or mixture in a solution that is capable of neutralizing both acids and bases.

■ GLOSSARY of
Food and Vitamin Label Terms

caffeine a central nervous system stimulant that, when used as a food additive, lends a bitter flavor note. See also *flavoring agents.*

calcium carbonate a calcium compound that, like many other calcium compounds, acts as a firming agent in frozen and canned goods. See *firming agents.*

calcium silicate see *anticaking agents.*

calorie a unit in which energy is measured. Food energy is measured in *kilocalories* (thousands of calories), abbreviated *kcalories* or *kcal*, or capitalized: *Calories*. Most people, even nutritionists, speak of these units simply as calories, but technically, on paper, they should be prefaced by a *k*. (The pronunciation of *kcalories* ignores the *k*.) This book uses the informal term and spelling, *calorie.*

carbohydrate an energy nutrient composed of monosaccharides; some types of fiber are also carbohydrates. See also Chapter 5.
　carbo = carbon
　hydrate = water

carotene see *beta-carotene.*

carrageenan see *stabilizers (thickeners).*

casein (KAY-seen) the main protein of cow's milk.

cell salts a mineral preparation sold in health-food stores, supposed to have been prepared from living, healthy cells. It is not necessary to take such preparations, and it may be dangerous.

cellulose (CELL-you-loce) see *fiber.*

chelating agents acids added to foods to prevent discoloration, flavor changes, and rancidity that might occur because of processing. Examples are citric acid, malic acid, and tartaric acid (cream of tartar).

cholecalciferol (COAL-ee-cal-SIFF-er-ol) the chemical name for vitamin D.

cholesterol one of the fats, a sterol. See Chapter 5.

choline a compound found in food, not an essential nutrient for human beings.

citric acid see *chelating agents.*

cobalamin (co-BAL-uh-min) vitamin B$_{12}$.
　cobal = cobalt containing
　amine = vitamin

collagen the characteristic protein of connective tissue.
　kolla = glue
　gennan = to produce

coloring agents substances used to enhance the colors and, for some, the attractiveness of foods. Vegetable dyes are extracted from vegetables such as beets and carrots. Food colors are a mix of vegetable dyes and synthetic dyes approved by the FDA for use in food. In recent years, in response to consumer demand, the number permitted for use has been reduced from over 100 to 33.

complex carbohydrates the polysaccharides (starch, glycogen, and cellulose).

confectioner's sugar finely powdered sucrose (table sugar).

convenience food a food prepared or packaged in such a way that it is easy to cook and serve at home.

corn sweeteners corn syrup and sugars derived from corn.

corn syrup a syrup produced by the action of enzymes on cornstarch. High-fructose corn syrup (HFCS) may contain as little as 42 percent or as much as 90 percent fructose; dextrose makes up the balance.

cyclamate a petroleum-derived artificial sweetener, many times sweeter than sugar; cyclamate is banned in the United States but is allowed in Canada because it has never been shown conclusively to cause cancer in human beings.

cysteine, cystine see *amino acid.*

desiccated liver dehydrated liver, a powder sold in health-food stores and supposed to contain in concentrated form all the nutrients found in liver. Possibly not dangerous, this supplement has no particular nutritional merit, and grocery store liver is considerably less expensive. *Desiccated* means "totally dried."

dextrins short chains of glucose formed by breaking down starch. The word sometimes appears on food labels, because dextrins can be used as an additive to thicken foods.

dextrose a form of glucose that is very soluble in water. See also *glucose, sugar.*

diet pills pills that depress the appetite temporarily, such as physician-prescribed amphetamines (speed). It is generally agreed that their use can cause a dangerous dependency. It is also agreed that these drugs are of little value for permanent weight loss.

diglyceride see *emulsifiers.*

dipeptide two amino acids bonded together, a protein fragment.
　di = two
　peptide = amino acid

disaccharide a pair of sugar units bonded together. Example: sucrose.
　di = two
　saccharide = sugar

electrolyte an electrically charged mineral ion, such as sodium (positively charged) and chloride (negatively charged). Electrolytes partially dissociate in water, helping to give it electrical conductivity. Electrolytes are among the minerals required for normal body functions.

empty-calorie food a popular term used to denote foods that contain no nutrients, only calories. Actually, almost all foods contain some nutrients. Therefore nutritionists prefer to say "food of low nutrient density."

emulsifiers chemicals that attract both fats and water, and act to help the two to mix (detergents are emulsifiers). Emulsifiers are used to incorporate fats into watery portions of foods. Examples are *lecithin, monoglycerides* and *diglycerides*, and *propylene glycol esters.*

engineered food a food subjected to a complex technical process, such as extraction of certain components.

enriched food a food to which nutrients have been added. Specifically, in the case of refined bread or cereal, four

■ GLOSSARY of
Food and Vitamin Label Terms

nutrients have been added: thiamin, niacin, and iron in amounts approximately equivalent to those originally present in the whole grain, and riboflavin in about twice the amount originally present. See also *fortified.*

enzyme a large protein molecule that facilitates a specific chemical reaction. Enzymes added to products usually appear on labels with chemical names ending in *-ase,* such as *amylase* (an enzyme that splits starch, or amylose). The ending *-ase* indicates an enzyme; the root tells what it digests. Other examples: *protease* (an enzyme that splits protein), or *lipase* (an enzyme that splits fats). Enzymes added to foods to "aid digestion" are of little value, because enzymes, being proteins, are broken down in the stomach, like any other proteins. Foods are sometimes treated with enzymes during processing; for example, milk can be treated with *lactase*—an enzyme that breaks down the milk sugar lactose, making it digestible by people who otherwise could not tolerate it. See also *meat tenderizer.*

Equal the trade name given to a household artificial sweetener, made from aspartame mixed in a lactose base. See also *aspartame, lactose.*

ergogenic a term intended to imply that a food or supplement gives energy; used especially with reference to products for athletes. Actually, no foods have special power to produce energy.

fabricated food a food put together from highly processed ingredients, such as substitute-meat burgers made from textured vegetable protein.

fast food food prepared quickly in a fast-food restaurant such as a hamburger stand or fried-chicken place.

fat lipids; triglycerides, cholesterol, and phospholipids. See Chapter 5.

fiber the portions of food human beings do not have the enzymes to digest. Names on labels might include *cellulose, hemicellulose, pectin,* or *lignin.* Fiber that occurs naturally in foods is not listed on the label. The terms *crude fiber* and *dietary fiber* are more precise, since they

distinguish between fiber left in food after chemical processing and that left in the body after digestion (intestinal flora digest only certain fibers, whereas chemical processes digest more).

firming agents substances added to processed fruits and vegetables to preserve firm texture through cooking or freezing.

fish oil see *omega fatty acids.*

flavoring agents substances used to add or enhance flavor. The flavoring agent most often added to food is sugar; second is salt. Monosodium glutamate, plant oils, herbs and spices, and a host of synthetic flavors are also in this group. See also *monosodium glutamate.*

folate, folic acid one of the B vitamins.

fortified a term referring to the addition of nutrients to a food, often not originally present, and often added in amounts greater than might be found there naturally. The term *enriched* sometimes also has this meaning (see also *enriched food*).

fructose a monosaccharide; sometimes known as *fruit sugar.* See also *sugar.*
    fruct = fruit

galactose a monosaccharide; part of the milk sugar, lactose.
    galakt = milk

ginseng one of a number of plants whose leaves, flowers, or other parts are popularly used for the making of herbal teas. Hazards are associated with this and many other plants.

gliadin (GLIGH-uh-den) a fraction of the gluten protein.

glucomannan (glue-co-MAN-an) a preparation derived from a vegetable (konjac tuber) used in Japanese cooking. In a controlled experiment reported in 1982, glucomannan was ineffective in controlling weight.

glucose a monosaccharide; sometimes known as *blood sugar,* sometimes as *grape sugar.* See also *dextrose.*

glutamic acid, glutamine see *amino acid.*

gluten (GLOOT-en) a protein found in wheat, oats, rye, and barley.

glycerol a small compound related to carbohydrates that is a part of the triglycerides and phospholipids.

glycine see *amino acid.*

granola a cereal made from oats and other grains that is often high in simple sugars and saturated fats.

granulated sugar crystalline sucrose.

GRAS (Generally Recognized As Safe) list a list of food additives, established by the FDA, that have long been in use and were believed safe before testing was required. The list is now subject to revision as new facts about additives become known.

green pills pills containing dehydrated, crushed vegetable matter. One pill contains nutrients equal to those in one small forkful of fresh vegetables—minus losses incurred in processing. Sixty pills costing $15 deliver vegetable matter worth about $1.50.

guar see *stabilizers (thickeners).*

gums see *stabilizers (thickeners).*

HCG, or human chorionic gonadotropin (core-ee-ON-ic go-nad-o-TROPE-in) a hormone excreted in the urine of pregnant women believed by some to enhance weight loss and reduce hunger. It does neither.

health food a misleading term used on labels, usually of organic or natural foods, to imply unusual power to promote health.

hemicellulose see *fiber.*

high-quality protein an easily digestible, complete protein whose amino acids fit the pattern needed by human beings.

histidine see *amino acid.*

honey invert sugar formed by an enzyme from nectar gathered by bees. Composition and flavor vary, but honey usually contains fructose, glucose, maltose, and sucrose. See also *invert sugar.*

humectants substances used to retain moisture in foods, and to improve their texture.

hydrolyzed protein protein treated with acids or enzymes to yield a combination

■ GLOSSARY of
Food and Vitamin Label Terms

of free amino acids and short peptide chains. See also *protein isolate*.

hypertonic   a term that describes a liquid solution more concentrated than blood serum.
  hyper = greater, more

hypotonic   a term that describes a liquid solution less concentrated than blood serum.
  hypo = less

imitation foods   foods created to replace familiar foods, but inferior in nutrient composition. Nutritional inferiority is defined as a reduction in the content of an essential vitamin or mineral, or of protein, that amounts to 10 percent or more of the U.S. RDA. In adjuncts, such as vanilla flavoring, the losses to the diet are inconsequential; in items of daily consumption, such as fruit juice, the nutrient differences become important.

inositol   a compound found in foods, not an essential nutrient for human beings.

invert sugar   a mixture of glucose and fructose formed by the splitting of sucrose in a chemical process. Sold only in liquid form, and sweeter than sucrose, invert sugar is used as an additive to prevent crystallization, to help preserve food freshness, and to prevent shrinkage.

irradiated food   a food preserved by a technique using ionizing radiation to kill microorganisms and prevent sprouting. See also *URPs*.

isoleucine   see *amino acid*.

isotonic   a formula with the same concentration as blood serum.
  iso = the same
  ton = tension

kcalorie   see *calorie*.

kelp   a kind of seaweed used by the Japanese as a foodstuff. Kelp tablets are made from dehydrated kelp. The urine of people who use kelp has been found to contain raised concentrations of arsenic, a poison and possible carcinogen.

kilocalorie   see *calorie*.

lactase   see *enzyme*.

lactose   a disaccharide composed of glucose and galactose, commonly known as milk sugar.
  lact = milk

laetrile (LAY-uh-trill)   substance isolated from apricot pits, advertised as a cancer cure and sold under the trade name "vitamin B$_{17}$" but actually not a vitamin and never shown to be either safe or effective as a cancer cure.

leavening agents   substances added to create bubbles of carbon dioxide in grain products to make them light in texture. Examples are yeast, bicarbonates, and phosphates.

lecithin   a fatty compound made by the body and found widely in foods. Magical properties are sometimes attributed to lecithin, and supplementation is recommended by faddists. No extra lecithin is needed; it is often added as an emulsifier in processed foods. See also *emulsifiers*.

leucine   see *amino acid*.

levulose   the technical name for fructose.

lignin   see *fiber*.

lipase   see *enzyme*.

lipoic acid   a compound found in food, probably not an essential nutrient for human beings.

locust bean gum   see *stabilizers (thickeners)*.

low fat   a term for a product that has less fat than the ordinary variety of the same product. It is used as a comparison measure, not an absolute descriptor.

low salt   a term for a product with less salt than the ordinary variety of the same product.

low sodium   a term designated by the FDA to mean a product with less than 140 milligrams of sodium per serving; *very low sodium* products contain less than 35 milligrams of sodium per serving.

lysine   see *amino acid*.

magnesium carbonate   see *anticaking agents*.

malic acid   see *chelating agents*.

maltitol   see *sugar alcohols*.

maltose   a disaccharide composed of two glucose units; sometimes known as malt sugar. See also *sugar*.

mannitol   see *sugar alcohols*.

maple sugar   although once a common sweetener, this sugar is rarely added to foods and is commonly replaced by sucrose and artificial maple flavoring. The only source of true maple sugar is the concentrated sap of the sugar maple tree. Maple sugar is expensive, compared with other sweeteners.

meat replacements   textured vegetable-protein products formulated to look and taste like meat, fish, or poultry. Many of these are designed to match the known nutrient contents of animal-protein foods, but sometimes they fall short.

meat tenderizer   a preparation of enzymes (proteases) that break down the tough connective tissues in meats, making them tender. The chief enzyme in a meat tenderizer is papain (PAP-ane).

menadione (men-uh-DYE-own)   a synthetic compound similar to vitamin K and sometimes used as a substitute for it.

methionine   see *amino acid*.

molasses   a thick, brown syrup, which tastes bitter and sour as well as sweet, created during cane sugar production. Molasses contains a few minerals, but is low in nutrient density (high in calories per nutrient). Like sugar, molasses promotes tooth decay.

monoglyceride   see *emulsifiers*.

monosaccharide (mon-oh-SACK-uh-ride)   a single sugar unit; for example, glucose.
  mono = one
  saccharide, ose = sugar

monosodium glutamate (MSG)   a bland-tasting substance that, when added to other foods, enhances their flavors. It is sold under the trade name Accent and included in almost all seasoning blends and mixes, and it can be a significant contributor of sodium to the diet. "Chinese restaurant syndrome," reported to include a burning sensation, chest and facial flushing, and headache, is reported, but not proved, to be a reaction to ingestion of large quantities of MSG. Legislation deems MSG safe for adults, but it is not permitted in infant foods. See also *flavoring agents*.

■ GLOSSARY of
Food and Vitamin Label Terms

monounsaturated fatty acid a fatty acid that has one point of unsaturation where hydrogens are missing; for example, oleic acid.

natural food a food that has been altered as little as possible from the original farm-grown state. An unprocessed food; a term often mistakenly used as synonymous with "good for you."

natural sweeteners any of the sugars listed in this glossary except sucrose.

niacin one of the B vitamins; active forms include *nicotinic acid, nicotinamide,* and *niacinamide.* (Earlier names were vitamin G or vitamin B₃.)

niacin equivalents the amount of niacin present in food, including the niacin that can theoretically be made by the body from tryptophan, one of the amino acids, present in the food.

nicotinamide, nicotinic acid see *niacin.*

nitrite a salt added to food to prevent the kind of bacteria from growing in food that can cause the deadly form of food poisoning known as botulism, and to color the food. **Nitrosamines** (nigh-TROHS-uh-meens) are derivatives of nitrites that may be formed in the stomach when nitrites combine with amines; nitrosamines are carcinogenic. See also *antimicrobial agents.*

nitrosamines see *nitrite.*

Nutrasweet the trade name given to a concentrated form of aspartame used to sweeten products. *Nutrasweet blend* includes both Nutrasweet and saccharin. See also *aspartame.*

nutrients on labels, substances added to food to improve nutritive value.

nutritional yeast a preparation of yeast cells, often praised for its high nutrient content. Yeast is a concentrated source of B vitamins, as are many other foods. Also called brewer's yeast. Not the yeast sold for baking; see *leavening agents* for baker's yeast.

nutritious food a food with high nutrient density.

omega fatty acids fatty acids that occur in oil from fish, possibly active in prevention of some kinds of heart disease, but also toxic if taken in large quantities. Also called *fish oil, alpha-omega fatty acids,* or *omega-three fatty acids.*

organic (chemist's definition) a substance that contains carbon atoms; by this definition, all foods are organic, as are petroleum products.

organic (popular definition) a term referring to foods produced without the use of chemical fertilizers, pesticides, or additives. (May also refer to nutrients extracted from natural sources as opposed to those that are chemically synthesized.) As used on labels, this term may misleadingly imply unusual power to promote health.

oyster shell powdered oyster shells, sold as a calcium supplement, but not well absorbed by the digestive system.

pangamic acid not an identifiable substance, a term used in quackery. Sometimes called "vitamin B₁₅," but such a vitamin does not exist.

pantothenic acid one of the B vitamins.

papain see *meat tenderizer.* Also called *papaya enzyme.*

para-aminobenzoic acid (PABA) a substance found in foods, probably not an essential nutrient for human beings.

pectin see *fiber.*

pepsin see *enzyme.*

peroxide see *bleaching agents.*

phenylalanine see *amino acid.*

phosphates see *leavening agents.*

polypeptide a chain of many amino acids bonded together, a protein fragment.
  poly = many
  peptide = amino acid

polysaccharide a chain of many sugar units bonded together.
  poly = many
  saccharide = sugar

polyunsaturated fatty acid (PUFA) a fatty acid with two or more points of unsaturation. Examples: linoleic acid (two such points) and linolenic acid (three). A *polyunsaturated fat* is composed of triglycerides containing a high percentage of PUFA.

processed food any food subjected to a process such as enrichment, refinement, fortification, alteration of texture, mixing, or cooking.

proline see *amino acid.*

propionic acid see *antimicrobial agents.*

propyl gallate See *antioxidant.*

propylene glycol esters see *emulsifiers.*

protein a compound composed of amino acids linked in a chain. See also Chapter 5.

protein isolate a protein with high biological value that has been chemically separated from a source containing a variety of proteins; different from hydrolyzed protein in that the protein is extracted whole.

pyridoxal, pyridoxamine, pyridoxine active forms of vitamin B₆.

raw sugar the residue of evaporated sugar cane juice, tan or brown in color. Raw sugar can only be sold in the United States if the impurities (dirt, insect fragments, and the like) have been removed.

refined food a food from which the coarse parts have been removed. Specifically, with respect to grains, a product from which the bran, germ, and chaff have been removed, leaving only the endosperm.

retinal, retinol, retinoic acid active forms of vitamin A; retinol is used as the standard for measuring vitamin A activity.

riboflavin (RYE-bo-flay-vin) a B vitamin, formerly known as vitamin B₂.

rose hips fruits of rose plants, high in vitamin C; they are used in herbal teas and other mixtures, and as a vitamin C source for the manufacture of supplements.

rutin one of the bioflavonoids, not an essential nutrient in human nutrition. See also *bioflavonoids.*

saccharin an intensely sweet petroleum derivative that is used as an artificial sweetener; saccharin is an inexpensive, heat-stable ingredient that is 200 times sweeter than table sugar. The safety of the sweetener has been questioned, and

■ GLOSSARY of
Food and Vitamin Label Terms

it is banned in Canada but allowed with warning labels in the United States (Canadians use cyclamate, banned in the United States because of similar safety questions). Saccharin causes a specific kind of bladder tumor in rats, but has been shown not to increase the incidence of any cancers in human beings to the limits of detection.

salt on labels, sodium chloride. See *sodium chloride,* Chapter 5.

saturated fat see *saturated fatty acid.*

saturated fatty acid a fatty acid with no points of unsaturation. A *saturated fat* is composed of triglycerides in which all, or virtually all, of the fatty acids are saturated.

selenium (se-LEEN-ee-um) a trace element that functions as part of an enzyme that acts as an antioxidant; selenium can substitute for vitamin E in some of that vitamin's antioxidant activities.

serine see *amino acid.*

sodium chloride table salt, a flavor additive and preservative second only to sugar in prevalence in foods. See *antimicrobial agents.*

sodium salts for compounds of sodium, see main constituent name. For example, for sodium saccharin, see *saccharin.*

sorbic acid see *antimicrobial agents.*

sorbitol see *sugar alcohols.*

spirulina a kind of alga ("blue-green manna") said to contain large amounts of vitamin B_{12} and to suppress appetite. It does neither.

stabilizers (thickeners) substances used to maintain foam, emulsions, or suspensions in products, or to thicken them. Examples are gums such as carrageenan, guar, locust bean, tragacanth, xanthan gum, gum arabic, agar (a seaweed extract), starch, and pectin.

starch a plant polysaccharide composed of glucose and digestible by humans. See also *stabilizers (thickeners)* and Chapter 5.

starch blockers products derived from kidney beans that are incorrectly credited with blocking starch digestion in humans. They were banned by the FDA

when they were found to cause nausea, diarrhea, and stomach pains, and not to block starch digestion.

sucrose a disaccharide composed of glucose and fructose; commonly known as table sugar, beet sugar, or cane sugar.

sugar technically, the monosaccharides and disaccharides; on labels, sucrose, maltose, dextrose, fructose, glucose, invert sugar, cane syrup, honey, beet sugar, corn syrup, corn sweeteners, and maple sugar. These are chemically similar and nutritionally identical substances. Pound for pound, sugar is the most widely used additive in the food supply. See also Chapter 5.

sugar alcohols sweet-tasting substances that can be extracted from fruits or produced from dextrose; absorbed and metabolized differently from sugar in the human body, and not usable by the ordinary mouth bacteria that cause dental caries.

sulfites salts containing sulfur, added to fresh and frozen fruits and vegetables to prevent spoilage, but that can cause a dangerous allergic reaction in people who have asthma and other allergies; their use is being limited, but they are currently allowed in beer, wine, and packaged foods without disclosure on the labels.

sulfur dioxide see *antimicrobial agents.*

supplement used on labels to denote a food to which nutrients have been added in amounts greater than 50 percent above the U.S. RDA.

tartaric acid see *chelating agents.*

tartrazine a food-coloring agent, also known as yellow dye no. 5; its presence must be declared on labels, because some people are allergic to it. See also *coloring agents.*

thiamin (THIGH-uh-min) a B vitamin, formerly known as vitamin B_1.

thickeners see *stabilizers (thickeners).*

threonine see *amino acid.*

tocopherol (toe-COFF-er-all) the chemical name for a class of compounds with vitamin E activity. Alpha tocopherol is the most active of these.

tragacanth see *stabilizers (thickeners).*

triglyceride a compound composed of glycerol with three fatty acids attached to it; the principal form of fat in foods and in the body.
  tri = three
  glyceride = a compound of glycerol

tryptophan see *amino acid.*

tyrosine see *amino acid.*

URPs (unique radiolytic products) chemicals formed in foods that have been irradiated. URPs are not radioactive, and they have been found to be harmless in toxicity tests. See also *irradiated food.*

valine see *amino acid.*

vitamin A a fat-soluble vitamin.

vitamin B_1 see *thiamin.*

vitamin B_2 see *riboflavin.*

vitamin B_3 see *niacin.*

vitamin B_6 one of the B vitamins; active forms include pyridoxal, pyridoxamine, and pyridoxine.

vitamin B_{12} one of the B vitamins, also known as cobalamin.

vitamin B_{15} not a true vitamin; see *pangamic acid.*

vitamin B_{17} not a true vitamin; see *laetrile.*

vitamin C a water-soluble vitamin, also known as ascorbic acid.

vitamin D a fat-soluble vitamin, also known as cholecalciferol.

vitamin E a fat-soluble vitamin, also known as alpha tocopherol.

vitamin G see *niacin.*

vitamin K a fat-soluble vitamin.

water miscible (MISS-ih-bul) a term used to describe fat-soluble compounds, such as vitamins, that readily mix with water and can be absorbed without fat.

wheat germ a part of the wheat grain, rich in nutrients.

whole grain a grain that retains its outside layers (except the chaff); one that has not been refined.

xanthan see *stabilizers (thickeners).*

xylitol see *sugar alcohols.*

When an emergency is at hand, fast, effective action can save a life, perhaps your own. On the other hand, attempts to help without knowledge of correct procedures can do more harm than no action at all. This appendix is inadequate to prepare you for administering emergency treatments, but is presented with the idea that it, alone, may some day be the only reference at hand in an emergency. The local Red Cross and hospitals offer first aid courses that can prepare you fully, so take one. Until then, here are techniques that can save a life until properly trained help arrives. In order of urgency—stop excessive bleeding, keep the person breathing, and treat for shock. In addition to these basics, there are tips specific to heart attack, burns, hypothermia (cold stress), poisonings, and emergency childbirth.

In a serious emergency, it is urgent that someone call for help at the earliest possible moment. If you are the only one available, give first aid first, then call. In most places in the United States, the emergency telephone number is 911. You may ask whoever answers to connect you with poison control, ambulance service, or whatever assisting organization you require.

Many people wonder what is considered an emergency. You need to see your health care provider if you have or have had:

- An oral temperature above 104 degrees Fahrenheit (41 degrees centigrade). (Between 102 and 104 degrees Fahrenheit, call and ask whether you should be seen, or control with aspirin, acetaminophen, or ibuprofen.)
- Any serious accident or injury, including animal bites, puncture wounds, wounds with much blood loss, severe burns, suspected breaks or fractures, or possible poisoning.
- Falls with possible injury to the head or spine, followed by headache; vision abnormality; vomiting; bleeding from the ears, nose, or mouth; unusual behavior or drowsiness; paralysis; or convulsions.
- Sudden, severe pain or cramps in the abdomen.
- Breathing difficulty.
- Loss of consciousness, even if brief.
- Persistent severe headache.
- Intense itch.
- Sudden high fever.
- Bleeding or loss of any fluid from any body opening with unknown cause. (Blood in vomit or stools may appear black or brown, like coffee grounds; blood in urine may make it appear pink, red, or smoky.)
- Possible internal bleeding, as indicated by faintness, dizziness, weak or rapid pulse, shallow or irregular breathing, cold or clammy skin, or a bluish cast to the lips or fingernails.
- Possible cardiovascular abnormality, as indicated by a noticeable increase or decrease in heart rate.

■ Possible nervous system damage, as indicated by impaired thought processes, vision (especially a halo effect), hearing, sense of touch, or ability to move.
■ Any adverse drug reaction.
■ Continuous diarrhea or vomiting.

■≡ The Medicine Chest

In order to offer emergency treatment, you must have access to supplies, or you must use makeshift substitutes for those that are not available. For example, freshly laundered clothing is an acceptable substitute for gauze used to cover wounds or burns. Each home medicine chest should be stocked with a variety of simple equipment, as listed in Table E–1. One of the simplest and most useful bandages is the "butterfly," made from strips of adhesive tape and used to close open wounds (see Figure E–1). Make a few of these in advance, and store them on the roll of adhesive tape. Also, a standard reference, such as the American Red Cross publication *First Aid and Personal Safety,* will help remind you of what to do in an emergency and should be kept close at hand.

Most accidents occur at home, but they occur on outings, too. Campers and hikers can carry a similar array of equipment, with the addition of a snake-bite kit that consists of a sharp instrument for lancing the bite (a shallow incision is made connecting the fang marks, just through the skin layers), a strap to tie around the limb between the bite and the heart to temporarily reduce blood flow to the bite (see later cautions on tourniquets), and a suction device to remove venom. Some people keep a medicine box in their car, so it goes wherever they go.

■≡ Treating Wounds and Controlling Bleeding

Prompt treatment of wounds is necessary to prevent excessive bleeding and infection. Everyone should know how to treat the five types of wounds: **abrasion, avulsion, incision, laceration,** and **puncture** (see Miniglossary of Wounds). Table E–2 shows how to treat each type. Wounds deeper than the outer layers of skin are serious and should be evaluated by a health care professional after first aid has been administered. Further, medical treatment is required for any wound that has spurted blood, even if first aid has controlled it. Medical treatment is also necessary for any wound that may have involved muscles, tendons, ligaments, or nerves (indicated by paralysis or numbness); any bite wound (animal or human); any heavily contaminated wound; or any wound that contains soil or object fragments.

In order to determine the type and severity of the wound, look at it carefully. If you can't see the wound because of clothing, cut or tear away the clothing. The treatments proceed in the order of urgency for the protection of life. First, stop the blood flow from a wound that is bleeding steadily until the person can receive professional emergency help. Figure E–2 shows how to stop bleeding. Notice that the figure doesn't list a tourniquet for controlling bleeding; a tourniquet almost always kills the limb to which it is applied and should be used rarely, if ever. In almost all cases,

TABLE E–1 ■ Standard Supplies for the Medicine Chest

Item	Purpose
Bandages and Dressings	
Rolled gauze bandages, 2- and 3-inch widths	Wound wrap to hold sterile dressings or splints in place
Ready-to-apply sterile first aid dressings, individually packaged, various sizes	Padding to be applied directly to open wounds or burns
Triangular bandages, 36 × 36 inches	Diagonally folded sling for fractured or broken arm or shoulder; wrap to hold dressings in place; folded compress
Adherent dressing strips, 2- and 3-inch widths	Covering to be cut to size for simple wounds
Individually packaged adhesive bandages, various widths and shapes	Covering for minor cuts and scrapes
Medicines	
Aspirin or aspirin substitute	Pain reliever
Antiseptic cream or petroleum jelly	Sterile application for dressings, to prevent sticking to minor wounds
Liquid antiseptic	Cleanser for skin surfaces in cases of minor wounds
Calamine lotion	Agent for relieving itching from insect bites or exposure to skin irritants
Table salt packets	Treatment of shock with salted fluids
Syrup of ipecac	Emetic to induce vomiting in certain cases of poisoning
Activated charcoal	Adsorbent to bind certain types of poisons
Epsom salts	Laxative to speed passage of certain poisons through the digestive tract
Miscellaneous	
Adhesive tape	Fastening for bandages or dressings
Large safety pins	Fastening for bandages or slings
Tweezers	Splinter or insect stinger remover
Blunt-tipped scissors	Implement for severing lengths of bandage, adhesive tape, and the like
Thermometer(s)	Rectal or oral temperature taking
Hypoallergenic soap	Wound cleanser
Absorbent cotton, paper tissues	Absorbent dressing; wipe for cleansing wounds

SOURCE: Adapted from *Good Housekeeping Family Health and Medical Guide* (New York: Hearst, 1980), p. 876; E. Kiester, Jr., ed., *Better Homes and Gardens New Family Medical Guide* (Des Moines: Meredith Corporation, 1982), p. 833.

bleeding can be controlled by direct pressure; just a few cases require the addition of indirect pressure. Like the tourniquet, indirect pressure that constricts an artery can damage the healthy tissue normally fed by that artery, and should be used only in cases of severe hemorrhage where direct pressure will not stop the flow. Elevate the injured part to encourage blood to drain back into the body and to slow the blood flow to it.

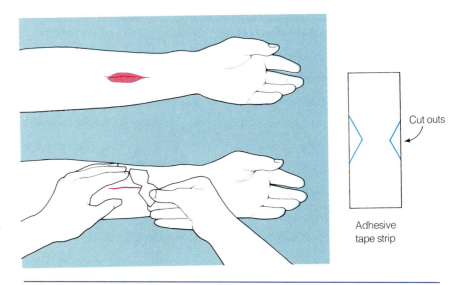

Cut outs

Adhesive
tape strip

FIGURE E–1 ■ **The butterfly bandage strip.**

To close an open wound, make butterfly strips from adhesive tape by cutting triangles from each edge halfway along the strip. Use one hand to close the wound, and the other to apply the butterfly.

■ MINIGLOSSARY of Wounds

abrasion a wound caused by rubbing or scraping the skin, such as rug or rope burns or skinned knees; typically, a thin layer of skin is removed over an area of flesh, leaving it open to infection.

avulsion a lifting or removal of a flap of skin and tissue, possibly involving torn veins and arteries; often caused by animal bites, motor vehicle and machinery accidents, gunshots, or explosions. This type of wound may bleed excessively and later may become infected.

Incision a straight-edged cut with clean edges resulting from contact with a sharp edge such as a knife or razor; if deeper than the top skin layers, it may bleed excessively and become infected later on.

laceration a cut that has jagged edges, with bruised, torn tissue, possibly involving veins and arteries; caused by blows from heavy blunt objects.

puncture a stab wound from a pointed object, such as a nail or stick; the long, narrow wound rarely bleeds excessively, but is most likely to become infected, possibly with anaerobic tetanus bacteria. (See Chapter 16 for more about infections.)

◼≡ Breathing Assistance

Second in urgency to controlling bleeding is restoring breathing. (A person can bleed to death from hemorrhage in just seconds, but can live for a minute or two without breathing.) People commonly choke on food at the table, and a person who is choking may need your help. First, ask this critical question: ''Can you make any sound at all?'' If the victim makes a sound, air is moving over the vocal cords, which means that some air can get into the lungs. In this case, the person might try bending over, coughing, and other self-help maneuvers before you intervene. Whatever you do, don't hit the victim on the back. If you do, the particle caught in the throat may become lodged in the air passage.

If the victim is unable to make a sound, you must act fast. To properly perform the techniques described here, a person should learn from a professional first aid instructor and practice on medical models. The objective of first aid is to clear the breathing passageway and to force air into and out of the lungs until spontaneous breathing resumes or professional emergency help arrives. It may take hours for help to arrive, but do not give up for at least four hours, even if the victim appears to be dead—the pulse may simply be weak, and recovery may be possible.

First, check inside the throat for tongue blockage or foreign matter, and clear the breathing passageway. Figure E–3 shows techniques for opening the airway and for cleaning out debris. After these measures, administer breathing assistance: kneel by the victim's head, tilt the chin up by pulling up on the back of the neck, pinch closed the nostrils, and blow into the mouth. (If the victim is a baby, cover both nose and mouth with your mouth, and blow small puffs of air.) Then listen closely for exhalation of air. If the air fails to enter the victim's lungs after a try or two, there may be an object lodged deep within the air passages. Quickly lift the person to standing or sitting on a chair, and perform the Heimlich maneuver as shown in Figure E–4 to remove lodged debris. Quickly return the person to the floor and begin again, clearing the mouth and throat, and start mouth-to-mouth

TABLE E–2 ■ Treatment of Wounds

	Abrasion	Avulsion	Incision or Laceration	Puncture
Minor Wound Treatment	Wash with soap, water, and sterile gauze, wiping away from the center of the wound with a new surface at each wipe. Bathe the wound in rubbing alcohol, and cover with sterile gauze. Change gauze frequently.	Wash with soap and water. Place torn tissue in its original location, and bandage with butterfly strips and sterile gauze. Seek prompt medical help.	Wash out cut with soap and water. Use adhesive tape butterfly strips to close the wound, and cover with sterile gauze.	Wash the surface with soap and water, and remove the object (sliver, pin, or small nail) that has punctured the tissue. Seek prompt medical help.
Serious Wound Treatment	See a physician if the wound contains dirt that can't be washed away, is deeper than the top layers of skin, or is located where scarring would be objectionable.	Stop bleeding with pressure. Preserve any pieces of tissue removed from the body in moist sterile gauze, and return flaps to original positions. Do not attempt to return a dislocated organ (such as an eyeball or loop of intestine) to the body cavity; lightly cover it with moist, sterile gauze, and obtain immediate emergency care.	Stop the bleeding. Close the wound with butterfly strips. Cover with sterile gauze, and obtain emergency medical help.	If the wound is deep or large, do not attempt to remove the object (to do so could cause further injury or allow profuse bleeding). If necessary, cut the object free from its attachments so that the person and the object may be transported to an emergency facility.

breathing again. If the person is large or unconscious, you can perform the maneuver by allowing the victim to remain lying on his or her back. Kneel astride the thighs, and place both hands as shown in Figure E–4 below the rib cage; press quickly and firmly upward. Be sure to make contact with your fist *before* the thrust—don't punch, but press suddenly. If it is you who is choking, you can be your own rescuer by thrusting your fist into your own abdomen, or thrusting your body forward forcefully against a firmly placed object—the back of a chair, side of a table, or edge of a sink or stove.

You can tell whether someone who is unconscious is breathing by placing your face close to his or hers and listening and feeling for air coming out of the mouth or nose. If the chest is not moving, the person is not breathing, but chest movements can also be caused by muscle spasms that mimic breathing, and should not be trusted as the sole indicator. Normal breathing rate is about 17 breaths per minute.

Early signs of inadequate breathing are dizziness; headache; memory problems; pounding in the ears; rapid pulse; and cold, clammy skin. A minute later a light-skinned person may start to appear blue; the blueness can be seen in dark-skinned people in the fingernails, or in the edges of the

A. Direct pressure

B. Indirect pressure

C. Indirect pressure points

FIGURE E–2 ■ **Using direct and indirect pressure to control bleeding.**

For direct pressure (A), use sterile gauze, if available, to cover the wound, and use your hand to apply pressure. Bleeding should stop or slow to oozing in under 30 minutes. For severe hemorrhage, indirect pressure (B) on an artery that feeds the damaged area can stop the flow. Select a place between the heart and the wound to apply indirect pressure. The points indicated here (C) are only a few of the possible pressure points. Like a tourniquet, indirect pressure robs healthy tissues fed by the artery, and may kill them; use indirect pressure only in severe hemorrhage when direct pressure fails to stem the flow of blood.

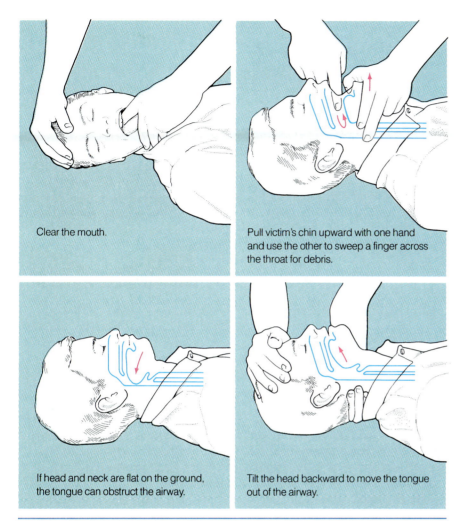

Clear the mouth.

Pull victim's chin upward with one hand and use the other to sweep a finger across the throat for debris.

If head and neck are flat on the ground, the tongue can obstruct the airway.

Tilt the head backward to move the tongue out of the airway.

FIGURE E–3 ■ **Clearing the airway.**
To clear debris from the mouth, turn the victim's head to the side, and use a finger to wipe out the debris. If the debris is lodged in the throat within finger's reach, try to catch an edge of the debris with a sweeping motion of a finger between the debris and the side of the throat, taking extreme care not to push the blockage further down toward the lungs. In children, use a small finger.

inner membranes of the lips and eyelids. Further, pupils may dilate, breathing and pulse may be stopped or irregular, heartbeat may cease, and the person may lose consciousness. Appearance may differ among individuals; some appear bluish black or pale. A cherry red color indicates carbon monoxide suffocation. Death occurs in over 50 percent of people within five minutes after breathing stops; all die within about ten minutes.

Drowning victims need breathing assistance. Before trying to move the victim completely out of the water, unless the water is so deep that you must do so, force air into the lungs with about ten breaths, using more pressure than normal to blow air past the water in the lungs. After the ten breaths have been delivered, move the victim out of the water, and undertake the breathing assistance as described above. The Heimlich maneuver has been recommended by some to reduce the amount of water in the lungs, but others consider it dangerous because it may cause vomiting, which can obstruct the lungs in an unconscious person. In any case, don't waste too much time trying to remove water while the lungs are starving for air. It is normal for the victim to vomit water from the stomach in the recovery from drowning; turn the victim's head to the side to prevent choking.

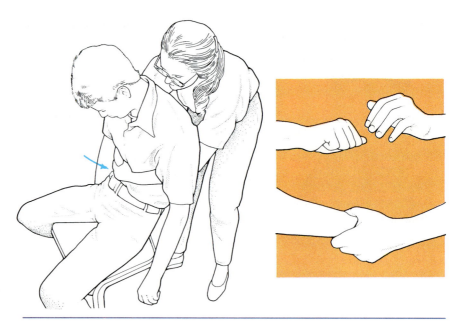

FIGURE E–4 ■ **How to perform the Heimlich maneuver.**

Sit or stand the victim in front of you, and wrap your arms around the waist. Make a fist with one hand, and cover it with the other. Place the fist against the victim's abdomen, just below the rib cage. Use a sudden squeezing motion to thrust your fist into the victim's abdomen with a quick, upward motion. Repeat four times in rapid succession. The food or debris should be ejected by the force of the air escaping from the lungs.

■ ☰ Treating for Shock

The condition called traumatic shock follows all injuries, including drownings. Its severity depends partly on the extent of physical injury and on the amount of blood lost, and partly on the victim's nervous system characteristics. Rough treatment, delayed treatment, emotional reactions, and pain worsen it. Every injury victim should be treated for shock as the third matter of business—bleeding first, then breathing, then treatment for shock.

Traumatic shock is not related to electric shock, diabetic shock, or others, but those medical conditions can certainly bring it on. Traumatic shock is a last-resort attempt by the body to save itself in the event of severe injury, to conserve the body's total blood supply by rerouting it from bleeding outer tissues to pools in the great vessels of the body. As circulation slows, vital organs become starved for blood and for the oxygen that it carries—a condition as dangerous as breathing obstruction. People whose injuries would not have killed them have died of shock.

In shock, the victim's pulse becomes weak and rapid, and the skin becomes pale or mottled or bluish, cold, and clammy. Breathing becomes irregular, and the person feels weak. The pupils may dilate. The treatment for shock is relatively simple, and Table E–3 gives the details.

■ ☰ Heart Attack Assistance

The three first aid measures described above are basic to almost any injury or sudden illness, but there is much more to know about specific injuries, binding fractured bones, transporting victims, administering aid to a heart attack victim, and other specifics. It is worthwhile to note that heart attack and stroke victims are especially in need of help, even though their pain

---

TABLE E–3 ■ **Treatment of Shock**

1. Lay the victim flat to facilitate circulation. Elevate only those body parts that have been treated for bleeding. The feet may be raised slightly by resting them on a folded blanket or other object.
2. Loosen any constricting clothing, particularly collars, belts, and waistbands.
3. Regulate the victim's body temperature by covering with blankets and inserting padding such as spare clothing between the victim's body and the surface beneath.
4. If the victim is conscious and has no abdominal or head injuries, and if help is not likely to arrive within an hour, giving room-temperature fluids can help. Give small amounts—no more than half a glass—every 15 minutes, for as long as the victim accepts them. If salt is available, add a light sprinkle (not more than 1/8 tsp) to each half glass of fluid.

---

may be slight, and they may deny that a heart attack or stroke is occurring. Most heart attack victims die within an hour of the onset of symptoms, before professional help can be delivered. If you notice any of the symptoms of heart attack or stroke listed in Chapter 18, you should:

■ Call an emergency rescue service, and tell them to bring oxygen (or transport the victim to an emergency treatment facility).
■ Administer the breathing assistance described above when necessary, and treat for shock. Those trained in the chest compression technique called cardiopulmonary resuscitation (CPR) can do much more to prolong life after heart attack until professional help is available, but *the untrained should not attempt it*.

This appendix will cover four more emergencies where special help is needed: burns, hypothermia (cold stress), poisoning (including drug overdose), and emergency childbirth. There are many more, and you would be wise to seek out a first aid course to teach you what to do in case something unforeseen should befall you or someone near you.

■≡ Treating Burns

Burns are classified by the depth of the tissue injury. First-degree burns injure just the top layers of skin and appear as redness, with mild swelling and pain; they heal rapidly. A light sunburn and a mild scald are examples. Second-degree burns involve deeper tissue damage and appear red or mottled, develop blisters, swell considerably, and are wet at the surface. A deep sunburn, flash burn from flammable fluid ignition, or contact with very hot liquid can cause second-degree burns. Third-degree burns involve deep tissue destruction and have a white or charred appearance; sometimes third-degree burns will appear to be second degree at first. Flame, ignited clothing, prolonged contact with hot fluids or objects, or electricity can all cause third-degree burns. Table E–4 shows the standard treatments for first-, second-, and third-degree burns.

TABLE E–4 ■ **Standard Treatments for Burns**

To treat first-degree burns:
- ■ Submerge the burned part in cold water, or apply gauze soaked in cold water.
- ■ Then, if exposure to soil is likely, layer dry gauze over the wet gauze to create a barrier to microbes.
- ■ Never apply grease of any kind to any burn.

To treat second-degree burns:
- ■ Treat as described above for first-degree burns, and seek medical treatment. Do not break blisters; remove tissue; or use antiseptic spray, cream, or any other product.
- ■ Elevate burned part.

To treat third-degree burns:
- ■ Elevate the burned part, especially the extremities.
- ■ Cover the burn with many layers of sterile gauze.
- ■ An ice pack with a dry surface may be applied to the burn, but do not apply water.
- ■ Treat for shock, and arrange transportation to an emergency medical facility.
- ■ Do not attempt to remove clothing or debris from the burn.

■ Treating Hypothermia

Hypothermia (literally, "low heat") is a condition marked by an abnormally low internal body temperature. It develops when body heat is lost to the environment faster than it can be replaced. A susceptible person in a cool room can develop hypothermia; the temperature of the surroundings does not have to be anywhere near freezing for the condition to occur. Susceptible people include older people who live alone, who do not shiver in response to cold, or who take certain medicines that interfere with their temperature-regulating mechanisms. Thousands of older people probably die of hypothermia each year; it affects about 10 percent of all persons over 65.

The signs of hypothermia include stiff muscles, with some trembling; shivering; puffy face; cold skin; problems with coordination; slowed breathing and heart rate; and pale or splotchy skin. As hypothermia progresses, the person may become confused and seem apathetic. If you suspect hypothermia, call an ambulance or rescue squad immediately; and while waiting for help, be careful not to do anything to make the victim's condition worse. Do *not* handle the person roughly (the heart is weak when the body is cold); do not attempt to rewarm the person with hot baths, electric blankets, or hot water bottles; and do not offer any food or drink. If the person is unconscious, do not raise the feet or legs, for the blood there is cooler than in other parts of the body and can further chill the body's core. Do wrap the person in available covering such as blankets, towels, pillows, scarves, or newspapers. Hypothermia is a dangerous, complicated medical problem, and the victim needs professional attention, so try to obtain help promptly.

■≡Treating Poisoning

Any adverse effect on the body from a chemical substance is considered poisoning, from an overdose of drugs to chemical burns of the eyes. Poisonings pose difficult problems for those administering first aid, because they vary in symptoms and treatments according to the substance involved.

The most common household poisonings involve overdoses of aspirin or other over-the-counter pain relievers, eaten by children or taken by mistake by adults. In this case, if the victim is conscious, administer syrup of ipecac to induce vomiting, then give activated charcoal and transport the victim to an emergency facility. This sequence is adequate for overdoses of most medications taken by mouth. If poisons are taken by injection, assistance in breathing may be required; it is always necessary to treat for shock and to seek immediate emergency assistance. Table E–5 lists the basic first aid steps for each type of poisoning, but there are hundreds of possible causes and treatments. An essential measure is to find out what chemical is involved, by reading the labels or by asking the person; then contact professionals at

---

TABLE E–5 ■ First Aid for Poisonings

If poisoning by mouth is suspected:
- ■ If the victim is conscious, administer a glass of milk or water to dilute the poison while you get information.
- ■ Try to identify the substance involved; read the labels of bottles or ask the person.
- ■ Call the nearest poison control center and ask how to treat the poisoning—what to administer, and when.
- ■ Save any containers, as well as samples of any vomited material, for inspection by emergency personnel.

If the poison was inhaled:
- ■ Remove the person from the source of the gas to fresh air.
- ■ Open all doors and windows.
- ■ Treat skin and eyes as necessary, and call for an emergency rescue unit.
- ■ Administer breathing assistance, if necessary.

If the poison is on the skin:
- ■ Remove clothing that has been contaminated, and flood the affected skin for ten minutes with water. A shower works well for large areas. While flooding the skin, call the emergency rescue unit.
- ■ After ten minutes, wash the affected area with soap and water.
- ■ For rashes from poisonous plants, wash the affected area and all clothing with soap and water, dry the rash, and apply calamine lotion. Seek medical treatment if the reaction is severe.

If the poison is in the eye:
- ■ Flood the eye with water (body temperature, if possible) for 15 minutes. Do this by having the victim lean over a water fountain or under a faucet or shower and allow a gentle flow to run through the affected eye, while blinking as much as possible. Direct the flow away from the nose. If no faucet is available, pour water from a cup or other object over the eye repeatedly for 15 minutes. After first aid has started, call an emergency rescue unit.

a poison control center for advice on how to proceed in each specific case. If the chemicals are illegally obtained drugs, do not try to protect the victim from legal action by not calling for help—the legalities are small when compared with loss of life.

■≡ Emergency Childbirth

If you are in the presence of a woman who is delivering an infant without health care assistance, and you are truly beyond reach of medical help, she may want you to assist her. First, be absolutely certain that you are indeed outside of reach of medical assistance. If you can, summon whatever medical professional you are able to contact. While waiting for help to arrive, remember: childbirth is not like drowning or other dangerous medical emergencies. It is a normal body function, and women deliver babies every day around the world, with or without help. Your main function is to offer comfort to the woman, make sure the newborn is breathing, and clean up. Here's how:

- ■ Childbirth is messy. Spread clean sheets, towels, or paper for the delivery.
- ■ Allow the woman to choose her own most comfortable position; provide props for her to lean on, if she desires them.
- ■ Once she is settled, encourage her to use a bedpan or other container for urinating or moving the bowels, rather than moving to a toilet. It is common for the woman to urinate or defecate during the delivery. If this happens, remove the soiled coverings or just cover them up with fresh ones.
- ■ Wash your hands with soap and water. Refrain from cleaning any part of the woman, especially around the vagina.
- ■ Expect the delivery to more or less follow the course described in Chapter 14. Do not interfere; do not pull or push on the infant; do not be upset if the woman yells out from her contractions. The condition is temporary and normal. Give encouragement.
- ■ Upon delivery, your first aid skills can come in handy. Make sure the newborn is breathing; clear away any obstruction blocking the airway. If the amniotic sac hasn't broken, break it gently, and uncover the baby's face. Use a clean cloth that doesn't leave particles, to wipe the baby's face, but don't wipe the rest of the body.
- ■ Chances are it won't happen, but if the umbilical cord has wrapped around the baby's neck during delivery, ask the woman to stop pushing so that you can unwrap it. Slip the loop over the baby's head. Observe the baby for breathing after birth, and provide mouth-to-mouth assistance if no breathing has begun.
- ■ Let the umbilical cord and the placenta be expelled naturally; put no tension on the cord. The cord contains blood that belongs to the baby and won't allow any back flow out of the baby's body, so you needn't cut it. Lightly wrap it up, with the infant and placenta, in a clean cloth for the health care professionals to deal with. If it will be a day or so before help arrives, wait until the cord stops pulsating to cut it (there's no hurry). Tie a clean string or strip of gauze tightly around it 6 inches from the infant's

body; place another tie an inch or so closer to the placenta, and cut between them with a clean knife.

■ Preserve the placenta for inspection by a health professional.

■ Place the baby near the mother; wipe the woman dry with clean cloth; and provide fluids or blankets if she requests them. Keep them both warm and dry. The baby may nurse and should be allowed to do so; nursing triggers contractions that shrink the woman's uterus and prevent excessive bleeding.

If you are convinced that the labor and delivery are not proceeding normally, make the woman as comfortable as possible, and transport her to the nearest emergency facility.

This appendix offers information on most of the foods people commonly eat. To present all the available data would require hundreds of pages, space not available here. Given limited space, we have chosen to present calories (because everyone wants to know them); the percentages of calories from protein, carbohydrate, and fat; fiber; cholesterol; and sodium contents of foods.

Keep a sense of perspective in using this table. Foods are not eaten singly, they are combined into diets—and diets may be beneficial or harmful. Foods, however, can pull diets in one direction or another, and the amounts eaten should be adjusted accordingly. For this reason, it can be useful to see what contributions individual foods make.

For a perspective on calories, remember that an average-sized adult man might require about 2,000 to 3,000 calories per day to maintain his weight, and a woman, about 1,200 to 2,200. With respect to the fat content of foods, remember (Chapter 5) that a widely accepted dietary goal is that no more than 30 percent of the day's calories should come from fat. Total dietary fiber for a day should perhaps add up to about 15 to 30 grams. Cholesterol recommendations probably need not be made for the general public, but people who are advised by their health care providers to restrict their cholesterol intakes may want to keep them below about 300 mg a day. As for sodium, current guidelines indicate that an intake of 2,000 to 3,000 mg a day might be desirable.

TABLE F–1 ■ **Food Composition**

Key	Name	Measure	Energy (calories)	Protein/ Carbohydrate/ Fat (%)	Fiber (g)	Cholesterol (mg)	Sodium (mg)
	BEVERAGES						
	Alcoholic:						
	Beer:						
1	Regular (12 fl oz)	1½ cups	146	2/36/0*	0.5	0	19
1	Light (12 fl oz)	1½ cups	100[1]	3/18/0*	0.5	0	10
	Gin, rum, vodka, whiskey:						
1	90 proof	1½ fl oz	110	0/0/0*	0	0	4
	Wine:						
1	Red	3½ fl oz	74	1/10/0*	0	0	6
1	White medium	3½ fl oz	70	1/5/0*	0	0	5
	Carbonated[3]:						
1	Cola beverage (12 fl oz)	1½ cups	151	1/100/0	0	0	14
1	Diet cola (12 fl oz)	1½ cups	2	40/60/0	0	0	21[4]
1	Ginger ale (12 fl oz)	1½ cups	124	1/100/0	0	0	25
1	Lemon-lime (12 fl oz)	1½ cups	149	0/100/0	0	0	41
	Coffee:[3]						
1	Brewed	1 cup	2[5]	8/90/2	t	0	5
	Fruit drinks,[6] noncarbonated:						
1	Fruit punch drink, canned	1 cup	118	0/99/1	0	0	56
1	Lemonade, prepared from frozen concentrate	1 cup	100	0/99/1	0.5	0	8
	Fruit and vegetable juices; see Fruit and Vegetable sections.						
	Tea:[3]						
1	Brewed	1 cup	2[5]	0/100/0	0	0	7
1	From instant, sweetened	1 cup	86	0/99/1	0	0	t
	DAIRY						
	Butter: see Fats and Oils						
	Cheese, natural:						
2	Blue	1 oz	100	24/3/73	0	21	39
2	Brie	1 oz	95	25/1/74	0	28	17
2	Camembert	1 oz	85	26/1/73	0	20	23
2	Cheddar, cut pieces	1 oz	114	25/1/74	0	30	17
	Cottage:						
2	Creamed, small curd	1 cup	215	50/11/39	0	31	85
2	Lowfat 2%	1 cup	205	63/17/20	0	19	91
2	Cream	1 oz	99	8/3/89	0	31	84
2	Gouda	1 oz	101	28/2/70	0	32	23
2	Monterey jack	1 oz	106	26/1/73	0	26	152
2	Mozzarella, made with part skim milk, low moisture	1 oz	80	40/5/55	0	15	150
2	Parmesan, grated	1 oz	129	37/3/60	0	22	528
2	Provolone	1 oz	100	29/2/69	0	20	248
2	Ricotta, made with whole milk	1 cup	428	26/7/67	0	124	207

*Alcohol contributes additional calories, bringing the total to 100%.

[1]Calories can vary from 78 to 131 for 12 fluid ounces.

[3]Sodium content varies depending on water source.

[4]Value for product sweetened with aspartame only; sodium is 32 mg if a blend of aspartame and sodium saccharin is used; 75 mg if just sodium saccharin is used.

[5]Calorie values are not available: this is a USDA estimate.

[6]Usually less than 10% fruit juice.

(For purposes of calculations, use "0" for t.)

Key: 1 = Bev 2 = Dairy 3 = Eggs 4 = Fat/Oil 5 = Fruit 6 = Bakery 7 = Grain 8 = Fish 9 = Meat 10 = Poultry 11 = Sausage 12 = Mixed Dishes 13 = Nuts/Seeds 14 = Sweets 15 .= Veg/Leg 16 = Misc 22 = Soup/Sauce 25 = Fast Foods by Brand Name

TABLE F–1 ■ Food Composition

Key	Name	Measure	Energy (calories)	Protein/ Carbohydrate/ Fat (%)	Fiber (g)	Cholesterol (mg)	Sodium (mg)
DAIRY (cont.)							
	Cheese, natural (cont.):						
2	Swiss	1 oz	107	30/4/66	0	26	74
	Pasteurized processed cheese products:						
2	American	1 oz	106	23/2/75	0	27	406
2	Swiss	1 oz	95	30/3/67	0	24	388
2	American cheese food	1 oz	93	24/9/67	0	18	337
2	American cheese spread	1 oz	82	24/12/64	0	16	381
	Cream, sweet:						
2	Half and half (cream and milk)	1 tbsp	20	8/14/78	0	6	6
2	Light, coffee or table	1 tbsp	30	5/8/87	0	10	6
2	Light whipping cream, liquid	1 tbsp	44	3/4/93	0	17	5
2	Heavy whipping cream, liquid	1 tbsp	51	2/3/95	0	20	6
2	Whipped cream, pressurized	1 tbsp	10	4/20/76	0	3	5
2	Cream, sour, cultured	1 tbsp	30	5/8/87	0	6	7
	Cream products-imitation and part dairy:						
	Coffee whitener:						
2	Frozen or liquid	1 tbsp	20	2/33/65	0	0	12
2	Powdered	1 tsp	11	0/39/61	0	0	4
2	Dessert topping, frozen	1 tbsp	15	0/29/71	0	0	1
2	Imitation sour cream	1 tbsp	29	4/12/84	0	0	14
	Milk, fluid:						
2	Whole milk	1 cup	150	21/30/49	0	33	120
2	2% Lowfat milk	1 cup	121	27/38/35	0	22	122
2	Skim milk	1 cup	86	39/56/5	0	4	126
2	Buttermilk	1 cup	99	33/47/20	0	9	257
	Milk, canned:						
2	Evaporated, whole	1 cup	340	20/29/51	0	74	267
2	Evaporated, skim	1 cup	200	39/59/2	0	10	293
	Milk, dried:						
2	Buttermilk	1 cup	464	36/51/13	0	83	621
2	Instant, nonfat	1 cup	244	40/58/2	0	12	373
	Milk beverages and powdered mixes:						
	Chocolate:						
2	Whole	1 cup	210	15/49/36	t	31	149
2	2% Fat	1 cup	180	18/57/25	t	17	151
2	Egg nog, commercial	1 cup	342	12/39/49	0	149	138

(For purposes of calculations, use "0" for t.)

Key: 1 = Bev 2 = Dairy 3 = Eggs 4 = Fat/Oil 5 = Fruit 6 = Bakery 7 = Grain 8 = Fish 9 = Meat 10 = Poultry 11 = Sausage 12 = Mixed Dishes 13 = Nuts/Seeds 14 = Sweets 15 = Veg/Leg 16 = Misc 22 = Soup/Sauce 25 = Fast Foods by Brand Name

TABLE F–1 ■ **Food Composition**

Key	Name	Measure	Energy (calories)	Protein/ Carbohydrate/ Fat (%)	Fiber (g)	Cholesterol (mg)	Sodium (mg)
	DAIRY (cont.)						
	Cream products (cont.):						
	Milk shakes:						
2	Chocolate (10 fl oz)	1¼ cups	360	11/63/26	0.5	37	273
2	Vanilla (10 fl oz)	1¼ cups	314	12/64/24	t	32	232
	Milk desserts, frozen:						
	Ice cream, regular (about 11% fat) vanilla:						
2	Hardened	1 cup	269	7/46/47	0	59	116
2	Soft Serve	1 cup	377	7/40/53	0	153	153
2	Ice cream, rich vanilla (about 16% fat), hardened	1 cup	349	6/44/50	0	88	108
	Ice milk, vanilla (about 4% fat):						
2	Hardened	1 cup	184	11/62/27	0	18	105
2	Soft serve (about 3% fat)	1 cup	223	14/68/18	0	13	163
2	Sherbet (2% fat)	1 cup	270	3/85/12	0	14	88
	Milk desserts, other:						
2	Custard, baked	1 cup	305	18/38/44	0	278	209
	Puddings, prepared from dry mix with whole milk:						
2	Chocolate, instant	1 cup	310	10/69/21	0.5	28	880
2	Rice	½ cup	155	10/67/23	t	15	140
2	Tapioca	½ cup	145	10/66/24	0	15	152
2	Vanilla, instant	½ cup	150	10/67/23	0	15	375
	Yogurt, lowfat:						
2	Fruit added[13]	1 cup	231	17/73/10	0.5	10	133
2	Plain	1 cup	144	33/45/22	0	14	159
2	Vanilla or coffee flavor	1 cup	193	23/64/13	0	11	150
2	Yogurt, made with nonfat milk	1 cup	127	42/55/3	0	4	173
2	Yogurt, made with whole milk	1 cup	138	23/30/47	0	29	104
	EGGS						
3	Raw, large, whole, without shell	1 ea	79	32/3/65	0	213	69
	Cooked:						
3	Fried in butter	1 ea	95	27/2/71	0	278	162
3	Hard-cooked, shell removed	1 ea	79	32/3/65	0	215	69
3	Scrambled with milk and butter (also omelet)	1 ea	95	26/6/68	0	282	176

[13]Carbohydrate and calories vary widely—consult label if more precise values are needed.

(For purposes of calculations, use "0" for t.)

Key: 1 = Bev 2 = Dairy 3 = Eggs 4 = Fat/Oil 5 = Fruit 6 = Bakery 7 = Grain 8 = Fish 9 = Meat 10 = Poultry 11 = Sausage 12 = Mixed Dishes 13 = Nuts/Seeds 14 = Sweets 15 = Veg/Leg 16 = Misc 22 = Soup/Sauce 25 = Fast Foods by Brand Name

TABLE F-1 ■ Food Composition

Key	Name	Measure	Energy (calories)	Protein/ Carbohydrate/ Fat (%)	Fiber (g)	Cholesterol (mg)	Sodium (mg)
	FATS and OILS						
	Butter:						
4	Tablespoon	1 tbsp	100	t/0/99	0	31	116[14]
4	Pat (about 1 tsp)[15a]	1 ea	34	0/0/100	0	11	41[14]
4	Fats, cooking (vegetable shortening)	1 tbsp	115	0/0/100	0	0	0
	Margarine:						
4	Imitation (about 40% fat) soft	1 tbsp	50	0/0/100	0	0	136[14]
	Regular, hard (about 80% fat):						
4	Tablespoon	1 tbsp	100	t/t/99	0	0	133[14]
4	Pat[15a]	1 ea	36	0/0/100	0	0	47[14]
4	Regular, soft (about 80% fat)	1 tbsp	100	4/0/96	0	0	153[14]
	Spread (about 60% fat), hard:						
4	Tablespoon	1 tbsp	75	0/0/100	0	0	139[14]
4	Pat[15a]	1 ea	25	0/0/100	0	0	50[14]
4	Spread (about 60% fat) soft	1 tbsp	75	0/0/100	0	0	139[14]
	Oils:						
	Corn:						
4	Tablespoon	1 tbsp	125	0/0/100	0	0	0
	Olive:						
4	Tablespoon	1 tbsp	125	0/0/100	0	0	0
	Peanut:						
4	Tablespoon	1 tbsp	125	0/0/100	0	0	0
	Salad dressings/sandwich spreads:						
4	Blue cheese:	1 tbsp	75	4/5/91	t	3	.3
	French:						
4	Regular	1 tbsp	85	0/5/95	t	0	188
4	Low calorie	1 tbsp	24	0/36/64	t	0	306
	Italian:						
4	Regular	1 tbsp	80	t/5/95	t	0	162
4	Low calorie	1 tbsp	5	0/26/74	t	0	136
	Mayonnaise:						
4	Regular	1 tbsp	100	1/2/97	0	8	80
4	Imitation	1 tbsp	35	0/23/77	0	4	75
4	Ranch style	1 tbsp	54	3/5/92	0	6	65
4	Salad dressing-mayo type	1 tbsp	58	1/24/75	0	4	105
4	Tartar sauce	1 tbsp	74	1/3/96	t	4	182
	Thousand Island:						
4	Regular	1 tbsp	60	1/15/84	t	4	110
4	Low calorie	1 tbsp	25	2/40/58	t	2	153
	Salad dressings, prepared from home recipe:						
4	Vinegar & oil	1 tbsp	70	0/0/100	0	0	0

[14]For salted butter or margarine; unsalted varieties contain 12 mg sodium per stick or ½ cup, 1.5 mg per tablespoon, or .5 mg per pat.
[15a]Pat is 1 in square, ⅓ in high; 90 per lb.

(For purposes of calculations, use "0" for t.)

Key: 1 = Bev 2 = Dairy 3 = Eggs 4 = Fat/Oil 5 = Fruit 6 = Bakery 7 = Grain 8 = Fish 9 = Meat 10 = Poultry 11 = Sausage 12 = Mixed Dishes 13 = Nuts/Seeds 14 = Sweets 15 = Veg/Leg 16 = Misc 22 = Soup/Sauce 25 = Fast Foods by Brand Name

TABLE F-1 ■ **Food Composition**

Key	Name	Measure	Energy (calories)	Protein/ Carbohydrate/ Fat (%)	Fiber (g)	Cholesterol (mg)	Sodium (mg)
	FRUITS and FRUIT JUICES						
	Apples:						
	Raw, with peel:						
	2¾″ diam (about 3 per lb						
5	with cores)	1 ea	80	1/94/5	4.5	0	1
	3¼″ diam (about 2 per lb						
5	with cores)	1 ea	125	1/94/5	6.5	0	2
5	Dried, sulfured	10 ea	155	1/98/1	9.0	0	56[20]
5	Apple juice, bottled or canned[21]	1 cup	116	1/97/2	0.5	0	7
	Applesauce:						
5	Sweetened	1 cup	195	1/97/2	3.5	0	8
5	Unsweetened	1 cup	106	1/98/1	5.0	0	5
	Apricots:						
	Canned (fruit and liquid):						
5	Heavy syrup	1 cup	214	2/97/1	4.5	0	10
5	Juice pack	1 cup	119	5/95/0	4.5	0	9
	Dried:						
5	Dried halves	10 ea	83	6/92/2	3.5	0	3
	Avocado, raw, edible part only:						
5	Mashed, fresh, average	1 cup	370	4/17/79	6.5	0	24
	Bananas, raw, without peel:						
5	Whole, 8¾″ long (weighs 175g						
	with peel)	1 ea	105	4/92/4	3.5	0	1
5	Blackberries, raw	1 cup	74	5/89/6	9.5	0	0
	Blueberries:						
5	Raw	1 cup	82	4/90/6	5.0	0	9
	Frozen, sweetened:						
5	Cup	1 cup	185	2/97/1	7.0	0	3
	Cherries:						
5	Sour, red pitted, canned water pack	1 cup	90	8/90/2	2.5	0	17
5	Sweet, raw, without pits	10 ea	49	6/83/11	1.5	0	0
	Cranberry juices:						
5	Cranberry juice cocktail	1 cup	145	0/99/1	1.0	0	5
5	Cranberry sauce, canned, strained	¼ cup	105	1/98/1	0.5	0	20
	Dates:						
5	Whole, without pits	10 ea	228	3/96/1	7.0	0	2
5	Figs, dried	10 ea	477	4/92/4	24.0	0	21
	Fruit cocktail, canned, fruit and liquid						
5	Heavy syrup pack	1 cup	185	2/97/1	2.5	0	15
5	Juice pack	1 cup	115	4/96/0	2.5	0	10
	Grapefruit:						
	Raw 3¾ in diam, whole fruit weighs 1 lb 1 oz with refuse (peel, membrane, seeds):						
5	Pink/red, half fruit, edible part	1 half	37	7/91/2	1.5	0	0

[20]Unsulfured product contains less sodium.
[21]Also applies to pasteurized apple cider.

(For purposes of calculations, use "0" for t.)

Key: 1 = Bev 2 = Dairy 3 = Eggs 4 = Fat/Oil 5 = Fruit 6 = Bakery 7 = Grain 8 = Fish 9 = Meat 10 = Poultry 11 = Sausage 12 = Mixed Dishes 13 = Nuts/Seeds 14 = Sweets 15 = Veg/Leg 16 = Misc 22 = Soup/Sauce 25 = Fast Foods by Brand Name

TABLE F–1 ■ Food Composition

Key	Name	Measure	Energy (calories)	Protein/ Carbohydrate/ Fat (%)	Fiber (g)	Cholesterol (mg)	Sodium (mg)
	FRUITS and FRUIT JUICES (cont.)						
	White, half fruit, edible						
5	part	1 half	39	7/91/2	1.5	0	0
5	Canned sections with liquid	1 cup	152	3/96/1	2.0	0	4
	Grapefruit juice:						
5	Raw	1 cup	96	5/93/2	0.5	0	2
	Canned:						
5	Unsweetened	1 cup	93	5/93/2	0.5	0	2
5	Sweetened	1 cup	115	5/94/1	0.5	0	5
	Frozen concentrate, unsweetened:						
5	Diluted with 3 cans water	1 cup	102	5/92/3	0.5	0	2
	Grapes, raw European type (adherent skin):						
5	Thompson seedless	10 ea	35	3/90/7	1.0	0	1
5	Tokay/Emperor, seeded types	10 ea	40	4/90/6	1.0	0	1
	Grape juice:						
5	Bottled or canned	1 cup	155	4/95/1	1.5	0	8
	Frozen concentrate, sweetened:						
5	Diluted with 3 cans water	1 cup	128	2/97/1	1.5	0	5
5	Kiwi fruit, raw, peeled (about 5 per lb with skin):	1 ea	46	6/89/5	1.5	0	4
5	Lemons, raw, without peel and seeds (about 4 per lb whole)	1 ea	17	9/84/7	1.5	0	1
	Lemon juice:						
	Fresh:						
5	Tablespoon	1 tbsp	4	0/100/0	t	0	.1
	Canned or bottled, unsweetened:						
5	Tablespoon	1 tbsp	5	0/100/0	t	0	3[33]
5	Mango, raw, edible part (weighs 300g with skin and seed)	1 ea	135	3/93/4	3.0	0	4
	Melons, raw, without rind and cavity contents:						
5	Cantaloupe, 5 in diam (2⅓ lb whole, with refuse), orange flesh:	½ ea	94	9/85/6	2.5	0	24
5	Honeydew, 6½ in diam (5¼ lb whole with refuse) slice = ¹/₁₀ melon	1 pce	45	5/94/2	1.5	0	13
5	Nectarines, raw, without pits, 2½ in diam	1 ea	67	7/86/7	3.0	0	0
	Oranges, raw:						
5	Whole without peel and seeds 2⅝ in diam (weighs about 180 g with peel and seeds)	1 ea	60	7/90/3	3.0	0	t
	Orange juice:						
5	Fresh, all varieties:	1 cup	111	6/90/4	0.5	0	2

[33]Sodium benzoate is added as a preservative.

(For purposes of calculations, use "0" for t.)

Key: 1 = Bev 2 = Dairy 3 = Eggs 4 = Fat/Oil 5 = Fruit 6 = Bakery 7 = Grain 8 = Fish 9 = Meat 10 = Poultry 11 = Sausage 12 = Mixed Dishes 13 = Nuts/Seeds 14 = Sweets 15 = Veg/Leg 16 = Misc 22 = Soup/Sauce 25 = Fast Foods by Brand Name

TABLE F–1 ■ Food Composition

Key	Name	Measure	Energy (calories)	Protein/ Carbohydrate/ Fat (%)	Fiber (g)	Cholesterol (mg)	Sodium (mg)
	FRUITS and FRUIT JUICES (cont.)						
5	Canned, unsweetened	1 cup	105	6/91/3	0.5	0	5
	Frozen concentrate:						
5	Diluted with 3 parts water by volume	1 cup	110	5/94/1	1.0	0	2
	Peaches:						
	Raw:						
5	Whole, 2½ in diam, peeled, pitted (about 4 per lb with peels and pits)	1 ea	37	6/94/0	2.0	0	0
	Canned, fruit and liquid:						
	Heavy syrup pack						
5	Half	1 ea	60	2/98/0	1.5	0	5
	Juice pack						
5	Half	1 ea	34	5/95/0	1.5	0	3
	Dried:						
5	Uncooked	10 ea	311	5/92/3	10.5	0	9
	Frozen, sliced, sweetened:						
5	Cup, thawed measure	1 cup	235	3/96/1	5.5	0	16
	Pears:						
	Raw, with skin, cored:						
5	Bartlett, 2½ in diam (about 2½ per lb, whole)	1 ea	98	2/92/6	5.0[36]	0	1
5	Bosc, 2½ in diam (about 3 per lb, whole)	1 ea	85	3/92/5	4.0[36]	0	t
5	D'Anjou, 3 in diam (about ½ lb, whole)	1 ea	120	2/93/5	6.0[36]	0	t
	Canned, fruit and liquid:						
	Heavy syrup pack:						
5	Half	1 ea	59	1/98/1	1.5[36]	0	4
	Juice pack:						
5	Half	1 ea	38	3/97/0	1.5[36]	0	3
5	Dried halves	10 ea	459	3/95/2	19.0	0	10
	Pineapple:						
5	Raw chunks, diced	1 cup	76	3/90/7	3.0	0	2
	Canned, fruit and liquid:						
	Heavy syrup pack:						
5	Slices	1 ea	45	2/98/0	0.5	0	1
	Juice pack:						
5	Slices	1 ea	35	2/98/0	0.5	0	1
5	Pineapple juice, canned, unsweetened	1 cup	140	3/96/1	1.0	0	3

[35]Dietary fiber data varies 2.4 to 3.4 grams per 100 grams for fresh pears; 1.6 to 2.6 grams per 100 grams for canned pears.

(For purposes of calculations, use "0" for t.)

Key: 1 = Bev 2 = Dairy 3 = Eggs 4 = Fat/Oil 5 = Fruit 6 = Bakery 7 = Grain 8 = Fish 9 = Meat 10 = Poultry 11 = Sausage 12 = Mixed Dishes 13 = Nuts/Seeds 14 = Sweets 15 = Veg/Leg 16 = Misc 22 = Soup/Sauce 25 = Fast Foods by Brand Name

TABLE F–1 ■ Food Composition

Key	Name	Measure	Energy (calories)	Protein/ Carbohydrate/ Fat (%)	Fiber (g)	Cholesterol (mg)	Sodium (mg)
	FRUITS and FRUIT JUICES (cont.)						
	Plums, without pits:						
	Raw:						
5	Medium 2⅛ in diam	1 ea	36	5/86/9	1.5	0	t
	Canned, purple, with liquid:						
	Heavy syrup pack:						
5	Plums	3 ea	98	2/97/1	2.0	0	21
	Juice pack:						
5	Cup	1 cup	146	3/97/0	5.5	0	3
5	Plums	3 ea	55	3/97/0	2.0	0	1
	Prunes, dried, pitted:						
5	Uncooked (10 prunes with pits weigh 97 g):	10 ea	201	4/94/2	13.5[40]	0	3
5	Prune juice-bottled or canned	1 cup	181	3/97/0	3.0	0	10
	Raisins, seedless:						
5	One packet, ½ oz	1 ea	41	4/96/0	1.0	0	2
	Raspberries:						
5	Raw	1 cup	60	7/84/9	9.0	0	0
	Frozen, sweetened:						
5	Cup, thawed measure	1 cup	255	3/96/1	13.5	0	3
	Strawberries:						
5	Raw, whole, capped	1 cup	45	7/82/11	3.5	0	2
	Frozen, sliced, sweetened:						
5	Cup, thawed measure	1 cup	245	2/97/1	5.5	0	8
	Tangerines, without peel and seeds:						
5	Raw (2⅜ in diam)	1 ea	37	5/91/4	1.5	0	1
	Watermelon, raw, without rind and seeds						
5	Piece, 1 in thick by 10 in diam (weighs 2 lb with refuse)	1 pce	152	7/82/11	2.5	0	10
5	Diced	1 cup	50	7/82/11	1.0	0	3
	BAKED GOODS: BREADS, CAKES, COOKIES, CRACKERS, PIES, PANCAKES, TORTILLAS						
6	Bagel, plain, enriched, 3½ in diam	1 ea	200	15/77/8	0.5	0	245
	Biscuits:						
6	From mix	1 ea	94	9/60/31	0.5	t	265
	Breads:						
	Cracked wheat bread (¼ cracked wheat flour, ¾ enr wheat flour):						
6	Slice (18 per loaf)	1 pce	65	14/75/11	1.5	0	106
	French/Vienna bread, enriched:						
6	Vienna, slice 4¾ × 4 × ½ in	1 pce	70	14/73/13	0.5	0	145
	French toast: see Mixed dishes, key 12						
	Italian bread, enriched:						
6	Slice 4½ × 3¼ × ¾ in	1 pce	83	13/84/3	0.5	0	176

[40]Dietary fiber data can vary to a lower value of approx 8.1 grams for 10 prunes.

(For purposes of calculations, use "0" for t.)

Key: 1 = Bev 2 = Dairy 3 = Eggs 4 = Fat/Oil 5 = Fruit 6 = Bakery 7 = Grain 8 = Fish 9 = Meat 10 = Poultry 11 = Sausage 12 = Mixed Dishes 13 = Nuts/Seeds 14 = Sweets 15 = Veg/Leg 16 = Misc 22 = Soup/Sauce 25 = Fast Foods by Brand Name

TABLE F–1 ■ **Food Composition**

Key	Name	Measure	Energy (calories)	Protein/ Carbohydrate/ Fat (%)	Fiber (g)	Cholesterol (mg)	Sodium (mg)
	BAKED GOODS (cont.)						
	Breads (cont.):						
	Mixed grain bread, enriched:						
6	Slice (18 per loaf)	1 pce	65	12/75/13	1.0	0	106
	Oatmeal bread, enriched:						
6	Slice(18 per loaf)	1 pce	65	13/72/15	1.0	0	124
6	Pita pocket bread, enr, 6½ in round	1 ea	165	15/80/5	0.5	0	339
	Pumpernickel break (⅔ rye flour, ⅓ enr wheat flour):						
6	Slice, 5 × 4 × ⅜ in	1 pce	80	14/74/12	1.5	0	277
	Raisin bread, enriched:						
6	Slice (18 per loaf)	1 pce	68	11/76/13	0.5	0	92
	Rye bread, light (⅓ rye flour, ⅔ enr wheat flour):						
6	Slice, 4¾ × 3¾ × 7/16 in	1 pce	65	13/74/13	1.5	0	175
	Wheat bread[45] (blend of enr wheat flour and whole wheat flour):						
6	Slice (18 per loaf)	1 pce	65	14/72/14	1.5	0	135
	White bread, enriched:						
6	Slice (18 per loaf)	1 pce	65	13/74/13	0.5	0	129
	Whole wheat bread:						
6	Slice (16 per loaf)	1 pce	70	16/69/15	3.0	0	180
	Bread stuffing, prepared from mix:						
6	Dry type	¼ cup	125	7/39/54	0.5	0	314
6	Moist type, with egg	¼ cup	105	8/38/54	0.5	17	256
	Cakes[46], prepared from mixes:						
6	Boston cream pie, ⅛ cake	1 pce	260	4/68/28	0.5	20	225
	Coffee cake:						
6	Piece, ⅙ cake	1 pce	230	8/65/27	0.5	47	310
	Devil's food with chocolate frosting:						
6	Piece, 1/16 of cake	1 pce	235	5/66/29	0.5	37	181
6	Cupcake, 2½ in diam	1 ea	120	5/64/31	t	19	92
	Gingerbread:						
6	Piece, ⅑ of cake	1 pce	174	5/73/22	0.5	1	192
	Yellow, with chocolate frosting, 2 layer:						
6	Piece, 1/16 of cake	1 pce	235	5/66/29	0.5	36	157
	Cakes from home recipes with enriched flour:						
	Carrot cake, cream cheese frosting:						
6	Piece, 1/16 of 9 × 13 in sheet cake 2¼ × 3¼ in	1 pce	385	4/48/48	0.5	74	279
	Fruitcake, dark, 7½ in diam tube-2¼ in high:						
6	Piece, 1/32 of cake, ⅔ in arc	1 pce	165	5/58/37	1.0	20	67

[45]A blend of white and whole wheat flour—no official ratio specified.

[46]Excepting angel food cake, cakes were made from mixes containing vegetable shortening, and frostings were made with margarine. All mixes use enriched flour.

(For purposes of calculations, use "0" for t.)

Key: 1 = Bev 2 = Dairy 3 = Eggs 4 = Fat/Oil 5 = Fruit 6 = Bakery 7 = Grain 8 = Fish 9 = Meat 10 = Poultry 11 = Sausage 12 = Mixed Dishes 13 = Nuts/Seeds 14 = Sweets 15 = Veg/Leg 16 = Misc 22 = Soup/Sauce 25 = Fast Foods by Brand Name

TABLE F–1 ■ **Food Composition**

Key	Name	Measure	Energy (calories)	Protein/ Carbohydrate/ Fat (%)	Fiber (g)	Cholesterol (mg)	Sodium (mg)
	BAKED GOODS (cont.)						
	Cakes (cont.):						
	Sheet cake, plain, unckd white frosting:						
6	Piece, 1/9 of cake	1 pce	445	4/68/28	0.5	70	275
	Pound cake:						
6	Piece, 1/17 of loaf	1 pce	120	7/53/40	t	32	97
	Cakes, commercial:						
	Snack cakes:						
6	Chocolate w/creme filling, 2 small cakes per package	1 ea	105	4/63/33	t	15	105
6	Sponge cake w/creme filling, 2 small cakes per package	1 ea	155	2/69/29	t	7	155
	White cake with white frosting, 2 layer cake, 8 or 9 in:						
6	Piece, 1/16 of cake	1 pce	260	5/64/31	0.5	3	176
	Yellow cake with chocolate frosting, 2 layer cake:						
6	Piece, 1/16 of cake	1 pce	245	4/59/37	0.5	38	192
	Cheesecake:						
6	Piece, 1/12 of cake	1 pce	278	7/37/56	0.5	170	204
	Cookies made with enriched flour:						
	Brownies with nuts:						
6	Commercial with frosting, 1½ × 1¾ × ⅞ in	1 ea	100	4/59/37	t	14	59
6	Home recipe, 1¾ × 1¾ × ⅞ in	1 ea	95	5/41/54	t	18	51
	Chocolate chip cookies:						
6	Commercial, 2¼ in diam	4 ea	180	5/56/39	t	5	140
6	Home recipe, 2⅓ in diam	4 ea	185	4/50/46	1.0	18	82
6	From refrigerated dough, 2¼ in diam	4 ea	225	4/54/42	t	22	173
6	Fig bars	4 ea	210	4/80/16	1.0	27	180
6	Oatmeal raisins cookies, 2⅝ in diam	4 ea	245	5/59/36	t	2	148
6	Peanut butter cookie, home recipe, 2⅝ in diam	4 ea	245	6/44/50	1.0	22	142
6	Sandwich-type cookies, all	4 ea	195	4/59/37	t	0	189
	Shortbread cookies:						
6	Commercial, small	4 ea	155	5/50/45	t	27	123
6	Sugar cookies from refrigerated dough, 2½ in diam	4 ea	235	3/52/45	t	29	261
6	Vanilla wafers	10 ea	185	4/62/34	t	25	150
6	Corn chips	1 oz	155	5/42/53	0.5	0	233
	Crackers:						
6	Cheese crackers	10 ea	50	7/44/49	t	6	112
6	Cheese crackers with peanut butter	4 ea	150	11/47/42	t	4	338
6	Graham crackers	2 ea	60	7/71/22	1.5	0	86
6	Melba toast, plain	1 pce	20	18/70/12	t	0	44
6	Rye wafers, whole grain	2 ea	55	8/75/17	1.5	0	115
6	Saltine crackers	4 ea	50	8/72/20	t	4	165
6	Snack-type crackers, Ritz	3 ea	45	5/47/48	t	0	90
6	Wheat cracker, thin	4 ea	35	11/55/34	0.5	0	69

(For purposes of calculations, use "0" for t.)

Key: 1 = Bev 2 = Dairy 3 = Eggs 4 = Fat/Oil 5 = Fruit 6 = Bakery 7 = Grain 8 = Fish 9 = Meat 10 = Poultry 11 = Sausage 12 = Mixed Dishes 13 = Nuts/Seeds 14 = Sweets 15 = Veg/Leg 16 = Misc 22 = Soup/Sauce 25 = Fast Foods by Brand Name

TABLE F–1 ■ **Food Composition**

Key	Name	Measure	Energy (calories)	Protein/ Carbohydrate/ Fat (%)	Fiber (g)	Cholesterol (mg)	Sodium (mg)
	BAKED GOODS (cont.)						
	Crackers (cont.):						
6	Whole wheat wafers	2 ea	35	11/53/36	0.5	0	59
6	Croissant, 4½ × 4 × 1¾ in	1 ea	235	8/46/46	0.5	13	452
	Danish pastry:						
6	Round piece, plain, 4¼ in diam, 1 in high	1 ea	220	7/46/47	0.5	49	218
6	Round piece with fruit	1 pce	235	6/46/48	0.5	56	233
	Doughnuts:						
6	Cake type, plain, 3¼ in diam	1 ea	210	5/45/50	0.5	20	192
6	Yeast-leavened, glazed, 3¾ in diam	1 ea	235	7/44/49	0.5	21	222
	English muffin:						
6	Plain, enriched	1 ea	140	14/79/7	1.5	0	378
	Muffins, 2½ in diam, 1½ in high:						
	From commercial mix:						
6	Blueberry	1 ea	140	7/62/31	1.5	45	225
6	Bran	1 ea	140	8/67/25	2.0	28	385
6	Cornmeal	1 ea	145	8/57/35	1.5	42	291
	Pancakes, 4 in diam:						
6	Buckwheat, from mix; egg and milk added	1 ea	55	36/48/16	1.5	20	125
6	Plain, from mix; egg, milk, oil added	1 ea	60	14/55/31	0.5	16	160
	Pies, 9 in diam; pie crust made with veg shortening, enriched flour:						
	Apple pie[55]:						
6	Piece, ⅙ of pie	1 pce	405	4/58/38	3.0	0	476
	Banana cream pie[56]:						
6	⅙ of pie	1 pce	320	8/57/35	1.5	15	422
	Cherry pie[55]:						
6	Piece, ⅙ of pie	1 pce	410	4/58/38	2.5	0	480
	Chocolate cream pie[57]:						
6	Piece, ⅙ of pie	1 pce	311	9/54/37	0.5	15	428
	Custard pie:						
6	Piece, ⅙ of pie	1 pce	293	11/46/43	0.5	148	333
	Lemon meringue pie[55]:						
6	Piece, ⅙ of pie	1 pce	355	5/59/36	1.0	137	395
	Peach pie[55]:						
6	Piece, ⅙ of pie	1 pce	405	3/59/38	3.0	0	423
	Pecan pie[55]:						
6	Piece, ⅙ of pie	1 pce	583	4/61/35	1.5	137	304
	Pumpkin pie[55]:						
6	Piece, ⅙ of pie	1 pce	375	9/54/37	2.5	109	325
	Pies, fried, commercial:						
6	Apple	1 ea	255	3/49/48	1.5	14	326
6	Cherry	1 ea	250	3/49/48	1.5	13	371
	Pretzels, made with enriched flour:						
6	Thin sticks, 2¼ in long	10 ea	10	10/82/8	t	0	48

[55]Recipes updated for latest USDA values for fruits/nuts/fruit juice.
[56]Recipe based on pie crust, cooked vanilla pudding, 2 bananas.
[57]Based on values for pie crust, cooked chocolate pudding with meringue.

(For purposes of calculations, use "0" for t.)

Key: 1 = Bev 2 = Dairy 3 = Eggs 4 = Fat/Oil 5 = Fruit 6 = Bakery 7 = Grain 8 = Fish 9 = Meat 10 = Poultry 11 = Sausage 12 = Mixed Dishes 13 = Nuts/Seeds 14 = Sweets 15 = Veg/Leg 16 = Misc 22 = Soup/Sauce 25 = Fast Foods by Brand Name

TABLE F–1　■　**Food Composition**

Key	Name	Measure	Energy (calories)	Protein/ Carbohydrate/ Fat (%)	Fiber (g)	Cholesterol (mg)	Sodium (mg)
	BAKED GOODS (cont.)						
	Pretzels (cont.):						
6	Thin twists, 3¼ × 2¼ × ¼ in	10 ea	240	10/82/8	1.5	0	966
	Rolls and buns, enriched:						
	Commercial:						
6	Hotdog bun	1 ea	115	12/71/17	1.0	0	241
6	Hamburger bun	1 ea	129	12/71/17	1.0	0	271
6	Hard roll, white, 3¾ in diam, 2 in high	1 ea	155	13/76/11	1.0	0	313
6	Submarine roll or hoagie, 11½ × 3 × 2½ in	1 ea	400	12/80/8	2.0	0	683
6	Toaster pastry, fortified	1 ea	210	4/71/25	0.5	0	248
	Tortillas:						
6	Corn, enriched, 6 in diam	1 ea	65	12/75/13	1.0	0	1
6	Flour, 8 in diam	1 ea	105	9/69/22	1.0	0	134
6	Taco shell	1 ea	48	7/56/37	0.5	0	50
	Waffles, 7 in diam:						
6	From home recipe	1 ea	245	11/42/47	1.5	102	445
6	From mix, egg/milk added	1 ea	205	13/52/35	1.5	59	515
	GRAIN PRODUCTS: CEREALS, FLOUR, GRAINS, PASTA and NOODLES, POPCORN						
	Barley, pearled:						
7	Cooked	1 cup	196	9/88/3	4.5	0	2
	Breakfast cereals, hot, cooked:						
	Corn grits (hominy) cooked:						
7	White, instant, prepared from packet	1 ea	80	10/88/2	0.5	0	343
	Cream of Wheat®, cooked:						
7	Regular, quick, instant	1 cup	140	11/85/4	0.5	0	5[64,65]
7	Mix 'n eat, plain, packet	1 ea	100	12/84/4	0.5	0	241
7	Malt-O-Meal® cereal, cooked	1 cup	122	12/86/2	0.5	0	2[65]
	Oatmeal or rolled oats, cooked:						
7	Regular, quick, instant, non-fortified	1 cup	145	16/69/15	9.0	0	1[65]
	Instant, fortified:						
7	Plain, from packet	¾ cup	104	17/69/14	7.0	0	285[60]
7	Flavored, from packet	¾ cup	160	12/77/11	6.5	0	254[60]
7	Whole wheat cereal, cooked	1 cup	110	15/79/6	5.5	0	3
	Breakfast cereals, ready to eat:						
7	All-Bran®	⅓ cup	70	15/81/4	8.5	0	320
7	Cheerios®	1 cup	89	15/71/14	1.0	0	246
7	Corn Flakes, Kellogg's®	1¼ cup	110	9/91/0	0.5	0	351
7	40% Bran Flakes, Kellogg's®	1 cup	125	13/83/4	5.5	0	363
7	Grape Nuts®	½ cup	202	20/79/1	3.5	0	394
7	Nature Valley® Granola	1 cup	503	9/57/34	7.5	0	232
7	Product 19®	1 cup	126	10/88/2	0.5	0	378
7	Raisin Bran, Kellogg's®	1 cup	211	9/85/6	6.0	0	386
7	Rice Krispies, Kellogg's®	1 cup	112	7/91/2	t	0	340
7	Puffed Rice	1 cup	56	6/92/2	t	0	t
7	Shredded Wheat	¾ cup	115	11/83/6	4.0	0	3

[60]Salt added.

[64]For regular and instant cereal. For quick cereal, sodium is 142 mg.

[65]Cooked without salt. If salt added as directed, sodium content is 390 mg for Cream of Wheat, 324 mg for Malt-O-Meal, 374 mg for oatmeal.

(For purposes of calculations, use "0" for t.)

Key: 1 = Bev　2 = Dairy　3 = Eggs　4 = Fat/Oil　5 = Fruit　6 = Bakery　7 = Grain　8 = Fish　9 = Meat　10 = Poultry　11 = Sausage　12 = Mixed Dishes　13 = Nuts/Seeds　14 = Sweets　15 = Veg/Leg　16 = Misc　22 = Soup/Sauce　25 = Fast Foods by Brand Name

TABLE F–1 ■ Food Composition

Key	Name	Measure	Energy (calories)	Protein/ Carbohydrate/ Fat (%)	Fiber (g)	Cholesterol (mg)	Sodium (mg)
	GRAIN PRODUCTS (cont.)						
	Breakfast cereals (cont.):						
7	Special K®	1½ cup	125	20/79/1	0.5	0	298
7	Sugar Frosted Flakes®	1 cup	133	5/94/1	0.5	0	284
7	Total®	1 cup	116	11/84/5	2.5	0	409
7	Wheaties®	1 cup	101	10/86/4	3.5	0	363
	Bulgar:						
7	Cooked	1 cup	246	17/79/4	7.0	0	3
	Cornmeal:						
7	Degermed, enriched, cooked	1 cup	120	9/87/4	1.0	0	1
	Macaroni, cooked:						
7	Tender stage, cold	1 cup	115	13/84/3	1.0	0	1
7	Tender stage, hot	1 cup	155	13/83/4	1.0	0	1
	Noodles:						
7	Egg noodles, cooked	1 cup	200	14/77/9	t	50	3
7	Chow mein, dry	1 cup	220	10/46/44	t	5	450
	Popcorn:						
7	Air popped, plain	1 cup	30	13/76/11	1.5	0	1
7	Popped in veg oil/salted	1 cup	55	7/43/50	1.5	0	86
7	Sugar syrup coated	1 cup	135	6/88/6	0.5	0	1
	Rice:						
7	Brown rice, cooked	1 cup	232	8/87/5	4.0	0	0
	White, enriched, all types:						
7	Cooked without salt	1 cup	223	7/92/1	1.0	0	0
7	Instant, prepared without salt	1 cup	180	8/91/1	0.5	0	0[66]
	White, parboiled/converted rice:						
7	Cooked, hot	1 cup	186	8/91/1	0.5	0	9
7	Wild rice, cooked	½ cup	92	16/82/2	2.5	0	2
	Spaghetti, cooked:						
7	Tender stage, hot	1 cup	155	13/84/3	1.0	0	1
7	Wheat bran	½ cup	38	18/70/12	8.0	0	3
	Wheat germ:						
7	Toasted	1 cup	431		3.0	0	2
7	Whole grain wheat, cooked	⅓ cup	28	13/81/6	1.0	0	2
	FISH and SHELLFISH						
	Clams:						
8	Canned, drained	3 oz	85	60/9/31	t	54	102
	Cod:						
8	Baked with butter	3½ oz	114	63/0/37	0	60	224
8	Batter fried	3½ oz	199	39/15/46	0	55	100
8	Poached, no added fat	3½ oz	94	89/0/11	0	60	110
8	Crab meat, canned	1 cup	135	75/3/22	0	135	1350
8	Fish sticks	2 ea	140	36/24/40	t	52	106
	Flounder/sole, baked with lemon juice:						
8	With margarine	3 oz	120	54/0/46	0	55	151
8	Without added fat	3 oz	80	88/0/12	0	57	101

[66]If prepared with salt as directed, sodium would equal 608 mg.

(For purposes of calculations, use "0" for t.)

Key: 1 = Bev 2 = Dairy 3 = Eggs 4 = Fat/Oil 5 = Fruit 6 = Bakery 7 = Grain 8 = Fish 9 = Meat 10 = Poultry 11 = Sausage 12 = Mixed Dishes 13 = Nuts/Seeds 14 = Sweets 15 = Veg/Leg 16 = Misc 22 = Soup/Sauce 25 = Fast Foods by Brand Name

TABLE F–1   ■   **Food Composition**

Key	Name	Measure	Energy (calories)	Protein/ Carbohydrate/ Fat (%)	Fiber (g)	Cholesterol (mg)	Sodium (mg)
	FISH and SHELLFISH (cont.)						
8	Haddock, breaded/fried[67]	3 oz	175	38/16/46	t	75	123
	Halibut, broiled with butter and						
8	lemon juice	3 oz	140	60/0/40	0	62	103
8	Ocean perch, breaded/fried	3 oz	185	33/15/52	t	66	138
	Oysters:						
	Raw:						
8	Eastern	1 cup	160	54/22/24	0	120	175
8	Pacific	1 cup	160	52/20/28	0	120	185
	Cooked:						
8	Eastern, breaded, fried	1 ea	90	24/24/52	0	35	70
8	Western, simmered	3½ oz	135	46/24/30	0	77	165
	Salmon:						
8	Canned pink, solids and liquid	3 oz	120	60/0/40	0	34	443
8	Broiled or baked	3 oz	140	65/0/35	0	60	55
8	Smoked	3 oz	150	50/0/50	0	51	1700
8	Atlantic sardines canned, drained	3 oz	175	49/0/51	0	85	425
8	Scallops, breaded, from frozen	6 ea	195	32/21/47	t	70	298
	Shrimp:						
8	Cooked, boiled	3½ oz	109	88/0/12	0	147	180
8	Canned, drained	3 oz	100	87/4/9	0	128	1955
8	Fried, 7 medium[69]	3 oz	200	32/22/46	t	168	384
	Trout, broiled with butter and						
8	lemon juice	3 oz	175	50/1/49	0	71	122
	Tuna, canned, drained solids:						
8	Oil pack	3 oz	165	60/0/40	0	55	303
8	Water pack	3 oz	135	93/0/7	0	48	468
	MEAT and MEAT PRODUCTS						
	Beef, cooked:[70]						
	Braised, simmered, pot roasted:						
	Relatively fat, like chuck						
	blade:						
9	Lean and fat, piece						
	2½ × 2½ × ¾ in	3 oz	325	27/0/73	0	87	51
9	Lean only	2.2 oz	170		0	66	44
	Relatively lean, like round:						
9	Lean and fat, piece						
	4⅛ × 2¼ × ¾ in	3 oz	220	48/0/52	0	81	43
9	Lean only	2.8 oz	175	58/0/42	0	75	40
	Ground beef, broiled, patty 3 × ⅝ in:						
9	Lean	3 oz	230	37/0/63	0	74	65
9	Regular	3 oz	245	53/0/47	0	76	70
9	Liver, fried	3 oz	185	51/15/34	0	410	90
	Roast, oven cooked, no added						
	liquid:						
	Relatively fat, rib:						
9	Lean and fat, piece						
	4⅛ × 2¼ × ½ in	3 oz	315	25/0/75	0	72	54

[67]Dipped in egg, milk and breadcrumbs; fried in vegetable shortening.
[69]Dipped in egg, breadcrumbs, and flour; fried in vegetable shortening.
[70]Outer layer of fat removed to about ½ in of the lean. Deposits of fat within the cut remain.

(For purposes of calculations, use "0" for t.)

Key: 1 = Bev 2 = Dairy 3 = Eggs 4 = Fat/Oil 5 = Fruit 6 = Bakery 7 = Grain 8 = Fish 9 = Meat 10 = Poultry 11 = Sausage
12 = Mixed Dishes 13 = Nuts/Seeds 14 = Sweets 15 = Veg/Leg 16 = Misc 22 = Soup/Sauce 25 = Fast Foods by Brand Name

TABLE F–1 ■ Food Composition

Key	Name	Measure	Energy (calories)	Protein/ Carbohydrate/ Fat (%)	Fiber (g)	Cholesterol (mg)	Sodium (mg)
	MEAT and MEAT PRODUCTS (cont.)						
	Beef (cont.):						
9	Lean only	2.2 oz	150	46/0/54	0	49	45
	Relatively lean, round:						
9	Lean and fat, piece						
	2½ × 2½ × ¾ in	3 oz	205	46/0/54	0	62	50
9	Lean only	2.6 oz	135	66/0/34	0	52	46
	Steak, broiled, sirloin:						
9	Lean and fat, piece 2½ × 2½ × ¾ in	3 oz	240	41/0/59	0	77	53
9	Lean only	2.5 oz	150	62/0/38	0	64	48
9	Beef, canned, corned	3 oz	185	49/0/51	0	80	802
9	Beef, dried, chipped	2.5 oz	145	73/0/27	0	46	3053
	Lamb, cooked:						
	Chops (3 per lb with bone):						
	Arm chop, braised:						
9	Lean and fat	2.2 oz	220	37/0/63	0	77	46
9	Lean only	1.7 oz	135	52/0/48	0	59	36
	Loin chop, broiled:						
9	Lean and fat	2.8 oz	235	38/0/62	0	78	62
9	Lean only	2.3 oz	140	58/0/42	0	60	54
	Leg, roasted:						
9	Lean and fat, piece						
	4⅛ × 2¼ × ½ in	3 oz	205	43/0/57	0	78	57
9	Lean only	3 oz	163	60/0/40	0	76	58
	Pork, cured, cooked (see also Sausages):						
9	Bacon, medium slices	3 pce	109	78/0/22	0	16	303
9	Canadian-style bacon	2 pce	86	55/3/42	0	27	719
	Ham, roasted:						
9	Lean and fat, 2 pieces						
	4⅛ × 2¼ × ¼ in	3 oz	207	36/0/64	0	53	1009
9	Lean only	3 oz	133	67/0/33	0	47	1128
9	Ham, canned, roasted	3 oz	140	52/1/47	0	35	908
	Pork, fresh, cooked:						
	Chops, loin (cut 3 per lb with bone):						
	Broiled:						
9	Lean and fat	3.1 oz	275	36/0/64	0	84	61
9	Lean only	1 ea	166	58/0/42	0	71	56
	Pan fried:						
9	Lean and fat	1 ea	334	25/0/75	0	92	64
9	Lean only	1 ea	178	44/0/56	0	71	57
	Leg, roasted:						
9	Lean and fat, piece						
	2½ × 2½ × ¾ in	3 oz	250	34/0/66	0	79	50
9	Lean only	3 oz	187	53/0/47	0	80	54

(For purposes of calculations, use "0" for t.)

Key: 1 = Bev 2 = Dairy 3 = Eggs 4 = Fat/Oil 5 = Fruit 6 = Bakery 7 = Grain 8 = Fish 9 = Meat 10 = Poultry 11 = Sausage 12 = Mixed Dishes 13 = Nuts/Seeds 14 = Sweets 15 = Veg/Leg 16 = Misc 22 = Soup/Sauce 25 = Fast Foods by Brand Name

TABLE F–1 ■ **Food Composition**

Key	Name	Measure	Energy (calories)	Protein/ Carbohydrate/ Fat (%)	Fiber (g)	Cholesterol (mg)	Sodium (mg)
	MEAT and MEAT PRODUCTS (cont.)						
	Pork (cont.):						
	Rib, roasted:						
9	Lean and fat, piece 2½ × 2½ × ¾ in	3 oz	270	32/0/68	0	69	37
9	Lean only	2½ oz	175	48/0/52	0	56	33
	Shoulder, braised:						
9	Lean and fat, 3 pieces, 2½ × 2½ × ¼ in	3 pce	295	31/0/69	0	93	75
9	Lean only	2.4 oz	165	55/0/45	0	76	68
	Veal, medium fat, cooked:						
	Veal cutlet, braised or broiled,						
9	4⅛ × 2¼ × ½ in	3 oz	185	52/0/48	0	109	56
	POULTRY and POULTRY PRODUCTS						
	Chicken, cooked:						
	Fried batter dipped:						
10	Breast (5.6 oz with bones)	1 ea	364	39/14/47	t	119	385
10	Drumstick (3.4 oz with bones)	1 ea	193	33/15/54	t	62	194
10	Thigh	1 ea	238	32/13/55	t	80	248
10	Wing	1 ea	159	25/14/61	t	39	157
	Fried, flour coated:						
10	Breast (4.2 oz with bones)	1 ea	218	60/3/37	t	88	74
10	Drumstick (2.6 oz with bones)	1 ea	120	45/3/52	t	44	44
10	Thigh	1 ea	162	42/5/53	t	60	55
10	Wing	1 ea	103	33/3/64	t	26	25
	Roasted:						
10	Dark meat	1 cup	286	56/0/44	0	130	130
10	Light meat	1 cup	242	75/0/25	0	118	108
10	Breast, without skin	½ ea	142	80/0/20	0	73	64
10	Drumstick	1 ea	76	69/0/31	0	41	42
10	Thigh	1 ea	153	42/0/58	0	58	52
10	Chicken meat, stewed, all types	1 cup	248	64/0/36	0	116	98
10	Chicken liver, simmered	1 ea	30	54/19/27	0	126	10
	Turkey, roasted, meat only:						
10	Dark meat	3 oz	159	64/0/36	0	72	67
10	Light meat	3 oz	133	81/0/19	0	59	54
	Poultry food products (see also Sausages):						
10	Canned, boneless chicken	5 oz	235	55/0/45	0	88	714
10	Gravy and turkey, frozen package	5 oz	95	36/28/36	0.5	26	787
10	Turkey loaf breast meat	2 pce	46	86/0/14	0	17	608
	SAUSAGES and LUNCHMEATS						
	Bologna:						
11	Beef and pork	1 pce	89	15/4/81	0	16	289
11	Turkey	2 pce	113	28/2/70	0	56	498
	Brown and serve sausage links,						
11	cooked	1 ea	50	15/1/84	0	9	105
	Frankfurter (see also Chicken Frankfurter):						
11	Beef and pork	1 ea	145	14/3/83	0	23	504

(For purposes of calculations, use "0" for t.)

Key: 1 = Bev 2 = Dairy 3 = Eggs 4 = Fat/Oil 5 = Fruit 6 = Bakery 7 = Grain 8 = Fish 9 = Meat 10 = Poultry 11 = Sausage
12 = Mixed Dishes 13 = Nuts/Seeds 14 = Sweets 15 = Veg/Leg 16 = Misc 22 = Soup/Sauce 25 = Fast Foods by Brand Name

TABLE F–1 ■ **Food Composition**

Key	Name	Measure	Energy (calories)	Protein/ Carbohydrate/ Fat (%)	Fiber (g)	Cholesterol (mg)	Sodium (mg)
	SAUSAGES and LUNCHMEATS (cont.)						
	Frankfurter (cont.):						
11	Turkey	1 ea	102	25/3/72	0	44	550
	Ham:						
11	Ham luncheon meat, canned						
	3 × 2 × ½ in	1 pce	70	15/2/83	0	13	271
11	Ham lunchmeat, regular	2 pce	103	40/7/53	0	32	746
11	Ham lunchmeat, extra lean	2 pce	75	62/3/35	0	27	810
11	Turkey ham	2 pce	75	61/1/38	0	32	565
11	Pork sausage link, cooked[75]	1 ea	50	22/1/77	0	11	168
	Salami:						
11	Pork and beef	2 pce	145	23/3/74	0	37	607
11	Turkey	2 pce	111	34/1/65	0	46	535
11	Dry, beef and pork	2 pce	85	22/2/76	0	16	372
11	Sandwich spread, pork and beef	1 tbsp	35	13/20/67	0	6	152
11	Vienna sausage, canned	1 ea	45	15/3/82	0	8	152
	MIXED DISHES						
12	Beef and vegetable stew, homemade	1 cup	220	29/27/44	3.5	71	292
12	Beef pot pie, homemade[76]	1 pce	515	16/31/53	1.0	42	596
12	Chicken and noodles, home recipe	1 cup	365	25/29/46	1.0	103	600
12	Chicken chow mein, canned	1 cup	95	26/66/8	5.0	8	725
12	Chicken pot pie, home recipe[76]	1 pce	545	17/31/52	1.5	56	594
12	Chili con carne with beans, canned	1 cup	339	22/37/41	5.0	28	1354
12	Chop suey with beef and pork	1 cup	300	34/17/49	2.5	68	1053
12	Cole slaw[78]	1 cup	84	6/64/30	2.5	10[145]	28
12	French toast, home recipe[143]	1 pce	156	16/40/44	1.0	140	257
	Macaroni and cheese:						
12	Canned[79]	1 cup	230	16/45/39	1.5	24	730
12	Home recipe[49]	1 cup	430	16/37/47	1.0	44	1086
12	Quiche lorraine[76], ⅛ of 8 in quiche	1 pce	600	9/19/72	0.5	285	653
	Spaghetti (enriched) in tomato sauce:						
	With cheese:						
12	Canned	1 cup	190	12/79/9	2.5	3	955
12	Home recipe	1 cup	260	14/56/30	2.5	8	955
	With meatballs:						
12	Canned	1 cup	260	19/46/35	3.0	23	1220
12	Home recipe	1 cup	330	22/36/42	3.0	89	1009
	Burrito[80]:						
12	Beef and bean	1 ea	390	21/40/39	5.0	52	516
12	Bean	1 ea	322	16/57/27	8.0	15	1030
	Cheeseburger:						
12	Regular	1 ea	300	20/36/44	1.5	44	672
12	4 oz patty	1 ea	524	21/28/51	2.5	104	1224

[49]Made with margarine.
[75]One patty (8 per pound) of bulk sausage is equivalent to 2 links.
[76]Crust made with vegetable shortening and enriched flour.
[78]Recipe: 41% cabbage, 12% celery, 12% table cream, 12% sugar, 7% green pepper, 6% lemon juice, 4% onion, 3% pimiento, 3% vinegar, 2% salt, dry mustard, and white pepper.
[79]Made with corn oil.
[80]Made with a 10½ inch diameter flour tortilla.
[143]Recipe: 35% whole milk, 32% white bread, 29% egg and cooked in 4% margarine.

(For purposes of calculations, use "0" for t.)

Key: 1 = Bev 2 = Dairy 3 = Eggs 4 = Fat/Oil 5 = Fruit 6 = Bakery 7 = Grain 8 = Fish 9 = Meat 10 = Poultry 11 = Sausage
12 = Mixed Dishes 13 = Nuts/Seeds 14 = Sweets 15 = Veg/Leg 16 = Misc 22 = Soup/Sauce 25 = Fast Foods by Brand Name

TABLE F–1 ■ **Food Composition**

Key	Name	Measure	Energy (calories)	Protein/ Carbohydrate/ Fat (%)	Fiber (g)	Cholesterol (mg)	Sodium (mg)
	MIXED DISHES (cont.)						
12	Chicken patty sandwich	1 ea	436	23/31/46	1.5	68	2732
12	Corn dog	1 ea	330	12/33/55	t	37	1252
12	Enchilada	1 ea	235	25/30/45	2.0	19	1332
12	English muffin with egg, cheese, bacon	1 ea	360	20/35/45	1.5	213	832
	Fish sandwich:						
12	Regular with cheese	1 ea	420	15/37/48	1.5	56	667
12	Large without cheese	1 ea	470	15/35/50	1.5	90	621
	Hamburger with bun:						
12	Regular	1 ea	245	27/18/55	1.5	32	463
12	4 oz patty	1 ea	445	23/34/43	1.5	71	763
12	Hotdog/frankfurter and bun	1 ea	260	13/33/54	1.0	23	745
12	Cheese pizza, ⅛ of 15 in round[76]	1 pce	290	20/53/27	2.0	56	699
12	Roast beef sandwich	1 ea	345	26/39/35	1.5	55	757
12	Beef taco	1 ea	195	18/31/51	1.0	21	456
12	Potato salad with mayonnaise and egg[81]	1 cup	358	8/35/57	3.5	170	1323
12	Tuna salad[83]	1 cup	375	35/20/45	2.5	80	877
	NUTS, SEEDS, and PRODUCTS						
	Almonds:						
	Whole, dried:						
13	Ounce	1 oz	167	13/13/74	3.0[85]	0	3[86]
13	Almond butter	1 tbsp	101	9/12/79	1.5	0	2[87]
13	Brazil nuts. dry (about 7)	1 oz	186	8/7/85	2.5	0	0
	Cashew nuts:						
	Dry roasted, salted:						
13	Ounce	1 oz	163	10/21/69	1.5	0	181[88]
	Oil roasted, salted:						
13	Ounce	1 oz	163	10/19/71	1.5	0	177[89]
	Coconut:						
	Raw:						
13	Shredded/grated[91]	1 cup	283	4/16/80	11.0	0	16
	Dried, shredded/grated:						
13	Unsweetened	1 cup	515	4/13/83	19.0	0	29
13	Sweetened	1 cup	466	2/37/61	19.0	0	244
	Filberts (hazelnuts), chopped:						
13	Ounce	1 oz	179	8/9/83	2.0	0	1
	Macadamia nuts, oil roasted, salted:						
13	Ounce	1 oz	204	4/7/89	1.0	0	74[92]
	Mixed nuts, salted:						
13	Dry roasted	1 cup	814	11/16/73	11.0	0	91[93]
13	Roasted in oil	1 cup	876	10/13/77	11.0	0	926[93]

[76] Crust made with vegetable shortening and enriched flour.

[81] Recipe: 62% potatoes, 12% egg, 8% mayonnaise, 7% celery, 6% sweet pickle relish, 2% onion, 1% each for green pepper, pimiento, salt, and dry mustard.

[83] Made with drained chunk light tuna, celery, onion, pickle relish, and mayonnaise-type salad dressing.

[85] Values reported for dietary fiber in almonds vary from 7.0 to 14.3 per 100 grams.

[86] Salted almonds contain 1108 mg sodium per cup, 221 mg sodium per ounce.

[87] Salted almond butter contains 72 mg sodium per tablespoon.

[88] Dry roasted cashews without salt contain 21 mg of sodium per cup or 4 mg per ounce.

[89] Oil roasted cashews without salt contain 22 mg sodium per cup or 5 mg per ounce.

[91] 1 cup packed = 130 grams

[92] Macadamia nuts without salt contain 9 mg sodium per cup or 2 mg per ounce.

[93] Mixed nuts without salt contain about 15 mg sodium per cup.

(For purposes of calculations, use "0" for t.)

Key: 1 = Bev 2 = Dairy 3 = Eggs 4 = Fat/Oil 5 = Fruit 6 = Bakery 7 = Grain 8 = Fish 9 = Meat 10 = Poultry 11 = Sausage 12 = Mixed Dishes 13 = Nuts/Seeds 14 = Sweets 15 = Veg/Leg 16 = Misc 22 = Soup/Sauce 25 = Fast Foods by Brand Name

TABLE F–1 ■ Food Composition

Key	Name	Measure	Energy (calories)	Protein/ Carbohydrate/ Fat (%)	Fiber (g)	Cholesterol (mg)	Sodium (mg)
	NUTS, SEEDS and PRODUCTS (cont.)						
	Peanuts:						
	Oil roasted, salted:						
13	Ounce	1 oz	165	17/12/71	2.0	0	123[94]
	Dried, unsalted:						
13	Ounce	1 oz	161	17/11/72	2.5	0	5
13	Peanut butter	1 tbsp	95	18/10/72	1.0	0	75[95]
	Pecans, halved, dried:						
13	Ounce	1 oz	190	4/10/86	1.5[96]	0	3[97]
13	Pine nuts/pinyon, dried	1 oz	161	7/11/82	1.5	0	20
13	Pistachio nuts, dried, shelled	1 oz	164	13/16/71	1.5	0	2[98]
13	Pumpkin kernels, dried, unsalted	1 oz	154	17/12/71	1.5	0	5[99]
13	Sesame seeds, hulled, dry	¼ cup	221	17/6/77	6.0	0	15
	Sunflower seed kernels:						
13	Dry	¼ cup	205	15/12/73	2.0	0	1
13	Oil roasted	¼ cup	208	13/9/78	2.0	0	205[100]
	Black walnuts, chopped:						
13	Ounce	1 oz	172	15/7/78	2.5	0	0
	English walnuts, chopped:						
13	Ounce	1 oz	182	8/11/81	2.0	0	3
	SWEETENERS and SWEETS (see also Dairy (milk desserts) and Baked Goods):						
14	Caramel, plain or chocolate	1 oz	115	3/74/23	t	1	64
	Chocolate (see also Syrups and Miscellaneous):						
	Milk chocolate:						
14	Plain	1 oz	145	5/42/53	0.5	6	23
14	With almonds	1 oz	150	7/36/57	1.0	5	23
14	With peanuts	1 oz	155	12/24/64	1.5	3	19
14	With rice cereal	1 oz	140	6/50/44	1.0	6	46
14	Sweet dark chocolate	1 oz	150	3/40/57	1.0	0	5
	Fondant candy, uncoated (mints,						
14	candy corn, other)	1 oz	105	0/100/0	0	0	57
14	Fudge, chocolate	1 oz	115	2/75/23	t	1	54
14	Hard candy, all flavors	1 oz	109	0/100/0	0	0	7
14	Marshmallows	4 ea	90	3/97/0	0	0	25
14	Gelatin salad/dessert	½ cup	70	10/90/0	t	0	55
	Honey:						
14	Tablespoon	1 tbsp	65	0/100/0	0	0	1
	Jam or preserves:						
14	Tablespoon	1 tbsp	54	1/99/0	t	0	2
	Jellies:						
14	Tablespoon	1 tbsp	49	0/100/0	0	0	4
14	Popsicle, 3 oz when fluid	1 ea	70	0/100/0	0	0	11
	Sugars:						
14	Brown sugar	1 tbsp	51	0/100/0	0	0	6

[94]Peanuts without salt contain 22 mg sodium per cup or 4 mg per ounce.
[95]Peanut butter without added salt contains 3 mg sodium per tablespoon.
[96]Dietary fiber data calculated/derived from data on other nuts.
[97]Salted pecans contain 816 mg sodium per cup and 214 mg per ounce.
[98]Salted pistachios contain approx 221 mg sodium per ounce.
[99]Salted pumpkin/squash kernels contain approx 163 mg sodium per ounce.
[100]Unsalted sunflower seeds contain 1 mg sodium per ¼ cup.

(For purposes of calculations, use "0" for t.)

Key: 1 = Bev 2 = Dairy 3 = Eggs 4 = Fat/Oil 5 = Fruit 6 = Bakery 7 = Grain 8 = Fish 9 = Meat 10 = Poultry 11 = Sausage
12 = Mixed Dishes 13 = Nuts/Seeds 14 = Sweets 15 = Veg/Leg 16 = Misc 22 = Soup/Sauce 25 = Fast Foods by Brand Name

TABLE F–1 ■ **Food Composition**

Key	Name	Measure	Energy (calories)	Protein/ Carbohydrate/ Fat (%)	Fiber (g)	Cholesterol (mg)	Sodium (mg)
	SWEETENERS and SWEETS (cont.)						
	Sugars (cont.):						
	White sugar, granulated						
14	Tablespoon	1 tbsp	45	0/100/0	0	0	t
	White sugar, powdered, sifted	1 tbsp	24	0/100/0	0	0	t
	Syrups:						
	Chocolate:						
14	Thin type	2 tbsp	85	5/90/5	1.0	0	36
14	Fudge type	2 tbsp	125	6/61/33	1.0	0	42
14	Molasses, blackstrap	2 tbsp	85	0/100/0	0	0	38
14	Pancake table syrup (corn and maple)	¼ cup	244	0/100/0	·0	0	38
	VEGETABLES and LEGUMES						
15	Alfalfa seeds, sprouted	1 cup	10	44/41/15	1.0	0	2
15	Artichoke, cooked globe (300 g with refuse)	1 ea	53	18/79/3	4.0	0	79
	Asparagus, green, cooked:						
	From raw:						
15	Cuts and tips	½ cup	22	33/57/10	1.5	0	4
15	Spears, ½ in diam at base	4 spears	15	34/56/10	1.0	0	2
	From frozen:						
15	Cuts and tips	1 cup	50	33/56/11	3.0	0	7
15	Spears, ½ in diam at base	4 spears	17	33/54/13	1.0	0	2
15	Canned, spears, ½ in diam at base	4 spears	11	35/42/23	1.5	0	278[101]
15	Bamboo shoots, canned, drained slices	1 cup	25	30/55/15	3.5	0	9
	Beans (see also Great northern beans, Kidney beans, Navy beans, Pinto beans, Refried beans, Soybeans):						
15	Black beans, cooked	1 cup	225	26/71/3	15.5	0	1
	Lima beans:						
	Thin-seeded (baby), cooked from						
15	frozen	½ cup	94	25/72/3	5.0	0	26
	Snap bean/green beans, cuts and french style:						
15	Cooked from raw	1 cup	44	18/75/7	3.0	0	4
15	Cooked from frozen	1 cup	36	17/79/4	3.5	0	17
15	Canned, drained	1 cup	26	20/77/3	2.0	0	340[104]
	Navy beans, canned:						
15	Pork and beans with tomato sauce	1 cup	311	20/61/19	18.5	10	1181
15	Pork and beans with sweet sauce	1 cup	383	16/56/28	18.0	8	969
15	Beans with frankfurters	1 cup	365	21/35/44	17.5	30	1374
	Bean sprouts (mung):						
15	Raw	1 cup	32	32/63/5	1.5	0	6
	Beets:						
	Cooked from fresh:						
15	Sliced or diced	½ cup	26	14/86/0	2.0	0	42
	Canned:						
15	Sliced or diced	½ cup	27	11/86/3	2.0	0	233[106]
15	Pickled slices	½ cup	74	5/94/1	2.5	0	301

[101]Special dietary pack contains 3 mg sodium.
[104]Dietary pack contains 3 mg sodium.
[106]Dietary pack contains 39 mg sodium.

(For purposes of calculations, use "0" for t.)

Key: 1 = Bev 2 = Dairy 3 = Eggs 4 = Fat/Oil 5 = Fruit 6 = Bakery 7 = Grain 8 = Fish 9 = Meat 10 = Poultry 11 = Sausage 12 = Mixed Dishes 13 = Nuts/Seeds 14 = Sweets 15 = Veg/Leg 16 = Misc 22 = Soup/Sauce 25 = Fast Foods by Brand Name

TABLE F–1 ■ Food Composition

Key	Name	Measure	Energy (calories)	Protein/ Carbohydrate/ Fat (%)	Fiber (g)	Cholesterol (mg)	Sodium (mg)
	VEGETABLES and LEGUMES (cont.)						
	Blackeyed peas, cooked:						
15	From fresh, drained	1 cup	179	29/65/6	7.0	0	7
15	From frozen, drained	1 cup	224	25/71/4	7.5	0	9
	Broccoli:						
	Raw:						
15	Chopped	1 cup	24	33/58/9	3.5	0	24
15	Spears	1 spear	42	33/59/8	5.5	0	41
	Cooked from raw:						
15	Spears	1 spear	53	32/61/7	7.5	0	20
15	Chopped	1 cup	46	32/62/6	6.5	0	16
	Cooked from frozen:						
15	Spears	1 spear	8	36/64/0	1.0	0	7
15	Chopped	1 cup	51	36/61/3	6.0	0	44
	Brussels sprouts:						
15	Cooked from raw	1 cup	60	28/64/8	5.5	0	17
15	Cooked from frozen	1 cup	65	28/65/7	5.0	0	36
	Cabbage, common varieties:						
15	Raw, shredded or chopped	1 cup	16	16/79/5	1.5	0	12
15	Cooked, drained	1 cup	32	15/76/9	4.0	0	29
	Chinese cabbage:						
15	Bok choy or pak-choi, cooked, drained	1 cup	20	41/48/11	3.5	0	57
	Carrots:						
	Raw:						
15	Whole, 7½ × 1⅛ in	1 carrot	31	8/89/3	2.0	0	25
	Cooked, sliced, drained:						
15	Cooked from raw	½ cup	35	9/89/2	3.0	0	52
15	Cooked from frozen	½ cup	26	13/87/0	2.5	0	43
15	Canned, sliced, drained	½ cup	17	18/74/8	2.0	0	176[108]
15	Carrot juice	¾ cup	73	9/88/3	2.5	0	54
	Cauliflower:						
15	Raw, flowerets	½ cup	12	29/71/0	1.5	0	7
	Cooked, drained, flowerets:						
15	From raw	½ cup	15	28/67/5	1.5	0	4
15	From frozen	1 cup	34	27/65/8	4.0	0	33
	Celery, pascal-type, raw:						
15	Large outer stalk, 8 × 1½ in (at root end)	1 stalk	6	18/82/0	1.0	0	35
	Chickpeas (see Garbanzo)						
	Collards, cooked, drained:						
15	From raw	1 cup	20	27/65/8	4.0	0	27
15	From frozen	1 cup	61	27/65/8	5.0	0	85
	Corn:						
	Cooked, drained:						
15	From raw, on cob, 5 in long	1 ear	83	11/80/9	3.5	0	13
15	From frozen, on cob, 3½ in long	1 ear	59	12/82/6	3.0	0	3
15	Kernels, cooked from frozen	½ cup	67	13/87/0	4.0	0	4

[108]Dietary pack contains 31 mg sodium.

(For purposes of calculations, use "0" for t.)

Key: 1 = Bev 2 = Dairy 3 = Eggs 4 = Fat/Oil 5 = Fruit 6 = Bakery 7 = Grain 8 = Fish 9 = Meat 10 = Poultry 11 = Sausage 12 = Mixed Dishes 13 = Nuts/Seeds 14 = Sweets 15 = Veg/Leg 16 = Misc 22 = Soup/Sauce 25 = Fast Foods by Brand Name

TABLE F–1 ■ Food Composition

Key	Name	Measure	Energy (calories)	Protein/ Carbohydrate/ Fat (%)	Fiber (g)	Cholesterol (mg)	Sodium (mg)
	VEGETABLES and LEGUMES (cont.)						
	Corn (cont.):						
	Canned:						
15	Cream style	½ cup	93	8/88/4	6.5	0	365[110]
15	Whole kernel, vacuum pack	1 cup	166	11/84/5	10.0	0	572[111]
	Cowpeas (see Blackeyed peas)						
15	Cucumber with peel, ⅛ in thick, 2⅛ in diam	6 slices	4	20/80/0	0.5	0	1
15	Eggplant, cooked	1 cup	45	10/83/7	6.0	0	5
15	Garbanzo beans (chickpeas), cooked	1 cup	270	22/65/13	8.5	0	11
15	Great northern beans, cooked	1 cup	210	26/70/4	12.5	0	13
15	Escarole/curly endive, chopped	1 cup	8	14/39/47	1.0	0	11
15	Kidney beans, canned	1 cup	230	25/72/3	20.0	0	968
15	Lentils, cooked from dry	1 cup	215	28/68/4	10.0	0	26
	Lettuce:						
	Butterhead/Boston types:						
15	Leaves, 2 inner or outer	2 leaves	2	40/60/0	0.5	0	t
	Iceberg/crisphead:						
15	Wedge, ¼ of head	1 wedge	18	29/57/14	2.5	0	12
15	Chopped or shredded	1 cup	7	30/59/11	1.0	0	5
	Romaine:						
15	Chopped	1 cup	9	37/54/9	1.0	0	4
	Mushrooms:						
15	Raw, sliced	½ cup	9	28/63/9	1.0	0	1
15	Cooked from raw, pieces	½ cup	21	26/61/13	2.0	0	2
15	Canned, drained	½ cup	19	26/67/7	2.0	0	332
	Mustard greens:						
15	Cooked from raw	1 cup	21	47/43/10	3.0	0	22
15	Cooked from frozen	1 cup	28	38/52/10	4.0	0	38
15	Navy beans, cooked from dry	1 cup	225	26/70/4	16.5	0	13
	Okra, cooked:						
15	From fresh pods	8 pods	27	20/77/3	3.0	0	4
15	From frozen slices	½ cup	34	19/74/7	3.0	0	3
	Onions:						
	Raw:						
15	Chopped	1 cup	54	13/81/6	2.5	0	3
15	Sliced	1 cup	39	13/81/6	2.0	0	2
15	Cooked, drained, chopped	½ cup	30	10/84/6	1.5	0	8
15	Dehydrated flakes	¼ cup	45	9/91/0	1.5	0	3
15	Onions, spring, chopped, bulb and top	½ cup	13	24/76/0	1.5	0	2
15	Onion rings, breaded, prepared from frozen	2 rings	80	5/40/55	t	0	75
	Parsley:						
	Raw:						
15	Chopped	½ cup	10	25/75/0	2.0	0	12
15	Freeze dried	¼ cup	4	40/60/0	0.5	0	5
	Peas (see also Blackeyed peas):						
15	Edible pods, cooked	1 cup	67	30/65/5	5.0	0	6
	Green:						
15	Canned, drained	½ cup	59	25/71/4	5.5	0	186[113]
15	Cooked from frozen	½ cup	63	26/71/3	7.5	0	70

[110]Dietary pack contains 4 mg sodium per ½ cup.
[111]Dietary pack contains 6 mg sodium per cup.
[113]Dietary pack contains 1.7 mg sodium.

(For purposes of calculations, use "0" for t.)

Key: 1 = Bev 2 = Dairy 3 = Eggs 4 = Fat/Oil 5 = Fruit 6 = Bakery 7 = Grain 8 = Fish 9 = Meat 10 = Poultry 11 = Sausage 12 = Mixed Dishes 13 = Nuts/Seeds 14 = Sweets 15 = Veg/Leg 16 = Misc 22 = Soup/Sauce 25 = Fast Foods by Brand Name

TABLE F–1 ■ **Food Composition**

Key	Name	Measure	Energy (calories)	Protein/ Carbohydrate/ Fat (%)	Fiber (g)	Cholesterol (mg)	Sodium (mg)
	VEGETABLES and LEGUMES (cont.)						
	Peas (cont.):						
15	Split, green, cooked from dry	1 cup	230	27/71/2	10.0	0	26
	Peppers, hot:						
	Hot green chili:						
15	Canned	½ cup	17	12/88/0	1.0	0	10
15	Raw	1 pepper	18	17/83/0	1.0	0	3
15	Jalapenos, chopped, canned	½ cup	17	11/70/19	2.5	0	995
	Peppers, sweet, green:						
15	Whole pod (90 g with refuse), raw	1 pod	18	12/75/13	1.5	0	2
15	Pinto beans, cooked from dry	1 cup	265	23/74/3	19.0	0	3
	Potatoes						
	Baked in oven, 4¾ × 2⅓ in diam:						
15	With skin	1 potato	220	8/91/1	4.5	0	16
15	Flesh only	1 potato	145	8/91/1	4.0	0	8
	Boiled, about 2½ in diam:						
15	Peeled before boiling	1 ea	116	8/91/1	1.5	0	7
	French-fried, strips 2 to 3½ in long, frozen:						
15	Oven heated	10 strips	111	6/59/35	1.5	0	15
15	Fried in veg oil	10 strips	158	5/49/46	1.5	0	108
15	Hashed brown, from frozen	1 cup	340	6/49/45	1.5	0	53
	Mashed:						
15	Home recipe with milk and margarine	1 cup	222	7/59/34	1.0	4[123]	619
15	Prepared from flakes; water, milk, butter, salt added	1 cup	237	6/51/43	1.0	4[123]	697
	Potato products, prepared:						
	Au gratin:						
15	From dry mix	1 cup	228	9/53/38	4.0	12	1076
15	From home recipe[119]	1 cup	322	15/34/51	4.5	56[120]	1064
	Potato salad (see Mixed foods)						
	Scalloped:						
15	From dry mix	1 cup	228	9/52/39	4.5	27	835
15	Home recipe[124]	1 cup	210	13/49/38	4.5	29[125]	821
15	Potato chips	14 chips	148	5/37/58	0.5	0	133[126]
15	Red radishes	10 radishes	7	14/76/10	1.0	0	11
15	Refried beans, canned	1 cup	295	24/67/9	22.0	0	1228
15	Sauerkraut, canned with liquid	1 cup	44	16/79/5	4.5	0	1561
	Soybean products:						
15	Miso	3 tbsp	88	23/53/24	1.0[128]	0	1534
15	Tofu, piece 2½ × 2¾ × 1 in	1 pce	86	40/12/48	2.0[128]	0	8
	Spinach:						
15	Raw, chopped	1 cup	12	40/49/11	2.5	0	44

[119]Recipe: 55% potatoes; 30% whole milk; 9% cheddar cheese; 3% butter; 2% flour; 1% salt.

[120]For butter; if margarine is used, cholesterol = 37 mg.

[123]For margarine; if butter is used, cholesterol = 25 mg for 29 total mg.

[124]Recipe: 59% potatoes; 36% whole milk; 2% butter; 2% flour; 1% salt.

[125]For butter; if margarine is used cholesterol = 15 mg.

[126]If no salt is added, sodium = 2 mg.

[128]Estimate based on cooked soybeans.

(For purposes of calculations, use "0" for t.)

Key: 1 = Bev 2 = Dairy 3 = Eggs 4 = Fat/Oil 5 = Fruit 6 = Bakery 7 = Grain 8 = Fish 9 = Meat 10 = Poultry 11 = Sausage 12 = Mixed Dishes 13 = Nuts/Seeds 14 = Sweets 15 = Veg/Leg 16 = Misc 22 = Soup/Sauce 25 = Fast Foods by Brand Name

TABLE F–1 ■ **Food Composition**

Key	Name	Measure	Energy (calories)	Protein/ Carbohydrate/ Fat (%)	Fiber (g)	Cholesterol (mg)	Sodium (mg)
	VEGETABLES and LEGUMES (cont.)						
	Spinach (cont.):						
	Cooked, drained:						
15	From raw	1 cup	41	40/51/9	6.0	0	126
15	From frozen (leaf)	1 cup	53	35/60/5	6.5	0	163
15	Canned, drained solids	1 cup	50	38/46/16	7.5	0	683[129]
	Squash, summer varieties, cooked slices:						
15	Crookneck	1 cup	36	16/78/6	3.0	0	2
15	Zucchini	1 cup	29	13/87/0	3.0	0	5
	Squash, winter varieties, cooked:						
15	Acorn, baked, mashed	1 cup	83	7/91/2	6.0	0	6
15	Butternut, baked cubes	1 cup	83	7/91/2	5.0	0	7
	Sweet potatoes:						
	Cooked, 5 × 2 in diam:						
15	Baked in skin, peeled	1 potato	118	7/92/1	3.0	0	12
15	Boiled without skin	1 potato	160	5/93/2	4.0	0	20
15	Candied, 2½ × 2 in	1 pce	144	2/78/20	2.0	0[131]	74
	Canned:						
15	Solid pack, mashed	1 cup	258	8/91/1	6.5	0	191
	Tomatoes:						
	Raw:						
15	Whole, 2⅗ in diam	1 tomato	24	16/75/9	2.0	0	10
15	Cooked from raw	1 cup	60	15/76/9	5.5	0	25
15	Canned, solids and liquid	1 cup	47	16/74/10	2.0	0	390[134]
15	Tomato juice, canned	1 cup	42	15/83/2	1.5	0	881[135]
	Tomato products, canned:						
15	Paste	1 cup	220	15/77/8	6.0	0	170[136]
15	Puree	1 cup	102	14/84/2	4.0	0	49[137]
15	Sauce	1 cup	74	15/81/4	3.0	0	1481[138]
	Turnip greens, cooked:						
15	From raw (leaves and stems)	1 cup	29	19/73/8	4.0	0	41
15	From frozen (chopped)	½ cup	24	37/54/9	2.5	0	12
15	Vegetable juice cocktail, canned	1 cup	46	12/85/3	1.5	0	883
	Vegetables, mixed:						
15	Canned, drained	1 cup	77	21/75/4	6.5	0	243
15	Frozen, cooked, drained	1 cup	107	18/80/2	7.5	0	64
	Water chestnuts, canned:						
15	Slices	½ cup	35	6/94/0	0.5	0	6
	MISCELLANEOUS						
16	Basil, ground	1 tbsp	11	18/70/12	1.0	0	2
	Catsup:						
16	Tablespoon	1 tbsp	18	7/93/0	t	0	156
16	Celery seed	1 tsp	8	17/37/46	0.5	0	4
16	Chili powder	1 tsp	8	12/54/34	0.5	0	26

[129]Dietary pack contains 58 mg sodium.
[131]For recipe using margarine; if butter is used cholesterol = 8 mg.
[134]Dietary Pack contains 31 mg sodium.
[135]If no salt is added, sodium content is 24 mg.
[136]If salt is added, sodium content is 2070 mg.
[137]If salt is added, sodium content is 998 mg.
[138]With salt added.

(For purposes of calculations, use "0" for t.)

Key: 1 = Bev 2 = Dairy 3 = Eggs 4 = Fat/Oil 5 = Fruit 6 = Bakery 7 = Grain 8 = Fish 9 = Meat 10 = Poultry 11 = Sausage 12 = Mixed Dishes 13 = Nuts/Seeds 14 = Sweets 15 = Veg/Leg 16 = Misc 22 = Soup/Sauce 25 = Fast Foods by Brand Name

TABLE F–1 ■ **Food Composition**

Key	Name	Measure	Energy (calories)	Protein/ Carbohydrate/ Fat (%)	Fiber (g)	Cholesterol (mg)	Sodium (mg)
	MISCELLANEOUS (cont.)						
	Chocolate:						
16	Baking	1 oz	145	8/17/75	2.0	0	1
	Semi-sweet, milk, and dark chocolates (see Sweets and Sweeteners)						
16	Cinnamon	1 tsp	5	0/100/0	0.5	0	1
16	Curry powder	1 tsp	5	10/58/32	0.5	0	1
	Garlic:						
16	Cloves	4 cloves	18	17/83/0	t	0	2
16	Powder	1 tsp	9	20/80/0	t	0	1
16	Gelatin, dry, plain	1 envelope	25	100/0/0	1.0	0	6
16	Ginger root, raw, sliced	5 slices	8	11/89/0	t	0	1
	Mustard, prepared, packet (1 packet = 1						
16	tsp)	1 tsp	4	21/32/47	t	0	63
16	Miso (see Vegetables, soybean products)						
	Olives:						
16	Green	10 olives	45	3/3/94	1.5	0	936
16	Ripe, pitted[140]	10 olives	50	3/22/75	1.5	0	410
16	Onion powder	1 tsp	5	10/90/0	t	0	1
16	Oregano, ground	1 tsp	5	12/61/27	t	0	t
16	Paprika	1 tsp	6	13/57/30	0.5	0	1
16	Pepper, black	1 tsp	5	12/88/0	0.5	0	1
	Pickles:						
16	Dill, medium, 3¾ × 1¼ in diam	1 pickle	5	24/66/10	1.0	0	928
16	Fresh pack, slices, 1½ in diam × ¼ in thick	4 slices	20	5/95/0	0.5	0	201
16	Sweet, small, about 2½ × ¾ in diam	1 pickle	20	0/100/0	t	0	107
16	Pickle relish, sweet	1 tbsp	20	0/100/0	0.5	0	107
	Popcorn (see Grains)						
16	Salt	1 tsp	0	0/0/0	0	0	2132
16	Vinegar, cider	1 tbsp	2	0/100/0	0	0	t
	SOUPS, SAUCES, and GRAVIES						
	Soups, canned, condensed:						
	Prepared with equal volume of whole milk:						
22	Clam chowder, New England	1 cup	163	23/41/36	2.5	22	992
22	Cream of chicken	1 cup	191	16/31/53	t	27	1046
22	Cream of mushroom	1 cup	205	12/29/59	0.5	20	1076
22	Tomato	1 cup	160	14/54/32	0.5	17	932
	Prepared with equal volume of water:						
22	Bean with bacon	1 cup	173	18/52/30	2.5	3	952
22	Beef broth, bouillon, consomme	1 cup	16	56/21/23	0	1	782
22	Beef noodle	1 cup	84	23/43/34	t	3	952
22	Chicken noodle	1 cup	75	21/49/30	t	7	1106
22	Chicken rice	1 cup	60	23/48/29	1.0	7	815
22	Clam chowder, Manhattan	1 cup	78	19/57/24	1.0	2	1808
22	Cream of chicken	1 cup	115	11/32/57	0.5	10	986
22	Cream of mushroom	1 cup	130	6/30/64	1.5	2	1032
22	Minestrone	1 cup	80	20/53/27	1.0	2	911
22	Split pea with ham	1 cup	189	21/58/21	0.5	0	1008

[140]This is the most recent tested data from the California Olive industry, October 1986.

(For purposes of calculations, use "0" for t.)

Key: 1 = Bev 2 = Dairy 3 = Eggs 4 = Fat/Oil 5 = Fruit 6 = Bakery 7 = Grain 8 = Fish 9 = Meat 10 = Poultry 11 = Sausage 12 = Mixed Dishes 13 = Nuts/Seeds 14 = Sweets 15 = Veg/Leg 16 = Misc 22 = Soup/Sauce 25 = Fast Foods by Brand Name

TABLE F–1 ■ Food Composition

Key	Name	Measure	Energy (calories)	Protein/ Carbohydrate/ Fat (%)	Fiber (g)	Cholesterol (mg)	Sodium (mg)
	SOUPS, SAUCES, and GRAVIES (cont.)						
	Soups (cont.):						
22	Tomato	1 cup	86	9/72/19	0.5	0	872
22	Vegetable beef	1 cup	79	28/51/21	1.0	5	956
22	Vegetarian vegetable	1 cup	70	11/66/23	1.0	0	823
	Soups, dehydrated:						
	Unprepared, dry products:						
22	Bouillon	1 packet	15	24/24/52	0	1	1019
22	Onion	1 packet	20	14/70/16	t	t	627
	Prepared with water:						
22	Chicken noodle	¾ cup	40	19/59/22	t	2	957
22	Onion	¾ cup	20	15/69/16	t	0	635
22	Tomato vegetable	¾ cup	41	14/71/15	0.5	0	856
	Sauces:						
	From dry mixes:						
22	Cheese sauce, prepared with milk	1 cup	305	20/30/50	t	53	1565
22	Hollandaise, prepared with water	1 cup	240	8/22/70	—	52	1564
22	White sauce, prepared with milk	1 cup	240	16/35/49	0.5	34	797
	Ready to serve:						
22	Barbeque sauce	1 tbsp	10	7/58/35	t	0	128
22	Soy sauce	1 tbsp	11	48/52/0	0	0	1029
	Gravies:						
	Canned:						
22	Beef	1 cup	124	27/35/38	0.5	7	117
22	Chicken	1 cup	189	9/27/64	t	5	1375
22	Mushroom	1 cup	120	10/44/46	0.5	0	1357
	FAST FOODS BY BRAND NAME						
	McDONALD'S[142]						
25	Chicken McNuggets®	—	323	24/17/59	—	56	512
25	Hamburger	—	263	19/43/38	—	37	506
25	Cheeseburger	—	328	19/36/45	—	53	743
25	Quarter Pounder®	—	427	23/27/50	—	86	718
25	Quarter Pounder® w/Cheese	—	525	23/23/54	—	118	1220
25	Big Mac®	—	570	17/28/55	—	103	979
25	Filet-O-Fish®	—	435	14/33/53	—	50	799
25	Mc D.L.T.®	—	680	18/23/59	—	109	1030
25	French fries, regular	—	220	5/48/47	—	0	109
25	Biscuit w/sausage, egg	—	585	14/25/61	—	275	1301
25	Egg McMuffin®	—	340	22/36/42	—	226	885
25	Hot cakes w/butter, syrup	—	500	6/75/19	—	21	1070
25	English muffin w/butter	—	186	11/63/26	—	9	310
25	Hash brown potatoes	—	125	5/45/50	—	9	325
25	Chocolate shake	—	383	10/69/21	—	10	300
25	Hot fudge sundae	—	357	8/65/27	—	6	170
25	Apple pie	—	253	3/46/51	—	0	398
25	McDonaldland® Cookies	—	308	5/64/31	—	0	358

[142]*Source:* McDonald's Corp, Oak Brook, Illinois. Nutrient analyses by Hazelton Laboratory of America (formerly Raltech Scientific Services Inc), Madison, Wisconsin.

(For purposes of calculations, use "0" for t.)

Key: 1 = Bev 2 = Dairy 3 = Eggs 4 = Fat/Oil 5 = Fruit 6 = Bakery 7 = Grain 8 = Fish 9 = Meat 10 = Poultry 11 = Sausage 12 = Mixed Dishes 13 = Nuts/Seeds 14 = Sweets 15 = Veg/Leg 16 = Misc 22 = Soup/Sauce 25 = Fast Foods by Brand Name

TABLE F–1 ■ **Food Composition**

Key	Name	Measure	Energy (calories)	Protein/ Carbohydrate/ Fat (%)	Fiber (g)	Cholesterol (mg)	Sodium (mg)
	FAST FOODS (cont.)						
	WENDY'S[143]						
25	Single hamburger, multigrain bun	—	340	30/24/46	—	67	290
25	Bacon cheeseburger, white bun	—	460	25/20/55	—	65	860
25	Chicken sandwich, multigrain bun	—	320	32/40/28	—	59	500
25	Chili, 8 oz	—	260	32/40/28	—	30	1070
25	French fries, regular	—	280	5/50/45	—	15	95
25	Taco salad	—	390	23/36/41	—	40	1100
25	Frosty dairy dessert	—	400	8/60/32	—	50	220
25	Hot stuffed baked potatoes	—	250	10/83/7	—	t	60
25	Ham & cheese omelet	—	250	29/10/61	—	450	405
25	Breakfast sandwich	—	370	18/36/46	—	200	770
25	French toast, 2 slices	—	400	11/46/43	—	115	850
25	Home fries	—	360	4/41/55	—	20	745
	COCA-COLA[144]						
25	Coca-Cola classic®	—	144	0/100/0	—	—	—
25	Coca-Cola®	—	154	0/100/0	—	—	—
25	Cherry Coke®	—	154	0/100/0	—	—	—
25	Diet Coke®**	—	1	0/100/0	—	—	—
25	Sprite®	—	142	0/100/0	—	—	—
25	Mr. Pibb®	—	142	0/100/0	—	—	—
25	Mello Yello®	—	172	0/100/0	—	—	—
25	Ramblin' Root Beer®	—	158	0/100/0	—	—	—
25	Fanta® Orange	—	164	0/100/0	—	—	—
25	Fanta® Grape	—	168	0/100/0	—	—	—
25	Fanta® Root Beer	—	158	0/100/0	—	—	—
25	Fanta® Ginger Ale	—	126	0/100/0	—	—	—
25	Hi-C® Orange***	—	152	0/100/0	—	—	—
25	Hi-C® Lemon***	—	142	0/100/0	—	—	—
25	Hi-C® Punch***	—	154	0/100/0	—	—	—
25	Hi-C® Grape***	—	164	0/100/0	—	—	—
25	Tab®**	—	1	0/100/0	—	—	—
25	Diet Sprite®**	—	3	0/100/0	—	—	—
25	Minute Maid® Orange	—	160	0/100/0	—	—	—
	ARBY'S[145]						
25	Roast beef, regular	—	350	25/36/39	—	39	590
25	Beef 'n Cheddar®	—	490	20/42/38	—	51	1520
25	Chicken breast sandwich	—	592	19/39/42	—	57	1340
25	French fries	—	211	4/62/34	—	6	30
25	Bac'n Cheddar Deluxe	—	561	20/26/54	—	78	1385

[143]*Source:* Wendy's International Inc, Dublin, Ohio. Nutrient analyses: entree items, Hazelton Laboratory of America (formerly Raltech Scientific Services Inc), Madison, Wisconsin; other items, US Department of Agriculture Handbook #8.
[144]*Source:* The Coca-Cola Co, Atlanta, Georgia.
Nutritive value of fountain products, 12-oz servings without ice. **Sweetened with an aspartame-saccharin blend. Bottled and canned versions of Diet Coke and Diet Sprite are sweetened with 100% NutraSweet, a registered trademark of The NutraSweet Co for aspartame. ***Hi-C soft drinks do not contain fruit juice and are not the same as Hi-C fruit-juice-containing drinks produced by Coca-Cola Foods, a division of The Coca-Cola Co. *Source:* The Coca-Cola Co, Atlanta, Georgia.
[145]*Source:* Arby's Inc, Atlanta, Georgia. Nutritional analyses by Arby's Laboratory and other independent testing laboratories.

Key: 1 = Bev 2 = Dairy 3 = Eggs 4 = Fat/Oil 5 = Fruit 6 = Bakery 7 = Grain 8 = Fish 9 = Meat 10 = Poultry 11 = Sausage 12 = Mixed Dishes 13 = Nuts/Seeds 14 = Sweets 15 = Veg/Leg 16 = Misc 22 = Soup/Sauce 25 = Fast Foods by Brand Name

TABLE F-1 ■ Food Composition

Key	Name	Measure	Energy (calories)	Protein/ Carbohydrate/ Fat (%)	Fiber (g)	Cholesterol (mg)	Sodium (mg)
	FAST FOODS (cont.)						
	ARBY'S (cont.):						
25	Hot Ham 'n Cheese	—	353	30/37/33	—	50	1655
25	Turkey Deluxe	—	375	25/34/41	—	39	850
25	Baked potato	—	290	11/88/1	—	0	12
25	Taco	—	619	15/46/39	—	145	1065
25	Vanilla shake	—	295	11/59/30	—	30	245
25	Chocolate shake	—	384	9/65/26	—	32	300
25	Jamocha shake	—	424	8/71/21	—	31	280
25	Roasted chicken breast	—	254	71/3/26	—	200	930
25	Roasted chicken leg	—	319	53/1/46	—	214	995
25	Chicken salad sandwich	—	386	19/34/47	—	30	630
	BURGER KING[146]						
25	Whopper Sandwich®	—	640	17/26/57	—	94	842
25	Whopper® w/cheese	—	723	17/24/59	—	117	1126
25	Double Beef Whopper®	—	850	21/24/55	—	—	1080
25	Double Beef Whopper® w/cheese	—	950	21/23/56	—	—	1535
25	Hamburger	—	275	21/41/38	—	37	509
25	Cheeseburger	—	317	21/37/42	—	48	651
25	French fries, regular	—	227	5/43/52	—	14	160
25	Onion rings, regular	—	274	6/41/53	—	0	665
25	Apple pie	—	305	4/60/36	—	4	412
25	Chocolate shake, medium	—	320	10/57/33	—	—	202
25	Vanilla shake, medium	—	321	11/61/28	—	—	205
25	Whaler® Fish Sandwich	—	488	15/36/49	—	84	592
25	Whaler® w/Cheese	—	530	16/34/50	—	95	734
25	Ham and cheese sandwich	—	471	20/37/43	—	70	1534
25	Chicken sandwich	—	688	15/33/52	—	82	1423
25	Chicken Tenders®	—	204	38/19/43	—	47	636
25	Scrambled egg platter w/bacon	—	536	14/25/61	—	378	975
	DAIRY QUEEN[147]						
25	Cone, regular	—	240	10/64/26	—	15	80
25	Dipped cone, regular	—	340	7/50/43	—	20	100
25	Sundae, regular	—	310	6/71/23	—	20	120
25	Shake, regular	—	710	8/68/24	—	50	260
25	Malt, regular	—	760	7/72/21	—	50	260
25	Float	—	410	5/80/15	—	20	85
25	Banana split	—	540	7/75/18	—	30	150
25	Parfait	—	430	8/74/18	—	30	140
25	Peanut Buster Parfait	—	740	9/50/41	—	30	250
25	Double Delight	—	490	7/56/37	—	25	150
25	Hot Fudge Brownie Delight	—	600	6/57/37	—	20	225
25	Strawberry shortcake	—	540	7/75/18	—	25	215
25	Freeze	—	500	7/71/22	—	30	180
25	Mr. Misty®, regular	—	250	0/100/0	—	0	10
25	Mr. Misty® Kiss	—	70	0/100/0	—	0	10
25	Mr. Misty® Freeze	—	500	7/72/21	—	30	140
25	Mr. Misty® Float	—	390	5/78/17	—	20	95
25	Buster Bar	—	460	9/35/56	—	10	175

[146]*Source:* Burger King Corp Inc. Nutritional analyses by Hazelton Laboratory of America (formerly Raltech Scientific Services Inc), Madison, Wisconsin, and Campbell Laboratories, Camden, New Jersey.

[147]*Source:* International Dairy Queen Inc, Minneapolis, Minnesota. Nutrient analyses by Hazelton Laboratory of America (formerly Raltech Scientific Services Inc), Madison Wisconsin.

Key: 1 = Bev 2 = Dairy 3 = Eggs 4 = Fat/Oil 5 = Fruit 6 = Bakery 7 = Grain 8 = Fish 9 = Meat 10 = Poultry 11 = Sausage 12 = Mixed Dishes 13 = Nuts/Seeds 14 = Sweets 15 = Veg/Leg 16 = Misc 22 = Soup/Sauce 25 = Fast Foods by Brand Name

TABLE F–1 ■ Food Composition

Key	Name	Measure	Energy (calories)	Protein/ Carbohydrate/ Fat (%)	Fiber (g)	Cholesterol (mg)	Sodium (mg)
	FAST FOODS (cont.)						
	DIARY QUEEN (cont.):						
25	Dilly Bar	—	210	6/39/55	—	10	50
25	DQ Sandwich	—	140	8/67/25	—	5	40
25	Single hamburger	—	360	23/37/40	—	45	630
25	Single w/cheese	—	410	24/32/44	—	50	790
25	Hot dog	—	280	16/31/53	—	45	830
25	Hot dog w/chili	—	320	16/28/56	—	55	985
25	Hot dog w/cheese	—	330	18/25/57	—	55	990
25	Fish filet sandwich	—	400	20/41/39	—	50	875
25	Chicken sandwich	—	670	17/28/55	—	75	870
25	French fries, small	—	200	4/51/45	—	10	115
25	Onion rings	—	280	5/44/51	—	15	140
	JACK IN THE BOX[148]						
25	Hamburger	—	276	18/43/39	—	29	521
25	Cheeseburger	—	323	20/39/41	—	42	749
25	Jumbo Jack®	—	485	21/31/48	—	64	905
25	Jumbo Jack® w/Cheese	—	630	20/29/51	—	110	1665
25	Moby Jack®	—	444	14/35/51	—	47	820
25	Regular taco	—	191	16/33/51	—	21	406
25	Club pita	—	284	31/43/26	—	43	953
25	Chicken Supreme	—	601	20/26/54	—	60	1582
25	Sausage Crescent	—	584	15/19/66	—	187	1012
25	Scrambled eggs breakfast	—	719	14/31/55	—	260	1110
25	Chicken strips dinner	—	689	23/38/39	—	100	1213
25	Sirloin steak dinner	—	699	22/43/35	—	75	969
25	Cheese nachos	—	571	11/34/55	—	37	1154
25	Taco salad	—	377	33/10/57	—	102	1436
25	French fries, regular	—	221	4/48/48	—	8	164
25	Onion rings	—	382	5/41/54	—	27	407
25	Hash brown potatoes	—	68	6/44/50	—	0	15
25	Vanilla shake	—	320	12/71/17	—	25	230
25	Strawberry shake	—	320	12/68/20	—	25	240
25	Chocolate shake	—	330	14/67/19	—	25	270
25	Apple turnover	—	410	4/44/52	—	15	350
	KENTUCKY FRIED CHICKEN[149]						
	Original Recipe®						
25	Center Breast*	—	257	40/12/48	—	93	532
25	Drumstick*	—	147	37/9/54	—	81	269
25	Thigh*	—	278	26/12/62	—	122	517
	Extra Crispy®						
25	Center Breast*	—	353	31/16/53	—	93	842
25	Drumstick*	—	173	29/14/57	—	65	346
25	Thigh*	—	371	21/15/64	—	121	766
25	Kentucky Nuggets (one)	—	46	25/19/56	—	12	140
	Kentucky Nugget Sauce (oz)						
25	Barbeque	—	35	3/82/15	—	1	450
25	Sweet and Sour	—	58	1/90/9	—	1	148
25	Kentucky Fries	—	268	7/50/43	—	2	89
25	Mashed potatoes	—	59	13/78/9	—	1	228

[148]*Source:* Jack in the Box Restaurants, Foodmaker, Inc, San Diego, California. Nutrient analyses by Hazelton Laboratory of America (formerly Raltech Scientific Services Inc), Madison, Wisconsin.

[149]*Source:* Kentucky Fried Chicken Corp. Nutrient analyses by Hazelton Laboratory of America (formerly Raltech Scientific Services Inc), Madison, Wisconsin.
  *edible portion

Key: 1 = Bev 2 = Dairy 3 = Eggs 4 = Fat/Oil 5 = Fruit 6 = Bakery 7 = Grain 8 = Fish 9 = Meat 10 = Poultry 11 = Sausage 12 = Mixed Dishes 13 = Nuts/Seeds 14 = Sweets 15 = Veg/Leg 16 = Misc 22 = Soup/Sauce 25 = Fast Foods by Brand Name

TABLE F–1 ■ **Food Composition**

Key	Name	Measure	Energy (calories)	Protein/ Carbohydrate/ Fat (%)	Fiber (g)	Cholesterol (mg)	Sodium (mg)
FAST FOODS (cont.)							
KENTUCKY FRIED CHICKEN (cont.):							
25	Chicken gravy	—	59	13/30/57	—	2	398
25	Buttermilk biscuit	—	269	8/47/45	—	1	521
25	Potato salad	—	141	5/36/59	—	11	396
25	Baked beans	—	105	20/70/10	—	1	387
25	Corn on the cob	—	176	11/73/16	—	1	21
25	Cole slaw	—	103	5/45/50	—	4	171
LONG JOHN SILVER'S[150]							
25	3 Pc Fish & Fryes	—	853	20/30/50	—	106	2025
25	Fish & More	—	978	14/33/53	—	88	2124
25	3 Pc Fish Dinner	—	1180	16/31/53	—	119	2797
25	4 Pc Chicken Planks Dinner	—	1037	16/32/52	—	25	2433
25	6 Pc Chicken Nuggets Dinner	—	699	13/30/57	—	25	853
25	Fish & Chicken	—	935	16/31/53	—	56	2076
25	Seafood platter	—	976	12/35/53	—	95	2161
25	Clam dinner	—	955	8/40/52	—	27	1543
25	Batter fried shrimp dinner	—	711	9/34/57	—	127	1297
25	Oyster dinner	—	789	8/40/52	—	55	763
25	2 Pc Kitchen-Breaded Fish Dinner	—	818	13/37/50	—	76	1526
25	Fish sandwich platter	—	835	15/40/45	—	75	1402
25	Seafood salad	—	426	18/20/62	—	113	1086
25	Hush puppies	—	145	8/49/43	—	1	405

[150]*Source:* Long John Silver's Inc, Lexington, Kentucky. Nutrient analyses by Department of Nutrition and Food Science, University of Kentucky.

Key: 1 = Bev 2 = Dairy 3 = Eggs 4 = Fat/Oil 5 = Fruit 6 = Bakery 7 = Grain 8 = Fish 9 = Meat 10 = Poultry 11 = Sausage 12 = Mixed Dishes 13 = Nuts/Seeds 14 = Sweets 15 = Veg/Leg 16 = Misc 22 = Soup/Sauce 25 = Fast Foods by Brand Name

Page 253, Reprinted with permission from the American College Health Association, Rockville, Maryland.

Page 279, Copyright 1985 by Herbert L. Gravitz and Julie D. Bowden.

Page 298, Table 11–1. Adapted from American Council on Science & Health, *Smoking or Health: It's Your Choice,* January 1984 (a report available from the American Council on Science and Healath, 1995 Broadway, 16th Floor, New York, NY 10023).

Page 318, M. Beattie, *Beyond Codependency* (New York; Harper and Row, 1989), pp. 151-164; © 1989, by Hazeldon Foundation, Center City, MN. Reprinted by permission.

Page 334, Fig. 12–5. Masters and Johnson Institue.

Page 335, Permission granted by Ann Landers and Creators Syndicate.

Page 342, List from *I Never Called It Rape* by Robin Warshaw, © 1988 by the Ms. Foundation for Educating and Communication, Inc. and Sarah Lazin books. Reprinted by permission of Harper Collins Publishers.

Page 349, Table 13–1. R. A. Hatcher, F. Stewart, J. Trussel, D. Lowal, F. Guest, G. K. Stewart, and W. Cates, *Contraceptive Technology* (1990–1992): 146. Used with permission.

Page 439, Fig. 16–1. Adapted by permission of Choice in Dying, formerly Concern for Dying/Society for the Right to Die, 250 W. 57th St., New York.

Page 444, Campbell Soup Company.

Page 450, Tallahassee Democrat.

Page 455, Table S16–1. Reprinted with permission from *Nursing Practice in the Care of the Dying,* © 1982, American Nurses Association, Kansas City, MO.

Page 482, Copyright 1990 by Consumers Union of United States, Inc.; Yonkers NY 10703. Adapted by permission from *Consumer Reports Health Letter/Consumer Reports on Health,* October 1990.

Page 489, Adapted with permission from R.A.Hatcher and coauthors, *Contraceptive Technology* (New York; Irvington, 1991), pp. 157–158.

Page 520, From *Priorities, The Quarterly Magazine of the American Council on Science.*

Page 539, Fig. 19–2. Courtesy of The Skin Cancer Foundation, New York, New York.

Page 548, Fig. 19–5. American Academy of Dermatology.

Page 549, Fig. 19–6. Courtesy of The Skin Cancer Foundation, New York, New York. From the brochure "The ABCD's of Moles and Melanomas," © 1985, The Skin Cancer Foundation.

Page 556, Adapted with permission from the University of Texas Lifetime Health Letter, Houston.

Page 569, Fig. 20–2. *New England Journal of Medicine.*

Page 578, Table 20–3. Metropolitan Life Insurance Company.

Page 594, Conservation International.

Chapter opening art credits

Chapter 1 "I'm Dancin' As Fast As I Can," 1984 by Miriam Schapiro. Collection of Dr. and Mrs. Harold Steinbaum. Courtesy of the Bernice Steinbaum Gallery, New York, New York.

Chapter 2 Bruce Wolfe.

Chapter 3 Douglas Bowles/The Image Bank.

Chapter 4 "New York City Marathon, 1987" by Tom Sciacca, © Tom Sciacca.

Chapter 5 Kristen Miller.

Chapter 6 John Martin/The Image Bank.

Chapter 7 Victor Stabin/The Image Bank.

Chapter 8 Douglas Struthers/The Image Bank.

Chapter 9 "The Hallucinogenic Toreador" (1969–1970). Oil on canvas, 157 x 119 inches. Collection of The Salvador Dali Museum, St. Petersburg, FL. © 1991 Salvador Dali Museum.

Chapter 10 "Adult Children of Alcoholics" by Daniel Zackroczemski.

Chapter 11 David Brendan Ryan.

Chapter 12 © Cathleen Toelke, 1990.

Chapter 13 "Men Exist For the Sake of One Another. Teach Them Then or Bear With Them," by Jacob Lawrence. National Museum of American Art, D.C./Art Resource, N.Y.

Chapter 14 Chris Burke/The Image Bank.

Chapter 15 Andy Zito/The Image Bank.
Chapter 16 "Untitled (1.5.88)," by Oliver Jackson. Courtesy of Ann Kohs and Associates.
Chapter 17 Douglas Struthers/The Image Bank.
Chapter 18 Kristen Miller.
Chapter 19 "People in the Sun," by Edward Hopper. National Museum of American Art, Smithsonian Institution. Gift of S.C. Johnson and Son, Inc.
Chapter 20 Joe Saffold/The Image Bank.
Chapter 21 "New Growth," by Jane R. Hofstetter.

Text photo credits

14 D.Degnan, H. Armstrong Roberts; **17** Seth Resnick, Stock, Boston; **18** Mary Kate Denny, Photo Edit; **20** Tony Freeman, Photo Edit; **22** Bob Daemmrich, Stock, Boston; **36** (*left*) Skjold, Photo Edit; (*middle*) Bob Daemmrich, Stock, Boston; (*right*) N. Grecco, Stock, Boston; **44** Mary Kate Denny, Photo Edit; **50** Alan Oddie, Photo Edit; **54** Brent Jones; **65** Jody Buren, Sygma; **76** Rhoda Sidney, Photo Edit; **77** Doug Plummer, Photo Researchers; **80** Tony Freeman, Photo Edit; **93** (top) Frank Siteman, Stock, Boston; **93** (bottom) International Stock Photography; **96** Ray Stanyard, Photo Edit; **103** David Frazier, Photo Researchers; **104** Ray Stanyard, Photo Edit; **105** (*all*) Ray Stanyard, Photo Edit; **111** (*all*) Ray Stanyard, Photo Edit; **114** (*all*) Tony Freeman, Photo Edit; **115** Gerard Vandystadt, Photo Researchers; **120** Richard Pasley, Stock, Boston; **121** (a & b) Courtesy of U.S. Department of Agriculture; (*c*) Four by Five; (*d-f*) Courtesy of U.S. Department of Agriculture; **128** Tony Freeman, Photo Edit; **133** Stacy Pick, Stock, Boston; **160** George S. Zimbel, Monkmeyer; **161** Felicia Martinez, Photo Edit; **173** Al Satterwhite, Image Bank; **174** Brent Jones; **177** Anna Baritista, Allsport; **178** Chevalier, Allsport; **191** A. Huharich, H. Armstrong Roberts; **195** Ray Stanyard, Photo Edit; **199** (*all*) Felicia Martinez, Photo Edit; **201** Douglas Struthers, Image Bank; **208** Barbara Alper, Stock, Boston; **212** Tony Freeman, Photo Edit; **213** Mary Kate Denny, Photo Edit; **218** Sam Abell, Woodfin Camp and Associates; **230** Thomas R. Fletcher, Stock, Boston; **232** Tony Freeman, Photo Edit; **235** Dr. Jeremy Burgess/Science Photo Library, National Audubon Society Collection, Photo Researchers; **240** Frank Siteman, Stock, Boston; **241** Tim Davis, Photo Researchers; **243** June Bug Clark, Photo Researchers; **249** A. Choisnet, the Image Bank; **252** Elizabeth Zuckerman, Photo Edit; **267** Myrleen Ferguson, Photo Edit; **275** Bob Daemmrich, Stock, Boston; **282** Kenneth Murray, Photo Researchers; **284** Richard Hutchings, Info edit; **301** Courtesy of American Cancer Society; **308** © 91, Joel Gordon; **321** Myrleen Ferguson, Photo Edit; **323** (left) Frank Siteman, Stock, Boston; (right) Charles Gupton, Stock, Boston; **340** José Ortega; **345** Nancy Durrell McKenna, Photo Researchers; **348** Tony Freeman, Photo Edit; **348** © 91, Joel Gordon; **372** Tony Freeman, Photo Edit; **388** (*a-c*) Petit Format/Nestle, Photo Researchers; (*d*) Anthony Vanelli; Photo Edit; **390** © 82, Joel Gordon; **398** Streissguth, A. P., Clarren, S.K. & Jones, K.L. (1985, July). Natural History of the Fetal Alcohol Syndrome: A Ten-year follow-up of eleven patients. *Lauret, II*, 89–92. **401** Explorer Pascale, Photo Researchers; **404** Charles Gupton, Stock, Boston; **407** Charles Gupton, Stock, Boston; **410** Myrleen Ferguson, Photo Edit; **412** Edward Lettau, Photo Researchers; **419** Barbara Alper, Stock, Boston; **422** Rhoda Sidney, Photo Edit; **427** Brent Jones; **436** Julie Houck, Stock, Boston; **443** David Young-Wolff, Photo Edit; **453** Herb Snitzer, Stock, Boston; **471** Alec Duncan, Taurus Photos; **495** Hank Morgan, Photo Researchers; **495** B. Martin, The Image Bank; **460** (*a–c*) Science Photo Library, Photo Researchers; **461** (*d*) Science Photo Library, Photo Researchers; (*e & f*) Centers for Disease Control, Atlanta, GA; © 91, **500** © 91, Joel Gordon; **511** ICI Pharmaceuticals; **520** Thomas S. England, Photo Researchers; **521** Bob Daemmrich, Stock Boston; **523** David Young-Woulff; Photo Edit; **525** Courtesy of the U.S. Department of Agriculture; **527** Seth Resnick, Stock, Boston; **530** Jean Claude Le Jeune, Stock, Boston; **539** (*a–c*) The Skin Cancer Foundation, Robert J. Friedman, M.D., Darrell S. Rigel, M.D., Alfred W. Kopf, M.D.; **541** (*top*) Ray Stanyard, Photo Eidt; (*bottom*) William Johnson, Stock, Boston; **549** The Skin Cancer Foundation, Robert J. Friedman, M.D., Darrell S. Rigel, M.D., Alfred W. Kopf, M.D.; **560** Kay Chernush, The Image Bank; **567** (*both*) Marilynne Hubert; **581** Blair Seitz, Photo Researchers; **585** David J. Farr, Imagesmythe, Inc.; **601** Myrleen Ferguson, Photo Edit; **615** Alan Oddie, Photo Edit; **617** Tony Freeman, Photo Edit; **619** NASA/Science Source, Photo Researchers; **621** Joseph Schuyler, Stock, Boston

Acceptable Weight for Height Based on Body Mass Index (BMI)

To determine your acceptable weight range, find your height in the top line. Look down the column below it and find the range represented by the color blue. Look to the left column to see what weights are acceptable for you.

Men

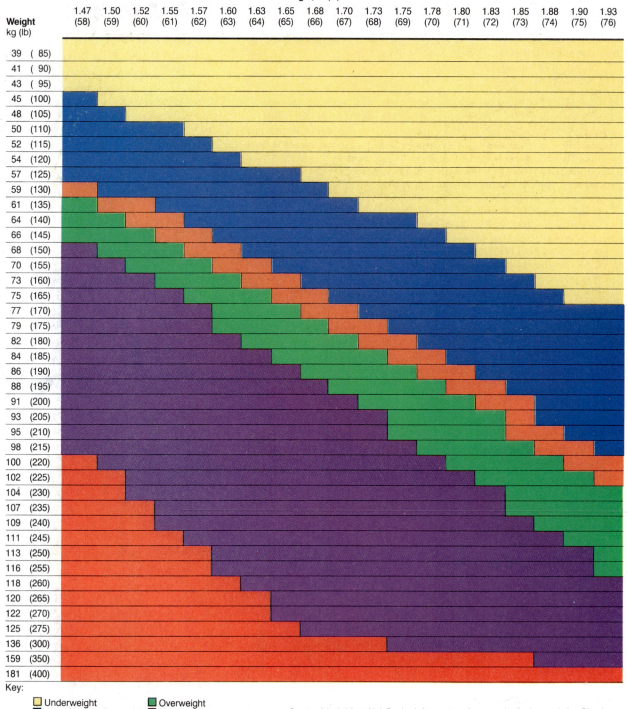

Height, m (in)

Weight kg (lb)	1.47 (58)	1.50 (59)	1.52 (60)	1.55 (61)	1.57 (62)	1.60 (63)	1.63 (64)	1.65 (65)	1.68 (66)	1.70 (67)	1.73 (68)	1.75 (69)	1.78 (70)	1.80 (71)	1.83 (72)	1.85 (73)	1.88 (74)	1.90 (75)	1.93 (76)

Weight values (kg / lb):
39 (85), 41 (90), 43 (95), 45 (100), 48 (105), 50 (110), 52 (115), 54 (120), 57 (125), 59 (130), 61 (135), 64 (140), 66 (145), 68 (150), 70 (155), 73 (160), 75 (165), 77 (170), 79 (175), 82 (180), 84 (185), 86 (190), 88 (195), 91 (200), 93 (205), 95 (210), 98 (215), 100 (220), 102 (225), 104 (230), 107 (235), 109 (240), 111 (245), 113 (250), 116 (255), 118 (260), 120 (265), 122 (270), 125 (275), 136 (300), 159 (350), 181 (400)

Key:

- Underweight
- Acceptable weight
- Marginal overweight
- Overweight
- Severe overweight
- Morbid obesity

Source: Adapted from M. I. Rowland, A nomogram for computing body mass index, Dietetic Currents 16 (1989): 9, used and reprinted with permission of Ross Laboratories, Columbus, OH 43216. Copyright 1989 Ross Laboratories.

Y